NEUROLOGY

Problems in Primary Care Series

Future volumes will include works on

Urology
Otolaryngology
Rheumatology
Cardiology
Gastroenterology
Pulmonary Medicine

NEUROLOGY

PROBLEMS IN PRIMARY CARE

JAMES L. BERNAT, MD
Associate Professor of Clinical Medicine (Neurology)
Dartmouth Medical School
Chief, Neurology Section
Veterans Administration Medical Center
White River Junction, Vermont

FREDERICK M. VINCENT, MD
Associate Professor of Medicine and Psychiatry
Chief, Neurology Section
Department of Medicine
Michigan State University College of Human Medicine
East Lansing, Michigan

Medical Economics Books
Oradell, New Jersey 07649

Acquisitions Editor: Thomas O. Bentz
Production Editor: Hattie Heavner
Art Director: Sharyn Banks
Text Design: Jim Bernard
Cover Design: Penina Wissner
Composition: Elizabeth Typesetting Company

Library of Congress Cataloging-in-Publication Data

Bernat, James L.
    Neurology: problems in primary care.

    Includes bibliographies and index.
    1. Nervous system—Diseases. 2. Family medicine.
I. Vincent Frederick M. II. Title. [DNLM: 1. Family
Practice. 2. Nervous System Diseases. WL 100 B524n]
RC 348.B47 1987   616.8   87-11010
ISBN 0-87489-407-7

ISBN 0-87489-407-7

Medical Economics Company Inc.
Oradell, New Jersey 07649

Printed in the United States of America

The authors and publisher have exerted every effort to ensure that drug selection, dosage,
and therapeutic modalities set forth in this text are in accord with current recommendations
and practice at the time of publication. However, in view of ongoing research, changes in
government regulations, and the constant flow of information relating to drug therapy and
drug reactions, the reader is urged to check the package insert for each drug for any change
in indications and dosage and for added warnings and precautions. This is particularly
important when the recommended agent is a new or infrequently employed drug.

Contents

Foreword

This is the best book I have read on neurology for the primary care physician. The authors have a sense of what is important and cover it in their writing.

Problem oriented, the book begins with the difficult topics of diagnostic tests and physical diagnosis, which are presented with ease and with interest to the reader. I literally read every word.

The sections on problems, diseases, and emergencies are equally good. They cover the field of neurological disorders for the primary practitioner, singling out the clinical problems that merit in-depth presentation and addressing only the basics on the others. The bibliography at the end of each chapter offers the reader an opportunity to go further if necessary.

I will keep this book in my library and use it as I do other key references when examining patients. It is a superb beginning for what promises to be a fine new series on Problems in Primary Care.

Thomas L. Stern, MD
Kansas City, Missouri

To Our Wives:
Judith Bernat and Tish Vincent
and Children:
Deborah and David Bernat
Michael, Joshua, and Melissa Vincent

Preface

In primary care practice, an estimated 20% of patients' complaints are referable to the nervous system. The majority of these patients do not require formal neurological consultation and can be well managed by the primary care physician. It is these physicians for whom we have written this book: to provide a clear account of the neurologist's own approach to the diagnosis and management of patients with symptoms and signs of nervous system disease.

This textbook is not intended to replace more comprehensive neurology textbooks and encyclopedias. Rather, we designed it to provide a terse, practical, and ready office and bedside guide to the common complaints and disorders likely to be encountered in primary care practice. We have limited the discussions of pathophysiology and anatomy to allow room for more practical advice. From our experience working closely with primary physicians in academic and community settings, we have chosen information that we judged should be of the greatest interest and value.

The book is organized in four sections: Assessment, Problems, Diseases, and Emergencies. In Assessment, we stress the relevant portions of the neurological examination and present a rationale for choosing neurological ancillary tests. In Problems and Emergencies, each chapter provides an approach to a specific neurological presenting syndrome, which recapitulates the thinking of the neurologist. In Diseases, the chapters contain a consistent internal structure permitting rapid reference. We include special chapters on the neurological complications of common medical conditions including diabetes, alcoholism, cancer, pregnancy, and drug effects. The Appendix lists the names, addresses, and services provided by various national agencies and philanthropies to patients with nervous system diseases.

We are grateful to Judith Bernat, Tish Vincent, and Mary MacIntosh for their much valued assistance in word processing. We appreciate the fine work of the editorial and production staffs at Medical Economics Books.

We hope that this book will prove useful to the busy practitioner and will contribute to the betterment of patient care.

James L. Bernat, MD
Frederick M. Vincent, MD

ONE

Assessment

The Neurological Examination

Neurology may be distinguished from other branches of medicine by its absolute reliance on a skillful physical examination for diagnosis. The brain and spinal cord cannot be inspected, palpated, percussed, or auscultated. The clinician must learn and perfect techniques to inferentially measure nervous system function. This chapter and the next two chapters present the techniques of the neurological examination of adults, children, and the elderly.

ASSESSMENT

The assessment of the patient with nervous system disease differs in one significant way from assessment in other branches of medicine. Before a differential diagnosis can be constructed on the basis of history, physical examination, and laboratory data, the clinician must localize the lesion to the affected area of the nervous system.

Consider the patient whose chief complaint is left-arm weakness. Lesions of the right hemisphere, brain stem, spinal cord, cervical nerve roots, brachial plexus, peripheral nerve, neuromuscular junction, and muscle can all produce left-arm weakness. But it would be absurd for the clinician to generate a differential diagnosis that includes hemispheric stroke, brain stem tumor, transverse myelitis, herniated cervical disc, brachial plexus neuropathy, diabetic mononeuropathy, myasthenia gravis, and polymyositis. The function of the history and, to a greater extent, of the physical examination is to localize the lesion in the nervous system. If the examination reveals a spastic left hemiparisis, left-sided multimodality sensory loss, mild lower-left facial weakness, and left homonymous hemianopia, the clinician can localize the lesion to the right hemisphere. This localization permits the clinician to exclude diseases of other parts of the nervous system from the differential diagnosis. The differential diagnosis is then constructed on the basis of the history, physical, and laboratory findings of disorders affecting that portion of the nervous system. In neurologic assessment, the clinician must *localize the lesion* before making a differential diagnosis.

HISTORY

In neurology, as in all of medicine, history is 80% to 90% of diagnosis. In paroxysmal disorders of the nervous system, including migraine and epilepsy, history is 100% of diagnosis. Neurologic histories include chief complaint, present illness, medical history, family history, social history, and review of systems.

When recording the chief complaint and present illness, it is particularly important to clarify the meaning of words used by the patient to describe his symptoms. Words such as "fit," "seizure," "dizziness," and "double vision" may mean different experiences to different patients. It is most helpful for the clinician to obtain a chronological history of the illness, its course, the effects of previous treatment, and the presence of exacerbating and ameliorating factors. In nervous system disorders that affect consciousness and cognition, it is necessary to obtain corroborating history from the spouse, relatives, fellow workers, and friends. It is necessary to contact eyewitnesses in cases of paroxysmal disorders that affect consciousness, such as seizures and syncope.

The medical history sets the stage for the present illness. In the patient with a presumptive diagnosis of stroke, it is necessary to inquire about past hypertension, angina, myocardial infarction, intermittent claudication, smoking, hyperlipidemia, and diabetes. Past major illnesses, operations, injuries, and hospitalizations should be reviewed.

Family history is particularly important. Hereditary transmission is seen in many diseases of the nervous system. Many otherwise undiagnosed polyneuropathy syndromes can be revealed as hereditary if a careful family history is obtained and if family members are interviewed and examined.

The social history should contain questions about tobacco, alcohol, and drug use; occupational traumas; toxin exposure; the patient's living arrangements and financial status; allergies; and current medications.

The review of systems in the neurologic patient should include questions about headache, dizziness, loss of consciousness, memory loss, confusion, visual and hearing disturbances, difficulty in speaking and swallowing, weakness, numbness, clumsiness, imbalance, falling, and trouble in walking.

The handedness of the patient always must be determined. Right-handed patients must be asked if they have always been right-handed or if they were forced to switch in childhood. The extent of handedness can be determined by inquiring with which hand the patient writes, eats, throws a ball, and threads a needle. Handedness and dominance is discussed further in Chapter 16.

NEUROLOGICAL EXAMINATION: GENERAL REMARKS

Conduct of the neurological examination is designed to answer the question: From which part of the nervous system does the patient's complaints originate?

The examination has both "horizontal" and "vertical" components. Horizontally, the physician always examines mental status, cranial nerves, motor and sensory functions, coordination, gait and station, and reflexes. In the vertical sense, the examiner assesses each function at a variable depth, depending on the findings and the nature of the problem.

In practice, most experienced clinicians evolve a screening neurological examination: a brief overview of the complete exam that can be performed in five to seven minutes. Any abnormalities found on screening can be pursued in more depth (vertically) by more sensitive supplementary methods of examination. The screening neurological examination should include:

1. Mental status: level of consciousness, attention, immediate memory, and language.
2. Cranial nerves: pupillary reflexes, visual acuity, visual fields, eye movements, facial movements, hearing, swallowing, phonation, shoulder shrug, and tongue movements.
3. Motor: sample of upper and lower limb tone, strength, and appearance.
4. Sensory: pain and vibration sensation in all four limbs.
5. Coordination: finger-to-nose and heel-to-shin tests.
6. Gait and station: ordinary walking and tandem gait.
7. Reflexes: deep-tendon reflexes of biceps, triceps, brachioradialis, knees, and ankles; abdominal cutaneous reflexes.

The order of components of the neurological examination is not critical. It is, however, necessary for the clinician to learn and follow one particular order so that no part of the exam will be omitted inadvertently. The above-listed order of the screening exam has a logical pattern. Mental status is assessed first. The interpretation of the remainder of the examination findings will be affected if the patient is confused or aphasic. Coordination follows mental status, cranial nerves, motor, and sensory function examination because it requires all these primary functions in addition to cerebellar function. Similarly, normal gait and station require all the preceding functions. Reflexes, the most objective part of the examination, may be performed following the motor exam or at the end of the exam.

The patient should be disrobed and wearing a hospital gown. The examining room should be warm and quiet. The clinician should try to relax the patient by gentle reassurance that the exam will be painless.

PHYSICAL EXAMINATION: PERTINENT FEATURES

The neurological examination does not exist in isolation from the general physical examination. Certain features of the general physical examination must be performed as part of every neurologic assessment. They include the examination of vital signs; optic fundi; facies, head, neck, and extremity pulses; color; and evidence of trophic limb changes.

Other portions of the general examination are also performed, depending on the presenting problem. For the patient in whom cerebrovascular disease is part of the differential diagnosis, a neurovascular examination should be performed, including palpation of carotid and facial arteries; listening for carotid, orbital, and subclavian bruits; detailed examination of the heart; and blood pressure determination in both arms. For the patient with acute sciatica, the clinician must examine the back for tenderness, range of movements, and muscle spasm; straight leg raising and inverse straight leg raising; hip mobility; and rectal examination.

MENTAL STATUS EXAMINATION

A complete mental status examination should assess level of consciousness, orientation, attention, language, recent and remote memory, higher integrative functions, thought, and behavior. Examiners vary greatly in mental status questionnaires. Experienced clinicians have evolved certain questions that they have validated internally on the basis of examinations of hundreds of patients, but few routine mental status questions in general use have been validated statistically, i.e., specific answers correlated with specific proved diagnoses.

Level of consciousness is assessed first. Normally, patients are "alert," showing full wakefulness and quick responsiveness to verbal questions and commands. The "lethargic" patient exhibits blunted wakefulness and impaired responsiveness to verbal questions and commands. The "stuporous" patient exhibits a pathological state of sleep-like unawareness and unresponsiveness from which he can be aroused to temporary responsiveness only by noxious stimuli. The "comatose" patient exhibits a pathological state of sleep-like unawareness and unresponsiveness from which he cannot be aroused despite the use of noxious stimuli. More subtle impairments of the level of consciousness are manifest by inability to maintain attention. Examination of the stuporous and comatose patient is considered in Chapter 35.

Orientation testing is performed next. Normal patients are oriented properly to name, age, birth date, home address, location of examination, and exact day, date, season, and general time of day of the examination. In confusional states, disorientation in time appears first, followed by disorientation of place.

Language testing is a very important part of the mental status examination. See Chapter 16 for a discussion of language testing, aphasia, apraxia, and agnosia.

Attention is next assessed—the ability to continue to respond to and continue thinking about a specific stimulus without distraction by other stimuli. Attention for at least 30 seconds is considered normal. Attention is assessed both by behavioral observations throughout the examination and by specific tests. In the digit repetition test, patients are asked to repeat a string of random numbers of increasing length. Normally, patients should be able to accurately repeat 6 integers. The serial sevens test requires patients to subtract 7 from 100, then 7 from the remainder, and so on. (Subtraction of serial threes from 20 is an alternative test if arithmetic ability or education is in question.) Patients should make no more than two errors in eight serial subtractions. Patients can be described as normally attentive or with grades of inattentiveness.

Memory assessment is a crucial component of the mental status exam. The clinician tests both new, short-term memory recording and the intactness of long-term memory traces. (So-called "immediate memory" is merely attention as discussed above.) The ability to record and recall new memory traces over the short term is tested by asking the patient to repeat and remember three unrelated words (eg, table, red, 53 Broadway), distracting him, then asking him to say the words after five or ten minutes. Normally, at least two of the words should be remembered without cues, and all three with cues (eg, "One was a street address").

More detailed, individual assessments of verbal and visual short-term memory can be made. For verbal memory, a short detailed story can be read to the patient; afterward, the patient is asked to repeat the story. He is scored on the percentage of individual parts of the story that he can recount. Visual memory can be tested by showing the patient a series of geometric designs, then hiding them and asking him to draw them from memory.

Remote memory is tested by asking the patient to recall the dates of significant life events, but the answers must be corroborated by the spouse or another family member. Alternatively, the patient can be quizzed about dates and facts in history that most people are expected to remember (eg, in the United States, recent Presidents, dates of recent wars, details of the assassination of John F. Kennedy).

Higher integrative functions are assessed following the assessment of the fundamental mental skills of attention, orientation, language, and memory. These tests are highly education-biased, hence must be interpreted in light of the patient's formal educational level and employment history. Tests of fund of knowledge and proverb interpretation are particularly education-biased and must be cautiously interpreted. Better are tests of similarities and differences. The patient is asked to name as many ways in which an apple and an orange are similar and different. The question is repeated for chair and table, then for painting and statue. The patient is asked the difference between a child and a midget; between a river and a canal.

Tests of calculation should be given. The patient can be asked: "How many nickels are there in $1.35." or "Apples cost 7 cents each. How much change should I get if I buy a dozen apples and pay a dollar?"

Thought and behavior should be assessed. The examiner first should make an assessment of the patient's mood. Is he apathetic, depressed, euphoric, or manic? Behavior should be assessed. Is there evidence for restlessness or agitation? Thought should be assessed. Is there anxiety? Are there morbid thoughts, illusions, hallucinations, delusions, obsessions, or compulsions?

Screening Mental Status Testing

The preceding tests are time-consuming and subject to varied interpretations. A statistically validated rapid screening mental status examination called the "Mini-Mental State" has been devised by Folstein et al. It can sensitively assess mental status in only five to ten minutes, and its results have been correlated with diagnostic syndromes. The format for the Mini-Mental State is presented in Table 1-1.

The highest possible score on the Mini-Mental State is 30. Its originators found that normal patients, including the elderly scored, 25 to 30; depressed or neurotic patients, 20 to 30; and demented patients, usually below 20. The test is useful for rapid dementia screening and for serial use in the delirious patient.

TABLE 1-1 MINI-MENTAL STATE EXAMINATION

Maximum Score	Score	
Orientation		
5	( )	What is the (year) (season) (date) (day) (month)?
5	( )	Where are we (state) (town) (country) (hospital) (floor)?
Registration		
3	( )	Name 3 objects (1 second to say each). Then ask the patient all 3 after you have said them. Give one point for each correct answer. Then repeat them until he learns all 3.
Attention and Calculation		
5	( )	Serial 7s. 1 point for each correct. Stop after 5 answers. Alternatively, spell "world" backwards.
Recall		
3	( )	Ask for the 3 objects repeated above. Give 1 point for each correct.
Language		
9	( )	Name a pencil and watch (2 points) Repeat: "No ifs, ands, or buts" (1 point) Follow a 3-stage command: "Take a paper in your right hand, fold it in half, and put it on the floor." (3 points) Read and obey: "Close your eyes." (1 point) Write a sentence. (1 point) Copy a design. (1 point)
TOTAL SCORE	_____	

Adapted from Falstein MF, Folstein FE, McHugh PR: Mini-Mental State. *J Psychiatr Res* 1975; 12:189-198. Used with permission.

CRANIAL NERVE EXAMINATION
I (Olfactory Nerve)

The olfactory nerves subserve the sense of smell and are a direct extension of the central nervous system (CNS) from the limbic region to the olfactory mucosa. Olfaction is tested by presenting an odoriferous substance to the patient with eyes closed—testing each nostril separately—and asking if he or she can smell and recognize the substance. The best test substances have an aroma but are not pungent. A bottle of oil of wintergreen or cloves is an ideal test substance. Pungent substances (eg, ammonia) irritate the nasal mucosa, producing trigeminal nerve stimulation, which makes them inadequate tests of olfaction.

The most common causes of anosmia are obstructive, and include occluded nasal passages from upper respiratory infection or deviated septum. Nonobstructive causes include occipital head trauma in which anosmia is often bilateral and permanent, vitamin B12 deficiency, and tabes dorsalis. Unilateral, nonobstructive, nontraumatic anosmia suggests an olfactory groove meningioma.

II (Optic Nerve)

The visual system, including eyes, optic nerves, optic tracts, optic radiations, and visual cortex are usually tested as a whole. A lesion of any one anatomic component produces a predictable pattern of impairment of visual acuity or visual fields, as shown in Figure 1-1.

The examiner begins by inspecting the surface of the visual apparatus and continues inspection by funduscopic examination. The lens is examined for opacities by setting the ophthalmoscope at positive 5 or 6 diopters and holding it several inches from the patient's cornea. Then the fundus is examined with the ophthalmoscope set at 0 to negative 4 diopters.

The examiner should inspect the optic disc and optic cup. The disc is normally pale pink, and the cup is a paler pink. The cup is 1 to 2 diopters in depth, the disc margins are normally sharp, and the temporal border is more well-defined than the nasal. Arteries and veins can be inspected as they cross the disc margin. Normally, 16 to 22 vascular structures can be counted, with an artery-to-vein ratio of 3:5.

Papilledema is said to be present when the disc margin is blurred, the normal spontaneous pulsations of the retinal veins are no longer seen, the vessel count across the disc margin exceeds 22, and the disc itself is raised above the surrounding retina by more than 1 diopter. Normal ophthalmic conditions, including drusen and myelinated nerve fibers, can be mistaken for papilledema. Optic atrophy is present when the disc is pale, is slightly smaller than usual, has a very sharply defined outline, and has a smaller vessel count than normal.

Figure 1-1. Visual field defects resulting from lesions in different regions of the visual system. (From Homans JA: *A Textbook of Surgery.* Courtesy of Charles C Thomas, Publisher, Springfield, Illinois.)

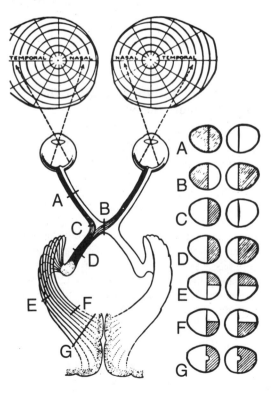

Visual acuity is best tested with a standard Snellen chart at 20 feet, with each eye tested individually at the best possible refractive correction. The patient may gaze through a pinhole if uncorrected myopia is present. A less adequate test is near visual acuity with a 14-inch card.

Visual fields are tested by the confrontation technique, with each eye tested separately. The patient covers one eye and gazes directly at the opposite eye of the examiner, who stands 2 to 3 feet away. The examiner slowly moves the test object from the periphery into the field of vision and compares the point where the patient first acknowledges seeing the test object with when the examiner sees it. A small, red test object (eg, a red match head) is most sensitive for disclosing subtle visual field defects. It is difficult but possible to plot the blind spots similarly.

For stuporous, confused, or uncooperative patients, the threat technique is used. The examiner makes a rapid flicking finger movement toward the patient's eye, quickly advancing sequentially from each quadrant of vision. A blink response usually signifies that the visual field is grossly intact. The examiner must take care not to touch the patient's eyelash or cornea, and not to move a standing column of air against the patient's cornea, thereby inducing a corneal blink reflex.

Visual fields are tested most accurately by formal means using a tangent screen or perimeter. The tangent screen examines the fields out to 30 degrees and is sufficiently sensitive to disclose field defects caused by CNS disease. The perimeter examines fields to 90 degrees; it can additionally disclose intra-ocular abnormalities. Blind spots can be measured accurately with both techniques. Many machines guarantee total visual fixation to eliminate poor fixation as a source of error. These machines also allow fields to be tested with different test object sizes and colors to detect the most subtle abnormalities.

III (Oculomotor Nerve), IV (Trochlear Nerve) VI (Abducens Nerve)

Tests of cranial nerves III, IV, and VI are commonly performed together. These nerves leave the rostral brain stem, traverse the cavernous sinus, and enter the orbit through the superior orbital fissure to innervate the eyelid and the ocular muscles. Dysfunction of the III, IV, and VI system can occur at the nuclear level in the brain stem by infarction, hemorrhage, or tumor; at the peripheral nerve level by nerve compression or infarction; at the neuromuscular junction level in myasthenia gravis; or at the muscle level in myopathic disorders, such as from thyroid disease. Complete assessment of III, IV, VI function includes testing pupillary reflexes, eye movements, and presence of ptosis and nystagmus.

The normal pupillary size is determined by the resting equilibrium between the sympathetic pupillodilating fibers and the parasympathetic pupilloconstricting fibers. The anatomy of the system and sites of common defects are shown in Figure 1-2.

Pupillary size, roundness, and symmetry are observed first. The pupil is usually 3.0 to 7.0 mm in diameter. It constricts to bright light, to accommodation, and with advancing age. Ordinarily, both pupils constrict consensually, even when a stimulus is applied to only one eye. Pupillary size is graded as follows:

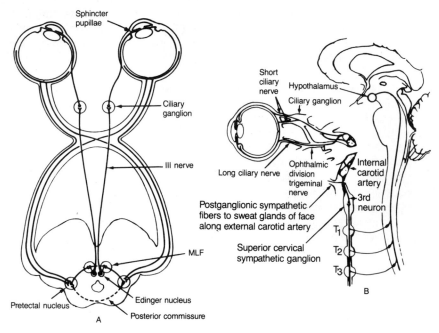

Figure 1-2. Anatomy of pupillary innervation. (A) The parasympathetic pupilloconstrictor pathway. (B) The sympathetic pupillodilator pathway. (Reproduced, with permission, from Plum F, Posner JB: *The Diagnosis of Stupor and Coma,* ed 3. Philadelphia, F.A. Davis, 1980, p 41.)

<1.0 mm	Pinpoint
1.0 to 3.0 mm	Small
3.0 to 7.0 mm	Mid-position
>7.0 mm	Large

Physiologic anisocoria is usually a pupillary diameter of less than 1.0 mm.

Pupillary light reflexes are tested by shining a point light source obliquely into one pupil and observing the rapidity and magnitude of the direct and consensual constriction. The light is not shined directly in front of the pupil because the patient may attempt to focus on it, perhaps producing an accommodation response. Both the direct and consensual reactions should be assessed in each eye. If anisocoria is present, the patient should be moved to a dark room, where it can be reassessed. In Horner's syndrome, the small pupil will not dilate in darkness, while the normal pupil will dilate; thus, the anisocoria will be amplified in darkness.

Pupillary reflex impairment can be the result of an afferent optic nerve lesion or to an efferent oculomotor nerve lesion. In an afferent optic nerve lesion caused by, say, optic neuritis, there is loss or delay in both the direct and consensual light reflexes from that eye. There is a normal direct and consensual pupillary light reflex from the unaffected eye. In an efferent oculomotor nerve lesion, the direct pupillary reflex is absent, but the consensual reflex persists. Shining the light in the unaffected pupil produces a direct, but not a consensual, reflex.

Pupillary reflexes to accommodation are part of the near reflex of convergence, pupilloconstriction, and change in lens shape for near vision. The patient is asked to look into the distance, then suddenly to focus on the examiner's finger, which is placed 10 to 15 inches from the patient's face. Detectable pupilloconstriction should be observed.

Several stereotyped pupillary abnormalities have been recognized in addition to the afferent and efferent pupillary lesions already described. The Argyll Robertson pupil is a small, slightly irregular pupil that constricts to accommodation but not to light. Tertiary syphilis was formerly the most common cause of Argyll Robertson pupils, but now diabetes is more common. Adie's or tonic, pupil is a midposition pupil that constricts incompletely and very slowly to sustained light or accommodation stimuli. Generalized hyporeflexia commonly accompanies Adie's pupil(s). Horner's pupil is part of the miosis, ptosis, anhidrosis, and enophthalmos of Horner's syndrome; it is caused by sympathetic denervation. Horner's pupil is small and reactive to light and accommodation but does not enlarge in darkness.

Evaluation of the abnormal pupil is not complete without pharmacologic stimulation with selected pupilloconstrictor or pupillodilator drops. See Mayo Clinic (1981), DeJong (1979), and Bickerstaff (1980) in the bibliography for further discussions of the use in practice of pharmacologic pupillary stimulation.

The presence of ptosis should be ascertained. There are two eyelid elevating muscles: (1) the levator palpebra, innervated by the oculomotor nerve, which is responsible for 90% to 95% of eyelid elevation; and (2) Müller's muscle, innervated by the sympathetic nervous system, which is responsible for 5% to 10% of elevation. Ptosis from a complete nerve III lesion is severe, with the eyelid dropped completely covering the eye. Ptosis from a sympathetic nervous system lesion (ie, Horner's syndrome) is mild, with a slight droop of the upper lid that covers more of the pupil than usual. Ptosis in myasthenia gravis and in ocular myopathies is usually of intermediate severity.

Assessment of extraocular movements sensitively tests most functions of nerve III and all functions of nerves IV and VI. Each eye is moved horizontally, vertically, or in rotation by the action of the six extraocular muscles. The functions of the extraocular muscles are listed in Table 1-2; their anatomic relationships are shown in Figure 1-3.

TABLE 1-2 FUNCTIONS OF THE EXTRAOCULAR MUSCLES

Muscle	Cranial Nerve	Primary Function	Secondary Function
Lateral rectus	VI	Abduction	—
Medial rectus	III	Adduction	—
Inferior rectus	III	Depresses when eye abducted	Extorts when eye adducted
Superior rectus	III	Elevates when eye abducted	Intorts when eye adducted
Inferior oblique	III	Elevates when eye adducted	Extorts when eye abducted
Superior oblique	IV	Depresses when eye adducted	Intorts when eye abducted

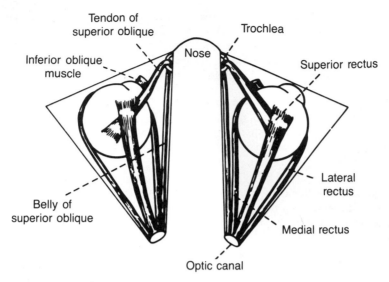

Figure 1-3. Anatomy of the extraocular muscles. (From: Baker AB: *Clinical Neurology.* Reproduced with permission from Lippincott/Harper & Row.)

Eye movements are tested best by having the patient gaze at a point light source about 3 feet away. The examiner can see the reflection of the light as a bright dot in the exact center of the patient's pupils during normal, conjugate-gaze "fovealization" of an image. If the least dysconjugation occurs, the examiner can see the dot move off center in the affected eye.

Primary gaze is tested first, with the examiner noting any dysconjugation or nystagmus. Horizontal gaze is tested next by having the patient look laterally to his extreme right and then to his extreme left. Vertical gaze is tested by asking the patient to look up and then down with eyes laterally deviated to the right; the test is repeated with eyes deviated to the left. These maneuvers are illustrated in Figure 1-4.

In a complete left nerve VI palsy, the affected eye is slightly adducted on primary gaze because of the loss of lateral rectus function. Right lateral gaze is normal. Left lateral gaze reveals normal adduction of the right eye and failure of abduction of the left eye. Vertical gaze is normal. The patient experiences horizontal diplopia that is worse on left lateral gaze.

In a complete left nerve III palsy, the eye is abducted and depressed ("down and out") on primary gaze. This position is achieved because of the resulting vector of the resting tone of the two remaining innervated muscles, the lateral rectus (VI) abducting the eye and the superior oblique (IV) depressing the eye. There is a failure of adduction because of medial rectus paresis, a loss of upward gaze because of superior rectus and inferior oblique paresis, and a loss of most downward gaze because of inferior rectus paresis. Additionally, there is profound ptosis because of loss of levator palpebra function, and a dilated, unreactive pupil

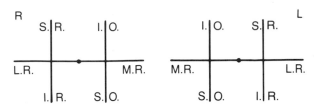

Figure 1-4. Actions of the extraocular muscles. (Reproduced from Mayo Clinic: *Clinical Examinations in Neurology,* ed 5. Philadelphia, 1981, with permission from W.B. Saunders.)

because of parasympathetic denervation. With the eyelid held open, the patient has profound vertical and horizontal diplopia that is worse on attempted upward gaze and when looking to the right.

In a complete left nerve IV palsy, there is inability to depress the eye in the adducted position. Patients develop vertical diplopia, which they learn can be compensated for somewhat by tilting their heads (Bielschowsky's sign).

For the patient who complains of diplopia, the history itself may be diagnostic. The examiner should ask if the diplopia is horizontal, vertical, or both (diagonal). Is it worse on gaze to the left, right, up, or down? Is it worse for near vision (eg, reading) or far vision?

In the case of a left nerve VI palsy, the patient should report that the diplopia is horizontal, worse on attempted left lateral gaze, and worse for far vision. Purely horizontal diplopia limits the dysfunction to the left or right medial or lateral rectus muscles. The fact that the diplopia is worse on left lateral gaze further limits the dysfunction to the left lateral rectus or the right medial rectus muscles. If the diplopia is worse on far gaze, the left lateral rectus muscle must be involved because it is more necessary for far gaze and because the medial rectus is more necessary for near gaze.

The examination for diplopia is directed toward the identification of the weak extraocular muscle(s). If the examiner cannot be confident which muscle is weak by the flashlight following test, the red glass test is performed. The examiner covers one of the patient's eyes with a red transparent glass or plastic cover and asks him to look at a flashlight point light source. Ordinarily, one red-and-white image is seen. In diplopia, the images are separated; one red and one white. The examiner can tell from which eye each image is seen. The examiner tests all nine cardinal fields of gaze, with results as shown in Figure 1-5.

There are several rules of thumb for identifying the affected eye and muscle.

1. The distance between diplopic images increases in the direction of action of the paretic muscle.

2. The more peripheral-lying image comes from the paretic eye.

3. In vertical diplopia, if the vertical distance between diplopic images is greatest with the affected eye adducted, the paresis is of the inferior or superior rectus; if the vertical distance between diplopic images is greatest with the eye adducted, the paresis is of inferior or superior oblique muscles.

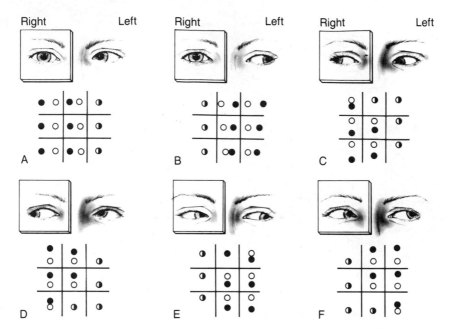

Figure 1-5. The red glass test to evaluate extraocular muscle paralysis. (From Cogan DG: *Neurology of the Ocular Muscles,* ed 2. Courtesy of Charles C Thomas, Publisher, Springfield, Illinois.)

4. If the primary function of an eye muscle cannot be assessed, the examiner should try to assess its secondary function. For example, detection of a nerve IV paresis in the setting of a nerve III paresis is difficult because the eye cannot be adducted (due to medial rectus paresis) to permit testing depression, the primary action of the superior oblique muscle. But because nerve IV is secondarily an intorter in the abducted position, attempted adduction–depression movements intort the eye in the presence of intact nerve IV function.

Nystagmus should be assessed. By convention, the direction of nystagmus is said to be in the direction of the fast component. Nystagmus may be purely horizontal, purely vertical, or rotatory. Types of nystagmus are listed in Table 1-3.

V (Trigeminal Nerve)

The trigeminal nerve has both motor and somatic sensory functions. It arises from the pons, wherein the motor nuclei lie, whereas the sensory nuclei reside in the Gasserian ganglion. The trigeminal nerve divides into ophthalmic (first), maxillary (second), and mandibular (third) divisions (Figure 1-6). The first division supplies sensation to the cornea and to the forehead up to the vertex of the head. The second division supplies sensation to the cheeks, nose, upper teeth, and palate. The third division supplies sensation to the lower teeth, mandible, tongue, and ear, and provides innervation to the muscles of mastication.

TABLE 1-3 NYSTAGMUS

CATEGORY	CHARACTERISTICS	CAUSE
Peripheral vestibular	Horizontal or rotatory; suppressed by fixation; worsened by head movement; impaired caloric response	Labyrinth imbalance
Central vestibular	Vertical, horizontal, or rotatory; poorly suppressed by fixation; smooth pursuit impaired	Central vestibular dysfunction
Gaze-evoked	Induced by eccentric eye positions; seen best in darkness; pursuit deficit; rebound nystagmus	Seen in myasthenia gravis and eye muscle paresis
Rebound	Evoked by sustained eccentric gaze	Neural mechanism
Dissociated	Nystagmus different in each eye (eg, internuclear ophthalmoplegia)	Unknown
Congenital	Horizontal, conjugate; variable amplitude; accompanied by head shaking; worse with attention and arousal	Blindness in some cases
Latent	Conjugate; evoked by covering one eye; the other eye drifts toward the nose	Unknown
Acquired pendular	No fast or slow component; has both horizontal and vertical components.	Cerebellar dysfunction in multiple sclerosis and palatal myoclonus
Voluntary	Rapid horizontal oscillation at 15-25 Hz, tending to converge	Voluntary
Pursuit	Solely horizontal or vertical; low velocity drift	Lesions of parietal lobes or cerebellum
Rare forms	Consult Leigh and Zee	

Adapted from Leigh RJ, Zee DS: *The Neurology of Eye Movements.* Philadelphia, F.A. Davis, 1983, pp. 192-193. Used with permission.

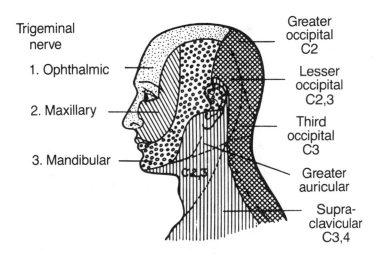

Figure 1-6. Trigeminal nerve sensory distribution. Adapted from Brash JC: *Cunningham's Textbook of Anatomy*, ed 9. New York, Oxford University Press.

Examination of the motor function of nerve V begins with observation of the temporalis muscles for evidence of hollowing. Palpation of the masseter muscle bulk can be performed with the patient clenching his teeth. The strength of the bite can be tested by having the patient bite down unilaterally on a tongue depressor placed between the molar teeth. The patient then slowly opens his jaw and the examiner looks for evidence of jaw deviation. In unilateral pterygoid weakness, the jaw deviates toward the side of the weak muscle. The examiner can then push laterally against the jaw as the patient opposes the force.

Sensation is tested with pin, light touch, vibration, position, and temperature stimuli as discussed in the section "Sensory Examination." The corneal reflex has the trigeminal nerve as the afferent limb and the facial nerve as the efferent limb. A light wisp of cotton is used as a stimulus. The tapered end of a cotton-tipped applicator, twisted to a cotton point, is an ideal stimulus. The patient is asked to gaze to his left. The examiner approaches the right eye from the right side and briefly touches the cotton tip on the right conjunctiva. This serves as a control stimulus because some people are so sensitive to touch anywhere about the eye that they blink even in response to this stimulus. Ordinarily, there should be no blink. The examiner then touches the right cornea and assesses the strength of the blink reflex. The process is repeated on the left with the eyes directed to the right and the examiner approaching from the left. The patient can be asked to compare the perceived sensations of the two stimuli.

VII (Facial Nerve)

The facial nerve has motor, parasympathetic, somatic sensory, and special sensory functions. The nerve arises from the pons, travels with nerve VIII through the internal auditory meatus, thence through the facial canal in the temporal bone, and exits the skull through the stylomastoid foramen. The motor portion innervates the muscles of facial expression and the stapedius muscle in the middle ear. The somatic sensory portion conducts sensation from a portion of the external ear canal and the mastoid region. The special sensory portion carries taste sensation from the anterior two-thirds of the tongue by way of the chorda tympani. The parasympathetic portion permits lacrimation by way of the superficial petrosal nerve, and salivation by way of the chorda tympani.

Motor function of nerve VII is tested first by observation of the patient's facies at rest, with spontaneous emotional expression, and with commands to "close your eyes," "raise your eyebrows," "blow out your cheeks," and "purse your lips." Subtle asymmetries in the depth of nasolabial folds, palpebral fissures, and the position of the corners of the mouth are sought. The symmetry of the platysma should be observed as the patient growls. The strength of the orbicularis oculi and orbicularis ori may be tested by the examiner forcefully attempting to open the patient's eyes and mouth with the patient opposing these actions.

Taste sensation on the anterior two-thirds of the tongue can be tested with a solution of salt or sugar painted on the lateral aspects of the outstretched tongue. The patient shakes his head "yes" or "no" to indicate whether the solution can be tasted—before bringing the tongue back into the mouth. Somatic sensation is not tested ordinarily because of the overlap of nerves V and IX and because of individual variation. Lacrimation can be tested with Schirmer's paper. Stapedius paralysis produces auditory hyperacusis, which can be determined by standard hearing tests, described under the discussion of cranial nerve VIII.

Facial hemiparesis is caused by a facial nerve lesion (lower motor neuron) such as Bell's palsy, or by a supranuclear lesion (upper motor neuron) such as contralateral corticobulbar tract damage from hemispheric stroke. The upper half of the face receives bilateral supranuclear innervation to each facial nerve, whereas the lower half receives only unilateral supranuclear innervation. In an upper motor neuron lesion, there is only lower-half facial paresis, whereas in a facial nerve lesion, the entire half of the face is paretic. Strength of the orbicularis oculus is the key to making the differentiation. There is trace weakness of this muscle in an upper motor neuron facial hemiparesis but profound weakness in a facial nerve lesion such as Bell's palsy.

Bell's palsy can impair other functions of the facial nerve in addition to causing muscular paresis, depending upon the location of the lesion. Consequently, the patient should be tested for taste, lacrimation, and auditory hyperacusis to survey whether these facial nerve functions are also affected.

VIII (Acoustic Nerve)

The acoustic nerve transmits the special sensations of hearing and balance from the inner ear to the brain stem. The acoustic nerve has a division for each function: the cochlear division for hearing and the vestibular for balance.

Hearing is tested clinically by placing a sound stimulus of known loudness and pitch before each ear. A softly ticking watch is an adequate stimulus, but a 512-Hz tuning fork is better because it has a high pitch and can be used to identify subtle hearing loss that especially affects high-frequency sounds. Furthermore, loudness can be regulated, and the patient's ability to hear can be compared with the examiner's ability. If unilateral hearing loss is detected, Weber's test can help classify the hearing loss as conductive or sensorineural. A 128-Hz tuning fork is sounded and placed in the center of the patient's forehead. If the unilateral hearing loss is conductive, the sound induced by the vibrating tuning fork will be heard loudest in the affected ear. If the hearing loss is sensorineural, the sound will be loudest in the normal ear.

The Rinne test measures the efficacy of air conduction of sound versus bone conduction. The 128-Hz tuning fork is sounded and placed on the mastoid process. The patient is instructed to indicate when he can no longer hear the sound. Then, the still vibrating tuning fork is placed next to the patient's ear and he indicates when he no longer hears the sound. Because air conduction is greater than bone conduction, the time the patient can hear the tuning fork by air conduction should be twice the time it can be heard by bone conduction. If air conduction time is less than twice bone conduction time, a conductive etiology to the hearing loss is suspected.

The precise pattern and often the etiology of hearing loss can be determined by formal audiometry. Standard pure-tone audiograms can be supplemented with more sophisticated tests to differentiate cochlear from retrocochlear lesions as well as types of conductive loss.

The vestibular division is not tested specifically in a general neurological examination, except when looking for nystagmus and for the extent to which the vestibular system contributes to coordination and gait. Vestibular imbalance produces vertigo. Vestibular system tests and evaluation of vertigo are considered in Chapter 6.

IX (Glossopharyngeal Nerve), X (Vagus Nerve)

The glossopharyngeal and vagus nerves are usually tested together. The former carries motor fibers from the medulla to the stylopharyngeus muscle, conducts somatic sensory input from the middle ear and eustachian tube, provides special sensory taste input from the posterior one-third of the tongue, and regulates parasympathetic secretory activity of the parotid gland. The vagus nerve conducts somatic motor impulses from the medulla to the pharynx, soft palate, and larynx; autonomic impulses to the heart, esophagus, stomach, and small intestine; somatic sensation from the ear; and special visceral sensation from thoracic and abdominal viscera.

Nerve IX and X testing begins with listening to the patient's voice. Pharyngeal paralysis increases the nasal quality of the voice. Unilateral vocal cord paralysis produces hoarseness. Bilateral vocal cord lesions produce a voice of reduced intensity, with an inability to make high-pitched sounds. Bilateral vocal cord paralysis in the adducted position produces cough, inspiratory stridor, and a brassy voice quality. Indirect laryngoscopy can be performed in cases of unexplained voice change to evaluate vocal cord movement.

The palate is examined as the patient says "Ahh." In unilateral pharyngeal weakness, the uvula and median raphe are deviated away from the paretic side to the normal side.

The swallowing of water is observed. Dysphagia is present with bilateral lesions of nerves IX and X (bulbar palsy) or with bilateral supranuclear corticobulbar lesions (pseudobulbar palsy). Fluids may be regurgitated through the nose in bilateral lesions of nerves IX and X.

The gag reflex is tested by touching each posterolateral pharyngeal wall sequentially with a wooden tongue blade. The normal response is contraction of the pharyngeal muscles, usually with gagging. Lesions of nerves IX and X produce loss of the gag reflex. Supranuclear corticobulbar lesions often have an exaggerated gag reflex.

It is possible, but difficult, to test taste on the posterior one-third of the tongue in a way that is analogous to taste testing for nerve VII. Most clinicians omit this test because it is very difficult to place the gustatory stimulus solution on the outstretched posterior one-third of the tongue without the solution diffusing onto the taste buds inside the mouth.

XI (Accessory Nerve)

This purely motor nerve, innervating the sternocleidomastoid and trapezius muscles, arises in the upper cervical spinal cord, ascends through the foramen magnum, and exits through the jugular foramen with nerves IX and X. Unilateral nerve XI lesions produce paralysis, atrophy, and fasciculations of the ipsilateral sternocleidomastoid and trapezius muscles. Upper motor neuron lesions produce only mild weakness because of bilateral supranuclear innervation, analogous to the upper face.

The examiner notes the size, shape, and symmetry of the sternocleidomastoid and trapezius muscles; both muscles can be easily palpated. Trapezius power is tested by having the patient shrug his shoulders against the examiner's resistance.

Sternocleidomastoid power is tested by having the patient turn his head in the direction *opposite* from the muscle tested, a useful point in the detection of factitious illness.

XII (Hypoglossal Nerve)

The hypoglossal nerve is a purely motor nerve that innervates the tongue. It arises in the medulla and passes through the hypoglossal foramen. It has primarily unilateral supranuclear control. Hypoglossal nerve lesions produce unilateral tongue weakness, atrophy, fasciculations, and dysarthria.

The examiner first observes the size and symmetry of the tongue as it rests on the floor of the mouth. Fasciculations should be sought in this position. The patient then protrudes the tongue. When there is weakness, the tongue deviates to the paretic side. Tongue deviation is usually more prominent in lower motor neuron lesions than in upper motor neuron lesions. The patient then pushes his tongue against the inside of his cheek while the examiner opposes this attempt with pressure on the outside of the cheek. The patient pronounces complicated phrases such as "Methodist-Episcopal" and "Commonwealth of Massachusetts" and repetitive lingual syllables such as "la-la-la..." and "the-the-the..." while the examiner listens for dysarthria.

MOTOR EXAMINATION

A complete motor examination includes tests and observations to assess muscle symmetry, size, shape, tone, and power; adventitious muscle movements; muscle coordination; mechanical muscle reactions; and muscle tendon reflexes. Examination of reflexes and coordination is discussed in other sections of this chapter.

Size, Shape, and Symmetry

The motor exam begins with the inspection of the limb and trunk musculature for evidence of atrophy and hypertrophy. Subtle degrees of asymmetric limb atrophy may be established by measuring left and right limb girths with a tape measure (at a constant distance proximal or distal to a joint) and comparing measurements. The patient's dominant arm may be 1 to 2 cm greater in circumference than his nondominant arm; asymmetries greater than 2 cm are significant.

Adventitious Movements

The limbs are inspected for evidence of involuntary, spontaneous, adventitious movements. Fasciculations are spontaneous synchronous contractions of the muscle fibers of a single motor unit as a result of denervation. They appear as minor muscle twitches not sufficiently strong to move a limb or to be obvious to the patient .They are seen in all denervating diseases of the lower motor neuron, but particularly in diseases of spinal cord anterior horn cells.

Myokymia is a continuous, regular, undulating, rippling fasciculation, usually of no pathologic significance.

Fibrillations are contractions of individual muscle fibers, also the result of denervation. Because an individual muscle fiber is so small, fibrillations usually cannot be seen or felt, except in the tongue. They can be detected easily by electromyography, however.

Tremor is a rhythmic, oscillatory dyskinesia, usually the result of sequential involuntary contractions of agonist, then antogonist, muscles. Tremor types, causes, and differential diagnosis are discussed in Chapter 12.

Chorea is a sudden, jerky, discrete, brief, irregular, purposeless, involuntary movement seen most often in the limbs and face. The amplitude of the dyskinesia is sufficient to move the part of the body affected. Movement occurs in an unpredictable pattern and disappears with sleep. The affected patient will often attempt to incorporate the choreiform movement into an ostensibly voluntary movement: A sudden jerk of the hand into the air may be followed by a voluntary smoothing down of the back of hair as if the entire gesture were volitional. Chorea is seen most often in Huntington's disease, Sydenham's chorea, side effects of medication (oral contraceptives, L-dopa), and unilaterally after strokes to the contralateral corpus striatum.

Athetosis is a distal, gross, slow, continuous, writhing movement in which there are varying degrees of tonic contraction of antagonistic muscles pulling the limb, face, or trunk in slow, contorted activity. It frequently coexists with chorea (choreoathetosis) in the disorders named above because both reflect damage to the corpus striatum. It is also seen as a type of cerebral palsy secondary to perinatal injury. Pseudoathetosis is a searching movement of the outstretched hands resulting from loss of proprioceptive input; it resembles athetosis only superficially.

Ballismus is a sudden, rapid, violent, involuntary flailing or flinging of a limb that requires so much muscular exertion that it exhausts the patient. It is often seen unilaterally involving an arm and leg, contralateral to a stroke in the subthalamic nucleus of Luys. As such, it is often associated with hemichorea.

Dystonia is a tonic, sustained involuntary muscular contraction of sufficient force to hold the affected body part in a "frozen," contorted state. The basal ganglia is the site of dysfunction in dystonias. Torticollis is a dystonia of the sternocleidomastoid muscles and sometimes other neck muscles. Dystonia musculorum deformans is a hereditary dystonia. Dystonias that include oculogyric crises often are seen as an idiosyncratic reaction to the first dose of a phenothiazine drug. Intravenous diphenhydramine (Benadryl) or benztropine mesylate (Cogentin) will quickly reverse neuroleptic-induced dystonia. Blepharospasm, another focal dystonia, is often associated with oromandibular dystonia (Meiges' syndrome).

Myoclonus is a sudden, rapid, muscle contraction of variable intensity. Multifocal myoclonus is an important sign of metabolic encephalopathy. It is often present in uremic and hypoxic encephalopathies, particularly after cardiac arrest. Nocturnal myoclonus, especially of the legs, awakens the patient many times nightly and disturbs sleep. The "hypnic jerk" is a single, synchronous myoclonic jerk that occurs normally as a person drifts off to sleep, particularly after an exhausting day. Palatal myoclonus is not true myoclonus, but a continuous tremor of the palate caused by brain stem-cerebellar disease of the pathways between the inferior olive, dentate nucleus, and red nucleus. It is the only type of tremor that persists during sleep.

Asterixis, or "flap," is an irregular, asynchronous movement of outstretched limbs in the patient with metabolic encephalopathies. When asked to hold hands or feet outstretched, he suddenly loses muscle tone; this is followed by a compensatory movement to return the limb to its outstretched position. It is often seen with tremor and multifocal myoclonus. Electrophysiologically, asterixis is an intermittent, sudden, brief lapse of extensor tone, during which there is electromyographic silence for less than 200 msec. The flap occurs just after the lapse of extensor tone.

Tics or habit spasms are learned, stereotyped, compulsive, complex movements, often of the face, that are under partial voluntary control. Patients asked to suppress them become anxious and are relieved only when they can resume performing the tic. In Gilles de la Tourette's syndrome, tics reach a magnitude in which they become socially and physically debilitating. There is partial improvement in Tourette's syndrome tics with haloperidol (Haldol).

Muscle Tone

The examiner tests muscle tone by assessing resistance to passive muscle stretching. The patient is instructed to "relax" and "go loose" to try to induce a state of resting muscle tone. Many anxious patients are unable to fully relax in this situation; further admonishment only makes the situation worse. Such patients should be given mental tasks to distract them during the assessment, such as to spell "world" backwards or to count backwards from 80 by seven.

While testing tone, the examiner notes the range of motion in joints, the presence of contractures, and the induction of pain on movement of the extremity. Resting tone can be described as normal, flaccid, spastic, or rigid. Normal resting tone produces the slightest resistance to passive stretch. In flaccidity, the limb is moved as dead weight with no opposition to movement. Flaccidity characterizes lower motor neuron syndrome when a lesion is present in the anterior horn cell of the spinal cord, peripheral nerve, root, or plexus.

Spasticity is caused by an upper motor neuron (corticospinal tract) lesion in which inhibitory descending control on the spinal reflex arc is eliminated. Hyperreflexia and increased muscle tone are produced by the disinhibition of the spinal reflex arc. Spasticity is a velocity-dependent increase in muscle tone, which is maximal at the onset of motion and decreases during motion. The "clasp-knife" quality is thus produced and a "giving way" is felt in the muscle during stretching. In very mild degrees of spasticity, only the spastic "catch" can be felt by the examiner when rapidly extending and flexing the patient's wrist or pronating and supinating the patient's arm. In severe spasticity, the arm tends to be held in a flexed posture at the elbow and wrist while the leg is held in extension at the knee and hip.

Rigidity is an extrapyramidal sign in which increased muscle tone is found throughout the range of passive movement. There is simultaneous contraction of agonist and antagonist muscles, often with tremor superimposed, producing "cogwheel" or "ratchety" rigidity. Limb rigidity has been called "lead-pipe" rigidity because of the increased tone throughout the range of movement.

A similar type of rigidity is seen in acute and chronic states of bilateral hemispheric dysfunction. Known as paratonia or *gegenhalten* (go–stop), it is marked by the patient's resistance to passive movement with an involuntary, antagonistic movement that is identical in force but opposite in direction to that made by the examiner.

Muscle Power

Testing the strength of individual muscles is a vital part of the neurological examination. It is necessary to identify the pattern of weakness to localize the disorder in the nervous sytem. For example, if only those muscles innervated by the radial nerve below the midhumerus are weak, the disorder is probably a radial mononeuropathy. Presenting syndromes of weakness are discussed in Chapter 10.

Muscle strength is tested by one of two techniques: (1) the patient is asked to hold a limb in a particular position and the examiner attempts to move it, or (2) the examiner begins to move a patient's limb and asks the patient to resist it. Experience dictates normal responses for age and sex. Women are generally significantly weaker than men, particularly in triceps power. Muscle power usually declines with age. The nondominant upper extremity is weaker than the dominant.

Muscle power is quantitated on a 0-to-5 scale as follows:

0   No contraction
1   Flicker or trace of contraction
2   Active movement with gravity eliminated
3   Active movement against gravity
4   Active movement against gravity and resistance
5   Normal power

To these numbers may be appended " + " or " − " to further describe the power. Alternatively, the terms slight, mild, moderate, and severe weakness may be applied. Specific techniques for examining each muscle are well described and illustrated in Mayo Clinic (1981), DeJong (1979), Bickerstaff (1980), Medical Research Council (1976), and Wolf (1981). The nerve root and peripheral nerve innervation of each muscle are listed in Table 1-4.

Subtle degrees of muscle weakness may be appreciated by testing for "drift." The patient extends both arms with hands supinated and eyes closed. In mild states of unilateral weakness, particularly in pyramidal lesions, there is a slow descent of the involved arm and pronation of the hand. In cases of factitious weakness, drift without pronation may be seen. Patients with parietal lobe lesions

TABLE 1-4 MUSCLE INNERVATIONS

MUSCLE	SEGMENTAL INNERVATION	PERIPHERAL NERVE
Head and Neck Movements		
Sternocleidomastoid	Cranial XI; C (1) 2-3	Spinal accessory nerve
Trapezius	Cranial XI; C (2) 3-4	Spinal accessory nerve
Scalenus anterior	C 4-7	
Scalenus medius	C 4-8	
Scalenus posterior	C 6-8	
Longus capitis	C 1-4	
Longus colli	C 2-6	
Rectus capitis	C 1-2	Suboccipital nerve
Obliquus capitis	C 1	Suboccipital nerve
Splenius	C 2-4 (1-6)	
Semispinalis capitis	C 1-4	
Semispinalis cervicis	C 3-6	
Spinalis cervicis	C 5-8	
Sacrospinalis	C 1-8	
Iliocostalis cervicis	C 1-8	
Longissimus	C 1-8	
Intertransversarii	C 1-8	
Rotatores	C 1-8	
Multifidi	C 1-8	
Shoulder Girdle and Arm Movements		
Trapezius	Cranial XI; C (2) 3-4	Spinal accessory nerve
Levator scapulae	C 3-4	Nerves to levator scapulae
	C 4-5	Dorsal scapular nerve
Rhomboideus	C 4-5	Dorsal scapular nerve
Serratus anterior	C 5-7	Long thoracic nerve
Deltoid	C 5-6	Axillary nerve
Teres minor	C 5-6	Axillary nerve
Supraspinatus	C (4) 5-6	Suprascapular nerve
Infraspinatus	C (4) 5-6	Suprascapular nerve
Latissimus dorsi	C 6-8	Thoracodorsal nerve (long subscapular)
Pectoralis major	C 5 - T 1	Lateral and medial anterior thoracic
Pectoralis minor	C 7 - T 1	Medial anterior thoracic
Subscapularis	C 5-7	Subscapular nerves
Teres major	C 5-7	Lower subscapular nerve

TABLE 1-4 *continued*

Muscle	Segmental Innervation	Peripheral Nerve
Subclavius	C 5-6	Nerve to subclavius
Coracobrachialis	C 6-7	Musculocutaneous nerve
Biceps brachii	C 5-6	Musculocutaneous nerve
Brachialis	C 5-6	Musculocutaneous nerve
Brachioradialis	C 5-6	Radial nerve
Triceps brachii	C 6-8 (T1)	Radial nerve
Anconeus	C 7-8	Radial nerve
Supinator brevis	C 5-7	Radial nerve
Extensor carpi radialis longus	C (5) 6-7 (8)	Radial nerve
Extensor carpi radialis brevis	C (5) 6-7 (8)	Radial nerve
Extensor carpi ulnaris	C 6-8	Radial nerve
Extensor digitorum communis	C 6-8	Radial nerve
Extensor indicis proprius	C 6-8	Radial nerve
Extensor digiti minimi	C 6-8	Radial nerve
Extensor pollicis longus	C 6-8	Radial nerve
Extensor pollicis brevis	C 6-8	Radial nerve
Abductor pollicis longus	C 6-8	Radial nerve
Pronator teres	C 6-7 (8)	Median nerve
Flexor carpi radialis	C 7 - T 1	Median nerve
Pronator quadratus	C 7 - T 1	Median nerve
Palmaris longus	C 7 - T 1	Median nerve
Flexor digitorum sublimis	C 7 - T 1	Median nerve
Flexor digitorum profundus (radial half)	C 7 - T 1	Median nerve
Lumbricales 1 and 2	C 8 - T 1	Median nerve
Flexor pollicis longus	C 8 - T 1	Median nerve
Flexor pollicis brevis (lateral head)	C 8 - T 1	Median nerve
Abductor pollicis brevis	C 8 - T 1	Median nerve
Opponens pollicis	C 8 - T 1	Median nerve
Flexor carpi ulnaris	C 7 - T 1	Ulnar nerve
Flexor digitorum profundus (upper half)	C 7 - T 1	Ulnar nerve
Interossei	C 8 - T 1	Ulnar nerve
Lumbricales 3 and 4	C 8 - T 1	Ulnar nerve
Flexor pollicis brevis (medial head)	C 8 - T 1	Ulnar nerve
Flexor digiti minimi brevis	C 8 - T 1	Ulnar nerve
Abductor digiti minimi	C 8 - T 1	Ulnar nerve
Opponens digiti minimi	C 8 - T 1	Ulnar nerve

Palmaris brevis	C 8 - T 1	Ulnar nerve
Adductor pollicis	C 8 - T 1	Ulnar nerve

Thorax and Abdomen Movements

Diaphragm	C 3-5	Phrenic nerve
Intercostal muscles (internal and external)	T 1-12	Intercostal nerves
Levatores costarum	C 8 - T 11	Intercostal nerves
Transversus thoracis	T 2-7	Intercostal nerves
Serratus posterior superior	T 1-4	Intercostal nerves
Serratus posterior inferior	T 9-12	Intercostal nerves
Rectus abdominis	T 5-12	Intercostal nerves
Pyramidalis	T 11-12	Intercostal nerves
Transversus abdominis	T 7 - L 1	Intercostal, ilioinguinal, and iliohypogastric nerves
Obliquus internus abdominis	T 7 - L 1	Intercostal, ilioinguinal, and iliohypogastric nerves
Obliquus externus abdominis	T 7 - L 1	Intercostal, ilioinguinal, and iliohypogastric nerves

Leg Movements

Psoas major	L (1) 2-4	Nerve to psoas major
Psoas minor	L 1-2	Nerve to psoas minor
Iliacus	L 2-4	Femoral nerve
Quadriceps femoris	L 2-4	Femoral nerve
Sartorius	L 2-4	Femoral nerve
Pectineus	L 2-4	Femoral nerve
Gluteus maximus	L 5 - S 2	Inferior gluteal nerve
Gluteus medius	L 4 - S 1	Superior gluteal nerve
Gluteus minimus	L 4 - S 1	Superior gluteal nerve
Tensor fasciae latae	L 4 - S 1	Superior gluteal nerve
Piriformis	S 1-2	Nerve to piriformis
Adductor longus	L 2-4	Obturator nerve
Adductor brevis	L 2-4	Obturator nerve
Adductor magnus	L 4-5	Sciatic nerve
Gracilis	L 2-4	Obturator nerve
Obturator externus	L 5 - S 3	Nerve to obturator internus
Obturator internus	L 5 - S 3	Nerve to obturator internus
Gemellus superior		

TABLE 1-4 *continued*

Muscle	Segmental Innervation	Peripheral Nerve
Gemellus inferior	L 4 - S 1	Nerve to quadratus femoris
Quadratus femoris	L 4 - S 1	Nerve to quadratus femoris
Biceps femoris (long head)	L 5 - S 1	Tibial nerve
Semimembranosus	L 4 - S 1	Tibial nerve
Semitendinosus	L 5 - S 2	Tibial nerve
Popliteus	L 5 - S 1	Tibial nerve
Gastrocnemius	L 5 - S 2	Tibial nerve
Soleus	L 5 - S 2	Tibial nerve
Plantaris	L 5 - S 1	Tibial nerve
Tibialis posterior	L 5 - S 1	Tibial nerve
Flexor digitorum longus	L 5 - S 1	Tibial nerve
Flexor hallucis longus	L 5 - S 1	Tibial nerve
Biceps femoris (short head)	L 5 - S 2	Common peroneal nerve
Tibialis anterior	L 4 - S 1	Deep peroneal nerve
Peroneus tertius	L 4 - S 1	Deep peroneal nerve
Extensor digitorum longus	L 4 - S 1	Deep peroneal nerve
Extensor hallucis longus	L 4 - S 1	Deep peroneal nerve
Extensor digitorum brevis	L 4 - S 1	Deep peroneal nerve
Extensor hallucis brevis	L 4 - S 1	Deep peroneal nerve
Peroneus longus	L 4 - S 1	Superficial peroneal nerve
Peroneus brevis	L 4 - S 1	Superficial peroneal nerve
Flexor digitorum brevis	L 4 - S 1	Medial plantar nerve
Flexor hallucis brevis	L 5 - S 1	Medial plantar nerve
Abductor hallucis	L 4 - S 1	Medial plantar nerve
Lumbricales (medial 1 or 2)	S 1-2	Medial plantar nerve
Quadratus plantae	L 5 - S 2	Lateral plantar nerve
Adductor hallucis	S 1-2	Lateral plantar nerve
Abductor digiti quinti	S 1-2	Lateral plantar nerve
Flexor digiti quinti brevis	S 1-2	Lateral plantar nerve
Lumbricales (lateral 2 or 3)	S 1-2	Lateral plantar nerve
Interossei	S 1-2	Lateral plantar nerve

Adapted from DeJong RN: *The Neurologic Examination,* ed 4. Hagerstown, Md, Harper & Row, 1979, pp. 339, 342, 360, 364. Used with permission.

affecting proprioceptive integration may elevate the affected hand when the eyes are closed.

Mechanical Muscle Reaction

Muscles should be palpated for consistency and tenderness. Increased consistency, with a feeling like hard rubber, is seen in muscular dystrophy and other primary myopathies. Muscle tenderness is often present in acute polymyositis and trichinosis. Denervating diseases and injuries produce muscles that are flabby and flaccid.

Muscle percussion normally induces the idiomuscular, or myotatic, response, a brief contraction that is akin to a deep-tendon reflex. This response is often absent in primary muscle diseases. If percussion of muscle induces a contraction that is sustained for several seconds or longer, percussion myotonia is said to be present. The muscles usually tested are the thenar eminence and the tongue. Contraction myotonia can be tested by having the patient sustain a contraction, then suddenly make a movement opposite to the contraction. For example, the patient squeezes his fingers tightly around the examiner's fingers for five seconds, then suddenly extends all his fingers. If myotonia is present, there is delayed and difficult finger extension that can take five seconds or longer. Myotonia is seen in myotonic dystrophy, myotonic congenita, and other primary diseases of muscle.

Myoedema is an unusual response of muscle to percussion, in which localized swelling persists for several seconds at the site of percussion. This finding has been described in severe hypothyroidism and other chronic illness.

SENSORY EXAMINATION

The sensory examination is the most tedious, subjective, and variable part of the examination of the nervous system. Many examiners perform it at the end of an already lengthy exam when both the patient and examiner are tired. Because the examination is totally subjective—with the results depending entirely upon the patient's perception of the applied stimuli—patients who are suggestible, histrionic, or embellishing can mislead the examiner. An adequate sensory examination requires an attentive and cooperative patient.

Testable sensory modalities can be divided into two groups: (1) the "primary" sensations of pain, temperature, light touch, vibration, and position; and (2) the "secondary," or higher cortical, sensations of stereognosis, barognosis, graphesthesia, two-point discrimination, and double simultaneous stimulation. The primary group requires the nervous system to be intact from the periphery to the thalamus; the secondary group requires intact thalamocortical connections as well.

There is an important anatomic separation of the primary sensory modalities that becomes important in assessment. At the peripheral nerve level, vibration and position sensations are carried along the heavily myelinated A fibers, whereas pain is carried by the unmyelinated C fibers. At the level of the spinal cord, the pain and temperature fibers ascend crossed in the lateral spinothalamic tracts. The fibers for position and vibration ascend uncrossed in the posterior columns.

At the brain-stem level, the pain and temperature fibers ascend in the spino-thalamic tracts of the lateral lemniscus, whereas position and vibration fibers form the medical lemniscus.

There are several principles of sensory examination. A screening exam is performed first over the trunk and limbs. Specific areas are tested further in detail if the patient's complaint is from that area (eg, "my hands are numb") or if the screening exam reveals an abnormality in that area. When a zone of decreased sensation is detected, the examiner should attempt to delineate the boundaries of the abnormality by marching repetitive sensory stimuli from the abnormal to the normal zones of sensation. Finally, if the primary modalities are markedly abnormal in an area, there is not much to be gained by testing the secondary modalities there.

Primary Sensory Modalities
Light Touch

Light touch is tested with a wisp of cotton applied to the skin in a nonrhythmic way. The patient closes his eyes and says "now" or "touch" when he perceives the light touch. The examiner should avoid stroking hairs because a stimulus of greater than intended magnitude is produced.

Pain

Pain sensation is best tested with an unused safety pin applied just to the point of being noxious but not to the point of piercing the skin or drawing blood. The clinician should not use the same pin over and over again because it gets dull and, more importantly, can transmit hepatitis virus between patients. Some experts advocate crisply breaking the stick of a cotton-tipped applicator and using the end as a sharp stimulus. The stick is cleaner than a used safety pin, but it is not as sharp. The clinician ideally should use a new safety pin for each patient. The patient indicates if the stimulus is felt to be sharp or painful.

Temperature

Ideally, temperature sensation is tested with glass tubes or metal disks containing hot and cold water. Because filling these containers is a nuisance, they are not commonly used. A simple and adequate test for temperature is to place one of the tines of a 128-Hz or 256-Hz tuning fork against the patient's skin and ask if it feels hot or cold, then to repeat the test with the end of a wooden tongue depressor. Because metal conducts heat well, its room temperature is felt as cool. Because the wood conducts heat poorly, it is perceived as a neutral thermal stimulus. Patients with normal temperature sensation can tell the "cold" from the "hot"; those with abnormal temperature sensation cannot.

Position

Joint position sensation is tested by the examiner moving the patient's distal finger or toe joint and asking him if the movement was up or down. The examiner must grasp the digit on the sides to minimize inadvertent cues provided to the patient.

If the digit is grasped above and below, the patient might feel pressure on the bottom as the joint is moved up. Normally, the patient should feel a distal finger movement of 2 degrees and a toe movement of 5 degrees. If position sensation in a given joint cannot be reported accurately, the next most proximal joint should be tested until the patient can report movement correctly.

Vibration

Vibration sensation can be tested on bony prominences or on the skin. A 128-Hz or 64-Hz tuning fork should be used; the 256-Hz fork does not impart a strong enough vibration to permit adequate testing. The examiner first applies the tuning fork to the patient's sternum to acquaint him with the feel of the stimulus. The tuning fork is then sounded and applied to the most distal bony prominences in the feet and hands. The patient reports when he can no longer feel the vibration stimulus. The examiner then applies the fork to the same part of his own body to use himself as a normal control. Allowances should be made for the decrease in vibration sensation that occurs with normal aging. If distal impairment is present, the stimulus should gradually be moved proximally until the limit of normal sensation is identified.

Secondary Sensory Modalities

If the primary sensory modalities are grossly intact and the examiner wants to assess the component of sensation served by hemispheric thalamocortical pathways, the secondary sensory modalities may be tested. Patients with parietal lobe lesions may have normal primary modality sensation but impaired secondary modality sensation on the side of the body contralateral to the lesion. Usually, performance on the two body sides is compared, using one side as a control for the other.

Two-point discrimination

The ability to discriminate between a single-point stimulus and two closely and simultaneously applied point stimuli is a parietal lobe function. The examiner may use the points of a drawing compass or of a commercially available device specifically designed to test two-point discrimination. A handy alternative is to crisply break the stick of a cotton-tipped applicator into two sharp fragments and to use the two resulting points. Normal two-point discrimination varies greatly over the skin surface. The lips and fingertips are most sensitive; the back is least sensitive. Whether a particular body part is adept at two-point discrimination depends not so much on the density or type of cutaneous receptors as it does on the amount of parietal cortex assigned to integrate the sensory input. Normal values for two-point discrimination over various body parts are:

     Fingertips: less than 4 mm
     Palms: less than 10 mm
     Toes: less than 10 mm
     Hand dorsum: less than 30 mm
     Back: less than 70 mm

It is crucial when testing two-point discrimination to apply the two stimuli simultaneously. An inadvertent, very slight time delay makes very simple the identification of the stimuli as two, even in the presence of impaired two-point discrimination. The examiner alternates between applying a single stimulus and two closely applied stimuli, each time asking the patient if he feels one or two points. The distance between the points is gradually increased until the threshold for accurate two-point discrimination is identified.

Double Simultaneous Stimulation

Thalamic lesions can produce extinction to double simultaneous stimulation on the side contralateral to the lesion. The patient is tested with his eyes closed. He responds verbally or by gesture to the exact location touched by the examiner. The examiner tests each hand and each side of the face separately. Then, without warning, the examiner touches homologous areas of both hands simultaneously and repeats the maneuver on other homologous body areas. Another type of extinction is "rostral dominance," the tendency to extinguish caudal stimuli in favor of rostral ones. Present in childhood, it may reappear in states of bilateral hemispheric dysfunction. The patient may extinguish the hand stimulus when hand and face are touched simultaneously.

Graphesthesia

Graphesthesia is the ability to recognize letters or numbers sketched on the skin. Like two-point discrimination, there is great variation in the size of characters that can be felt in different areas of the skin. The examiner draws numbers or letters 0.5 to 1 cm in height on the fingertips. The process can be repeated on the palms with 4-cm characters.

Stereognosis

Stereognosis is the ability to recognize common objects just by touching them. Test objects include coins, a safety pin, a paper clip, a key, and a rubber band. Test objects are placed in each hand one at a time, and the patient names them. He is not allowed to transfer objects from one hand to the other. The test can be made more sensitive by double simultaneous presentation of test objects in both hands.

Barognosis

Barognosis is the ability to discriminate the weight of objects by holding them. With the patient's eyes closed, objects of similar shapes and sizes but different weights are placed in his hands. The patient tells which object is heavier. With parietal lobe damage, the contralateral hand usually feels the object as lighter, even if it is heavier.

Sensory Localization

If abnormalities are disclosed on the sensory exam, the clinician next must interpret their significance. The presence of normal primary modalities with abnormal secondary modalities suggests parietal lobe dysfunction. If the primary modalities are impaired, the clinician first must consider which modalities are affected. If the sensory loss is "dissociated" (abnormal pain and temperature with normal position and vibration) the lesion is probably in the spinal cord (eg, syringomyelia) or in the peripheral nerves (eg, amyloid neuropathy). Abnormal position and vibration sensation with intact pain and temperature sensation suggests a lesion of the posterior columns of the spinal cord or of the periphered nerves.The clinician must compare the pattern of sensory loss he detects with anatomic charts of known nerve root and peripheral nerve sensory distributions (Figures 1-7 and 1-8).

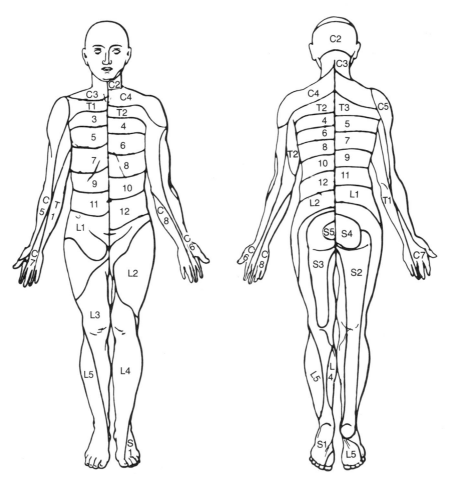

Figure 1-7. Dermatomal sensory patterns. (From Ford FR: *Diseases of the Nervous System in Infancy, Childhood and Adolescence*, ed 3. (Courtesy of Charles C Thomas, Publisher, Springfield, Illinois.)

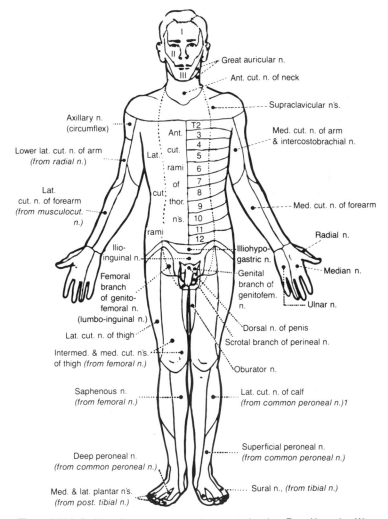

Figure 1-8(a). Peripheral nerve sensory patterns, anterior view. From Haymaker W. Woodall B: *Peripheral Nerve Injuries: Principles of Diagnosis.* (Reproduced with permission from W.B. Saunders.)

COORDINATION

Coordination testing ordinarily is performed to examine the cerebellar contribution to motor functioning. But normal coordinated movements require the proper functioning of sensory input systems in addition to the motor and cerebellar system. Vision is necessary to precisely guide the intended movement; vestibular and proprioceptive inputs provide spatial orientation cues necessary for fine motor control. Because normal cerebellar function depends on inputs from these sensory systems, impairments of coordination can arise from impaired visual,

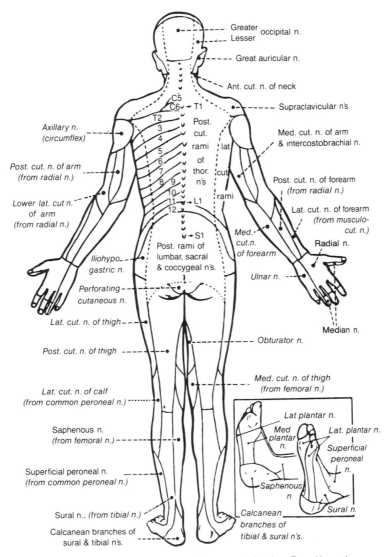

Figure 1-8(b). Peripheral nerve sensory patterns, posterior view. From Haymaker W, Woodhall B: *Peripheral Nerve Injuries: Principles of Diagnosis.* (Reproduced with permission from W.B. Saunders.)

vestibular, or proprioceptive inputs as well as from intrinsic cerebellar dysfunction. Coordination testing can be interpreted correctly only after examinations of visual, vestibular, motor, and proprioceptive functioning.

Coordination is tested by observing the accuracy, grace, and facility of fine movements of the extremities. In the finger-to-nose test, the patient extends his right forefinger and touches his nose. The examiner then holds his own right forefinger about 2 feet in front of the patient's nose. The patient alternately touches his own nose and the examiner's finger. The examiner moves his own finger into several different positions for the patient to gauge and reach in successive attempts. The left side is tested similarly. The speed, accuracy, and finesse of each movement is assessed by the examiner.

The heel-to-shin test makes a similar assessment of leg coordination. While supine, the patient raises his right leg and lightly places his right heel on his left knee, then makes even hops with the right heel being moved about 2 inches down the shin and distally to the foot. Once at the foot, the process is performed in reverse back to the knee. It is then repeated for the left heel and right knee.

Rapid rhythmic alternating limb movements are assessed in upper and lower extremities. The patient repetitively slaps his right palm on his right knee as quickly and accurately as possible; then he alternately slaps the palm and the dorsum of his hand against his knee. A similar test is to touch the thumb and forefingers rapidly and repetitively, or the thumb and all fingertips in succession. Leg movements are tested by having the patient repetitively tap the floor with each foot.

In cerebellar ataxia, there is decomposition of movement, slowness, clumsiness, overshooting the mark, and action tremor. The more fine and rapid the movement, the worse the ataxia. Dysmetria, the inability to judge distances by limb movement, and dysdiadochokinesia, the inability to perform rapid, rhythmic movements, are classic cerebellar signs.

In cerebellar dysfunction, frequently there are hypotonia and also a loss of checking movements. Checking movements are assessed by having the patient contract the biceps muscle against resistance; the examiner then suddenly removes the resistance. Normal checking is present when the sudden release of the limb is recognized and stopped after only about 30 degrees of inadvertent elbow flexion. In loss of checking caused by cerebellar disease, the hand may continue flexion movement when released, to the extent of striking the patient in his face. The examiner must guard the patient's face with his forearm to prevent injury. The legs can be similarly tested.

Cerebellar ataxia also may be assessed by observing phonation and the movements of eyelids, tongue, and lips. The patient makes rapid repetitive movements and the examiner watches for irregularity and decomposition of movement. To test for labial and lingual ataxia, the patient alternately moves the tongue from side to side and says "la la la...," "pa pa pa...," "me me me...," etc. Phonation ataxia is tested by having the patient hold a note (eg, middle C) while saying "eeee..." for at least five seconds. With phonation ataxia, the pitch and the volume of the sustained note fluctuate, producing an exaggerated vibrato.

GAIT AND STATION

Tradition has it that nineteenth century clinicians needed only to watch a patient walk to make a correct neurological diagnosis. Normal gait requires the proper functioning of almost all the components of the nervous system: adequate consciousness, praxis, and spatial orientation; visual fields, acuity, and vestibular functioning; and motor, proprioceptive, and cerebellar functioning. Gait examination, therefore, supplements the examination of each subsystem and confirms the findings.

The patient is taken to a hallway or large room where objects do not encumber the path and there is at least a 30 foot space to walk. The patient is asked to walk normally. The examiner notes the balance, ease, grace, poise, presence of associated arm movements, symmetry, confidence, freedom, and bounciness of gait. The patient is then observed walking on his toes, then on his heels. Tandem gait is tested by having the patient walk in a straight line with heel touching toe. Then the patient walks on the lateral surfaces of his feet in a waddling fashion. Heel, toe, tandem, and lateral foot gait tests are designed to stress the nervous system to magnify minor asymmetries and amplify minor signs. For example, the patient with mild pyramidal dysfunction of the left arm may have normal ordinary walking but may have abnormal posture and may not swing the left arm normally during stressed gait testing.

Station is tested by observing the patient while sitting for evidence of "titubation," a swaying ataxia seen in advanced midline cerebellar disease. While the patient stands, the clinician observes the width of his base. Ataxic patients tend to adopt a wide base to prevent themselves from falling. The patient is asked to stand with his feet together, toes and heels touching. This position is very difficult for ataxic patients.

If the narrow-base position can be assumed, the patient is asked to close his eyes. The normal person may exhibit a trace of swaying, but he can usually stand with feet together and eyes closed for 30 seconds. In cases of sensory ataxia, there is absolute reliance on visual input to compensate for impaired proprioceptive input. Here, Romberg's sign is positive as the patient sways and falls when the eyes are closed but not when the eyes are open. In cerebellar ataxia, the patient has great difficulty standing with feet together with his eyes open *or* closed. Unilateral vestibular disease can also produce swaying and falling with eyes closed. The examiner must take care to guard the patient with his hands to prevent injury while testing for Romberg's sign.

In young patients with subtle forms of ataxia, the sharpened Romberg's sign can be performed. The patient stands with his feet in the tandem position, with heel touching toe in a straight line. Normal young people should be able to stand in this position for 20 seconds with eyes closed.

A number of classic abnormal gait patterns have been described. More than one pattern can coexist; for example, the multiple sclerosis patient often has both spastic and ataxic components to his gait. Various degrees of severity may be present in all types.

1. *Hemiplegic gait.* Unilateral upper-extremity and lower-extremity pyramidal dysfunction produces hemiplegic or hemiparetic gait. The leg is extended at the knee and circumducted at the hip, with the toe scraping the floor. The arm is flexed at the elbow and wrist and associated swinging movement is decreased. Hemispheric stroke is the most common cause of hemiplegic gait.

2. *Spastic gait.* Bilateral leg pyramidal dysfunction produces the spastic "scissors" gait. The patient walks slowly and with effort with the knees extended

and the hips moved in adduction movements with pelvic tilting movements. The thighs scraping each other in adduction produces a scissorlike movement. Cerebral palsy and multiple sclerosis are common causes of spastic gait.

3. *Sensory ataxic gait.* Impairment of proprioceptive input produces sensory ataxia. The patient may say he "does not know where the floor is" and slaps and stamps his feet as he walks. The gait is mildly wide-based and the feet are lifted high and uncertainly. The patient relies entirely on visual cues and his eyes are fixed to the ground. Gait impairment is much worse in the dark.

Normal people occasionally experience sensory ataxia when descending stairs. If a person is not looking and incorrectly expects one more step, he is surprised as his foot suddenly stamps the floor. This is what patients with sensory ataxia experience all the time. Disorders of peripheral nerves and posterior columns can produce sensory ataxia.

4. *Cerebellar ataxic gait.* This disorder is produced by dysfunction of the midline cerebellum (anterior superior vermis). The gait is erratic, irregular, reeling, imbalanced, and very wide-based. Attempted compensatory movements often exacerbate the state of imbalance. This gait is seen in patients with cerebellar degeneration and midline cerebellar neoplasms.

5. *Steppage gait.* Patients with unilateral or bilateral foot drop must pick up their knee very high to avoid dragging the foot. There is a slapping quality as the foot is placed toe-first on the floor. There is an inability to walk on the heels. The gait is often called "equine" because it is similar to that of a prancing horse. Foot drop may be the result of common peroneal mononeuropathy, hereditary motor-sensory neuropathy (Charcot–Marie–Tooth disease), or ruptured lumbar intervertebral disc with L5 root compression.

6. *Waddling gait.* In patients with primary muscle disease, proximal pelvic girdle muscle weakness produces characteristic walking called waddling or dystrophic gait. While walking, the patient's pelvis tilts inappropriately, producing swaying of the trunk that resembles a duck waddling. Myopathic diseases, including the muscular dystrophies and polymyositis, produce the waddling gait.

7. *Parkinsonian gait.* The patient with idiopathic or drug-induced parkinsonism walks with short steps (*marche à petit pas*), shuffling feet, stooped trunk, flexed head, arms flexed at the elbows and wrists, and fingers adducted and flexed at the metacarpophalyngeal joints while extended at the interphalangeal joints. This patient also has decreased or absent arm swing, and acceleration (festination), as if he were trying to chase his own center of gravity that somehow got ahead of him. The patient often cannot initiate walking and exhibits retropulsion and rigid and clumsy *en bloc* turning.

8. *Apraxic gait.* Although perhaps a misnomer, patients with frontal lobe gait, particularly that resulting from bifrontal tumors or hydrocephalus, exhibit a distinct gait disorder. It is also called "Bruns' apraxia" and "glue-footed gait." The patient cannot initiate walking—as if his shoes were stuck to the floor. Once walking, he shuffles and is clumsy. He cannot skip or hop. Disorders producing apraxic gait also produce urge urinary incontinence and subcortical dementia.

9. *Senile gait.* With advancing age, the gait begins to resemble mild parkinsonism, with short steps, flexion, and some loss of associated movements. This gait is discussed in Chapter 3.

10. *Hysterical gait.* A variety of bizarre, inconsistent, and exaggerated gait types are seen in conversion and malingering. Generally, the gait appearance does not fit a characteristic syndrome and is inconsistent with findings on the rest of the exam. Often there is much lurching and exaggerated compensatory movements without falling. The clinician should exercise caution in assigning this diagnosis.

REFLEXES

Reflex assessment is the most objective part of the examination of the nervous system. In addition to the cranial nerve reflexes already discussed, three types of reflex activity are commonly assessed: (1) deep-tendon (muscle stretch) reflexes; (2) cutaneous superficial reflexes; and (3) pathologic (regressive) reflexes.

Deep-Tendon Reflexes

Deep-tendon reflexes can be elicited from any muscle by suddenly stretching the muscle tendon. These monosynaptic reflexes receive descending inhibitory input from the corticospinal tract. Lesions of the lower motor neuron (anterior horn cell, nerve root, peripheral nerve) interrupt the reflex arc and cause hypoactivity or ablation of the reflex. Lesions of the corticospinal tract in the brain or spinal cord produce disinhibition and hence hyperactivity of the reflex arc. The most severe form of deep-tendon reflex hyperactivity is clonus, wherein a persistently applied stretch to the tendon produces continuous rhythmic phasic muscle contraction. Deep-tendon reflexes increase with anxiety, hyperthyroidism, hypocalcemia, and increases in muscle tone caused by injury and pain. There is a spectrum of normal reflex amplitude that each clinician must learn. Comparison between left and right sides is mandatory.

The clinician ordinarily assesses deep-tendon reflexes of the biceps (C5-C6), triceps (C7-C8), and brachioradialis (C5-C6) muscles in the arm, and of the quadriceps (L3-L4) and gastrocnemius (L5-S1) muscles in the leg. Other muscles easily tested include pectorals (C5-C6), finger flexors (C7-C8, T1) hamstrings (L5-S1), and leg adductors (L2-L4). The clinician usually taps the muscle tendon directly, but for biceps, pectorals, hamstrings, and leg adductors it is easier for the examiner to tap his own finger tip placed over the muscle tendon.

Deep-tendon reflex activity is graded as follows:

0 Absent
1 Hypoactive
2 Normal
3 Hyperactive
4 Hyperactive with sustained clonus

Subtle intermediate grades can be created by the addition of plus (+) and minus (−) qualifiers.

Complete relaxation and correct positioning are necessary for the proper assessment of reflexes. All arm reflexes can be tested with the arm flexed at 90 degrees to 120 degrees. The gastrocnemius reflex (ankle jerk) requires the examiner to actively dorsiflex the foot to its maximum extent.

If a reflex cannot be obtained despite proper technique, positioning, and relaxation, methods of reinforcement should be attempted. These measures are designed to increase the general state of body tone and amplify the reflexes. Reinforcement of upper-extremity reflexes is obtained by having the patient clench his teeth just before and during the tendon tap. Reinforcement of lower-extremity reflexes is obtained with Jendrassik's maneuver: The patient pronates one arm and supinates the other, locking the fingers of each hand together; just before and during the reflex, he pulls the left hand against the right. Only if no reflex can be obtained during reinforcement can the deep-tendon reflex in question be said to be absent.

Superficial Reflexes

In addition to corneal and gag reflexes, the superficial abdominal (T6-T12) and cremasteric (L1-L2) reflexes are ordinarily tested. The superficial abdominal reflexes are lost in pyramidal lesions, unlike the deep tendon reflexes, which become hyperactive. The superficial abdominal reflexes are tested with the patient supine, relaxed, and warm. Each quadrant of the abdomen is stroked briskly with a particularly noxious stimulus. The ideal stimulus is a sewing pattern tracer, which is a device with a handle and a rotating circular head that contains radially oriented straight pins and that rolls across the skin as the device is moved. The clinician should take care to have the patient relax properly and should observe the abdomen carefully on the first stroke because the superficial abdominal reflexes often extinguish in normal people. The reflex is present when the umbilicus moves in the direction of the stimulated quadrant. In a young person, the absence of abdominal reflexes is an important sign of bilateral pyramidal dysfunction (usually of spinal cord origin) and is commonly seen in multiple sclerosis.

In men, the cremasteric reflex is tested by stroking the medial superior aspect of the thigh of the supine patient with a mildly noxious stimulus, such as the sewing pattern tracer, the edge of a broken tongue blade, or a cotton-tipped applicator. Normally there is reflex contraction of the ipsilateral cremasteric muscle and elevation of the testicle. If the patient is cold, the testicles will already be elevated and the reflex cannot be appreciated.

The cutaneous anal reflex (S3-S5), (anal wink) is occasionally tested in patients with presumed spinal cord lesions. The left, then right, perianal skin is stroked once briskly with the broken edge of a cotton-tipped applicator. There should be reflex contraction of the external anal sphincter, which can be seen or can be felt by the gloved finger.

Pathologic ("Regressive") Reflexes

A group of reflexes seen in normal neonates later become inhibited with maturation and pyramidal tract myelination. In disease of the pyramidal tracts, these reflexes become disinhibited and may reappear in their infantile form. The clinician should test for Babinski's sign and Wartenberg's sign in patients with suspected pyramidal tract lesions. Tests for suck, snout, glabellar, palmomental, and grasp reflexes (see below) are performed in any patient with suspected bilateral hemispheric dysfunction. These may be present in the normal elderly person.

Babinski's sign is a time-honored sign that nearly always indicates corticospinal tract dysfunction. The clinician strokes the most lateral portion of the supine patient's sole with a blunt object from the heel to the base of the fifth toe, then across the ball of the foot to the base of the great toe. A key, the broken edge of a wooden tongue blade, or two broken edges of a cotton-tipped applicator make good stimuli. The normal response to this plantar stimulation is flexion of the great toe. The pathologic response (positive Babinski's sign) is extension of the great toe and fanning of the remaining toes. It is often difficult to distinguish between an extension response and a voluntary withdrawal response. If voluntary withdrawal is suspected, the clinician should stroke more lightly.

In the presence of continued withdrawal responses, the clinician can test the same reflex with several alternative methods of stimulation. The lateral foot can be stroked (Chaddock's reflex), or both Babinski's and Chaddock's reflexes can be tested simultaneously with the tines of a 128-Hz tuning fork: one tine on the lateral foot, the other on the lateral sole. The anterior tibial surface can be stroked from proximally to distally (Oppenheim's reflex) or the calf muscle can be squeezed (Gordon's reflex).

Wartenberg's hand sign is the upper-extremity equivalent of Babinski's sign in the lower extremity. It is highly suggestive of corticospinal tract disease. The clinician bends his fingers 2 through 5 into partial flexion and places his fingertips against those of the patient, which are in the same position. The clinician and patient pull against each other and movements of the thumb are observed. Normally, there is no movement or slight flexion. The positive pathologic response is adduction of the thumb across the hand.

It has been incorrectly stated that Hoffman's sign necessarily has pathological significance. When the examiner briskly flicks the distal phalanx of the patient's middle finger, Hoffman's sign is said to be present if there is reflex flexion of the distal phalanx of the thumb and forefinger. This sign only represents hyperactivity of the finger flexor reflex (C7-C8, T1). This hyperactivity may or may not be pathological.

Suck, snout, and grasp reflexes may indicate bilateral hemispheric dysfunction in the nonelderly patient. The suck response is tested by placing a tongue depressor in the patient's closed lips. Sucking or swallowing movements are the pathologic response. Snouting is tested by lightly tapping the closed lips with a tongue depressor or the middle phalanx of the examiner's flexed index finger. Reflex pursing of the lips is the positive response. Grasping is tested by stroking the patient's palm with the examiner's fingers. If the patient grasps the examiner's hand, he should be asked to let go. Grasping itself is not necessarily abnormal, but forced grasping in which the patient cannot let go suggests bilateral hemispheric dysfunction.

The palmomental reflex is tested by firmly stroking the patient's thenar eminence with a tongue blade and observing the ipsilateral mentalis muscle for evidence of contraction. The sign is said to be positive if, after five consecutive stimuli, there is no extinction and each stimulus continues to provoke a response. This sign is seen in 10% to 20% of normal people.

The glabellar reflex is tested by tapping the midline supraorbital ridge (glabella), approached from behind with the examiner's index fingertip. A positive response is the absence of extinction of the blink response after the fifth stimulus. This sign is present in parkinsonism (Myerson's sign) and in some normal elderly patients.

The glabellar, palmomental, and snout reflexes may be normal in the elderly population (Chapter 3). Their significance must be interpreted in the context of the entire examination.

AUTONOMIC EXAM

Assessment of respiratory rate and pattern is considered in Chapter 35. Assessment of blood pressure is discussed in Chapter 7. Assessment of bowel, bladder, and sexual dysfunction is discussed in Chapter 17.

Bibliography

Bickerstaff ER: *Neurological Examination in Clinical Practice,* ed 4. Oxford, Blackwell Scientific Publications, 1980. (A terse, concise, clear, well-illustrated book; a briefer competitor of the Mayo Clinic book.)

DeJong RN: *The Neurologic Examination,* ed 4. Hagerstown, Md, Harper & Row, 1979. (A large reference work to be consulted for detailed explanations, obscure signs, and all eponyms.)

Folstein MF, Folstein FE, McHugh PR: Mini-mental state: A practical method for grading the cognitive state of patients for the clinician. *J Psychiatr Res* 1975; 12:189-198. (The source of Table 1-1; describes a useful screening mental status exam.)

Leigh RJ, Zee DS: *The Neurology of Eye Movements.* Philadelphia, F.A. Davis, 1983. (An old adage states: "He who knows neuro-ophthalmology knows neurology." This book contains an excellent and authoritative account of the clinical neurology of eye movements.)

Mayo Clinic: *Clinical Examinations in Neurology,* ed 5. Philadelphia, Saunders, 1981. (The best short work devoted to the neurologic examination; highly recommended.)

Medical Research Council: *Aids to the Examination of the Peripheral Nervous System.* London, Her Majesty's Stationery Office, 1976. (Small, portable, indispensable reference for examination of muscle weakness; very well-illustrated.

Spillane JD: *An Atlas of Clinical Neurology,* ed 3. London, Oxford University Press, 1984. (Beautifully illustrated and written picture book of neurologic exam findings, collected by a master clinician.)

Strub RL, Black FW: *The Mental Status Examination in Neurology,* ed 2. Philadelphia, F.A. Davis, 1984. (Authoritative reference work on the mental status examination.)

Wartenberg R: *Diagnostic Tests in Neurology.* Chicago, Year Book Publishers, 1953. (A classic book by the master neurologist of this century; long out of print and packed with clinical pearls.)

Wolf JK: *Segmental Neurology.* Baltimore, University Park Press, 1981. (Recent and able competitor to the Medical Research Council book. Well-organized and well-illustrated discussion of motor and sensory examination.)

The Neurological Examination of Neonates and Children

The principles of clinical diagnosis developed in adult neurology also apply to the neonate and older child. A careful history, detailing the neurological problem, must be obtained. Most often the chief complaint is given by the parents. It is important to obtain information from both parents, if possible, because they may have different perspectives on the child's illness. Careful attention must be paid to the history of the mother's pregnancy, labor and delivery, and the neonatal period. Attention must be paid to the developmental history and past medical history of the child. The family history should be obtained, in part to ascertain if the neurological problem is hereditary. An immunization history is also necessary. A standard medical history should be obtained, with emphasis on the relationship of medical illness to the child's neurological problem.

NEONATE

A gestation of 38 to 42 weeks usually results in a neurologically mature infant. It is usually best to perform a neurological examination on the second or third day after birth. There are several means of determining the gestational age of a newborn, including the date of the mother's last menstrual period, the child's head circumference, and certain developmental or neurophysiological functions. Examination of certain external characteristics, including the resilience of the ear cartilage and its reflection on ear position, the quantity of breast tissue, the presence of creases on the plantar surface of the foot, and the characteristics of the external genitalia all help determine gestational age. An infant with a normal length of gestation, tends at birth to have a firm pinna of the ear that stands erect from the head. Breast tissue amounts to a 6- to 7-mm nodule; external genitalia demonstrate (in the male) descended testes and a pendulous scrotum covered with rugae; (in the female) the clitoris is covered by the labia majora. Examination of the foot reveals plantar surface creases on the sole.

In the first part of the examination, the physician observes the recumbent infant. Most congenital abnormalities of the cranium, face, limbs, spine or skin are easily visible. Midline areas (face, spine, palate, cranium) should be carefully observed because defects in these areas are usually associated with anomalies of neural tube closure. The infant's level of alertness should also be determined. The full-term infant exhibits periods of attention to visual and auditory stimuli and is easily aroused. Sleep–waking cycles are evident, and crying is often observed during wakefulness. The typical newborn posture at rest is a symmetrically increased flexor tone with the arms and legs flexed and the hands fisted. In the prone position the infant maintains the flexed posture and elevates the pelvis with flexion of the hips and the knees. Spontaneous limb motions tend to be asymmetric and jerky. The alert newborn's eyes are usually symmetrically open; however, at times, only one eye is open. Conjugate horizontal ocular movements can be observed. Mild degrees of convergence or divergence are not unusual.

Cranial Nerves

I. Olfaction testing is rarely necessary in the newborn. Changes of various aromas can be noted by the newborn; in one study, those of greater than 32 weeks' gestational age responded (by sucking and/or arousal–withdrawal) to a cotton pledget soaked with peppermint abstract.

II. The estimated visual acuity in the newborn infant is 20/100 to 20/150. At term, he or she is capable of visual fixation and of following a bright object. An object (such as the examiner's face) can be placed 6 to 8 inches from the infant's face and moved slowly. Visual tracking should normally occur, although visual attention is usually brief. The funduscopic examination of the newborn may be difficult to perform; the optic disc has a pale greyish-white appearance, and has a less vascular appearance than that of an older child. In 20% to 40% of all newborns, retinal hemorrhages are evident, predominantly in infants delivered vaginally.

III, IV, VI. The symmetry of the pupils and the degree of pupillary reaction are often difficult to assess in the newborn because the eyes are often closed and difficult to open. Also, the color differences between the pupil and the iris are subtle. The size of the pupils in the newborn ranges from 4 to 5 mm. In some term infants, the eyes are slightly dysconjugate at rest. Spontaneous roving eye movements are present at term. Following movements can be tested with a bright moving object, although tracking movements are usually difficult to obtain in the newborn. The oculocephalic response can be produced by gentle passive movement of the head to one side then the other; normally, the eyes deviate conjugately in the direction opposite the movement of the head. The response to vertical movements can be tested by passive upward and downward head motions.

V. Facial sensation can be tested by touching the infant's face with a sharp object such as a sterile pin. The normal response is a facial grimace on the side stimulated. The motor function of the trigeminal nerve can be tested by observing how the infant sucks (for example, by sucking the examiner's clean finger).

VII. The position of the face at rest and the symmetry of facial movement when crying are easily determined components of facial nerve function. Attention should be paid to the symmetry of the palpebral fissures and the nasolabial folds.

Taste (also mediated by cranial nerve IX) is rarely evaluated in the neonate. Sweet and salty substances placed on an object for the baby to suck may be associated with a change in the rate of sucking and respiration, or may cause him to cry.

VIII. The neonate should respond to loud noises. Although a startle response is usually evident, he may respond to the sounds by opening his eyes, by becoming quiet, by changing his respiratory pattern, or by turning toward the noise. The baby so tested should be alert, not agitated or hungry, and free of significant ear wax. More sophisticated tests can be performed on the infant with suspected hearing loss.

IX-X. Movement of the palate can be observed during crying or gagging; a small cotton-tipped swab can be used to elicit a gag reflex as in the adult. Observation of the child feeding also provides information regarding the IX-X complex. Because feeding requires both sucking and swallowing, multiple cranial nerves are tested when the infant is observed feeding. Sucking motions require integrated functions of cranial nerves V, VII, and XII; swallowing utilizes cranial nerves IX and X; and tongue function relies on cranial nerve XII.

XI. The function of the spinal accessory nerve is difficult to test in the neonate. Sternocleidomastoid muscles should look and feel symmetrical, but it is often difficult to test these muscles individually. As the infant flexes and rotates his head to the opposite side, ipsilateral sternocleidomastoid muscles contract.

XII. Tongue movement can be assessed when the neonate sucks the examiner's fingertip; crying also permits observation of tongue movements.

Motor Reflexes
Tone

Muscle tone in a term neonate is increased, with a flexor predominance. Tone is best assessed by passive movements of all limbs at each joint. Careful observation of the infant's posture is also valuable when examining tone. Muscle tone must be evaluated with the infant's head held in midposition; deviation to either side can produce a tonic neck reflex (see below), which results in pseudoasymmetry of tone. Another means of estimating tone is to observe the posture of the limbs and body with the newborn held in horizontal suspension. The normal newborn maintains a flexed fetal position, whereas the hypotonic infant droops limply, with the limbs hanging downward, and the hypertonic infant assumes a very rigid extensor posture. There is a definite preference among newborns for the head to be held to the right. Studies have shown that almost 90% of infants at term spend 80% of their time with their heads to the right.

Movement and Power

The term infant who is awake is active if stimulated. The limbs tend to move in an alternating manner. Extensor and flexor power of the neck is apparent when the infant is pulled to a sitting position, as the head is held on the same plane as the rest of the body for a few seconds. When an irritable infant is stimulated, jittery or tremulous movements of the limbs or lower jaw may develop. These movements tend to persist until the infant falls asleep or stimulation ceases.

Tendon Reflexes

Deep-tendon reflexes (DTR) are usually easily obtained in the newborn, although on the first day after birth approximately one-quarter of infants have generalized areflexia. The triceps and brachioradialis reflexes are difficult to obtain, however. The patellar reflex is often associated with a crossed adductor response, which is normal in the first few months of life. DTRs are often brisk, especially when the infant is excited. Crying increases DTRs, and central nervous system (CNS) depression decreases them. DTRs are normally symmetrical; asymmetrical reflexes are often caused by unilateral CNS or peripheral nervous system lesions. Unilateral depression of reflexes in the arm is common with traumatic brachial plexus injuries, whereas increased DTRs are often the result of hemiparetic states. Ankle clonus (symmetrical) of five to ten beats is a normal finding in the neonate if there are no other associated neurological signs. Ankle clonus is usually more prominent in hyperexcitable states. It usually disappears rapidly, so that more than a few beats at 1 or 2 months of age is abnormal.

The plantar response in the newborn is usually symmetrically flexor, even though the response is usually stated to be extensor. If the test is carefully performed, over 90% of normal neonates have a flexor plantar response. When evaluating the plantar response, the examiner should realize that extensor withdrawal secondary to pain (often accompanied by a triple flexion response at the hip, knee, and ankle) or contact avoidance may develop and cause a false-positive response.

Neonatal Developmental Reflexes

A number of infantile developmental reflexes are present at or soon after birth but ultimately disappear within 6 to 12 months of life. These reflexes are used to demonstrate depression of CNS function or asymmetry of CNS function. Table 2-1 lists some of the useful developmental reflexes. Of those listed, the Moro reflex, tonic neck response, and palmar grasp response are the most useful.

Moro Reflex

With the infant supine, his head is lifted off the examining table and is allowed to fall from approximately 30 degrees to the angle of the trunk. Normally, abduction

TABLE 2-1   DEVELOPMENTAL REFLEXES

Reflex	Age of Appearance	Age of Disappearance
Moro	Birth	5 to 6 months
Palmar grasp	Birth	6 months
Plantar grasp	Birth	9 to 10 months
Rooting	Birth	3 months
Tonic neck response	Birth	5 to 6 months
Parachute	8 to 9 months	Persists
Landau reflex	10 months	24 months

Adapted from Volpe JJ: *Neurology of the Newborn.* Philadelphia, Saunders, 1981, p. 72. Used with permission.

and extension of the arms, followed by adduction of the upper extremities associated with crying, develops. The Moro reflex may be elicited in infants up to 6 months of age. By 2 months of age, the reflex becomes asymmetric and incomplete; the first phase of the response to disappear is the arm adduction. A depressed Moro reflex may be seen in any condition that causes depression of CNS activity. An asymmetric response may be seen in infants with brachial plexus lesions or in those with infantile hemiplegia.

Palmar Grasp

The palmar grasp is assessed by placing one's finger (or an object) in the palm of the infant's hand from the ulnar side. This results in flexion of the fingers and grasping of the object. The palmar grasp usually disappears within two to three months of age and is replaced by voluntary grasping. Its persistence is one of the early signs of infantile hemiplegia.

Tonic Neck Response

The tonic neck response is usually well developed by 1 to 2 months of age, and disappears 5 to 6 months after birth. It is elicited by rotating the head to one side (with the child in the supine position with the shoulders fixed). Extension of the arms and legs on the side toward which the face is rotated and flexion of arms and legs on the side of the occiput is a normal response. The response is never sustained in the normal infant because he can break the posture by struggling. The response is abnormal if it can be elicited beyond the sixth month of age. The reflex may be unilaterally or bilaterally abnormal. It usually arises as the result of cerebral dysfunction, usually greatest in the hemisphere opposite the direction in which the face is turned.

Traction Response

With the infant supine, the examiner grasps his hands and gently pulls him up to a sitting position. In the neonate the head lags while the infant is being pulled forward. When he is upright, the head falls forward and then briefly extends. By 3 to 5 months of age, the infant often is able to keep his head and trunk in a straight line and is able to assist actively in being pulled upright; the head neither lags nor drops forward. Head lag beyond 5 months of age is usually a result of hypotonia. Under 3 months of age the infant flexes the arms; after this period, there is symmetrical flexion of the forearms at the elbow, with the infant actively pulling toward the sitting position. Asymmetrical arm traction suggests weakness of the arm (eg, from brachial plexus palsy). A marked traction response (with the infant being pulled into a direct standing posture) suggests the presence of moderate spasticity.

Sensory Examination

Detailed evaluation of sensory function is usually not performed as part of the neonatal examination because sensation is difficult to assess. The response to multiple pinpricks over the extremities gives gross evidence of intact sensory functions. The latency of the response to pain, the degree of limb and facial movement, and crying are noted. Most normal, full-term newborns usually cry or attempt to avoid further stimuli, and they withdraw the limbs stimulated.

Cranium

The head circumference should always be measured. Increased head circumference is a function of an increase in intracranial contents; diminished circumference is associated with a decrease in intracranial contents (microcephaly). The occipitofrontal head circumference in a full-term newborn is 32.5 to 35 cm, with a 2-cm increase expected in the first month of life.

Transillumination of the skull is part of the neonatal neurologic examination. The degree of transillumination is greater frontally (2 cm maximum) and is more pronounced in lightly pigmented infants. Positive transillumination is seen in any situation in which there is a large fluid compartment overlying the meninges or brain or within the brain (eg, hydrocephalus, porencephaly, subdural effusion).

EXAMINATION BEYOND THE NEONATAL PERIOD

Many neurological examination techniques performed on the newborn apply to the child beyond the neonatal period. The cranial nerve examination is no different, except that as the child matures, cooperation is better. As with the neonate, the child should be observed first, then examined.

Observation of the child's limb and facial movements, level of alertness, and speech capacity can be carried out easily. It is best for the younger child to sit in the parent's lap during this phase of the examination. As the history is being taken the child is being observed constantly. The cranial nerve examination can then be performed, usually evaluating all areas that are evaluated in the adult. A brightly colored ball or other object can be used to test gross vision and oculomotor functions. Hearing can be tested grossly with a tuning fork or musical toy; the facial nerve, by observing the child's facial features.

Motor Examination

Motor examination is performed by looking for symmetry of movements, strength, muscle bulk, and tone. Muscle tone may be tested by passively shaking the child's hands and feet to detect limitation or excesses of movement. Strength is also tested by observing spontaneous movements of the child's extremities. A brightly colored object can be held to one side. The child usually attempts to grab the object permitting a determination of the child's dexterity, agility, and ability to grasp. Voluntary whole-hand grasping is present at 4 to 5 months of age, thumb and two-finger grasp at 7 months, and a thumb and forefinger pincer grasp at 9 to 11 months. The arms and legs may be moved passively in an entire range of motion, looking for resistance to passive movement (such as with spasticity) or active resistance. Definite hand preference before 18 months of age suggests difficulty with the opposite arm.

The *Landau* reflex is elicited when the infant is held prone in horizontal suspension and his head is flexed; flexion of the legs and trunk is the normal response. The Landau reflex usually appears at 3 months of age and disappears by 24 months.

The *parachute* response is present in the infant beyond 8 months of age. It is elicited by holding the infant in horizontal suspension, then thrusting him in a head-first direction toward the floor. Normally, the arms extend and abduct slightly and the fingers spread. Asymmetry of the response is seen in infants with unilateral limb weakness or spasticity.

The ages of acquisition of various motor and developmental skills vary greatly in the normal child. The normal pattern of child development is listed in Table 2-2. *Vocalization* begins at approximately 7 weeks of age or earlier, mainly with the production of vowel sounds. By 12 to 16 weeks the baby seems to be

TABLE 2-2 DEVELOPMENTAL MILESTONES AND REFLEXES
(Newborn to 24 Months)

AGE (MONTHS)	NORMAL FUNCTIONS
Newborn period	Blinking, tonic deviation of eyes on turning head, sucking, rooting, swallowing, yawning, grasping, brief extension of neck in prone position Moro response, flexion postures of limbs Biceps reflexes present, others variable Infantile type of flexor plantar reflex Periods of sleep and arousal Vigorous cry
2-3 months	Supports head Smiles Makes vowel sounds Adopts tonic asymmetric neck postures (tonic neck reflexes) Large range of movements of limbs, tendon reflexes usually present Fixates on and follows a dangling toy Suckles vigorously Period of sleep sharply differentiated from awake periods
4 months	Good head support, minimal head lag Coos and chuckles Inspects hands Tone of limbs moderate or diminished Turns to sounds Rolls over from prone to supine Grasping, sucking and tonic neck reflexes subservient to volition
5-6 months	Babbles Reaches and grasps Vocalizes in social play Discriminates between family and strangers Moro and grasp responses disappear Tries to recover lost object Begins to sit Positive support reaction Tonic neck reflexes gone Begins to grasp objects with one hand, holds bottle

TABLE 2-2 *continued*

Age (months)	Normal Functions
9 months	Creeps and pulls to stand, stands holding on Sits securely Babbles "mama," "dada," or equivalent Sociable, plays "pat-a-cake," seeks attention Drinks from cup Landau reflex present Parachute response present Grasps with thumb to forefinger
12 months	Stands alone May walk, or walks if led Tries to feed self May say several single words, echoes sounds Plantar reflexes definitely flexor Throws objects
15 months	Walks independently, falls easily Moves arms steadily Says several words Scribbles with crayon Requests by pointing Interest in sounds, music, pictures, and animal toys
18 months	Says at least 6 words Feeds self; uses spoon well May obey commands Runs stiffly, seats self in chair Hand dominance Throws ball Plays several nursery games Uses simple tools in imitation Removes shoes and stockings Points to two or three parts of body, common objects, and pictures in book
24 months	Says 2- or 3-word sentences Scribbles Runs well, climbs stairs one at a time Bends over and picks up objects Kicks ball Turns knob Organized play Builds tower of six blocks Occasionally toilet trained

Adapted from Adams RD, Victor M: *Principles of Neurology*, ed 3, New York, McGraw-Hill, 1985, p 28.

conversing with its mother by gurgling or cooing, eventually uttering a few consonants. At 32 weeks, syllables are combined, producing sounds like "dada." Words with meaning are usually not spoken until the child is about a year old, but just prior to this the child is able to comprehend and obey simple commands. The child usually will have two to six spoken words at 15 months of age; jargon speech is common between 15 and 18 months. Two- and three-word phrases and the pronouns "me," "I," and "you," are spoken by 21 to 24 months. By 2 years of age, the child may have a vocabulary of 50 words.

Cranium

The child's head should be carefully examined as described above. Head circumference should be charted against normal values because head size normally increases at a predictable rate. The circumference increases approximately 1 cm per month during the first six months of life and 1 cm every few months for the remaining six months of the first year. By the age of 3 years, 90% of the adult circumference can be expected.

The skull should also be auscultated. Audible systolic bruits occur in 50% to 75% of infants and young children, but they are uncommon after 6 years of age. Most bruits are easily heard over the orbits, and most are without clinical significance.

Developmental Milestones of the Older Child

Developmental milestones for the older child are listed in Table 2-3. The examination of the child greater than 4 years of age is much like that of the adult (Chapter 1). As always, a relaxed, nonthreatening environment is necessary. The child of this age is able to cooperate better so that the cranial nerve examination may be more complete. Motor functions, including strength and gait assessment, are easier to elicit, and cooperation is better with the sensory examination. Intellectual functions can also be tested; initiating the child in conversation can be quite revealing.

TABLE 2-3 DEVELOPMENTAL MILESTONES (age 2 to 5)

AGE (YEARS)	OBSERVED ITEMS	CLINICAL TESTS
2 years	Runs well Goes up and down stairs, one step at a time Climbs on furniture Opens doors Helps to undress Feeds well with spoon Puts three words together Listens to stories with pictures	Scribbles, imitates horizontal stroke Folds paper once Builds tower of six blocks
2 1/2 years	Jumps Walks on tiptoes if asked Knows full name; asks questions Refers to self as "I" Helps put away toys and clothes	Copies horizontal and vertical line Builds tower of eight blocks
3 years	Climbs stairs, alternating feet Talks constantly, recites nursery rhymes Rides tricycle Stands on one foot momentarily Plays simple games Helps in dressing Washes hands Identifies five colors Knows age and sex	Builds nine-cube tower Builds bridge with three cubes Imitates circle and cross with pencil

TABLE 2-3 *continued*

AGE (YEARS)	OBSERVED ITEMS	CLINICAL TESTS
4 years	Climbs well; hops and skips on one foot; throws ball overhand; kicks ball Uses scissors to cut out pictures Counts four pennies Tells a story; plays with other children Goes to toilet alone	Copies cross and circle Builds gate with five cubes Builds a bridge from model Draws a man with two to four parts other than head Distinguishes short and long line
5 years	Skips Names four colors Counts 10 pennies Dresses and undresses Asks questions about meaning of words	Copies square and triangle Distinguishes heavier of two weights More detailed drawing of a human figure

Adapted from Adams RD, Victor M: *Principles of Neurology,* ed 3, New York, McGraw-Hill, 1985, p 28. Used with permission.

Bibliography

Baird HW, Gordon EC: *Neurological Evaluation of Infants and Children. Clinics in Developmental Medicine No 84/85.* Philadelphia, Lippincott, 1983, no 84/85. (An updated edition of the Paine and Oppe text.)

Brown SB, Sher PK, Wright FK: Neurologic examination in children, in Swaiman KF, Wright FB (eds): *The Practice of Pediatric Neurology,* ed 2. McGraw-Hill, St. Louis, 1982, vol 1, pp 9-51. (Summarizes nicely the neurological examination from birth to adolescence.)

Paine RS, Oppe TE: *Neurological Examination of Children, Clinics in Developmental Medicine Vol 20/21.* Philadelphia, Lippincott, 1966, vol 20/21. (The definitive reference on the neurological examination of children.)

Volpe JJ: *Neurology of the Newborn (Major Problems in Clinical Pediatrics* Ser vol 22.) Philadelphia, Saunders, 1981, ch 3. (Concise chapter on the neurological examination of the neonate.)

3

The Geriatric Patient

The cycle of human development that begins in fetal life and infancy ends in senescence. Just as there are features unique to the neurological examination of the infant and child, so are there features unique to the neurological examination of the elderly patient. In normal senescence, there is a progressive impairment of general and special senses, fine motor control, certain cognitive abilities, and gait. Because of these characteristics, the neurological examination of the normal octogenarian yields different baseline findings than does the examination of the normal young adult. This chapter describes the findings of the neurological examination of the normal elderly patient. We use the Katzman and Terry (1983, p. 15) definition of normal aging of the nervous system: "Aging changes that occur in individuals free of overt disease of the nervous system."

History

It is particularly important to assess educational and occupational histories in the elderly patient. The older patient is more likely to have had less formal education than the younger patient and is less likely to have English as his first language. Thus, an educational bias may be inadvertently introduced if the examiner does not take background experiences into account.

Mental Status

There is a progressive decline of certain spheres of intellect and memory with normal aging. The most obvious example of this phenomenon is that the normal results for most of the Wechsler Adult Intelligence Scale (WAIS) performance subtests are scaled for age. If an 80-year-old achieves the same raw score (percentage correct) as a 20-year-old, the octogenarian is given a higher scaled score performance IQ than the younger person. The octogenarian is expected to perform more poorly than the younger adult because of the subtle, but inevitable, decline of intellect and memory occurring with normal aging.

Studies of intellectual functioning in aging disclose that on the WAIS, the performance tasks deteriorate more quickly than the verbal tasks. The octogenarian has more difficulty with the subtests of Picture Arrangement, Picture Completion, Object Assembly, Block Design, and Digit Symbol than on subtests of Vocabulary and Similarities. This same pattern in a younger patient would suggest right hemispheric dysfunction. Performance tasks begin to deteriorate at about 50 years of age and continue to worsen. Verbal tasks remain stable until the mid-70s when they, too, begin to deteriorate. The speed of central processing of information, which declines the most with aging, is sensitively disclosed by timed tests.

Studies of memory in normal aging have disclosed impairments in all three fundamental memory processes: (1) the acquisition–initial registration step of encoding and storing items to be remembered; (2) the retention of stored items over a time interval; and (3) the retrieval or recall of information at a later time. Of all these tasks, recall seems to be the most impaired. Again, it is likely that age-related increases in central processing time underlie the short-term learning and memory impairment of aging.

Clinically, mild intellectual and memory impairments may be manifest by several symptoms: (1) mental slowness in learning new ideas and in following lines of reasoning; (2) forgetfulness, particularly of names, addresses, telephone numbers, and other routine items; (3) inefficiency in planning and executing daily tasks; (4) a generalized slowing-down of movement and living; and (5) reluctance to attempt new activities and to consider new ideas. At the bedside, the clinician may detect slowness of thought and some impairment in recording and retrieving new memories.

Most elderly people are aware of a subtle decline in their intellect and memory, and some become distressed by it. The clinician can reassure the patient that a certain degree of memory loss is an inevitable consequence of aging and that he can help compensate for the loss by keeping written lists to supplement the memory. This subtle normal decline in memory and intellectual functioning must be distinguished from the pathological state of dementia in which there is a profound loss of intellect, memory, personality, orientation, and affect. The differential diagnosis of dementia and normal aging is considered in Chapter 13.

Language

A very subtle deterioration in language skills is another feature of normal aging. The normal aged person uses a more elaborate syntax with more verbal detail, commentary, and judgmental phrases than does the younger adult, who has a more concise declarative speech pattern. The elderly person has impaired naming skills, as tested in a timed trial to name as many animals, vegetables, etc, as possible in 30 seconds. A third area of language impairment in the elderly is comprehension, primarily the result of a deterioration of memory, attention, and timing. These subtle findings are not usually disclosed on the screening neurological examination.

Cranial Nerves

It is universally known that impairment of near visual acuity occurs with aging. Visual impairment, primarily caused by glaucoma, cataracts, and macular degeneration, grows from a prevalence of 6% in the under-65 age group to a prevalence of greater than 46% in the over-85 group. There is also a progressive impairment of pupillary reflexes to light and accommodation. By the age of 80, the pupillary light reflex is reduced or absent in 81% of healthy persons. The pupillary size diminishes with age to the extent that after the age of 70 years the diameter is normally 2.5 to 4.5 mm. This "miosis of the elderly" results from reduced preganglionic sympathetic tone. Pupillary irregularity (ie, not round) is also seen in normal aging. Impairments in upward gaze, convergence, and smooth visual tracking movements are other findings of normal aging. Upward gaze diminishes from 37 degrees above the horizontal meridian at age 15 to 16 degrees at 75 years.

Other special senses become impaired with age. Olfaction becomes impaired, although not usually to the point of total anosmia. Auditory acuity often deteriorates with age. Loss of cochlear hair cells and auditory nerve dysfunction produces serious hearing impairment in 25% of those over the age of 65. The sense of taste also deteriorates with age.

Motor and Cerebellar Function

The clinician frequently detects atrophy of distal muscles in normal aging, most often the dorsal interossei. There may be concomitant mild distal weakness of the involved muscles. Patients in their eighth decade have 60% to 80% of the muscle power of patients in their third decade. Muscle tone is often increased, resulting from both pyramidal and extrapyramidal dysfunction. The increased tone often is of the paratonic type: an involuntary opposition to passive stretch throughout the range of movements, with a force directly proportional to the velocity of attempted passive movement. Rapid fine finger movements and coordination also become impaired.

Gait and Station

The gait of the older person is so characteristic that comic impersonators can perform a credible caricature of an elderly person solely by imitating it. There is a slight forward flexion and stooped stance, a loss of associated arm swinging movements, and rapid short steps, sometimes with a broad base. Of course, this is also the description of the parkinsonian patient. With increasing age, there is the development of an extrapyramidal gait impairment that mimics parkinsonism.

The gait of elderly patients is also affected by sensory ataxia. Loss of proprioceptive input from the legs, loss of vestibular functioning, and poor vision all contribute to spatial disorientation which impairs well-coordinated gait.

Sensory Function

Cutaneous sensory modalities become impaired with aging. Distal vibration sense loss, which has been well-studied, clearly begins to deteriorate after the age of 50. Vibration sense loss is most severe in the legs. Proprioception, touch, pain, and temperature sensations are reduced to a lesser extent. The pattern of distal sensory loss in the elderly mimics that of a large-fiber polyneuropathy. There is a "stocking-and-glove" distribution of sensory loss, with the vibration and position senses most impaired.

Reflexes

It is generally accepted that distal deep-tendon reflexes become hypoactive with aging. Most studies have revealed reduction or loss of ankle jerk reflexes by the eighth decade, although a recent study (Impallomeni et al, 1984) contradicted these findings by disclosing only a 6% absence of ankle jerks in a group of patients over 65 years of age. The authors pointed out that it is hard to test for ankle jerk reflexes in the elderly because most of them cannot relax properly. Nevertheless, commonly there is an apparent loss of ankle jerks in the elderly in the hands of most examiners.

Abdominal cutaneous reflexes also are often reduced or lost in the elderly. Signs of frontal lobe release or "regressive reflexes" have an increased incidence with advancing age. Snout, glabellar, and palmomental reflexes may be present. The presence of these signs in the octogenarian does not necessarily have the same pathological significance as if all were present in the younger patient. Their presence must be interpreted within the context of the presenting syndrome.

The extensor plantar or Babinski's sign is found more often in the aged. Rather than being a normal concomitant of aging, this sign is probably the result of an otherwise asymptomatic cervical spondylotic myelopathy, which has a high incidence in the elderly.

Sleep

Changes in sleep patterns occur with aging. Elderly persons go to sleep earlier and awaken earlier. The total duration of sleep is shorter, with frequent midsleep awakenings. Less time is spent in slow-wave sleep. The signs and symptoms of sleep disorders in the elderly are considered in Chapter 29.

Significance of Impairment

The clinician must be cautious in interpreting neurological signs in the elderly; normal aging impairs nearly all spheres of nervous activity in a predictable pattern. Only when the impairment is greater than that expected for the person's age can the seemingly positive neurologic signs be afforded definite pathological significance. To a great extent, confidence in the interpretation of findings must be a function of experience.

Bibliography

Albert ML: *Clinical Neurology of Aging.* New York, Oxford University Press, 1984. (Authoritative and thorough, with practical information.)

Critchley M: The neurology of old age. *Lancet* 1931; 1:1119-1127, 1221-1230, 1331-1336. (The classic work by the master.)

Impallomeni M, Kenny RA, Flynn MD, et al: The elderly and their ankle jerks. *Lancet* 1984; 1:670-672. (The paper that shows that failure to obtain ankle jerks in the elderly may be caused primarily by deficiencies in technique.)

Jenkyn LR, Reeves AG, Warren T, et al: Neurologic signs in senescence. *Arch Neurol* 1985; 42:1154-1157. (Describes the frequency of "regressive reflexes" and other signs in normal elderly persons.)

Joynt RJ (ed): Neurology of aging. *Semin Neurol* 1981; 1:1-60. (A useful compendium of papers, somewhat less complete than Katzman and Terry, 1983. Good chapters include "Neurologic signs in uncomplicated senescence," "Mental status changes with aging," and "Changes in language with aging.")

Katzman R, Terry RD (eds): *The Neurology of Aging.* Philadelphia, F.A. Davis, 1983. (The best single source of current information. Excellent chapters include "Normal aging of the nervous system" and "The neurologic consultation at age 80." Well referenced throughout.)

Neurodiagnostic Tests

The physician who attempts to diagnose diseases of the nervous system faces an ever-increasing array of esoteric and expensive diagnostic tests. Most newly developed technologies are designed to sensitively and specifically survey one particular aspect of nervous system structure or function. Which test to perform for which clinical situation remains the essential diagnostic decision.

This chapter outlines an approach to the choice of neurological diagnostic tests and emphasizes newer technologies, and specifically, those that are the least invasive and that can be ordered in an outpatient setting. After the physician has decided that the patient's symptoms are the result of dysfunction of the central or the peripheral nervous system, he must choose tests designed to measure the structure or function of the particular part of the nervous system in question. Rather than ruling out diagnoses by ordering numerous tests, the clinician should order the single test that can prove that his clinical diagnosis is correct.

CENTRAL NERVOUS SYSTEM
Brain Scans
CT Scan

A computed tomography (CT) scan provides the most information about brain structure of any widely available test. It offers very high resolution and is painless and safe. The patient's radiation exposure is about the same as that of a routine skull series of x-rays. If a contrast-enhanced scan is also performed, the risk of intravenous injection of diatrizoate meglumine-ditrizoate sodium (Renografin-76, Angiovist-282) is the same as that of an intravenous pyelogram (IVP). A CT scan is expensive ($250 to $500).

The resolution of a CT scan depends on discrimination of differential densities. Thus, tiny flecks of calcium less than 1 mm in diameter are easily visualized, whereas 2 mm to 3 mm zones of recent infarction, with densities only slightly less than that of a normal brain, may not be seen.

A CT scan should be performed to document a suspected focal structural brain lesion such as a tumor, infarction, hemorrhage, or abscess (Figure 4-1). Patients with major head injury, suspected subdural hematoma, and suspected subarachnoid hemorrhage should be scanned. So should patients worked up for treatable causes of dementia. Patients with uncomplicated headaches, dizziness, syncope, or generalized weakness should be further assessed clinically before a scan is considered.

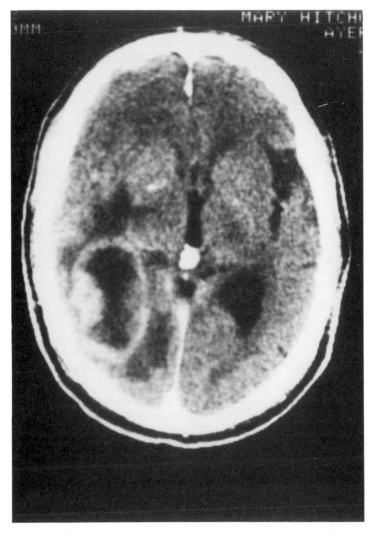

Figure 4-1. Enhanced CT scan of the brain showing a large left parietal lobe malignant glioma. A ring of enhancement encloses a cystic area, and there is surrounding edema with mass effect.

Radionuclide Scan

The advent of the CT scan has relegated the radionuclide scan to obsolescence in most medical centers. Yet radionuclide units are the only brain scanning units available in many smaller hospitals, and they maintain an occasionally useful screening value. They are less expensive than CT scans ($100 to $250) and very safe, but yield considerably less information.

Radionuclide scans have the following indications when CT scans are not available: documentation of routine cerebral hemispheric infarctions in stroke patients; screening for chronic subdural hematomas in the face of equivocal clinical evidence; and screening the patient who has a first convulsive seizure and has a normal neurological examination (Figure 4-2). They may be more sensitive than the CT scan in the early diagnosis of herpes simplex virus encephalitis and subdural empyema. Most units can perform flow studies that roughly measure internal carotid artery blood flow, which is not possible with CT.

Radionuclide scans have very poor resolution in the posterior fossa and do not provide sufficient information in the evaluation of dementia because neither the cerebral cortex nor the ventricular system is visualized. A positive finding on a radionuclide scan that is inconsistent with the clinical suspicion or is not itself diagnostic should be followed by a CT scan. As with the CT scan, the patient with uncomplicated headaches, dizziness, syncope, or weakness should not be scanned. If CT is available, there are very few indications for a radionuclide brain scan.

Radionuclide "cisternography" after lumbar intrathecal injection of radioisotope can document the direction of cerebrospinal fluid flow. Brain scans at 4, 24, and 48 hours can show reversal of direction of normal CSF flow, which is characteristic of communicating hydrocephalus.

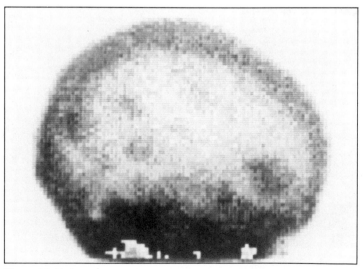

Figure 4-2. Technetium-99 radionuclide brain scan. Left lateral view discloses numerous spherical areas of increased uptake from metastatic bronchogenic carcinoma.

Magnetic Resonance Scans

Nuclear magnetic resonance imaging (MRI) scans are now available in many large medical centers. These devices are entirely noninvasive and are believed to be safe. Giant magnets are used to spatially label brain protons; the movement of the protons to fluxes electrically induced in the magnetic field are then measured. The technique is more sensitive than CT scan for differentiating gray and white matter. Subtle plaques of multiple sclerosis are visualized beautifully by MRI in cases when they might be inapparent on CT. The units are presently very expensive ($1 million to $2 million), which limits their availability, but in some areas they will probably replace CT. Compared to CT, MRI is generally more sensitive and does not expose patients to radiation. The technique is particularly sensitive for visualizing lesions of the posterior fossa and performing sagittal examinations (Figure 4-3).

PET Scans

Although not yet available for routine clinical use, positron emission tomography (PET) scans promise to be more sensitive than CT or MR scans in certain disorders. Following intravenous injection of fluorodeoxyglucose labeled with fluorine 18, the rate of glucose metabolism can be very sensitively measured in specific areas of the brain. Subtle areas of hypometabolism can be visualized prior to the anatomic alteration required by CT or scans for visualization. In early dementia, frontal cortical areas often show hypometabolism before CT or MR scanning reveals atrophy. The need for an on-site particle accelerator will restrict availability of these units in the future to large medical centers. The PET scan is currently a research tool.

Spinal Studies
Myelography

The myelogram remains the time-honored test to assess intrinsic or extrinsic lesions of the spinal cord and cauda equina. It is ordered to diagnose lumbar or cervical nerve root compression by herniated intervertebral discs or by spondylosis. It documents epidural spinal cord compression by metastatic carcinoma, abscess, or hematoma. It is diagnostic for intrinsic spinal cord tumor.

When only the lumbar subarachnoid space is to be examined, one of the water-soluble contrast agents, metrizamide (Amipaque), iohexol (Omnipaque), or iopamidol (Insovue), is usually chosen. Once injected, the spinal needle may be removed because the dye will be subsequently excreted in the urine. Complications include seizures and encephalopathy with asterixis if the dye reaches the brain in a high concentration. To ensure against this occurrence, the patient's head is maintained in an extended position during the procedure and should remain elevated for several hours afterward. Many radiologists also use the water-soluble contrast agents for cervical myelograms by cervical puncture.

When the thoracic or cervical area is to be examined, many radiologists prefer the water-insoluble dye iophendylate (Pantopaque). The spinal needle must

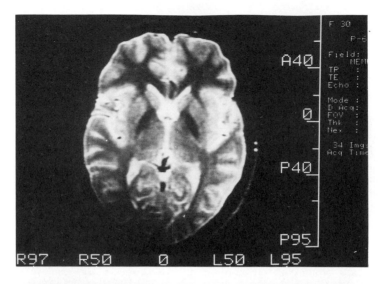

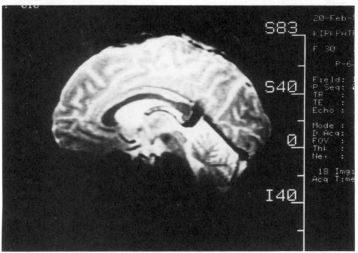

Figure 4-3A, B. MRI of the brain (spinecho technique, T_2 weighted images) in axial (A) and sagittal (B) planes. In this sequence CSF appears white, and there is excellent contrast between the gray and white matter.

remain in place during the procedure so that the dye can be removed at its conclusion. Complications include the rare occurrence of adhesive arachnoiditis, which is somewhat more common in patients with multiple sclerosis and much more common when the myelogram is performed after a traumatic lumbar puncture.

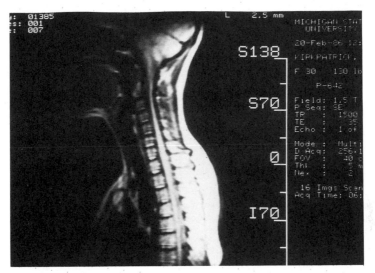

Figure 4-3C. MRI of the spinal cord. The spinal cord is easily visualized within the spinal canal; the cervicomedullary junction is quite distinct.

CT Scan

A spinal CT scan can be performed instead of a myelogram to diagnose compressions of the spinal cord and cauda equina by herniated intervertebral discs, spondylosis, or tumors. The CT scan offers speed and noninvasiveness, but requires the clinician to roughly localize the vertebral segments to be scanned. The CT scan is more valuable in the lumbar spine than in the cervical spine. Though the myelogram is more invasive, it permits a longitudinal radiographic evaluation of the spine. Thus, if the level of the lesion cannot be predicted clinically within a few spinal segments, the myelogram is the procedure of choice. For the diagnosis of herniated lumbar intervertebral discs, CT has replaced the myelogram in many medical centers.

MRI

MR scans have proved to be exceedingly sensitive in imaging the spinal cord. When a spinal cord lesion is suspected, MR scanning has largely replaced myelography in those medical centers where it is available. Because MR can scan in the sagittal plane, the clinician does not have to localize the exact spinal segment, which is necessary for CT scans of the spine.

Electrical Potential Recording
EEG

The electroencephalogram (EEG) measures the electrical "output" of the brain from the surface of the skull. Routine EEGs are entirely safe and relatively inexpensive ($75 to $150), but are cumbersome and time-consuming, and they provide relatively little information. An EEG should be ordered whenever an epileptic seizure is suspected to look for interictal seizure discharges (Figure 4-4). In idiopathic epilepsy, these discharges are present in two-thirds of patients. This frequency is lower with post-traumatic and other types of seizures. However, in a patient who has episodic unconsciousness, EEG findings cannot themselves establish or deny the diagnosis of epilepsy, which is a purely clinical diagnosis based on the history taken from those who have observed the patient's spells.

EEG should also be performed on the patient with memory and cognitive impairment. In general, early reversible dementias (drug intoxication or withdrawal, vitamin B_{12} deficiency, hypothyroidism, portosystemic or uremic encephalopathy) have diffusely slow EEG rhythms, whereas a patient with early Alzheimer's disease usually has a normal EEG. If focal brain lesions are suspected, a brain CT scan is more sensitive and specific. Episodic syncope is better studied with a Holter cardiac monitor than with an EEG. Rarely do EEGs performed in the workup of headaches or dizziness disclose any specific abnormalities that aid diagnosis.

Cortical Evoked Responses

Computer averaging techniques have made possible the study of specific cortical electrical responses evoked by visual, auditory, and somatesthetic stimuli. The visual evoked response (VER) is best recorded by stimulating the visual system in each eye by having the patient gaze at an alternating checkerboard pattern and recording the computer-averaged evoked response over the contralateral occipital cortex (Figure 4-5). This procedure is safe, painless, and not time-consuming, but is moderately expensive ($100 to $250). The VER is essentially a measurement of nerve conduction velocities in the visual system. This test should be ordered for

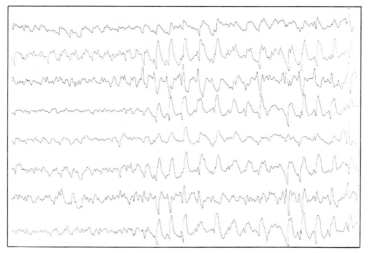

Figure 4-4. Eight-channel EEG recording over the surface of the temporal lobes. Left temporal lobe is top four channels, right temporal lobe is bottom four channels. A synchronous bitemporal atypical spike and wave seizure discharge begins at "d."

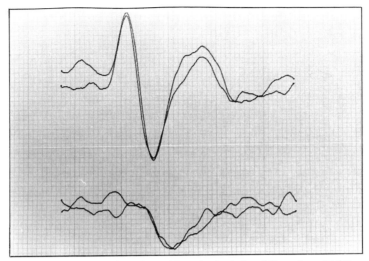

Figure 4-5. Visual evoked responses. Upper tracing is from left eye, lower tracing from right eye. This patient who has multiple sclerosis, had a known history of right optic neuritis. There is increased latency and decreased amplitude of the right-sided wave forms, corresponding to delayed nerve conduction through the right optic nerve. These findings confirm a history of right optic neuritis. (Duration of tracing is 250 msec; positivity is downward.)

all patients in whom the diagnosis of multiple sclerosis is seriously entertained and who have not had a known episode of optic neuritis. The identification of a defect in optic nerve conduction suggests the previous occurrence of an asymptomatic optic neuritis, and it may establish the classic multiple sclerosis diagnostic criterion of "dissemination of CNS lesions in space and time."

Brain stem auditory evoked responses (BAER) are the auditory analogue of VER. A long series of click sounds are presented to the subject, and the computer-averaged auditory evoked responses are recorded over the temporal and occipital lobes. A complex series of waves is produced, each corresponding to the transmission of the sound-induced electrical impulses through the brain stem (Figure 4-6). A local brain stem disturbance produced by demyelination in multiple sclerosis, brain stem tumor, or brain stem stroke may be reflected by abnormalities of these waves. The primary outpatient use of this examination is for assessing multiple sclerosis and central auditory disorders.

The somatosensory evoked potential (SSEP) is generated by stimulating a limb peripheral nerve (eg, the median nerve at the wrist) and averaging the evoked response over the contralateral hemisphere. It has numerous wave components corresponding to sites of transmission in the posterior columns of the spinal cord, medical lemniscus of the brain stem, thalamus, and somatosensory cortex. The full range of clinical application of SSEP is only now being realized, but it is useful for the diagnosis of diseases of the spinal cord and brain stem, particularly multiple sclerosis. Proximal portions of the peripheral nervous system (eg, cervical and lumbar nerve roots and plexuses), which are otherwise difficult to assess, can be studied accurately with SSEP.

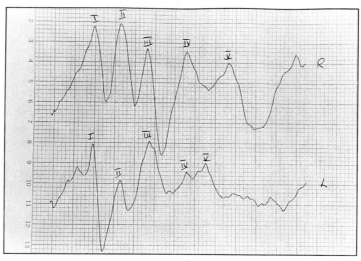

4-6. Brain stem auditory evoked responses. Upper tracing is from right ear, lower tracing from left ear. There are bilateral abnormalities in this patient with multiple sclerosis. The right III-V interwave latency is increased and the left IV and V amplitudes are decreased, compatible with brain stem conduction disturbances from demyelination. (Duration of tracing is 10 msec; positivity is upward.)

Vascular Studies
Noninvasive Carotid Battery

Evaluating the patient with suspected cerebrovascular disease often requires assessment of the carotid artery and its branches. Carotid arteriography is the "gold standard" examination, thanks to its high sensitivity and specificity, but its combined risks of stroke and death (0.5% to 2.0%) demand a safer procedure for this common problem. Accordingly, numerous noninvasive carotid artery tests have been proposed to fill this void.

No single test provides the information of arteriography; consequently, most medical centers with this capability have devised a battery of noninvasive tests to be used for screening purposes. Included are tests of the deep orbital circulation through the internal carotid, such as oculoplethysmography (OPG) and ophthalmodynamometry (ODM), carotid bruit evaluation with phonoangiography, real-time B-mode ultrasound imaging of the carotid bifurcation, and Doppler studies of arterial blood flow. OPG and ODM measure delays in circulation time from the carotid to eye, and therefore are indirect indicators of major hemodynamic alterations of the carotid artery. Conversely, B-mode ultrasound provides a direct image of the carotid bifurcation, analogous to angiography (Figure 4-7). OPG, ODM, and Doppler detect hemodynamic changes, but only B-mode ultrasound detects nonstenosing ulcerated plaques. The battery is very safe and moderately expensive ($200 to $400).

In general, the sensitivity and specificity of the noninvasive carotid battery are poorer than that of angiography. In particular, the battery often cannot identify a

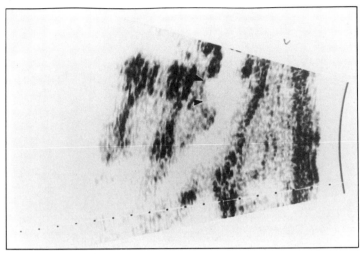

Figure 4-7. B-mode "real-time" ultrasonography of the internal carotid artery just distal to the bifurcation. There is concentric artherosclerotic narrowing of the vessel with a large ulcer crater (arrows) in the plaque.

tiny ulcerated plaque and may not be able to differentiate a tight carotid stenosis from a complete carotid occlusion. Indications for when this battery should be ordered are controversial. For patients with classic carotid transient ischemic attacks who are candidates for carotid endarterectomy, the carotid battery should be skipped and arteriography performed directly. The battery may be ordered to follow the progress of a known carotid lesion in a nonsurgical candidate or to evaluate the carotid artery when signs and symptoms of carotid disease are equivocal. The battery may also be ordered for patients with central retinal artery occlusion as a way of screening for concomitant carotid artery disease. Its value in the management of asymptomatic carotid bruits remains controversial.

Digital Subtraction Angiography

When this new technique becomes available to more physicians, it will greatly reduce the number of carotid arteriograms and will probably replace the noninvasive battery in many patients. Intravenous digital subtraction angiography (DSA) involves an intravenous injection of Renografin-76 in the forearm, followed by computer-assisted x-rays of the carotid and vertebral arteries and their branches. The computer detects the faint presence of the highly diluted Renografin-76 in the carotid and vertebral arteries and produces an image analogous to a combined carotid and vertebral arteriogram (Figure 4-8). The procedure carries the same risk as an intravenous pyelogram (IVP), and cost varies widely ($200 to $800). Intravenous DSA should definitely be ordered instead of a carotid arteriogram if the surgeon is willing to perform carotid endarterectomy solely on the basis of its images. Where available, it can be ordered instead of a carotid battery in the workup of suspected carotid artery disease.

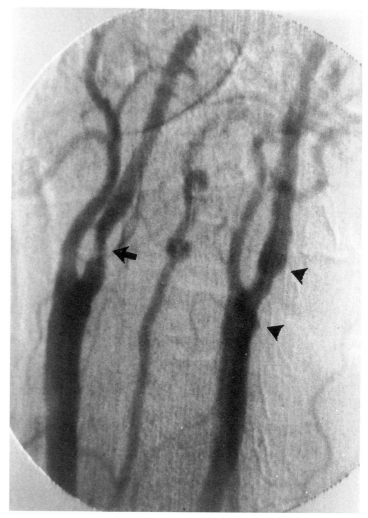

Figure 4-8. Intravenous digital subtraction angiogram of both carotid systems and the right vertebral artery. The left internal carotid has a high-grade stenosis (arrow); the right internal carotid has a nonstenotic ulcerated plaque (between arrowheads). Note the similarity in resolution to standard arteriography.

Cerebrospinal Fluid Studies

Two relatively new studies on the cerebrospinal fluid (CSF) are worthy of mention for their aid in the diagnosis of multiple sclerosis. (See Chapter 5 for the role of lumbar puncture in neurodiagnosis.)

CSF Immunoelectrophoresis

There is an elevation of the CSF oligoclonal IgG bands in 90% of patients with active multiple sclerosis (MS). This 90% figure is an improvement over the 66% of

MS patients who have an elevation of CSF gamma globulin on routine CSF protein electrophoresis.

CSF Myelin Basic Protein

Myelin basic protein is elevated in the presence of acute demyelination, most often from active multiple sclerosis. It can be elevated in other acute neurologic diseases but is usually normal in inactive MS. Both of these tests should be ordered in the evaluation of the patient with suspected multiple sclerosis. Their combined cost is $100 to $125.

PERIPHERAL NERVOUS SYSTEM
Electroneuromyography

When the lesion is localized to the peripheral nervous system, the choice of neurologic tests becomes limited to electroneuromyography (ENMG) and nerve/ muscle biopsy. ENMG includes several related studies designed to test the integrity of the motor and sensory units of the peripheral nervous system.

Electromyography

In electromyography (EMG), concentric needle electrodes are inserted into various skeletal muscles. Resting and volitional muscle action potentials are displayed on an oscilloscope and plotted on a voltage versus time graph (Figure 4-9).

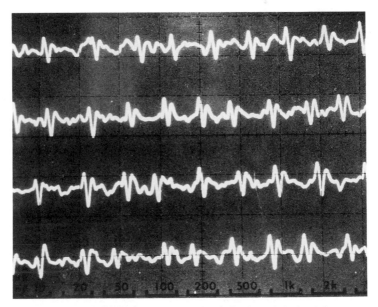

Figure 4-9. EMG recordings from a concentric needle electrode in the abductor pollicus brevis muscle in a case of motor neuron disease. A high firing rate confirms maximal effort. There is a dropout of motor unit potentials showing denervation.

Electroneurography

In electroneurography (ENG), an electrical stimulus is applied to a nerve. The motor or sensory conduction velocity of the applied potential is calculated by dividing the distance between successive stimulation points by the time latencies of their evoked responses (Figure 4-10).

Neuromuscular Transmission Studies

Neuromuscular transmission studies (NTS) consist of repeatedly stimulating a motor nerve at varying frequencies and recording the resulting train of compound muscle action potentials from the surface of a target muscle innervated by that nerve (Figure 4-11). All these studies are somewhat painful (particularly EMG and NTS). They are very safe but moderately time consuming and expensive ($150 to $600) depending on the extent of the examination.

When to Order ENMG

Electroneuromyography (ENMG) is ordered for the workup of compression mononeuropathies such as those affecting the median, ulnar, radial, and common peroneal nerves. These are easy diagnoses to confirm electrically. In the patient with polyneuropathy, ENMG can distinguish the etiology as axonal degeneration (eg, vitamin deficiency, toxic), segmental demyelination (eg, trauma), or both (eg, diabetes). ENMG is ordered for evaluation of primary muscle diseases, such as polymyositis and muscular dystrophy, as well as for diseases of the neuromuscular junction, such as myasthenia gravis. Many, but not all, ENMG laboratories also

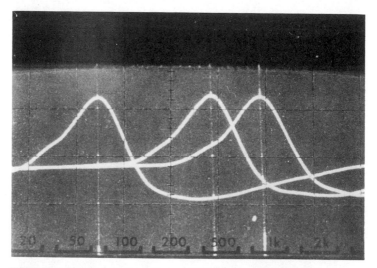

Figure 4-10. Nerve conduction velocity measured by recording the compound muscle action potentials over the abductor digiti minimi following electrical stimulation of the ulnar nerve at the wrist, below the elbow, and at the axilla. Amplitudes and latencies are normal, documenting normal ulnar nerve conduction velocities.

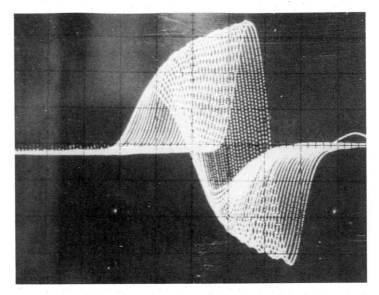

Figure 4-11. Neuromuscular transmission studies (NTS) obtained by supramaximal stimulation of the ulnar nerve at the wrist and recording the compound muscle action potential (CMAP) over the abductor digiti minimi. A train of 32 stimuli is delivered at 10 Hz. There is progressive enlargement of the CMAP with successive stimuli, to 250% of original amplitude, diagnostic of Eaton–Lambert (myasthenic) syndrome.

evaluate suspected cervical and lumbar radiculopathies (eg, from herniated discs)—but unequivocal diagnoses often require the use of more sophisticated techniques such as F-wave and H-reflex testing or somatosensory evoked potentials.

ENMG evaluations are an extension of the neurological examination. They are not ordered purely for screening purposes but rather to answer a specific question, such as "Is my patient's hand numbness caused by carpal tunnel syndrome?" Only rarely can electroneuromyography shed light on the diagnoses of patients who are referred with only pure neck or back pain or with leg cramps.

Muscle and Nerve Biopsy

Limb muscles and peripheral sensory nerves are the only convenient tissues to biopsy in diseases of the nervous system. Muscle biopsy is usually performed on the biceps or quadriceps muscles (Figure 4-12) and nerve biopsy on the sural nerve in the distal calf. Both can be performed under local anesthesia in an outpatient setting. There is moderate pain but little morbidity, other than permanent anesthesia of the heel after sural nerve biopsy. The tests are quite expensive ($500 to $1,000 in direct costs).

Muscle biopsy is ordered to establish treatability and prognosis if the patient's signs and symptoms point to a primary muscle disorder. In general, inflammatory

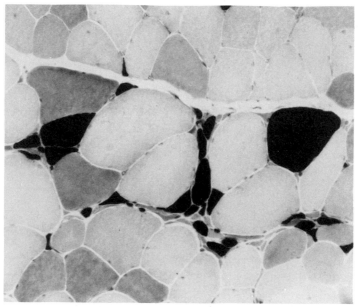

Figure 4-12. Gastrocnemius muscle biopsy stained with ATPase at pH 4.6. Differential staining shows type I fibers (black), type IIA fibers (white), and type IIB fibers (gray). The patient had type I fiber atrophy and type IIA and type IIB fiber hypertrophy, an uncommon sequela to chronic partial denervation.

and some metabolic myopathies are treatable, although the remainder are not. Even when a myopathy is not treatable, establishing the exact pathological diagnosis (eg, type of muscular dystrophy) is important to define the prognosis and the need for genetic counseling. If the question is merely one of differentiating inflammatory and noninflammatory myopathies, routine staining with hematoxylin and eosin is often sufficient. To make a more precise pathological diagnosis, it is usually necessary for the pathologist to additionally perform histochemical stains and often electron microscopy. Nerve biopsy should probably be ordered only by a neurologist, who can order specific tests on the nerve specimen.

Although most of the neurodiagnostic tests discussed present little risk to the patient, they are expensive and should be ordered only to answer specific questions. In neurological diagnosis, the proper use of expensive technology is not to rule out possible disorders by screening but to carefully arrive at a clinical diagnosis and order the one laboratory test that can prove that the clinician is correct.

Bibliography

Abrams HL, McNeil BJ: Medical implications of computed tomography. *N Engl J Med* 1978; 290:255-261, 310-318. (A sensible and still current summary of the role of CT scans in medical diagnosis.)

Ackerman RH: A perspective on non-invasive diagnosis of carotid artery disease. *Neurology* 1979; 29:615-622. (A balanced account of the usefulness and limitations of the "non-invasive carotid battery".)

Alderson PO, Mikhael M, Coleman RE, et al: Optimal utilization of computerized cranial tomography and radionuclide brain imaging. *Neurology* 1976; 26:803-807. (Outdated, but still the best study comparing the sensitivity and specificities of brain CT scans with radionuclide scans.)

Brownell GL, Budinger TF, Lauterbur PC, et al: Positron tomography and nuclear magnetic resonance imaging. *Science* 1982; 215:619-626. (An introduction to PET and NMR scanning principles and techniques.)

Chiappa KH: *Evoked Potentials in Clinical Practice.* New York, Raven Press, 1983. (Encyclopedic reference book for cortical evoked potentials; boring, but authoritative.)

Dubowitz V, *Muscle Biopsy*, ed 2. 1986. Philadelphia, Saunders, 1986. (The reigning text and reference for all aspects of muscle biopsy.)

Earnest F, Houser OW, Forbes GS, et al: The accuracy and limitations of intravenous digital subtraction angiography in the evaluation of atherosclerotic cerebrovascular disease: Angiographic and surgical correlation. *Mayo Clin Proc* 1983; 58:735-746. (Just what it says; authoritative and readable.)

Goodgold J, Eberstein A: *Electrodiagnosis of Neuromuscular Disease*, ed 3. Baltimore, Williams & Wilkins, 1983. (A good reference for all electromyographic and electroneurographic examinations.)

Keiffer SA, Cacayorin ED, Sherry RG: The radiological diagnosis of herniated lumbar intervertebral disk. A current controversy. *JAMA* 1984; 251:1192-1195. (The pros and cons of lumbar spine CT scan versus myelography for the diagnosis of herniated lumbar intervertebral disk.)

Klass DW, Daly DD (eds): *Current Practice of Clinical Electroencephalography.* New York, Raven Press, 1979. (An excellent reference for EEG indications, techniques, and interpretations.)

Williams A, Haughton V: *Cranial Computer Tomography: A Comprehensive Text.* St. Louis, Mosby, 1985. (The premier CT scan textbook.)

5

The Lumbar Puncture

Of the many neurodiagnostic procedures available, the lumbar puncture (LP) is the only one that the generalist, himself, will perform frequently. In the nearly 100 years since Quincke introduced the technique of LP, it has achieved an important place in the repertoire of most physicians. Yet LP should never be performed in a casual or purely routine manner. The physician must have in mind an appropriate indication, and he must be familiar with the contraindications and complications. Before performing LP, he must always ask, "Does the information to be gained justify the risk of the procedure?"

INDICATIONS

Most LPs are performed for diagnostic purposes. Rarer indications include therapeutic removal of cerebrospinal fluid (CSF) to lower CSF pressure in cases of benign intracranial hypertension or subarachnoid hemorrhage. Other unusual indications include the intrathecal infusion of substances for diagnosis (eg, myelography) or for therapy (eg, intrathecal gentamicin for gram-negative meningitis and intrathecal methotrexate for carcinomatous meningitis).

The principal indications for LP are to obtain information about the CSF that cannot be obtained from any other test. In cases of suspected meningitis, CSF examination must be performed to identify the organism by stain and culture. In cases of suspected subarachnoid hemorrhage from ruptured intracranial aneurysm, it is preferable to first obtain a computed tomography (CT) scan if any focal neurologic signs are present, but LP provides the most immediate information if there are no lateralizing signs. In cases of suspected benign intracranial hypertension, after a CT scan has excluded an intracranial mass lesion, only the demonstration of raised CSF pressure can establish the diagnosis. In cases of presumed multiple sclerosis, abnormalities of CSF immunoelectrophoresis and myelin basic protein help solidify the diagnosis.

The LP should not be the procedure of first choice in the evaluation of suspected brain tumor, brain abscess, subdural hematoma, stroke, head injury, epilepsy, or dementia. In such cases, a CT scan should be performed first and consideration given to LP later.

CONTRAINDICATIONS

Lumbar puncture should not be performed in any patient with an infection over or abutting the site of puncture because of the risk of introducing infection into the CSF. Known or strongly suspected intracranial or intraspinal mass lesions contraindicate LP except for the most pressing indications. Incipient cerebral herniations and spinal subarachnoid blocks may be made manifest by the sudden hydrodynamic change produced by the withdrawal of CSF. In such a case, a CT scan of the appropriate region should be performed instead. Severe thrombocytopenia (less than 50,000 platelets) and anticoagulation increase the bleeding complications of LP. In such a patient, LP should be performed only if bacterial meningitis must be excluded. In each case, the physician must weigh the possible indications against the possible contraindications before deciding to perform the procedure. He must always ask if there is an alternative, safer way to establish the diagnosis.

TECHNIQUE

Before beginning the LP, the physician should obtain informed consent and document that he has done so in the medical record. A careful, sensitive explanation is not only good medicine, it will also improve patient cooperation, aid relaxation, and improve comfort.

An intervertebral entry space is then chosen, in adults usually at L3-L4. This is most easily achieved by palpating the superior margins of the iliac crests and identifying the intervertebral space lying on the line connecting the two crests. It is also acceptable to insert the needle in the L4-L5 or L5-S1 interspaces, but the physician should not use the L2-L3 interspace or higher for fear of accidentally injuring the spinal cord. In infants, because the cord extends further caudally, the lowest possible interspace should be chosen.

Ordinarily, the LP is performed in the lateral decubitus position. If this fails, the sitting position can be used, but here the measurement of opening pressure is sacrificed. In the lateral decubitus position, the critical requirement, which often separates the successful from the unsuccessful LP, is adequate body flexion. If the patient cannot cooperate to provide adequate body flexion, an assistant should be recruited to hold the patient's head and legs flexed tightly against his abdomen and chest. For an accurate reading of opening pressure, the patient's head should not be elevated.

A #20 or a #22 spinal needle is ordinarily chosen. The #20 is easier to use because it bends less and the "pop" is more easily appreciated as it pierces the dura. The #22 produces a lower incidence of subsequent spinal headaches; therefore, many physicians prefer to use it. The bevel of the needle should be lined up in a longitudinal orientation to slide between rather than to interrupt the longitudinally oriented dural connective tissue fibers.

After gloving, suitable antisepsis, and sterile draping are completed, the skin overlying the entry position should be infiltrated with lidocaine or procaine, with most of the anesthetic placed in the dermis. The spinal needle is held with the hilt against both thumbs and the needle between both index fingers. This allows maximal control and proprioceptive input to help the operator guide the needle. The needle is inserted in the true midline, entering the skin halfway between the spinous processes and aimed 20 to 30 degrees superiorly, roughly toward the umbilicus. After the dura and arachnoid are pierced, the needle should be advanced a few more millimeters to ensure that the entire bevel is within the subarachnoid space. The needle then may be rotated to a position that permits the easiest egress of CSF. Next, the patient is instructed to relax and extend the legs somewhat just before opening pressure is measured. Otherwise, a falsely elevated pressure may result from Valsalva maneuver. The meniscus of CSF in the manometer should bob up and down during deep respirations or abdominal compression. The absence of these respirophasic fluctuations suggests that the needle tip is partially obstructed by a nerve root and indicates that the needle should be rotated. At least 12 mL of CSF, preferably more, is withdrawn, depending upon the clinical situation and the number of tests to be ordered. The stylet need not be replaced when withdrawing the needle, but care must be exercised to prevent inadvertent aspiration of a spinal nerve root as the needle is removed.

Although there is no agreement upon post-LP instructions, most neurologists suggest that the patient lie prone for the first three hours with the head slightly down, then supine and horizontal for at least another 12 hours. There is no evidence that fluid intake during the immediate post-LP period affects the frequency of subsequent headache.

INTERPRETATION

Normal CSF is clear, colorless and has an opening pressure of 65 to 195 mm of water. It should be acellular, although a few RBCs and fewer than three lymphocytes per mm^3 are normally seen in the counting chamber. Normal CSF obtained by LP has a total protein concentration of 15 to 45 mg/dL , of which 6% to 14% is gamma globulin and 5% to 12% is IgG. The CSF fasting glucose concentration is normally 45 to 80 mg/dL, which is 60% to 80% of the normal fasting serum glucose of 70 to 120 mg/dL. The differential diagnosis of CSF abnormalities are presented in Tables 5-1 through 5-6. Table 5-7 lists miscellaneous tests of CSF.

Normal CSF in infancy differs from that in adulthood. Neonates often have xanthochromic CSF because of hyperbilirubinemia. Often there are 2 to 20 WBC/mm^3 and up to 100 RBC/mm^3. The CSF protein in neonates averages 50 to 130 mg/dL, and the CSF glucose averages 40 to 90 mg/dL. These levels gradually reach adult levels by about 3 years of age. Distinguishing the CSF of an early stage of neonatal meningitis from the CSF of a normal neonate may be difficult.

COMPLICATIONS
Post-LP Headache

Post-LP headaches are encountered in 10% to 15% of patients after routine LP. The incidence is higher with myelography, with larger spinal needles, and with multiple attempts to insert the needle. Characteristically, the headache is bifrontal, has both aching and throbbing qualities, and usually lasts four to eight days. The distinguishing feature of this disorder is its exacerbation by sitting or standing and its improvement with recumbency. When severe, there may be postural vertigo, nausea, and vomiting.

Spinal headache is produced by the persistent leakage of CSF through the needle hole in the meninges after the completion of the LP, inducing CSF

TABLE 5-1 CONDITIONS THAT AFFECT CEREBROSPINAL FLUID PRESSURE

Elevated

Intracranial or intraspinal mass lesion
Elevated venous pressure
    Poor relaxation
    Valsalva maneuver
    Obesity
    Congestive heart failure
    Venous sinus thrombosis
    Chronic obstructive pulmonary disease
Hydrocephalus
Benign intracranial hypertension
Cerebral edema of any cause

Depressed

Poor needle placement
    Against nerve root
    In subdural space
CSF block by neoplasm or other condition
CSF leaks from prior LP
Ventriculosystemic shunting

TABLE 5-2 CAUSES OF ELEVATED CEREBROSPINAL FLUID PROTEIN LEVELS

Elevation of total protein

Meningitis
Brain and spinal cord tumor
Subarachnoid hemorrhage
CNS degenerative diseases
Brain infarction and hemorrhage
Diabetes mellitus
Herniated intervertebral discs
Peripheral polyneuropathies
Hypothyroidism

Elevation of Gamma Globulin or IgG

Multiple sclerosis
Herpes simplex encephalitis
Guillain-Barré syndrome
CNS syphilis
Subacute sclerosing panencephalitis

TABLE 5-3   CAUSES OF CEREBROSPINAL FLUID XANTHOCHROMIA

Hemolyzed RBC (begins 2 hours after bleeding)
Elevated serum bilirubin level
Elevated serum carotene level
Elevated CSF protein level (over 150 mg/dL)
Presence of serum protein when hematocrit over 1%

TABLE 5-4   CAUSES OF CEREBROSPINAL FLUID PLEOCYTOSIS

Infection

Bacterial meningitis
  WBC usually >2000
  Protein elevated
  Mostly PMN leucocytes
  Glucose depressed
Viral meningoencephalitis
  WBC usually <500
  Protein mildly elevated
  Mostly lymphocytes
  Glucose normal
Chronic meningitis
  Tuberculous, fungal, or other type
  Variable WBC, protein, glucose

Other causes of inflammation

Structural lesion near ventricles or subarachnoid space
  Tumor
  Infarction
  Demyelination
  Abscess
  Hemorrhage
  Arteritis
Intrathecally injected drugs
Radiation therapy in region of subarachnoid space
Recent seizure

hypotension. When the patient sits or stands, the brain "sinks" in the skull, putting traction on pain-sensitive structures at the base of the brain and producing the headache.

The headache is avoided by performing the LP carefully, with the smallest-bore needle possible. Lying prone for the first three hours is believed to promote tamponade of the meningeal tear by disallowing the apposition of dural and arachnoid needle holes. There is some evidence that lying with the head below the rest of the body after the LP is associated with a lower incidence of headache.

If the patient develops post-LP headache, the physician should order him to lie in bed for several days and to take a mild analgesic. He should reassure the patient that the problem will resolve within a week. Only if the headache persists for more than two weeks should the invasive treatment, the "blood patch" be offered. This involves the lumbar epidural injection of 10 mL of the patient's venous blood at the same interspace where the LP was performed earlier. This technique cures the headache in 80% to 90% of cases and is safe if adequate sterile technique is used and if blood is kept out of the subarachnoid space.

Cerebral Herniation

The most feared and lethal complication of LP is transtentorial and foramen magnum brainstem herniation. Herniation occurs in expanding hemispheric mass lesions in which surrounding edema is already displacing the ventricles and brain stem by downward pressure. Cerebral herniation occurs in a small percentage of brain tumors and hemorrhages and in a somewhat larger percentage of brain abscesses. Lumbar puncture should not be performed in these cases except for the most urgent reasons, such as diagnosing concomitant bacterial meningitis. Instead, a CT scan should be used to make the diagnosis. Cerebral herniation does not occur after LP in benign intracranial hypertension because intracranial contents do not undergo a lateralized shift, despite the raised intracranial pressure.

If LP must be performed in the presence of lateralized increased intracranial pressure, a small-bore needle should be used, only a small amount of CSF should be removed, and pressure should be reduced by the intravenous administration of furosemide or mannitol one hour before the LP. Should herniation occur during the LP—as evidenced by sudden coma, apnea, or unilateral pupillary dilatation—IV mannitol and furosemide should be administered immediately. The stylet should be returned to the needle and the needle left in place until intracranial pressure is reduced.

A similar event can occur in spinal mass lesions in which decompression from

---

TABLE 5-5 CAUSES OF DEPRESSED CEREBROSPINAL GLUCOSE LEVELS

Bacterial meningitis
Fungal meningitis
Parasitic meningitis
Carcinomatous, leukemic, or lymphomatous meningitis
CNS sarcoidosis
Subarachnoid hemorrhage
Subarachnoid spinal block
Hypoglycemia

TABLE 5-6 CAUSES OF BLOODY CEREBROSPINAL FLUID

Traumatic tap

Tenfold reduction in number of RBCs from tubes 1 to 4
No xanthochromia in supernatant fluid
CSF pressure normal
WBC/RBC ratio that of peripheral blood
Normal corrected CSF protein level
No crenated RBCs present
Spontaneous coagulation may occur

Subarachnoid hemorrhage

No reduction in number of RBCs from tubes 1 to 4
Xanthochromia present in supernatant fluid
CSF pressure often elevated
WBC/RBC ratio greater than in peripheral blood
Elevated corrected CSF protein level
Crenated RBCs often present
Spontaneous coagulation does not occur

TABLE 5-7   MISCELLANEOUS TESTS OF CEREBROSPINAL FLUID

Cryptococcal antigen	Much more sensitive than India ink stain for cryptococcal meningitis.
VDRL	Very sensitive for general paresis and meningovascular syphilis. Insensitive for tabes dorsalis.
Glutamine	Sensitive for portosystemic encephalopathy.
Myelin basic protein	May be elevated in acute multiple sclerosis and other acute destructive CNS processes.
Counterimmunoelectrophoresis	Allows rapid diagnosis of even partially treated common bacterial meningitides.
Cytology	Malignant cells and some infectious agents may be identified by examining cells in CSF.
Chloride	Don't order; it only reflects the state of hydration and is not specific for tuberculous meningitis.

below by LP may produce incipient spinal block. If the suspicion of cord tumor is high, a CT scan of the spinal region in question should be obtained or a myelogram performed and CSF examined from that procedure.

Spinal Hematoma

In patients who are anticoagulated or whose platelet counts are less than 50,000/μL spinal bleeding may complicate LP. Bleeding can be into the epidural, subdural, or subarachnoid space and can produce the clinical syndrome of acute paraplegia. Lumbar puncture should be performed only for the most pressing reasons on anticoagulated or thrombocytopenic patients. When that is the case, the most skilled operator available should perform the LP with the smallest-bore needle possible and with much effort to remain in the true anatomic midline to avoid the paired, paramedian epidural veins. Consideration should be given to the feasibility of reversing a patient's anticoagulated state before performing LP. If the patient is on IV heparin, the LP should not be performed if possible until four hours after the last heparin dose. If he has a platelet count below 20,000/μL or between 20,000 and 50,000/μL but rapidly falling (eg, after cancer chemotherapy), platelets should be transfused prior to LP. The use of "minidose heparin" (5,000 U every 12 hours subcutaneously) does not contraindicate LP.

Rare Complications

Occasionally a patient complains of double vision after LP, usually in association with spinal headache. This is probably horizontal diplopia caused by a sixth cranial nerve palsy that produces weakness of the lateral rectus muscle. Post-LP sixth nerve palsies may persist for a few months, but usually spontaneously resolve.

Nearly every type of infectious meningitis has been reported following LP, as a result of poor sterility. This complication is entirely avoidable with proper antisepsis and sterile technique. In children with bacteremia, LP has been associated with the production of meningitis, presumably by blood-borne bacteria gaining access to the CSF when the needle introduces a few drops of bacteremic blood. An analogous mechanism has been suggested for the spread of acute leukemia to the CSF.

During LP, a lumbar nerve root in the cauda equina may be accidentally impaled by too deep penetration of the spinal needle. The patient complains of a sudden jabbing pain radiating down the leg or into the groin or buttocks. This is usually a transient problem, but it may persist for a few days.

In an infant, a spinal epidermoid tumor may be iatrogenically introduced if the LP is performed without a stylet in the spinal needle. Presumably, a fragment of meninges or other connective tissue enters the CSF, inciting subsequent tumor formation.

Occasionally, a repeat LP at a previously tapped interspace yields an unexpectedly low pressure, high protein level, low glucose content, and a few cells. The likely cause is that the physician has tapped into an enlarged subdural space that was created when CSF leaked from the subarachnoid space into the potential subdural space during a previous LP. If this occurs, the LP should be repeated at a different interspace. Cervical or cisternal puncture may be necessary if the enlarged subdural space fills the entire lumbosacral region.

Bibliography

Breuer AC, Tyler HR, Marzewski DJ, et al: Radicular vessels are the most probable source of needle-induced blood in lumbar puncture. Significance for the thrombocytopenic cancer patient. *Cancer* 1982; 49:2168-2172. (Good diagrams of the mechanism of traumatic lumbar puncture.)

Duffy GP: Lumbar puncture in the presence of raised intracranial pressure. *Brit Med J* 1969; 1: 407-409. (A retrospective study of 30 patients who suffered cerebral herniation after LP.)

Fishman RA: *Cerebrospinal Fluid in Diseases of the Nervous System.* Philadelphia, Saunders, 1980. (The "bible" of LP performance and interpretation; the first reference to consult for any question.)

Marton KI, Gean AD: The spinal tap: a new look at an old test. *Ann Intern Med.* 1986; 104: 840-848. (Recent review of LP description, safety efficacy and interpretation. A similar "position paper" was adopted by the American College of Physicians: *Ann Intern Med* 1986; 104: 880-885.)

Pearce JMS: Hazards of the lumbar puncture. *Brit Med J* 1982; 285:1521-1522. (A recent review of LP complications.)

Petito F, Plum F: The lumbar puncture. *N Engl J Med* 1974; 290:225-227. (A brief but authoritative account of selected LP topics.)

Sarff LD, Platt LH, McCracken GH: Cerebrospinal fluid evaluation in neonates: Comparison of high-risk infants with and without meningitis. *J Pediatr* 1976; 88:473-477. (Points out the difficult differential diagnosis of normal neonatal CSF and neonatal meningitis.)

Tourtellotte WW, Haerer AF, Heller GL, et al: *Post-Lumbar Puncture Headaches.* Springfield, Il, Charles C Thomas, 1964. (All a physician could want to know about post-LP headaches.)

TWO

Problems

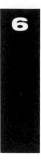

6

Dizziness and Vertigo

Dizziness is one of the most common complaints heard in outpatient practice. It can be defined as a nonspecific term describing a sensation of altered spatial orientation. Dysfunction of any of the body's spatial orienting systems can produce dizziness. Most often, dizziness is caused by dysfunction of the vestibular, visual, or proprioceptive systems, or by diffuse impairment of blood flow to the brain, which disturbs all orienting systems.

CLASSIFICATION

When a patient complains of dizziness, the physician must rejoin: "What exactly do you mean by dizziness?" Because a complaint of dizziness can refer to a variety of sensations produced by a large number of disorders, the physician must first attempt to classify the type of dizziness. Drachman's classification of dizziness into four cardinal types (Drachman and Hart, 1972) is now widely accepted.

Type I: Sensation of movement

The patient complains that he or his environment is moving in a rotational or translational fashion. He may have nausea, vomiting, and diaphoresis. The patient must hold on to a stable object to keep from being propelled to the floor. This type of dizziness strongly suggests vestibular dysfunction on a central or peripheral basis.

Type II: Sensation of impending faint

The patient feels that he is becoming lightheaded and is about to lose consciousness. There is often a "graying-out" of vision, pallor, and a roaring sound in the ears. This type of dizziness suggests global brain hypoperfusion caused by hypotension or impaired cardiac output secondary to mechanical obstruction or arrhythmia. This is the syncopal attack and is the subject of Chapter 7.

Type III: Dysequilibrium

This type of dizziness occurs only while standing or walking. It is an unsteadiness or a loss of balance without a peculiar sensation in the head. A patient says that the dizziness is in the feet, not in the head. This type of dizziness is seen in a variety of neurological disorders that impair gait, including parkinsonism, cerebellar ataxia, hydrocephalus, multisensory deprivation syndrome, and frontal lobe neoplasms.

Type IV: Other

This class is for dizziness not classifiable into Types I, II, or III. The most common causes include chronic hyperventilation syndrome, new eyeglasses, acute ophthalmoplegia, and phobic disorders.

HISTORY

The first and most important step in the evaluation of the dizzy patient is the history. The character of the dizziness allows the physician to classify the complaint into one of Drachman's groups: vertigo (Type I), lightheadedness (Type II), or unsteadiness (Type III).

The time course of dizziness should be ascertained. Sudden onset of vertigo with gradual resolution is seen in acute vestibular lesions such as vestibular neuronitis. Recurrent bouts of vertigo are characteristic of chronic vestibular lesions such as Ménière's disease. Continuous dizziness is unusual in vestibular lesions.

Precipitating factors should be sought. Dizziness when standing suddenly is characteristic of orthostatic hypotension. Dizziness with head movement is characteristic of a vestibular problem because head movement in certain directions exacerbates an already existing vestibular imbalance. A particularly common pattern in benign positional vertigo is for patients to become dizzy when rolling over in bed. A sudden Valsalva maneuver during coughing or sneezing acutely exacerbates vertigo in a perilymph fistula because the increased venous pressure accelerates endolymph. In Meniere's disease, loud noises can trigger vertigo (Tulio's phenomenon) because the cochlear endolymph flow stimulates the vestibular system.

The physician should inquire about associated symptoms. Nausea and vomiting are common with vertigo but uncommon in other types of dizziness. Hearing loss, tinnitus, and a fullness in the ear are also common with vestibular lesions because many peripheral and some central vestibular disorders affect the auditory system simultaneously. Concomitant brain stem symptoms such as diplopia, dysarthria, and dysphagia suggest a central vestibular process. Blurred vision while moving the head (oscillopsia) suggests bilateral vestibular damage, most often the result of ototoxic medications taken in the past. Such patients cannot read while walking. Facial pallor and progressive dimming of vision are common in lightheadedness (Type II).

The medical history may disclose important information. Any acute illness, even a viral upper respiratory infection, can produce dizziness caused by a general disturbance in all body spatial orienting mechanisms. Past head and ear trauma and surgery should be questioned because such events can cause permanent labyrinthine dysfunction. There is a higher incidence of vestibular dysfunction with a vascular basis in subacute bacterial endocarditis, hypertension, and syphilis.

Current and past medications must be reviewed, particularly any ototoxic medication, such as aminoglycoside antibiotics, salicylates, and furosemide. Barbiturates and benzodiazepines can produce dizziness by suppressing all orienting mechanisms. Antihypertensive medications are notorious for producing orthostatic hypotension. Alcohol and phenytoin produce a dose-related vestibular dysfunction, with nystagmus and vertigo in higher doses. The patient who experiences an acute attack of vertigo while on anticoagulant medication should be suspected of having a spontaneous inner ear hemorrhage.

EXAMINATION

The examination of the dizzy patient is conducted in three phases: the neurological exam, the otological exam, and the dizziness simulation battery.

Neurological Exam

Certain features of the neurological exam must be performed carefully in the dizzy patient. Eye movements are observed, particularly for the presence of nystagmus. Unilateral peripheral vestibular dysfunction produces nystagmus that is mostly horizontal, but that has a slight rotational component. The slow direction of the nystagmus is toward the side of the ablative vestibular lesion. The nystagmus is worse when gazing in the direction opposite the lesion, and is suppressed by visual fixation.

Hearing should be tested and any impairment evaluated by Weber test and Rinne test to assess whether the loss is conductive or sensorineural (Chapter 1). Visual acuity should be assessed and other cranial nerves tested to assess brain stem functioning.

Sensory examination is performed to assess proprioception. Dizziness and sensory ataxia can result from polyneuropathies or spinal cord posterior column degeneration that impair proprioceptive input.

Testing of past-pointing can assess subtle vestibular imbalance. The examiner stands about 6 feet in front of, and facing, the patient. Examiner and patient stand with their right arms extended and their index fingers extended in a pointing position such that they touch each other. The patient elevates his right arm above his head as if pointing to the ceiling, then lowers the arm to again touch the examiner's finger with his own. The patient closes his eyes and repeats the procedure several times. Without visual compensation and with repeated attempts, the patient with a unilateral vestibular dysfunction slowly rotates his hand in the direction of the impaired labyrinth.

A similar test can be performed with the patient walking. The patient walks in place with his eyes closed or takes three small steps forward, three backward, three forward, etc. with his eyes closed. If the patient has a unilateral vestibular lesion, he will begin to rotate the axis of his gait in the direction of the impaired labyrinth.

Romberg's sign should be assessed. The patient who falls with eyes closed and feet together either lacks proprioceptive input (sensory ataxia) or has a unilateral vestibular lesion. The patient with a vestibular lesion falls toward the damaged side. To disclose subtle vestibular lesions, the test can be sharpened by having the patient stand in a heel-on-toe tandem position with arms folded across his chest.

Otological Exam

The ears should be examined with an otoscope. Impacted cerumen should be removed carefully. Occasionally, an episodic vestibular disturbance is cured merely by removing impacted cerumen.

The tympanic membrane is examined and the response to pressures induced by a pneumatic bulb are tested. With perforation of the tympanic membrane, the suddenly increased pressure in the external auditory canal is transferred to the labyrinth, inducing sudden vertigo (fistula sign). A lesser degree of vertigo may be similarly induced in patients with Ménière's disease (Hennebert's sign).

Dizziness Simulation Battery

The cause of dizziness may remain elusive even after a careful history and neurological and otological examination. Then, a dizziness simulation battery should be performed. This is a series of tests designed to trigger dizzy spells or to reproduce various sensations of dizziness. If one of the tests produces a type of dizziness, the patient remarks, "That's exactly like one of my dizzy spells!" then the clinician has a diagnosis.

1. *Caloric testing.* Vestibular function is most easily assessed at the bedside by cold caloric testing. Cold water irrigated into the external canal establishes ampullofugal endolymph convection currents in the labyrinth, producing tonic eye deviation to the side of the cold water and horizontal nystagmus to the opposite side. From 1 to 10 mL of ice water is used, with the patient supine and his head at 30 degree elevation. The degree and duration of nystagmus evoked from stimulating each ear (with a five-minute rest between tests) are recorded. Vestibular dysfunction is evidenced by asymmetry of greater than 20%, with the affected ear producing less severe or less prolonged nystagmus. When nystagmus is produced, the patient experiences transient true vertigo. It is desirable to ask the patient if the induced vertigo is identical to his usual dizziness.

2. *Nylan–Bárány maneuver.* Many patients suffer positional vertigo. It is useful to attempt to reproduce an attack by suddenly altering the head position. The patient is seated on the edge of an examining table with his feet dangling off one side. The examiner grasps the patient's head and pulls it down over the far side of the examining table until the head is 10 to 30 degrees below the horizontal plane. The patient's head is then suddenly turned to the right. The patient is asked to look to the right, then to the left, and the examiner looks for evidence of nystagmus and vertigo. There is often a latency of 10 to 20 seconds before symptoms begin. The patient is then sat up and the maneuver is repeated with the head pulled down and turned to the left.

3. *Neck Twisting*. Rotation of the head, even in the erect posture, produces vertigo in certain patients. In some older patients, neck turning kinks and occludes a vertebral artery, inducing brain stem ischemia. Cervicogenic vertigo and nystagmus may also be induced by a sudden neck twist.

4. *Orthostatic Hypotension*. Measurement of blood pressure in the supine, standing-immediate, and standing-delayed positions are part of every dizziness evaluation. A systolic blood pressure drop of 15 to 20 mm Hg or more is significant, particularly if it is accompanied by symptoms of dizziness. If findings are equivocal, the patient can be placed on an x-ray tilt table, where blood pressure is measured at several degrees of tilt. Type II dizziness is common with orthostatic hypotension.

5. *Cardiovascular Reflexes*. Carotid sinus massage, Valsalva maneuver, and other cardiovascular reflexes are used to assess Type II dizziness (see Chapter 7).

6. *Walking and Turning*. Patients with Type III dizziness are best assessed while walking because only then is their dizziness present. They walk clumsily, with a parkinsonian gait or an apraxic gait (see Chapter 1). They have difficulty turning quickly and become unsteady and dizzy.

7. *Hyperventilation*. All patients in whom the diagnosis of dizziness is uncertain should undergo hyperventilation for three minutes by the clock. The patient should lie supine and be encouraged to breathe quickly and deeply. Hyperventilation performed properly for three minutes induces dizziness in everyone. The question for patients, however, is: "Does this dizziness feel like the dizziness you complain of?"

LABORATORY EVALUATION

After the clinician has performed the history and complete examination, he should be able to classify the dizziness into one of the Drachman types. Laboratory evaluation may then be helpful for an exact diagnosis. There is no "cookbook approach" to laboratory diagnosis of dizziness; each case should be individualized. The clinician should order a laboratory test only to answer a particular question.

Type I Dizziness

Audiometry is often useful for defining the nature of hearing loss that accompanies vestibular symptoms. Although rarely specific, audiometric tests, including pure tone studies, speech reception threshold, speech discrimination, loudness recruitment, and tone decay, can often localize an auditory lesion to the middle ear, cochlea, or retrocochlear regions. More specificity can be obtained by laboratories that perform tests of impedance audiometry, including static measurements, tympanometry, and acoustic reflex. Generally, the physician refers a patient with hearing loss and vertigo for audiometric evaluation, and the audiologist decides which tests to perform to evaluate the particular problem.

Brain stem auditory evoked responses (BAER) should be ordered only when vertigo and hearing loss are believed to be from lesions that are retrocochlear (nerve VIII) or in the central nervous sytem. This sophisticated test measures auditory conduction through the cranial nerve VIII and the central auditory pathways. It is useful in the diagnosis of acoustic neuroma and brain stem disorders.

Electronystagmography directly assesses vestibular function by electrically measuring eye movement responses to induced vestibular stimuli. Nystagmus can be quantitated and studied. Volitional saccadic (rapid) and tracking eye movements are studied first, optokinetic nystagmus next, and finally bithermal caloric testing with highly quantitated and exact thermal caloric stimuli. The side of the lesion can be determined as well as whether the lesion is central or peripheral.

In patients for whom clinical assessment and BAER make acoustic neuroma an important diagnostic consideration, a cranial computed tomography (CT) scan should be ordered as well as plain polytomography of the internal auditory canals. Stenver's skull views are a less acceptable alternative to polytomograms. If the CT scan is normal but the tomograms reveal erosion or enlargement of the internal auditory canal, an intrathecal air CT scan should be performed by a trained radiologist to look for an intracanalicular acoustic neuroma.

In rare cases of cervicogenic vertigo, cervical spine x-rays can be ordered to look for cervical spondylosis or other abnormalities. Hyperthyroidism, hyperglycemia, and hyperlipidemias have been associated with vertigo in rare cases. Epilepsy that produces vertigo (vestibular epilepsy) or is induced by vertigo (vestibulogenic epilepsy) should be investigated by electroencephalography (EEG). Otherwise, the greatest value of EEG in the dizzy patient is the cardiac rhythm strip it provides.

Other Dizziness Types

Laboratory evaluation of Type II dizziness is discussed in Chapter 7. There is little laboratory workup of value for patients with Types III and IV dizziness. If the cause of Type III dizziness is localized to a frontal lobe or cerebellar disorder, a cranial CT scan is probably indicated. Phobic patients with chronic hyperventilation syndrome that produces Type IV dizziness may have abnormal findings on the Minnesota Multiphasic Personality Index (MMPI).

DISEASES THAT PRODUCE TYPE I DIZZINESS

Peripheral Vestibular Disorders

By far the most common cause of acute and chronic vertigo are disorders of the peripheral vestibular apparatus. Vertigo and nystagmus of peripheral origin can be differentiated clinically from vertigo and nystagmus of central origin by several features. Nystagmus in peripheral disorders is usually unidirectional and horizontal, often with a slight rotational component. Central nystagmus is more coarse, often changes direction with different eye movements, and frequently has a vertical component. Nystagmus of peripheral vestibular origin is improved by visual fixation, whereas nystagmus of central origin is unchanged. Positional nystagmus of peripheral origin usually has a latency of several seconds after head movement, whereas positional nystagmus of central origin is immediate.

Acute Vestibular Neuronitis

Also known as acute labyrinthitis this is a monophasic, purely vestibular, disorder that is probably of viral origin. The patient experiences a sudden, prolonged attack of severe incapacitating vertigo with nausea and vomiting. Many patients report a viral upper respiratory illness within the preceding two weeks, and several family members may be simultaneously affected. Hearing is unimpaired, but gait is severely impaired because of the overwhelming rotational sensation. Nystagmus is marked and beats horizontally to the side opposite the vestibular dysfunction. Patients lie very still with their eyes closed because any movement worsens the vertigo. The disorder lasts as briefly as a few hours or as long as a few days and then gradually resolves. Several months later, however, there may be transient dizziness induced by sudden movements. Occasionally, there is a recurrence, but the vertigo is less than that of the initial episode.

Benign Positional Vertigo

This syndrome affects middle-aged and elderly patients in whom sudden head movements induce a brief attack of vertigo. Common offending movements are turning over in bed and looking up with the neck hyperextended. There is several seconds' latency after the movement before the vertigo begins. The vertigo usually lasts for less than 30 seconds. Examination discloses normal eye movements without nystagmus. On sudden head movements elicited by Nylan–Bárány maneuvers, however, several seconds' latency is followed by a brief burst of horizontal nystagmus and vertigo. Idiopathic benign positional vertigo usually resolves spontaneously within six months, whereas positional vertigo following head injury or labyrinthine infarction may persist longer.

Ménière's Disease

Also called endolymphatic hydrops, this is the tetrad of sensorineural hearing loss, tinnitus, attacks of vertigo, and a feeling of pressure or fullness in the ear. There is swelling and dilatation of the endolymph-containing structures in the cochlea and labyrinth. Many cases follow an inner-ear infection, and a familial predisposition exists. Attacks of vertigo in Ménière's disease are severe and last minutes to hours. Untreated, many cases proceed to complete deafness.

Examination discloses sensorineural hearing loss, no nystagmus (unless the patient is examined during an attack), a positive Hennebert's sign with the otoscope, and pain or vertigo induced by loud noises. Audiometric testing may be diagnostic, with characteristic findings of decreased low-frequency recruitment, poor speech discrimination, and abnormalities of the short-increment sensitivity index.

In addition to symptomatic treatment of vertigo, patients may benefit from diuretic therapy and a low-sodium diet. Surgical treatment by tack insertion and endolymphatic-subarachnoid shunt is often curative.

Toxic Vestibulopathy

This dose-related disorder is potentially reversible if offending drugs are withdrawn early in the course. Aminoglycoside antibiotics are particularly ototoxic. Streptomycin and gentamicin produce the most vestibulotoxicity, whereas neomycin, kanamycin, and tobramycin cause mostly auditory toxicity. Bilateral vestibular damage from aminoglycoside antibiotics produces loss of vestibulo-ocular reflexes and consequent oscillopsia (blurred vision and inability to focus during head movements). Salicylates produce a dose-related reversible syndrome of tinnitus, hearing loss, and dizziness. Furosemide and ethacrynate sodium are principally toxic to the auditory system. Alcohol produces reversible positional nystagmus and some positional vertigo in the dose range of 50 to 100 mg/dL.

Traumatic Vestibulopathy

Skull fracture directly through the temporal bone or by trauma at a distance from the labyrinth that induces labyrinthine concussion can cause traumatic vestibulopathy. The most common syndrome resulting from trauma is positional vertigo, believed to result from dislocation of the otolith from the macula of the utricle. A perilymph fistula may result, which can be detected by a positive fistula sign on otoscopy.

Other Disorders

Less common causes of vertigo result from peripheral vestibular dysfuntion. Labyrinthine and cochlear infarctions may produce sudden vertigo and deafness. Labyrinthine hemorrhages may produce similar symptoms and should be considered if the patient is anticoagulated. Tumors of the middle ear (cholesteatoma, glomus body) and of the inner ear (acoustic neuroma) produce vertigo, but sensorineural hearing loss is a more constant feature. Otosclerosis and Paget's disease produce vertigo in rare instances. Herpes zoster of the geniculate ganglion (Ramsay Hunt syndrome) produces ipsilateral Bell's palsy, hearing loss, and vertigo. Cervical spondylosis may produce vertigo as may sudden cervical flexion–extension (whiplash) injuries.

Treatment of Vertigo

The patient with an acute bout of prolonged vertigo needs bed rest, sedation, hydration, explanation, reassurance, and an antivertigo medication with antiemetic properties. He should lie still and rest until the acute phase subsides. Medications for treating vertigo are listed in Table 6-1. We have had the most success with prochloperazine and perphenazine in the acutely vertiginous patient.

In chronic vertigo and in the convalescent phase of acute vertigo, medications are of limited value. Instead, vestibular exercises are most useful. These exercises, listed in Table 6-2, extinguish vertigo induced by head movements. Some patients with frequent bouts of vertigo on a prolonged basis derive some benefit from meclizine. Drugs of choice to prevent motion sickness are meclizine, 25 to 50 mg

TABLE 6-1 DRUG TREATMENT OF VERTIGO

CLASS	DRUG	DOSAGE	SEDATION	ANTIEMETIC	DRYNESS OF MUCOUS MEMBRANES	EXTRAPYRAMIDAL SYMPTOMS
Anticholinergic	Scopolamine	0.6 mg orally q 4-6 h 0.5 mg transdermally q 3 d	+	+	+++	–
	Atropine	0.4 mg orally or intramuscularly q 4-6 h	–	+	+++	–
Monoaminergic	Amphetamine	5 or 10 mg orally q 4-6 h	–	+	+	+
	Ephedrine	25 mg orally q 4-6 h	–	+	–	–
Antihistamine	Meclizine	25 mg orally q 4-6 h	+	+	–	–
	Cyclizine	50 mg orally or intramuscularly q 4-6 h or 100 mg suppository q 8 h	+	+	++	–
	Dimenhydrinate	50 mg orally or intramuscularly q 4-6 h or 100 mg suppository q 8 h	+	+	+	–
	Promethazine	25 or 50 mg orally or intramuscularly, or suppository q 4-6 h	++	+	++	+
Phenothiazine	Prochlorperazine	5 or 10 mg orally or intramuscularly q 6 h or 25 mg suppository q 12 h	+	+++	+	++
	Perphenazine	2-4 mg orally or 5 mg intramuscularly q 6 h	+++	++	+	+++
	Chlorpromazine	25 mg orally or intramuscularly q 6 h	+++	++	+	+++
Benzodiazepine	Diazepam	5 or 10 mg orally, intramuscularly, or intravenously q 4-6 h	+++	+	–	–
Butyrophenone	Haloperidol	1.0 or 2.0 mg orally or intramuscularly q 8-12 h	+++	++	+	++
	Droperidol	2.5 or 5 mg intramuscularly q 12 h	+++	++	+	++

Adapted from Baloh RW: *Dizziness, Hearing Loss, and Tinnitus: The Essentials of Neurology.* Philadelphia, F.A. Davis, 1984. Used with permission.

TABLE 6-2 VESTIBULAR EXERCISES OF CAWTHORNE AND COOKSEY

In Bed

Eye movements (at first slow, then quick)
    up and down
    from side to side
    focusing on finger, moving it from 3 feet to 1 foot away from face
Head movements (at first slow, then quick; later with eyes closed)
    bending forwards and backwards
    turning from side to side

Sitting

Eye and head movements as performed in bed (above)
Shoulder shrugging and circling
Bending forwards and picking up objects from the ground

Standing

Eye and head movements as performed in bed (above) and shoulder shrugging and
    circling
Changing from sitting to standing position with eyes open and shut
Throwing a small ball from hand to hand (above eye level)
Throwing ball from hand to hand under knee
Change from sitting to standing and turning round in between

Moving About

Form a circle around a center person, who will throw a large ball and to whom it will be
    returned
Walk across room with eyes open and then closed
Walk up and down slope with eyes open and then closed
Walk up and down steps with eyes open and then closed
Play any game involving stooping, stretching, and aiming, such as skittles, bowling or
    basketball

Adapted from Baloh RW: *Dizziness, Hearing Loss, and Tinnitus: The Essentials of Neurotology.* Philadelphia,
F.A. Davis, 1984.

orally every four to six hours, or transdermal scopolamine, one patch every three days. Only in the most intractable and untreatable instances of vertigo should consideration be given to surgical section of the vestibular nerve or labyrinthectomy.

Central Vestibulopathy

These disorders are relatively rare in general practice. They should be suspected only if the patient's nystagmus has characteristics of central nystagmus (discussed above) and if there are also signs of other cranial nerve or motor-sensory long tract dysfunction to pinpoint the lesion to the brain stem.

Brain Stem Stroke

Either infarction or hemorrhage involving the vestibular nuclei or central vestibular pathways can produce acute vertigo. The lateral medullary syndrome (Wallenberg's syndrome), the most common stroke in this regard, usually results from vertebral artery occlusion. It produces a unique array of signs, including vertigo, marked nystagmus (often with a rotatory component), dysphagia, ipsilateral Horner's syndrome, ipsilateral limb ataxia, and ipsilateral facial and contralateral body sensory loss of pain and temperature sensations.

Multiple Sclerosis

Not infrequently, multiple sclerosis produces nystagmus and vertigo, but rarely as a presenting syndrome. Some vertigo accompanies acute internuclear ophthalmoplegia, as described in Chapter 23.

Migraine

Migraine can produce vertigo, particularly in children, on a central or a peripheral basis. A common childhood migraine "equivalent" is cyclic vertigo, nausea, and vomiting. Such children, as well as most other migraine patients, also have an increased propensity to develop motion sickness.

Epilepsy

Epilepsy can be caused by, or may induce, vertigo. Some temporal lobe seizure foci produce vertigo during the seizure ictus (vestibular epilepsy). It is believed that in these cases, the cortical representation of the vestibular system is the seizure focus. In vestibulogenic epilepsy, a bout of vertigo, of whatever cause, precipitates a seizure by reflex. This type of seizure disorder is analogous to other forms of reflex epilepsy, such as reading epilepsy and hot water epilepsy.

DISEASES THAT PRODUCE TYPE II AND TYPE III DIZZINESS

Diseases that produce Type II dizziness are discussed in Chapter 7. Those that produce Type III dizziness follow.

Multisensory Deprivation Syndrome

This is a very common disorder of late life. All bodily orienting systems become impaired, and the elderly patient feels insecure walking and fears falling. There is impairment of vision, hearing, proprioception, and vestibular functioning. Often, an intercurrent illness heralds the complaint of dizziness. We have seen many such patients complain of dizziness in the hospital just after cataract surgery. An eye being patched is the minor event that is sufficient to decompensate them for walking. Multisensory deprivation syndrome also often contributes to other causes of dizziness in the older patient. It is best treated by issuing the patient a cane or walker. This permits him just enough extra proprioceptive input and a third pivoting point to permit walking with confidence. For these patients, a simple cane may spell the difference between fear of walking and freedom.

Bifrontal Disorders

These disorders include bilateral frontal lobe tumors, strokes, and hydrocephalus. They produce an apraxia of gait (described in Chapter 1) as if the patient has forgotten how to walk. Accompanying signs include dementia, urinary urge incontinence, pseudobulbar palsy with pathologic laughing and crying, and regressive reflexes (Chapter 1).

Parkinsonism

This is diagnosed by the clinical criteria of bradykinesia, rigidity, static tremor, and loss of associated movements (see Chapter 24).

Cerebellar Vermis Lesions

These lesions produce ataxia of stance and gait. Common causes are alcohol-nutritional cerebellar degeneration, hereditary cerebellar degeneration, and primary and metastatic tumors of the midline cerebellum.

Bilateral Vestibular Disorder

After acute symptoms have resolved, bilateral vestibular disorders may feature dysequilibrium and oscillopsia. Aminoglycoside toxicity is the most common cause.

DISEASES THAT PRODUCE TYPE IV DIZZINESS

Chronic Hyperventilation Syndrome

Fully 25% of Drachman's original series of referred, previously undiagnosed, dizzy patients, had this syndrome. Most had no idea that they were hyperventilating. In addition to dizziness, most hyperventilators also complain of fatigability, headaches, dyspnea, tingling of fingertips and around the mouth, and chronic anxiety. The clinician should suspect chronic hyperventilation syndrome when the patient makes many deep "thoracic" breaths while relaxed, frequently moistens his lips and clears his throat, and has a nonproductive cough.

The hyperventilation provocation test should be performed as part of the dizziness simulation battery. If positive, symptoms can be reversed by rebreathing into a lunch-size brown paper bag. Other useful therapies are relaxation exercises and the use of beta-adrenergic blockade with propranolol or metoprolol. The identification of the problem and the support of the physician are important ameliorating factors.

Other causes

These include new eyeglasses, various phobias, height dizziness, and diplopia from extraocular muscle palsy.

Bibliography

Baloh RW: *Dizziness, Hearing Loss, and Tinnitus: The Essentials of Neurotology.* Philadelphia, F.A. Davis, 1984. (A concise summary of the subject by a premier neurotologist; the source of Tables 6-1 and 6-2.)

Brandt T, Daroff RB: The multisensory physiological and pathological vertigo syndromes. *Ann Neurol* 1980; 7:195-203. (A good review of the physiology of vertigo.)

Drachman DA, Hart CW: An approach to the dizzy patient. *Neurology* 1972; 22:323-334. (A classic paper that forms the basis for modern classification of dizziness into Types I to IV.

This paper is worth reading, but more current and complete writings on dizziness by Drachman are found in the 15th and 16th editions of *Cecil Textbook of Medicine*).

Magarian GJ: Hyperventilation syndrome: Infrequently recognized common expressions of anxiety and stress. *Medicine* 1982; 61:219-236. (A thorough description of clinical, psychologic, and biochemical aspects of chronic hyperventilation syndrome.)

Snow JB, Jr: Positional vertigo. *N Engl J Med* 1984; 310:1740-1741. (A brief, current editorial review of syndromes that produce positional vertigo.)

Troost BT: Dizziness and vertigo in vertebrobasilar disease. I and II. *Stroke* 1980; 11:301-303, 413-415. (An excellent account of central versus peripheral vascular etiologies of dizziness and vertigo.)

Wolfson RJ, Silverstein H, Marlowe FI, et al: Vertigo. *Ciba Clinical Symposia* 1981; 33 (6):1-32. (Clearly written and superbly illustrated. A very useful adjunct to other references.)

Syncope

Syncope is a sudden, reversible loss of consciousness and postural tone that results from temporary global cerebral ischemia. Consciousness is regained after the ischemia has been reversed. Although the loss of consciousness is from temporary brain failure, syncope is rarely a manifestation of an intrinsic brain disorder. More often it is precipitated by a failure of the cardiovascular system to provide the brain with a continuous, plentiful supply of oxygenated blood.

Disorders that induce syncope are paroxysmal, so the susceptible person has syncopal "attacks," which do not necessarily result in total loss of consciousness. Often, an attack begins with lightheadedness, graying-out of vision, and pallor, but it is aborted before consciousness is lost. Such a mild attack, termed "presyncopal," represents noncritical global cerebral ischemia. Many patients refer to their presyncopal sensations as dizziness. This complaint would count as Drachman Type II dizziness (see Chapter 6).

The exact prevalence of syncope has been difficult to ascertain, but it is an exceedingly common phenomenon. Some surveys of college students and young Air Force recruits have shown a prevalence rate as high as 47%. It is likely that most people have felt presyncopal at some time, and with the proper conditions, most could also develop true syncope.

The prognosis for patients with syncope is variable. In young adults with common vasodepressor syncope, it is rare for any serious complications to occur, although they may have a slightly increased rate of sudden death. In middle-aged patients admitted to the hospital for syncope of unknown cause, there was a 5% mortality nine months later (Kapoor et al, 1983). Patients with syncope of cardiovascular cause had the worst prognosis: as many as 24% died suddenly within one year. The same study found a 4% one-year mortality in patients with syncope of noncardiovascular origin and a 3% one-year mortality in patients with syncope of unknown cause.

MECHANISMS AND CLASSIFICATION

Syncope may be produced by any disorder that critically interferes with an adequate supply of oxygen or glucose to neurons. To provide adequate oxygen and glucose, the brain requires a cerebral blood flow rate of 55 mL/100 g of brain per minute under normal conditions. Consciousness is lost if the global cerebral blood flow rate falls below 20 mL/100 g per minute. The two major mechanisms by which there may be such a global drop in cerebral blood flow are hypotension and impaired cardiac output. Cardiac output, in turn, may be impaired by cardiac arrhythmia, conduction block, failure, or mechanical flow obstruction.

Even with adequate cardiovascular function, syncope may result from severe hypoxemia, anemia, or hypoglycemia. Hypocapnia may induce syncope by a secondary reduction of cerebral blood flow.

Epilepsy and vertebrobasilar arterial insufficiency may produce transient loss of consciousness, but these episodes are usually distinguishable from true syncope by an adequate description of the attacks. Table 7-1 classifies the disorders that produce syncope by pathophysiological mechanisms.

Syncope in the elderly is most often multifactorial. Lipsitz (1983) has pointed out that such patients often suffer from one or more of the following disorders: congestive heart failure, chronic renal failure, angina pectoris, anemia, chronic obstructive pulmonary disease, arterial and venous insufficiency in the legs, diabetes mellitus, and multiple drug regimens. These disturbances may work synergistically to reduce cerebral functioning. Often, the patient's cerebral functioning is already marginal, and a seemingly trivial additional event or stress is sufficient to induce syncope.

HISTORY

The evaluation of syncope begins with a detailed description of the attack itself. Did the patient feel a "graying out" with several seconds' sense of impending faint, or was there no premonitory warning? True syncope is usually marked by a presyncopal sense of impending faint with giddiness, graying out of vision, roaring in the ears, and diaphoresis. How did the patient look to an observer? When the common cardiovascular causes are responsible, the patient appears pale gray or white. What did the patient do when unconscious? In the typical syncopal attack, the patient slumps to the floor and lies limp and motionless for seconds to minutes. If true recumbency is not quickly achieved, an episode of tonic or clonic muscular activity of several seconds may occur as a rudimentary ischemic seizure is produced. How quickly was full consciousness regained? In syncope, normal mentation returns when consciousness recovers, unlike seizures in which postictal confusion lasting many minutes is the rule.

The clinician must discover what the patient was doing when the attack occurred. Syncope from orthostatic hypotension usually occurs several seconds after arising from bed or a chair, catching the patient midway across a room. Patients with such attacks frequently report many similar, but not so severe, attacks under similar circumstances. Vagovagal reflex syncopes, such as those that

TABLE 7-1 CLASSIFICATION OF SYNCOPE

Hypotension

Vasomotor failure
    Orthostatic hypotension
    Reflex syncope
        Micturition
        Defecation
        Cough
        Swallow
        Instrumentation
    Carotid sinus hypersensitivity
    Vasodepressor (vasovagal)
    Peripheral polyneuropathy
    Autonomic insufficiency
    Drug-induced
Hypovolemia

Decreased Cardiac Output

Cardiac arrhythmias
    Tachyarrhythmias
        Ventricular fibrillation
        Ventricular tachycardia
        Supraventricular tachycardia
    Bradyarrhythmias
        Asystole
        Sinus bradycardia
        Sinus arrest
    Heart block
    Sick sinus syndrome
    Glossopharyngeal neuralgia
Mechanical outflow obstruction
    Aortic stenosis
    Hypertrophic cardiomyopathy
    Cardiac myxoma
    Cardiac tamponade
    Prolapsed mitral valve
Pump failure
    Myocardial infarction
    Pulmonary embolism

Blood and Metabolism Disorders

Anemia
Hypoxemia
Hypoglycemia
Hypocapnia

Central Nervous System Disorders

Seizures
Cerebrovascular insufficiency

occur during urination, coughing, swallowing, or straining, can be diagnosed by the history. Exertional syncope may be seen in patients with aortic stenosis, hypertrophic cardiomyopathy, arrhythmias, and angina. Carotid sinus syncope should be considered when the attacks are associated with tight-fitting neckties, shaving, or extreme neck rotation. Syncope caused by vertebral artery mechanical occlusion is suggested if the attacks occur with neck hyperextension or extreme rotation. Syncope with arm and hand exercising suggests the subclavian steal syndrome.

The history of medication use is a critical part of the evaluation. Drug effects, interactions, and adverse responses are common provocative factors in syncope in the elderly. Many classes of drugs produce orthostatic hypotension. Sympatholytic drugs can block reflex tachycardias compensating for the hypotension, or they may induce heart block themselves. It is advisable to simplify in number and reduce in dose the medication regimen of any patient with recurrent syncope.

PHYSICAL EXAMINATION

In the ideal situation, the pulse and blood pressure will have been measured during the syncopal episode. In many patients with vasodepressor syncope, reflex syncope, or orthostatic hypotension, there will be both hypotension and relative or absolute bradycardia. Such a patient will become diaphoretic from excess parasympathetic discharge during the attack; his or her clothes may become ringing wet. The regularity of the pulse should be determined to assess cardiac arrhythmia. The heart should be examined carefully for murmurs and gallops. The carotid artery upstroke should be assessed by palpation, and auscultation for carotid and subclavian bruits should be performed. A screening neurological examination (Chapter 1) should be sufficient to discover focal signs suggestive of cerebrovascular disease or evidence of parkinsonism, which is often associated with orthostatic hypotension.

Attempts to provoke cardiac arrhythmias and hypotension form an important battery of ancillary tests to the physical examination in syncope. Orthostatic (postural) blood pressure and pulse change are always measured. The pulse and blood pressure are first assessed while the patient is lying down. He is then requested to stand quickly, and the measurements are repeated. The patient stands for two to three minutes and the measurements are again taken. In symptomatic orthostatic hypotension, there is both a drop in systolic blood pressure when the patient stands and a failure of reflex tachycardia to compensate for the hypotension, causing a critical deficit in cerebral perfusion.

In patients with suspected carotid sinus syncope, carotid sinus massage should be performed under electrocardiographic monitoring. The test is contraindicated in the presence of overt carotid atherosclerosis. In the elderly, it is safest to begin an intravenous infusion and to have a syringe of atropine ready in the event of sinus arrest or heart block.

The autonomic response to Valsava's maneuver can be assessed similarly. In the supine patient with normal sympathetic function after Valsalva's maneuver, the pulse slows and the blood pressure rises 10 to 30 torr. The absence of these responses suggests the presence of autonomic insufficiency.

LABORATORY TESTS

The specific laboratory investigations that are appropriate in the evaluation of syncope depend on the clinical features. In syncope with obvious cause (eg, fainting of blood donors or military recruits standing at attention) laboratory evaluation is probably unnecessary. In the usual case in which the etiology is not obvious, all patients should undergo a complete blood count, a serum glucose test, and a full ECG with a rhythm strip. Chest x-ray and arterial blood gases may be desirable if the diagnosis of pulmonary embolism is being entertained. If the cause of syncope remains elusive, a 24-hour taped ECG (Holter monitor) should be examined to assess for paroxysmal cardiac arrhythmia.

Kapoor et al (1982) have shown that screening assessments of syncope with five-hour glucose tolerance tests, radionuclide or CT brain scans, lumbar punctures, and skull x-rays do not help identify the underlying etiology. Electroencephalograms are rarely useful because, although often abnormal, they do not provide data of specific diagnostic value.

In patients with manifest cardiac disease and syncope, it is cost-effective to perform echocardiography and cardiac electrophysiologic studies. Such studies should also be considered for the patient without manifest cardiac disease but with recurrent syncope of unknown cause. If electrophysiologic studies disclose cardiac conduction abnormalities, cardiac pacing is usually indicated and frequently is curative. Despite all investigations, as many as 50% of patients with syncope will remain undiagnosed.

Thus, the patient with syncope should have a careful history and physical examination, complete blood count, serum glucose test, and ECG. Further testing, if any, should be based on the clinical findings. Specific treatment is based upon the final diagnosis. If there is no diagnosis, the patient should have any drug regimen scrutinized and simplified, and contributing disorders identified and treated. The patient with recurrent syncope of unknown cause should probably have cardiac electrophysiologic testing.

DISORDERS PRODUCING SYNCOPE

Syncope may be caused by a variety of disorders, which are classified by mechanism in Table 7-1. A detailed review of the more common causes follows.

Orthostatic Hypotension

Reduced cerebral perfusion pressure that results from a drop in systemic blood pressure on standing is the most common cause of syncopal and presyncopal symptoms in outpatient practice. Orthostatic hypotension readily results from a drop in blood volume (acute blood loss, dehydration), but much more often it is caused by an impairment in sympathetic vasomotor tone. Symptomatic orthostatic hypotension can usually be traced to the effects of aging, concomitant diseases, and/or use of medication.

The elderly are particularly prone to develop orthostatic hypotension. A quarter of normal persons over the age of 65 experience a drop in systolic pressure of 20 torr or more upon standing. In 9% of these persons, the systolic blood pressure drops more than 30 torr; and in 5%, more than 40 torr. Advancing age alone impairs the carotid body baroreceptor system for maintaining blood pressure on standing and impairs the ability to generate a reflex tachycardia to compensate for the hypotension.

Concomitant disease is often a contributory factor. Patients who have peripheral polyneuropathies from diabetes, alcohol abuse, nutritional deficiencies, or other causes have impaired postural blood pressure maintenance mechanisms. Patients with varicose veins have an increase in the capacitance vessels in the legs which, when filled upon standing, produce a drop in blood pressure. Patients who have Addison's disease, diabetes mellitus, diabetes insipidus, hypercalcemia, hypokalemia, or hypoalbuminemia, or who use diuretics chronically may have chronic intravascular volume depletion. Orthostatic hypotension may result also from certain central nervous system disorders, including idiopathic autonomic insufficiency (Shy–Drager syndrome), parkinsonism, and chronic bilateral diseases of the brain stem and spinal cord.

Drug use is an all-too-common contributory factor. All antihypertensives, antianginals, vasodilators, tricyclic antidepressants, neuroleptics, and diuretics produce orthostatic hypotension. Other drugs with similar hypotensive effects include levodopa, bromocriptine, and monoamine oxidase inhibitors.

Patients usually become symptomatic when they rise suddenly from a sitting or lying position, but the symptoms may be delayed for several minutes. In some patients, the usual feeling of faintness and lightheadedness are not as prominent as feelings of confusion, tremulousness, and staggering. The presence of orthostatic hypotension can be documented by showing a fall in blood pressure greater than 15 torr upon standing. The presence of autonomic insufficiency can be further documented by showing an absent or blunted reflex tachycardia in response to the hypotension.

Orthostatic hypotension is treated by eliminating offending medications or by reducing their dosage. Elastic stockings or pantyhose should be worn. Underlying contributing medical disorders should be sought and treated. Patients should be instructed to change positions very slowly and to sit with their feet elevated or to lie down at the first sign of impending faint. Resting vasomotor tone can be strengthened by sleeping with the head elevated on 6- or 8-inch blocks and by a program of frequent physical activity including walking. If necessary, intravascular volume can be increased by increasing dietary sodium intake or with the careful use (watching for signs of congestive heart failure) of fluorinated steroids.

Vasodepressor Syncope

The common faint in the otherwise healthy young patient is often vasodepressor (vasovagal) syncope. It has been known for many years that these attacks tend to occur in certain stereotyped situations: seeing blood (particularly one's own) during venipuncture, fear of bodily mutilation, and severe pain. After many years of study, Engel (1978) pointed out that the common psychologic theme in vasodepressor syncope is "the need to exaggerate bravery, strength, aggressiveness, and other culturally defined attributes of manliness and to deny, minimize, or at least not acknowledge fear, coupled with shame for failure to live up to such standards...." The patient may experience syncope when he feels that there is no escape from the frightening situation. Hunger, warmth, and crowding exacerbate the situation.

Engel showed that the circulatory changes in vasodepressor syncope are biphasic. In the first phase, occupying the initial minute or two, heart rate, blood pressure, systemic resistance, and cardiac output increase. The patient may appear apprehensive. The second phase then begins abruptly with a fall in heart rate, systemic and pulmonary blood pressures and resistances, and cardiac output. If the patient is standing, all the drops in cardiovascular functions are magnified. The cardiac rate may fall to such an extent that sinus arrest and escape rhythms occur. Atropine given at this time will correct the bradycardia but not the hypotension. The patient will become presyncopal with pallor, blurred vision, yawning, diaphoresis, lightheadedness, nausea, and weakness in the legs. If he does not lie down quickly, he will lose consciousness when the systolic blood pressure drops below 70 to 80 torr. Bradycardia and hypotension may persist for several minutes after he faints.

Vasodepressor syncope is common and is often recurrent. Patients so predisposed should be instructed to lie down immediately at the first sign of syncopal symptoms. Predisposition to vasodepressor syncope is a trait that tends to run in families. In such patients, extensive workups for the etiology of syncope should be avoided.

Reflex Syncopes

In addition to vasovagal syncope, there are other reflex syncopes in which afferents as well as efferents are vagally mediated (vagovagal syncopes). The diagnosis of most such attacks may be made by taking a careful history.

Micturition syncope tends to occur in two settings. The first is in healthy young men who awaken in the early morning with full bladders after a night's drinking. The sudden bladder evacuation while standing induces vagal afferent impulses. These impulses stimulate medullary vasodepressor centers to produce hypotension and vagal parasympathetic centers to reflexly slow the heart. Occasionally, heart block can be induced during micturition. A second clinical type of micturition syncope is present in middle-aged and elderly patients, especially women, who have preexisting causes of orthostatic hypotension.

Cough syncope was described by Charcot in 1876 as "laryngeal vertigo." It has since been called "tussive" or "post-tussive" syncope. In the usual case, a middle-aged, overweight, smoking man with chronic obstructive pulmonary disease has an episode of uncontrolled coughing that culminates in syncope within seconds to minutes. In 10% of cases, there may be abortive clonic seizure activity lasting a few seconds. Both hypotension and bradycardia occur, and cardiac output drops from those factors as well as from impaired venous filling due to the associated Valsalva's maneuver. Asthmatic children can develop cough syncope that may be mistaken for a seizure disorder.

Reflex syncope can also occur in other states of visceral dilatation. Defecation syncope has been described in elderly patients after a large bowel movement or following manual disimpaction. Instrumentation syncope can complicate air insufflation during proctosigmoidoscopy or colonoscopy. Swallow syncope can be seen in patients with esophageal or vagal lesions and may respond to anticholinergic treatment. Glossopharyngeal neuralgia, a disorder analogous to trigeminal neuralgia that is characterized by paroxysmal excruciating throat pain, may be complicated by sinus bradycardia, sinus arrest, and complete heart block on a vagovagal basis.

Carotid Sinus Syncope

Mechanical pressure on the carotid sinus normally induces a degree of reflex bradycardia and hypotension. In some people, who have hypersensitivity of the carotid sinus, a mechanical pressure can induce true syncope. Carotid sinus hypersensitivity increases with age and is more common in men. It has a higher incidence in persons with atherosclerotic vascular disease and with its chief risk factors, diabetes and hypertension. Mass lesions (tumors, lymph nodes) overlying the carotid sinus and aneurysmal dilatation of the internal carotid artery also correlate with carotid sinus hypersensitivity. The carotid sinus may be accidentally stimulated by neck turning and tight fitting collars. Medications, including digitalis, propranolol, and alpha-methyldopa, are also believed to predispose to carotid sinus hypersensitivity.

The diagnosis is made by massaging the right and left carotid sinuses sequentially for five seconds each, allowing at least a 30 second pause between sides. The ipsilateral superficial temporal artery should be palpated during massage to ensure that the carotid is not being totally occluded. Electrocardiographic and constant blood pressure monitoring are performed. If carotid sinus massage induces a sinus pause greater than three seconds or a drop in systolic blood pressure of greater than 50 torr, the diagnosis of carotid sinus hypersensitivity can be made. Carotid sinus massage is contraindicated in the presence of overt carotid artery atherosclerosis.

Carotid sinus hypersensitivity is treated with anticholinergic drugs, which block the vagal bradyarrhythmias but not the vasodepressor response. Atrioventricular sequential cardiac pacemaking is reserved for patients who are unresponsive to or intolerant of anticholinergic drugs.

Cardiac Arrhythmias

Although cardiac syncope is less common than the vascular causes just discussed, recognizing it is very important because it strongly suggests the presence of serious underlying cardiac disease and it increases the risk of sudden death. Electrical disturbances of the heart that produce syncope can be classified as arrhythmias, conduction disturbances, or sinus node disorders. Both tachyarrhythmias and bradyarrhythmias of supraventricular and ventricular origin may produce syncope, but bradyarrhythmias are the most common offenders.

Transient cardiac arrhythmias, including atrial, ventricular, and junctional premature beats, are common in adults and increase in frequency with aging. Even runs of paroxysmal atrial tachycardia, sinus bradycardia, and coupled or multifocal ventricular premature beats are common and usually asymptomatic. Interpreting certain arrhythmias on 24-hour Holter monitored electrocardiograms is difficult. Beyond making a presumptive association, to diagnose syncope as being caused by cardiac arrhythmia requires the temporal correlation of symptoms of syncope or presyncope with recorded ECG paroxysmal disturbances that are sufficient to induce those symptoms.

There is an increased incidence of cardiac conduction disturbances, including right and left bundle-branch blocks, bifascicular block, and trifascicular block in patients with syncope. Fortunately, the marker of conduction disturbances in syncopal patients does not infer a higher incidence of sudden death. As with arrhythmias, before conduction block can be blamed for syncope, it must be temporally related to the syncopal symptoms. Cardiac electrophysiological studies can pinpoint the location of the conduction disturbance.

Sick sinus syndrome is a relatively common cardiac cause of syncope. The syndrome is caused by an intrinsic disturbance of the automaticity of the sinus node, hence its competence as a pacemaker is jeopardized. The affected patient develops episodic sinus bradycardia, sinus arrest, or sinus node exit block and supraventricular tachyarrhythmias. Syncope most often occurs during the prolonged sinus node recovery time (the asystole following the cessation of the supraventricular tachycardia), but it can also occur during sinus arrest, severe bradycardia, and high-grade sinoatrial block. Medications (digitalis, propranolol, lidocaine, procainamide, quinidine, phenytoin, and lithium) have been reported to exacerbate sick sinus syndrome.

Treatment of the disturbances of cardiac rhythm and conduction includes antiarrhythmic medications and cardiac pacemaking. Cardiology texts should be consulted for details of these treatments, but, generally, pacemakers are preferred in cases of symptomatic bradyarrhythmias caused by sick sinus syndrome and heart block. A pacemaker will prevent syncope in these disorders and will help prevent sudden death in the patient who becomes syncopal from complete heart block (Stokes–Adams attack).

Cardiac Outflow Obstruction

Mechanical interference with cardiac output is a relatively uncommon cause of syncope. However, for the patient who complains of exertional syncope, the question should be raised of cardiac outflow obstruction by aortic stenosis or hypertrophic obstructive cardiomyopathy.

With angina and exertional dyspnea, syncope is a cardinal feature of critical aortic stenosis and calcific aortic sclerosis. Because their clinical features and murmurs are similar, echocardiography may be needed to differentiate them. In the patient with critical aortic stenosis in whom cardiac catheterization discloses a significant pressure gradient across the aortic valve, aortic valve replacement cures syncope and prolongs life.

As with aortic stenosis, hypertrophic obstructive cardiomyopathy (idiopathic hypertrophic subaortic stenosis) presents with syncope, angina, and exertional dyspnea. Syncope is caused by both left ventricular outflow obstruction and arrhythmias. Digitalis can make the obstruction worse, and beta-adrenergic blockade can improve it. Echocardiography is diagnostic.

Pump failure from myocardial infarction or cardiomyopathy with or without arrhythmia may produce syncope. Massive pulmonary embolism can also present with syncope. Atrial myxoma can produce episodic syncope which may be positional.

Blood and Metabolic Disorders

Abnormalities in the blood concentrations of hemoglobin, oxygen, carbon dioxide, and glucose usually are not solely responsible for syncopal attack. Rather, the marginally hypotensive or bradycardic patient who also has severe anemia or a low PO_2 may become syncopal. Thus, these disturbances may contribute to multifactorial syncopal attacks. Consciousness abnormalities induced by critical degrees of hypoglycemia, hypoxemia, hypercapnia, and anemia are not spontaneously reversible, hence they present clinically as confusion, stupor, or coma and not as a syncopal attack.

Central Nervous System Disorders

Transient ischemic attacks (TIAs) of the vertebrobasilar system, and more rarely of the carotid system, may produce syncope. Usually, the patient reports premonitory symptoms of focal brain dysfunction, such as hemiparesis, quadriparesis, hemianesthesia, quadrianesthesia, diplopia, dysarthria, aphasia, or hemianopia. Ordinary TIAs produce a transient focal brain disturbance without affecting consciousness.

"Drop attacks" are a curious syndrome in which the (usually) middle-aged patient suddenly drops to the floor without an alteration in consciousness. Most such spells do not have an identifiable cause, but some are probably caused by vertebrobasilar transient ischemic attacks. Prolonged attacks with paralysis persisting for minutes to hours may result from potassium-related periodic paralysis. Similar attacks in children and young adults may be epileptic seizures.

Seizure disorders are seen in about 25% of patients who come to the hospital emergency room with transient loss of consciousness (Day et al 1982). The distinction between seizures and true syncope is usually made with confidence on the basis of the history and particularly the accounts of eyewitnesses.

Difficulties may arise in the patient who, during a vasovagal syncopal episode, does not lie down. In such a case, a "helpful" friend or passerby may have held the person in a sitting position, or the attack may have occurred in a public toilet stall or in a telephone booth in which the patient slumped against the wall. If the brain is continuously deprived of oxygen because of sustained hypotension, tonic or clonic convulsive activity lasting 5 to 60 seconds may complicate syncope. Such patients are not epileptic and do not merit a seizure disorder evaluation. Similar episodes have been described in blood donors during venipuncture when the head of the reclining chair was not lowered sufficiently during a vasovagal episode.

Bibliography

Day SC, Cook EF, Funkenstein H, et al: Evaluation and outcome of emergency room patients with transient loss of consciousness. *Am J Med* 1982; 73:15-23. (Of some value epidemiologically, but intake criteria were arbitrary.)

DeMaria AA, Westmoreland BF, Sharbrough FW: EEG in cough syncope. *Neurology* 1984; 34:371-374. (Reviews the pathophysiology of cough syncope and the EEG findings in syncope.)

Engel GL: Psychologic stress, vasodepressor (vasovagal) syncope, and sudden death. *Ann Intern Med* 1978; 89:403-412. (Dr. Engel's more current thoughts are well worth reading. He shows a correlation between vasovagal syncope and sudden death.)

Kapoor WN, Karpf M, Levey GS: Issues in evaluating patients with syncope. *Ann Intern Med* 1984; 100:755-757. (An editorial that outlines diagnostic workup recommendations from the Pittsburgh group.)

Kapoor WN, Karpf M. Maher Y, et al: Syncope of unknown origin: The need for a more cost-effective approach to its diagnostic evaluation. *JAMA* 1982; 247:2687-2691. (The study showing that only the history, physical exam, and ECG [and, in selected patients, cardiac catheterization and electrophysiologic studies] are cost-effective in the workup of patients with syncope.)

Kapoor WN, Karpf M, Wicand S, et al: A prospective evaluation and follow-up of patients with syncope. *N Engl J Med* 1983; 309:197-204. (The study showing a higher incidence of sudden death in patients whose syncope has a cardiovascular cause.)

Kapoor WN, Peterson JR, Karpf M: Micturition syncope: A reappraisal. *JAMA* 1985; 253:796-798. (Shows that micturition syncope in the elderly usually is complicated by orthostatic hypotension.)

Klein GJ, Gulamhusein SS: Undiagnosed syncope: Search for an arrhythmic etiology. *Stroke* 1982; 13:746-749. (Reviews the role of cardiac arrhythmia in syncope and discusses Holter monitoring.)

Lipsitz LA: Syncope in the elderly. *Ann Intern Med* 1983; 99:92-105. (An excellent, thorough account of the mechanisms, causes, and treatment of syncope, upon which much of this chapter was based; well-referenced.)

Sugrue DD, Wood DL, McGoon MD: Carotid sinus hypersensitivity and syncope. *Mayo Clin Proc* 1984; 59:637-640. (Reviews pathophysiology of carotid sinus syncope.)

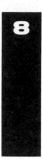

Headache

Headache is the most common outpatient complaint referable to the nervous system. Currently, at least 5% to 10% of the population of the United States seek medical attention for the relief of severe head pain. At least 40% of North Americans have experienced severe headache at some point in their lives. More than 15,000 tons of aspirin are consumed annually in the U.S., most of it being for the relief of head pain. The cost of evaluation and treatment of the patient with headache consumes millions of dollars a year, and days lost to the work force because of headache are considerable. A logical and orderly approach to headache will facilitate the prompt diagnosis and treatment of the various kinds of head pain. It is most important to treat any pain in its initial phase in an attempt to prevent a chronic pain syndrome from developing.

Headache may originate from various sources within the cranium, as a result of malfunction, displacement, or encroachment of pain-sensitive structures. These pain-sensitive areas are, for the most part, vascular. They include the proximal portion of the cerebral arteries, and the large veins and venous sinuses. The meninges, upper cervical nerve roots, and the scalp and neck muscles are also involved in the origin of head pain. Paradoxically, the brain itself and the ventricular surfaces are insensitive to pain.

Approximately 50% of patients evaluated at headache clinics suffer from migraine; 30% to 40% suffer from muscle contraction-tension headaches. Post-traumatic headache is seen in 3% to 5%, and brain tumor is seen in 1% to 2%. Vascular headache is the most common type, with migraine and its subgroups occurring most often. Cluster headache is also vascular, but its incidence is far lower than that of migraine. Muscle contraction-tension headache may frequently occur in isolation but may be associated with vascular headache.

Headache can be a symptom of a wide variety of diseases. *Fever* commonly produces head pain, which is usually throbbing in quality, often constant, and commonly located in the frontal and bitemporal areas, although occipital-nuchal pain may occur in 50% of patients. Eye pain may occur and often remains for a few days after the headache clears. Eye movement worsens the pain, and the globe may be tender to touch. In approximately 10% of patients, the eye pain is lateralized. Occasionally, some patients continue to experience pain after the remission of their febrile episode. This pain is frequently nonthrobbing and constant and may last for years. Mild analgesic medications are most effective for the pain associated with fever; tricyclic antidepressants (amitriptyline) seem to be the best agents for treating the more chronic headache.

Although frequently implicated as a cause of headache, *hypertension* is rarely a singular cause of head pain. In the past, an occcipital headache that was present on awakening and disappeared as the day progressed was believed to be an indicator of symptomatic essential hypertension. More recent studies, however, have shown that headache upon awakening without definite localization is more common in untreated hypertensive patients than in treated hypertensives or in a control group of patients without hypertension.

Paroxysmal throbbing headache, which usually awakens the patient from sleep, occurs in 80% of patients with *pheochromocytoma*. The pain usually reaches its zenith within a few minutes then gradually subsides. Other common manifestations of pheochromocytoma—palpitation, perspiration, nausea, and tremor— are often associated with headache. The duration of the headache is less than 15 minutes in 50% of patients, and less than one hour in 70%. Headache is often bifrontal in location. Coughing, straining, or sneezing often increases the pain, and the patient prefers not to remain supine. Precipitating factors may be exertion, straining, defecation, urination, emotional excitement, or moving in bed. Headache is the only complaint in 10% of patients. Blood pressure during the headache may range from 200/100 to 300/160 mm Hg. Patients who have sustained hypertension experience less frequent headache, and marked paroxysmal elevations of blood pressure may be seen in patients without headache.

MUSCLE CONTRACTION-TENSION HEADACHE

More than 40% of people who seek medical attention for headaches are diagnosed as having muscle contraction-tension headache. Muscle contraction headache is an ache or sensation of tightness, pressure, or constriction widely varied in intensity, frequency, and duration. Sometimes it is long lasting and often it is suboccipital. Headache is associated with sustained contraction of skeletal muscles in the absence of permanent structural change, usually as part of the individual's reaction to life stress. The term tension is used primarily to describe muscle tension rather than emotional stress. The traditional description of muscle contraction headache is much less clear than that of migraine. There are overlapping features between muscle contraction headache and migraine; as many as 40% of migraine *and* muscle contraction headache patients describe a throbbing quality to their pain, and 50% report a family history of headache. One-third of patients with muscle contraction headache also develop nausea and vomiting. The age of onset, gender predominance, and family history of patients with muscle contraction headache is not unlike that of patients with migraine.

Symptoms begin before the age of 20 in 40% of patients with muscle contraction headache. The headache tends to be bilateral in 90%, and is usually described as bandlike, dull, and pressing. It may wax and wane during the day, but in the classic case it reaches maximum intensity toward evening. About 10% of patients are awakened from sleep by a throbbing head pain. It is less likely to be present on weekends or during vacations, unlike migraine. The pain is predominantly occipital-nuchal in location, and is sometimes described as piercing, occasionally radiating to the vertex of the head (frequently described as though a nail were being driven into the skull). Nausea, lightheadedness, and photophobia may accompany muscle contraction headache.

Headache that is always present and never goes away is suggestive of muscle contraction headache. Depression may be the cause; 85% of patients with depression have some sort of head pain. The diagnosis is made by the history. Chronic muscle contraction headache is frequently unremitting and present for years, although episodic muscle headache is common. Most patients never see a physician because they are helped by simple analgesics.

The treatment of muscle contraction-tension headache is best directed toward psychological factors that may contribute to the pain, although physical factors that promote muscle contraction should be investigated also. If the headache is intermittent, mild analgesics are the primary medications, although nonsteroidal anti-inflammatory agents may be of some benefit. Heat and massage may also be beneficial. Muscle spasm can be relieved with muscle relaxants such as the benzodiazepines or cyclobenzaprine (Flexeril). They can cause tolerance and possibly psychological or physical dependence with chronic use, so they should be used only for a brief period of time. Tricyclic antidepressants are probably the most useful pharmacologic agents, especially if there is associated depression. Amitriptyline is most effective, given at bedtime in doses ranging from 75 to 150 mg. Propranolol is sometimes helpful (40 to 160 mg/day) especially when combined with amitriptyline. The use of chronic analgesic medications and other over-the-counter drugs should be avoided.

Reassuring the patient that there is not a serious cause for the headache is sometimes therapeutic. If there appears to be a psychological problem or stress, then these problems should be discussed with the patient as the most likely reason for the head pain. Physical therapy, relaxation techniques, massage, and hot showers may also be beneficial. Biofeedback can be of great value, especially in the patient who is not depressed.

MIGRAINE

Migraine is a hereditary recurrent throbbing headache of probable vascular origin. Prevalence rates for migraine are in the 20% to 25% range, although it has been suggested that these are underestimates of its true prevalence. Although the prevalence of migraine really does not differ with regard to race, social class, or educational background, it is by far a more common disease in women, who comprise as many as 75% of the patients in some series. There is a parental history of migraine in 60% of patients, and the incidence of migraine in children of migraineurs is increased if both parents have migraine.

More than 90% of patients with migraine report that their first attack occurred before the age of 40 years. Children may be affected; 20% to 35% of children with migraine were younger than 5 years of age when their headaches began. Under age 10, the sex ratio for migraine is reversed, with boys accounting for 60% of the childhood cases. The appearance of menarche is not a significant factor for the initial onset of migraine, nor for the frequency or severity of the headache. Migraine may be related to the menstrual cycle, and exacerbations may be seen in women at menopause, including women without a prior migraine history. Although most women are free of migraine during pregnancy, some may have their first attack then (so-called gestational migraine). Migraine attacks tend to occur less frequently and are less intense after middle age, although migraine can occur after the age of 55. Migraine can be classified into three varieties: common, classic, and complicated.

Common Migraine

Common migraine is characterized by episodic unilateral or bilateral headache, frequently associated with nausea, vomiting, and photophobia, but without overt neurological symptoms and signs. Headache commonly begins upon awakening, but may occur at any time of the day. It may be principally nocturnal, awakening the patient from sleep. During severe attacks, the headache is lateralized in 50% of patients. Either side of the cranium may be involved; the side may vary from attack to attack. However, the entire head is painful in as many as 25% of patients. Thus, the localization of pain is a relatively insensitive criterion for diagnosis: fewer than 50% of patients have true hemicrania.

Headache is usually gradual in onset, reaching its peak in a few minutes to a few hours, and persisting for several hours to several days. About two-thirds of patients report that the headache lasts for less than a day, even more report that it lasts less than four hours. Pain is initially dull and steady, becoming pulsatile when more severe. Movement or postural changes may turn a dull headache into a throbbing one. Half of patients complain of pulsatile head pain; one-third also note sharp, jabbing pains (ice pick-like). Pressure on an artery overlying the site of the headache, or over the ipsilateral carotid artery, may decrease the pain. Any type of rapid head motion, coughing, or straining aggravates migraine. A period of brief sleep may abort the spell, and lying still may reduce the pain.

Nausea occurs in the vast majority of patients, and vomiting occurs in more than 50%. Diarrhea may also occur; some patients experience only diarrhea with the headache. Blurred vision is common, and there may be heightened sensitivity to light, sounds, and smells. Vague lightheadedness is common, and syncope occurs in 10% of patients, more frequently in children. Scalp tenderness is common during or after the headache and may involve any portion of the head or neck. Fluid retention and weight gain may occur; nasal stuffiness may occur in 10% to 20%. Alterations of mood occur in most patients, sometimes before, but usually during the headache.

Precipitating factors for migraine include emotional and physical stress, loss of sleep, fatigue, skipped meals, and hormonal changes. Emotional stress is one of the most frequent precipitants. Frequently, migraine does not develop during the period of stress, but rather during the "letdown" period thereafter, such as on weekends or during vacations. Certain foodstuffs (aged cheeses, chocolate, and Chinese foods) may precipitate migraine because they contain vasoactive substances. In women, migraine may be strongly associated with the menstrual cycle; almost two-thirds note that at least some of their attacks are limited to menses. Headache that occurs only at the time of menstruation, so-called menstrual migraine, is much less common, but may be a manifestation of the premenstrual syndrome.

There is an increased incidence of migraine in women who use oral contraceptives; headache frequency seems to correlate with the estrogen content of the formulation. Approximately half of the women who develop headache in association with oral contraceptive use have had prior migraine attacks. When stopping the oral contraceptive, there may be a few months' delay before improvement of the headaches. Headache may develop from a few months to a few years after the oral contraceptive is started, but most women who experience headache as a side effect do so within the first few months of its use. Of the women who develop headache after starting oral contraceptives, 30% to 40% improve after the drug is stopped. Occasionally, headache will improve in women using oral contraceptives.

More than 60% of migraine attacks are associated with transient disturbances of cerebral function, visual disturbances being the most common (40%). The most common migrainous visual symptom is the scintillating scotoma, with "scintillating" referring to any kind of luminous visual display. Visual disturbances tend to be stereotyped in the same individual. In over 75% of patients visual hallucinations appear in both visual fields and are of unformed objects such as light, stars, or spots. The visual symptoms are monocular in 5% of patients. In 15%, there are illusions of altered size, shape, or position of objects (metamorphopsia) or hallucinations of structured objects. Unformed hallucinations suggest a disturbance of the occipital lobes within the distribution of the posterior cerebral artery; formed visual hallucinations suggest dysfunction of the posterior temporal lobe, which is in the distribution of the middle cerebral artery.

These visual hallucinations frequently occur in the central portions of the visual fields. Their margins are often poorly defined, and they persist with eye closure. Typical of the scotomata of migraine is the gradual enlargement of the scotoma, beginning in a small field and spreading to much of the visual field, then migrating to the periphery. This typical march of spectral figures occurs in approximately 10% of migraine patients. The scintillating scotoma appears to expand and spread as it grows larger, until it eventually disappears. This entire process may take as long as half an hour, and it may be followed by a headache that is usually contralateral to the involved visual field.

Classic Migraine

In patients with classic migraine, visual symptoms may also take the form of blindness, homonymous hemianopia, blurred vision, or altitudinal defects. It may be difficult to differentiate monocular visual disturbances from hemianopias, but if the visual change appears lateral in the temporal field, occipital involvement is likely. If the eyeball is displaced with the fingertip and the visual abnormality moves, then it is of retinal origin and not from the calcarine cortex.

Approximately one-third of patients with migraine complain of unilateral paresthesias with their migraine attacks. These sensory symptoms are characterized by paresthesias or numbness, which often begins in the fingers and hand (usually on the ulnar side), spreads to the forearm, skips the arm and shoulder, involves the corner of the mouth and is present in half of the tongue, lips, and buccal mucosa. This march of sensory symptoms may take as long as 30 minutes and may cross to the opposite side of the body. This slow spread (also called the sensory march of migraine) is comparable to the progression of visual scotomata and is much slower than that caused by a sensory seizure. It does not occur in thrombotic or embolic cerebrovascular disease. The sensory symptoms occurring during the sensory march of migraine characteristically resolve initially in the area that was first involved, with the last area affected by symptoms being the one that clears last. This is the opposite of what is seen in transient cerebrovascular ischemia and is a way of differentiating the two conditions.

Complicated Migraine

Complicated migraine is associated with transient or, rarely, permanent deficits of sensory or motor function. Subtypes of complicated migraine include the hemiplegic and ophthalmoplegic varieties. Complicated migraine usually commences before the age of 20, although it can occur at any age. Paralysis of one or all of the limbs in association with headache is uncommon. Such paralysis may occur as a prodrome to the actual migraine, with recovery in 30 minutes (usually as the cephalgia begins); the weakness may vary from side to side. Another type of paralysis may occur in which the hemiparesis usually affects the same side, usually persisting for hours to days, long after the headache subsides. It is frequently associated with a family history of similar attacks and is called familial hemiplegic migraine.

Ophthalmoplegic migraine is a rare form of complicated migraine characterized by episodes of orbital or periorbital head pain that radiates to the ipsilateral hemicranium and is associated with nausea and vomiting. As the pain begins to subside, ptosis and complete third-nerve palsy develop, sometimes associated with involvement of cranial nerve V (numbness in the ophthalmic division) and weakness of the lateral rectus muscle (cranial nerve VI). The ophthalmoplegia may persist for hours to months, and attacks may alternate between sides. Ophthalmoplegic migraine is so uncommon that other causes of painful ophthalmoplegia should be considered, including internal carotid artery aneurysm, diabetic ophthalmoplegia, cavernous sinus or orbital tumor, and meningeal inflammation. Computed tomography (CT) and cerebral angiography may be necessary to exclude some of these more sinister causes of painful ophthalmoplegia.

Many patients with migraine suffered from attacks of motion sickness during early childhood. Mitral valve prolapse may be associated with migraine, and in one series one-third of the patients with mitral valve prolapse also had a history of migraine. Classical migraine has been reported in patients with systemic lupus erythematosus as well as in patients with prosthetic heart valves. In studies of those with a prosthetic heart valve, transient neurological signs and symptoms that were highly characteristic of migraine developed with or without headache. Anticoagulation did not help, and the syndrome was self-limited to a period of several weeks.

Headache occurs in as many as 70% of patients undergoing hemodialysis, with the most common form being the precipitation of migraine in patients with a history of migraine. Others, without prior headache, experience cephalgia only in association with hemodialysis, usually felt as a bilateral throbbing pain .The headache may disappear after nephrectomy or successful renal transplant. If the transplant is rejected, a headache may occur as a manifestation of the rejection episode.

DIFFERENTIAL DIAGNOSIS

As with all neurological problems, the diagnosis of migraine depends upon a carefully obtained history that emphasizes the clinical manifestations of the headache. Migraine usually begins between the ages of 5 and 55. The attacks are episodic, usually lasting for hours. They may persist for a few days but almost never continue for many days or weeks. Migraine pain frequently begins as a mild, dull ache that increases to a throbbing discomfort that may become incapacitating. Pain is often lateralized but may be generalized. The presence of an aura or prodromal symptoms suggests migraine. During the attack, most patients seek a quiet place to rest because they are often hypersensitive to light and noise, and sometimes odors.

If the pain consistently recurs on the same side of the head, if symptoms or signs persist or develop following cessation of the headache, or if the neurological examination is abnormal, then the physician should evaluate the patient for a possible structural lesion.

Transient cerebrovascular ischemic attacks may simulate migraine; unilateral headache may occur in as many as one-third of patients with transient ischemic attacks. Headache and visual loss in the elderly patient should suggest the possibility of giant cell arteritis. Seizures must be differentiated from migraine, especially if the epileptogenic focus is in the sensory or visual cortex.

TREATMENT

Nonpharmacologic

Most patients with migraine can be helped. Because some note an increase in the frequency of migraine in relation to smoking, drinking alcoholic beverages, lack of sleep, stress, fatigue, or diet, the modification of those factors may control the headache. Anxiety and depression should be identified and treated with medication, counseling, or psychotherapy. Stopping oral contraceptives (after an alternative method of contraception has been selected) may be curative. Relaxation training combined with biofeedback may be quite helpful; in one series, the frequency of migraine attacks were reduced by one-third in a group employing biofeedback.

Pharmacologic

The pharmacologic regimen for migraine can be separated into drugs used to abort the attack, those used to prevent the attacks from occurring, and those used to treat the symptoms.

Abortive Treatment

The earlier the acute migraine attack is treated, the greater the likelihood that it can be aborted. Thus the patient with classic migraine can begin therapy at the start of the prodrome, whereas the patient with common migraine usually must wait until the onset of the headache. If the headache has been established for a period of hours, there is little value in the use of an abortive agent.

The treatment of choice for a migraine attack is one of the ergot alkaloids, principally ergotamine tartrate. Ergotamine may be administered alone or in combination with sedatives, analgesics, or antiemetics. Many ergotamine preparations contain caffeine, which produces cerebral vasoconstriction and potentiates the action of ergotamine. The absorption of ergotamine is rapid: about two-thirds of the dose is absorbed in 30 minutes. The ergotamines have many side effects (nausea, vomiting, diarrhea, abdominal cramps, intermittent claudication, acute arterial occlusions). Mild side effects, usually nausea and vomiting, occur in about one-third of the patients who use ergots. A number of ergotamine preparations are commercially available; they may be given orally, sublingually, by inhalation, parenterally or rectally. An adequate dose should be taken as soon as possible after onset, and a subnauseating dosage should be determined. The impaired absorption of oral agents together with the vomiting that may accompany migraine may lead the physician to prescribe ergots in forms other than oral tablets.

A coated tablet of ergotamine for oral administration is the least expensive and least effective, usually only of benefit for patients with a clear-cut prodrome of a few minutes before the headache. The usual dosage is 2 mg initially, with an additional 1 mg in 30 minutes if no relief was obtained from the initial dose. No more than a total of 6 mg should be used per attack, with a weekly total not to exceed 10 mg.

Sublingual ergotamine is probably more effective than the coated oral tablet. It is easier to use and is faster-acting, but it tends to cause slightly more nausea than the oral preparation. The usual dosage is one tablet at the onset of the headache and another in 30 to 45 minutes, if no relief was obtained. Maximum dosage recommendations are the same as for the oral form.

A 2-mg rectal suppository can be used, but if nausea develops, the second dose should be half of the original amount. Ergotamine tartrate aerosol (0.36 mg per inhalation) can also be utilized, with an initial dosage of 1 or 2 puffs. The patient should be instructed to exhale completely then deeply inhale, and once to establish a good inward flow of air. The patient should again exhale, then inhale while producing the "puff" by pressing on the canister. The inhalation should proceed to maximum capacity and be held as long as possible. A dose can be inhaled every four minutes, up to a maximum of six doses per day.

Ergotamine preparations are contraindicated in the presence of coronary or peripheral artery disease, hepatic or renal disease, hypertension, and pregnancy. If 1 to 2 mg daily does not help abort the headache, another form of therapy should be prescribed. Problems with ergotamine begin when it is used continuously in doses that exceed 20 mg per week, especially with the suppository form, and less frequently with the oral form. The most common serious side effect is gangrene of the extremities. Serious vasoconstriction usually preferentially affects the lower limbs bilaterally and is manifested initially by distal paresthesia, coldness of the digits and claudication. When ergotamine is taken frequently, it may increase the frequency of migraine because of rebound headache. Tolerance to ergotamine develops at a variable rate. Physical dependence on ergotamine parallels the tolerance phenomenon and often is expressed as worsening headache; this tends to occur in patients using daily dosages of greater than 20 mg. The cessation of ergotamine intake results in a severe withdrawal headache, which responds to an increase in the dose of the ergotamine.

Isometheptane mucate (Midrin), another vasoconstrictor, is somewhat less effective than ergotamine but has fewer side effects. The usual dosage is two capsules at the start of the headache, then one capsule every hour, to a maximum of five capsules in 12 hours.

When migraine is mild, aspirin or another analgesic combined with rest may be enough to abort the attack. The combination of a vasoconstrictor and an antiemetic agent, such as metoclopramide (Reglan), 10 to 20 mg orally, promethazine (Phenergan), 12.5 to 50 mg orally or rectally, or chlorpromazine (Thorazine), 12.5 to 50 mg rectally, may be of benefit in aborting the attack or controlling the nausea from the migraine itself, or from other medications.

Occasionally, for the patient with a definite prodrome, the use of a beta-blocker (propranolol, 40 to 60 mg) at the start of the prodrome combined with an analgesic may be enough to abort the migraine. Sublingual nifedipine (10 mg), a calcium-channel blocker, may have some effect in the abortive treatment of migraine, especially in the patient with classic migraine. Isoproterenol aerosol has also been reported to be effective in reducing or aborting classic migraine.

Prophylactic Treatment

Daily prophylactic medication to reduce the frequency and severity of migraine should be considered in patients who have more than one attack a week or in whom abortive therapy is ineffective (Table 8-1). The person who has only one attack per month may also be a candidate for prophylactic therapy if the attack lasts a few days and is not helped by abortive therapy.

Beta-Blocking Agents. Propranolol, 40 to 360 mg per day in divided doses, has been used with variable success to prevent migraine (Table 8-1). The mechanism of action of beta-blocking agents in the prevention of headache is uncertain, but may be related to central effects rather than beta-adrenergic mediated effects. The average effective daily dosage of propranolol is 120 mg. Asthma, congestive heart failure, and renal insufficiency are contraindications to the use of propranolol and most of the other available beta-blockers. They should be avoided in the patient with diabetes mellitus who requires insulin. Fatigue,

TABLE 8-1 PROPHYLACTIC DRUGS FOR MIGRAINE

CLASSIFICATION	DOSAGE (MG/DAY)
Beta-Blockers	
Propranolol (Inderal)	80-320
Atenolol (Tenormin)	50-100
Nadolol (Corgard)	40-160
Timolol (Blocadren)	20-40
Metoprolol (Lopressor)	100-200
Calcium-Channel Blockers	
Verapamil (Isoptin, Calan)	320-480
Nifedipine (Procardia)	40
Nimodipine	NR
Antidepressants	
Amitriptyline (Elavil, Endep)	75-150
Doxepin (Adapin, Sinequan)	25-100
Anti-inflammatory Drugs	
Indomethacin (Indocin)	75-200
Ibuprofen (Motrin, Rufen, Advil)	1,200-1,800
Naproxen sodium (Anaprox)	1100
Serotonin Antagonists	
Methysergide (Sansert)	4-8
Cyproheptadine (Periactin)	6-8
Lithium	
Lithium Carbonate (Eskalith, Lithobid)	600-900

NR = Not released.

orthostatic lightheadedness, and gastrointestinal complaints are common side effects, but tolerance to these side effects may occur over a few weeks. Beta-blocking drugs may also cause depression, mental confusion, and vivid dreams. For the patient with mild chronic obstructive pulmonary disease, metoprolol (50-100 mg daily) is effective and will have fewer pulmonary side effects. Beta-blocking drugs should not be withdrawn suddenly because rebound migraine may occur, just as rebound angina or hypertension occurs in patients who suddenly stop beta-blockers prescribed for those conditions. Recently a long-acting propranolol has been released that has been shown to be effective in the prophylaxis of migraine. Its main advantage is that it can be taken only once or twice a day; it can be substituted for regular propranolol on a milligram-for-milligram basis.

Tricyclic Antidepressants. Amitriptyline is quite effective in the prophylaxis of migraine, independent of its antidepressant action. The effective dosage of amitriptyline varies from 25 to 175 mg daily, with 90% of patients achieving a good effect with 50 to 100 mg daily. Excessive sedation, the most common side effect, seems to be dose related. It is best to start with 25 mg at bedtime, gradually increasing the dosage by 25 mg increments every five to seven days, reaching a total of 75 to 100 mg at bedtime. Approximately two-thirds of patients who experience a beneficial effect from amitriptyline usually note that the improvement started within seven days, but the range varies from one to 42 days. Dry mouth, tremor, nervousness, lightheadedness, and orthostatic hypotension are common side effects; they may respond to a reduction in the dosage of amitriptyline. Amitriptyline should be avoided in patients with cardiac arrhythmias or congestive heart failure and in men with signs of urinary outflow obstruction. Amitriptyline has no apparent direct effect on the cerebral arteries, but rather it exerts its effect through action on the serotonergic system by blocking the reuptake of serotonin. Occasionally, other antidepressants, such as doxepin or imipramine, may be effective for the prophylaxis of migraine, but amitriptyline is the most effective.

Calcium-Channel Blockers. Calcium-channel blocking drugs are quite effective in the prophylaxis of migraine. Verapamil (80 mg tid) or nifedipine (20 mg tid) reduce the monthly frequency of migraine. Nimodopine (60 to 120 mg per day) is the most effective calcium-channel blocker for migraine prophylaxis and has the fewest side effects, but it has not yet been released for use in the United States. These agents are effective for treating the prodromes and headaches of classic and complicated as well as common migraine. It may take two to four weeks for the beneficial effects to be noticed. The most frequent side effects are dizziness, edema, skin rash, and, occasionally, increased headache. Marked cardiac arrhythmia or the concomitant use of beta-blocking agents are relative contraindications to the use of the calcium-channel blockers.

Serotonin Antagonists. Methysergide (Sansert) is not a first-line drug for the prophylaxis of migraine because of its potentially serious side effects. It is a peripheral serotonin antagonist and has vasoconstrictor properties affecting the external carotid circulation. Methysergide in a dose of 2 to 8 mg daily (divided doses given at mealtime) is effective in 50% to 75% of patients. Those who have taken methysergide for a prolonged period may develop a fibrotic syndrome, including pleuropericardial, retroperitoneal, or endocardial fibrosis. In most cases the fibrosis is reversible if the drug is discontinued. Gastrointestinal pain, nausea and vomiting, diarrhea, dizziness, drowsiness, hallucinations, and psychotic reactions are side effects that may occur in as many as one-third of patients using methysergide. It is contraindicated in patients who are pregnant, in the presence of cardiac valvular, collagen vascular, coronary artery, or peripheral vascular disease, and in patients with fibrotic disease. A drug-free interval of four weeks after each six-month course of treatment is mandatory; the dosage should be reduced gradually during the last two to three weeks of each treatment course to prevent rebound headache.

Cyproheptadine (Periactin) is an antihistamine that has antiserotonin and platelet-antiaggregating properties. It is sometimes useful for migraine prophylaxis (more so for the pediatric patient), but is less effective than methysergide. The dosage varies from 8 to 24 mg per day, in divided doses. Sedation and weight gain are the most common side effects; fibrotic complications have not been reported.

Anticonvulsants. Phenytoin (Dilantin) and primidone (Mysoline) are effective occasionally in the treatment of migraine; there is a subpopulation of adults whose migraine is responsive to anticonvulsants. Children with migraine have a better response to phenytoin. The usual dosage of these medications is the same as that for seizure control (phenytoin 300 to 400 mg per day; primidone 250 to 270 mg per day, both in divided doses). Sedation, dizziness, and gastrointestinal upset are the most common side effects, although phenytoin in the child can induce hirsutism and gingival hypertrophy.

Anti-inflammatory Agents. Indomethacin (Indocin) 25 mg tid or qid, or ibuprofen (Motrin), 600 mg tid, are anti-inflammatory agents that may have some limited benefit in the prevention of migraine. They probably act to block prostaglandin effects on the cerebral vasculature, but overall they are not as effective as the agents discussed previously. Naproxen sodium (Anaprox), 550 mg bid, has recently been shown to be effective for the prophylaxis of migraine; it is superior to other anti-inflammatory medications.

Symptomatic Treatment

Headache and its associated manifestations can be treated with a combination of abortive agents and mild analgesic or anti-inflammatory medications. Occasionally, Fiorinal or propoxyphene are necessary to control head pain. Severe headache can be treated with codeine, usually in combination with acetaminophen or aspirin, but it may cause nausea. Nausea and vomiting can be produced by the headache itself, or it may be secondary to the use of ergotamines or codeine. Vomiting can be controlled with metoclopramide, 10 to 20 mg; promethazine, 25 to 50 mg; chlorpromazine, 25 to 75 mg; or compazine, 5 to 10 mg, usually in suppository form.

Occasionally, parenteral narcotics (meperidine, morphine) are necessary to control the pain of a severe migraine, but frequent use of parenteral medications as well as oral narcotic medications should be avoided. Occasionally, prolonged migraine, referred to as status migrainosus, occurs. It is usually best to hospitalize such a patient, to withdraw all vasoactive medications including ergotamine, and to support with analgesics, sedatives, intravenous fluids, and antiemetics. A short course of prednisone, 40 to 60 mg daily for seven to ten days, may be of benefit, and lithium carbonate, 300 mg tid, has been shown to be effective in some cases of status migrainosus.

POST-TRAUMATIC SYNDROME

For weeks or months following head trauma, many patients complain of headache, vertigo or dizziness, memory impairment, and difficulty with concentration. Because the affected patient does not have to be rendered unconscious by the head trauma to develop these symptoms the designation postconcussive syndrome is a misnomer. Post-traumatic syndrome is a more accurate designation.

Headache that persists for more than two months occurs in 40% to 60% of patients who have been hospitalized because of a closed head injury. There is no convincing data that the degree of brain injury is correlated with the incidence of the severity of the resultant headache. Some authors have emphasized that the incidence of headache is less frequent after major head trauma than after minor trauma.

Headache is the dominant symptom of the post-traumatic syndrome. It usually begins within 24 hours of the head injury, although approximately 6% of patients do not experience headache until several days or weeks later. The headache usually intensifies over a period of several days to weeks. It may wax and wane in intensity, sometimes becoming worse several months after it had all but subsided. The vast majority of patients suffer from a constant, dull aching sensation, frequently in a cap-like distribution or in an area removed from the site of the injury. At times the pain is throbbing, and it is often made worse by exertion, coughing, straining, postural changes, or rapid movements of the head. Nausea may accompany severe headache, and vomiting may occur. Recurring attacks of migraine may occur as a sequela of head trauma; these attacks may be indistinguishable from classic or common migraine.

Chronic post-traumatic headache is more likely to develop in patients with psychopathological conditions prior to the accident, in those seeking compensation, or in those who have had a marked emotional reaction to the injury. Vertigo and lightheadedness occur almost as frequently as headache. Vertigo is usually produced or accentuated by movement of the head or rapid change in body position. Impaired memory and concentration as well as fatigability and irritability occur in most patients with other post-traumatic symptoms, although they may occur independent of headache. Patients who have had true concussive head injuries are, for a time, unable to process information at a normal rate. Secondary psychological reactions are not uncommon; hypochondriasis, depression, and anxiety may result.

TREATMENT

Patients with post-traumatic syndrome should be evaluated to exclude any resultant brain lesion; however, most patients with chronic post-traumatic headaches have no intracranial abnormalities to account for the pain. A careful explanation of the cause, mechanisms, and natural history of the post-traumatic syndrome should be discussed with the patient. Compensation should be resolved as quickly as possible, for the longer the legal or compensation issues continue, the longer the headache will continue.

Ergotamine may be used in the patient with post-traumatic vascular headaches. The combination of amitriptyline (75 to 100 mg at bedtime) and propranolol (40 mg bid to tid) is useful in most patients with chronic generalized pain that has a vascular quality. Propranolol may also serve to reduce any associated anxiety. Depressive symptoms may require psychotherapy, in addition to tricyclic anti-depressants. Fortunately, a majority of patients with the post-traumatic syndrome return to work and experience an eventual remission of symptoms.

CLUSTER HEADACHE

Cluster headache is a periodic and paroxysmal headache disorder. There are two types of cluster headache: episodic and chronic. The episodic type is more common (occurring in 80% of patients) and is defined by periods of head pain (the cluster) alternating with periods of no headache (remission). Chronic cluster headache describes the condition in which remissions have not occurred for at least 12 months. Approximately 50% of chronic cluster patients have never experienced a remission. The incidence of cluster headache is 2% to 9% that of migraine, and males are affected more than females, with a ratio of 4.5 to 1. Most persons begin experiencing cluster headache between the ages of 20 and 50 (mean 35 years), although it can occur in children and as late as the eighth decade of life. The average duration of the episodic cluster is six to eight weeks, with remissions lasting 9 to 12 months. Attacks occur mostly in the spring and fall and are brief, usually lasting less than an hour. They can occur once or many times during the day, usually at nighttime, often awakening the patient from sleep. Attacks may be precipitated by alcohol, nitrites, and high altitude. The pain is usually in an orbital–periorbital location, occasionally radiating frontotemporally. The pain is described as excruciating, constant, and often boring or searing, or as though "a knife was cutting into my eye or head." In contrast to a migraine patient, one with cluster is frequently agitated and may pace or walk during the attack, sometimes striking the head against a wall or hard object in an attempt to relieve the pain. Associated symptoms are on the same side as the head pain and include lacrimation, rhinorrhea, conjunctival infection, nasal stuffiness, and a partial Horner's syndrome. The differential diagnosis includes migraine, trigeminal neuralgia, cranial arteritis, pheochromocytoma and glaucoma.

TREATMENT

Drug selection will depend on the type of cluster headache (chronic or episodic), its frequency, and the age of the patient. All patients should be advised to avoid alcoholic beverages during the cluster.

In patients under the age of 30, methysergide is the drug of choice, often in a dosage of 2 mg tid or qid with meals. Because episodic cluster lasts for less than eight weeks, fibrotic complications are not a problem. In the age range of 30 to 45 years, the patient is usually refractory to methysergide, especially if it had been used in the past. Prednisone, 40 to 50 mg per day in divided doses with a slow taper over three weeks, will result in marked headache reduction in 75% of patients, but only 40% of patients with chronic cluster will achieve benefit.

Lithium carbonate, 300 mg tid, is the best drug to use for patients with chronic cluster or for those with episodic cluster who are over the age of 45. Side effects are not common after the first dose, although tremor is common with dosages about 600 mg daily. Nausea, vomiting, paresthesias, renal dysfunction and hypothyroidism are side effects of chronic lithium therapy, and may be dose-related. Levels should be measured periodically and should be kept below 1.2 μg/mL.

Calcium-channel blockers may actually be the most effective drugs for the treatment of cluster in all age groups. Nimodopine, 60 to 120 mg in divided doses, and verapamil, 80 mg tid, have been reported to be quite effective for the control of cluster (both episodic and chronic), with nimodopine being superior to the other calcium-channel blockers.

Oral ergotamine is also an effective prophylactic agent for patients who have one attack a day, particularly those with nocturnal attacks. A 2-mg tablet should be taken approximately two hours before a nocturnal attack is expected.

Oxygen, inhaled at 7 to 10 liters/minute, is occasionally effective in aborting an acute cluster attack. It also may reduce the frequency of headache during the cluster period when used for five to ten minutes, three to four times a day. As many as 80% of patients improve with this form of therapy. Sublingual or aerosol ergotamine may be effective when used at the onset of an attack, and can be repeated in 15 minutes.

Chronic paroxysmal hemicrania is a variant of cluster in which there are daily attacks of head pain, usually 10 or more episodes, each lasting 10 to 30 minutes, and at times associated with rhinorrhea, lacrimation, and ptosis. Chronic paroxysmal hemicrania responds dramatically to indomethacin, 25 mg three to four times daily; characteristically the medications used to treat cluster are not effective for this cluster variant.

COITAL HEADACHE

Sudden, suboccipital headache, usually throbbing in nature and occasionally accompanied by vomiting, may be related to sexual activity. Such headaches may be divided into two varieties. The first type frequently develops as sexual excitement mounts and has the characteristics of a muscle contraction headache. The second type, occurring at the time of orgasm, is more severe, usually explosive in onset with throbbing pain. Occasionally, this second type of headache is caused by a ruptured intracranial aneurysm or an arteriovenous malformation, but these lesions are uncommon. Such headaches related to sexual activity, whether orgasmic or not, are best classified as a type of exertional headache, but are better known as sex headaches. If the headache is benign, indomethacin, (25 to 100 mg/day), as used for other exertional headaches, may be of benefit. Because sex headaches may occur in migraine patients with an increased incidence, a beta-blocking drug (eg, propranolol, 40 mg bid) may help prevent the headache. Such headaches can occur for no apparent reason, however, and then cease spontaneously. If the headache is recurrent and untreated, sexual dysfunction may ultimately develop. Patients who develop focal signs or recurrent headache should have a CT scan performed to exclude an obvious vascular lesion. If the patient is evaluated in the acute setting in which a CT scan is normal, a lumbar puncture is sometimes necessary to exclude subarachnoid bleeding not visible on CT.

FOOD-INDUCED HEADACHE

Ice cream headache is probably the best known of the food-induced head pains. When cold foods or liquids contact the oropharynx, an intense midfrontal pain, which is occasionally pulsatile, may occur; it lasts only a few seconds. Such a headache occurs in more than 90% of patients with migraine, and 30% of migraine-free patients have reported having had ice cream headache at some time during their lives.

Common foods that may increase or cause head pain in certain individuals include alcohol, chocolate, cheeses, and certain other dairy products. There is evidence that implicates tyramine and phenylethylamine (contained in cheese and chocolate, respectively) as chemical agents that may precipitate head pain. Other chemicals that can induce headache include sodium nitrite and monosodium glutamate.

Headache may be experienced after eating hot dogs because of the nitrite content. Such headaches are frequently bitemporal or bifrontal in location and may be associated with facial flushing. Almost one-third of those who eat Chinese food experience some sort of adverse reaction, with headache and chest tightness the most common ones. Monosodium glutamate, a principal ingredient of soy sauce, is the chemical cause of these symptoms. Those who experience headache after ingesting certain foods are more likely to develop spontaneous migraine.

TRIGEMINAL NEURALGIA

Trigeminal neuralgia (*tic doloreaux*) is characterized by brief paroxysms of high-intensity facial pain restricted to the sensory innervation of the 5th cranial nerve. Women are affected more than men. The condition occurs more often on the right side of the face than on the left; 14% of cases are bilateral. The pain occurs most commonly in the area supplied by both the second and third divisions of the trigeminal nerve (lower jaw and cheek), and less commonly in the forehead (first division). In 90% of patients, this disorder begins after the age of 40. Trigeminal neuralgia in the younger patient is often the result of multiple sclerosis with associated brain stem demyelination.

Trigeminal neuralgia by definition is paroxysmal, and in most cases each paroxysm lasts from a few seconds to a few minutes. The pain may recur with only brief intervals of freedom for a period of hours, so that the patient interprets it as continuous. Attacks of trigeminal neuralgia characteristically occur in bouts lasting a few days or weeks, or sometimes months, followed by remissions, which tend to be completely pain-free. The length of the remission can vary from a few weeks to years. The pain is described as excruciating, often like an electric shock or searing as if a red-hot poker were placed on the face. Usually there is no warning of an attack, and after the pain has passed, a feeling of warmth over the face may persist for a brief time.

Trigeminal neuralgia can be precipitated by eating, talking, shaving, washing or rubbing the face, as well as by cleaning the teeth. Cutaneous trigger points from which the episode of trigeminal neuralgia can be provoked often develop during the course of the disease. The upper lip, ala naris, and the angle of the mouth account for most of the trigger points. A trigger point in the ophthalmic division of cranial nerve V is uncommon, occurring in only 8% to 10% of patients.

Abnormal physical signs are absent in the idiopathic variety of trigeminal neuralgia. The discovery of sensory or motor deficits should raise the suspicion of "symptomatic" trigeminal neuralgia, possibly caused by a posterior fossa tumor, demyelination, or a vascular lesion. Trigeminal neuralgia with hemifacial spasm on the same side is known as tic-convulsif, and is usually caused by a mass (tumor or vascular) compressing cranial nerves V and VII.

The diagnosis of trigeminal neuralgia rests essentially on the history and the absence of abnormal findings on the neurological examination. Few conditions give rise to such severe paroxysmal pain, so the differential diagnosis is limited. Cluster headache, atypical migraine, and chronic paroxysmal hemicrania may involve the face, but the frequency of the pain is of much longer duration then that which is seen with trigeminal neuralgia, and the location of the pain is usually in the first division of cranial nerve V, rather than in the second or third divisions. Associated symptoms (lacrimation, rhinorrhea, and ptosis) do not occur with trigeminal neuralgia. Temporomandibular joint dysfunction causes more of a constant pain, which is often increased by chewing and cannot be provoked by tactile stimulation. Dental pain usually does not cause such intense paroxysmal pain. Glossopharyngeal neuralgia (cranial nerve IX) may at times be difficult to distinguish from trigeminal neuralgia. Coughing and swallowing, common triggers of glossopharyngeal neuralgia, rarely precipitate trigeminal neuralgia. The tonsillar area, a common site of pain in glossopharyngeal neuralgia, is rarely involved in trigeminal neuralgia.

MEDICAL TREATMENT

Analgesics or narcotics do not control the severe pain of trigeminal neuralgia; if they are used, the potential for addiction is high. Carbamazepine (Tegretol), an anticonvulsant related structurally to tricyclic antidepressant drugs, is the drug of choice for trigeminal neuralgia; it controls the pain in 80 % of patients. The age of the patient, duration of the trigeminal neuralgia, or the division of the nerve involved do not appear to influence the initial effects of carbamazepine. Pain is usually controlled within 12 to 48 hours. Carbamazepine is started at a dosage of 200 mg per day (100 mg bid), and the dose is increased slowly (in 100 mg increments) until relief is obtained—usually with a maximum daily dosage of 600 to 1200 mg—or toxic side effects are observed. Therapeutic blood levels are frequently required to control the pain. The principal side effects that limit the therapy are gastrointestinal upset, lightheadedness, ataxia, and drowsiness. Rare complications from carbamazepine include leukopenia, thrombocytopenia, and liver function abnormalities, necessitating withdrawal of the medication in 5% to 19% of patients. Initially, frequent monitoring (weekly or biweekly for the first six weeks of therapy) of the white blood count, platelet count, and liver function should be performed. Some reports suggest that phenytoin provides a degree of relief in some patients, perhaps as many as 20%. If carbamazepine does not control the pain, neither will phenytoin. Occasionally phenytoin is added to carbamazepine, but this rarely produces any additional benefit and often causes increased side effects of the medications.

Baclofen (Lioresal), an analog of the inhibitory neurotransmitter gamma aminobutyric acid (GABA), has been shown to prevent the painful paroxysms of trigeminal neuralgia. Although it is not as effective as carbamazepine, it does have synergistic action with carbamazepine and phenytoin. In patients who are no longer controlled by carbamazepine, the addition of baclofen often leads to the control of the paroxysms of trigeminal neuralgia. Baclofen may also be used as a first-line drug. The initial dose is 5 to 10 mg tid, with a gradual increase to 20 mg qid as necessary. Side effects include nausea, vomiting, and drowsiness. Baclofen should not be discontinued suddenly after long-term administration because hallucinations, seizures, or both can follow abrupt dosage reduction or discontinuation after more than two months of therapy. Baclofen is excreted primarily through the kidneys, so it should be given with caution in reduced doses to patients with impaired renal function.

SURGICAL TREATMENT

Despite the drugs that are available to treat trigeminal neuralgia, 25% to 50% of patients fail to respond to drug therapy and need some form of neurosurgical treatment. Various surgical procedures have been used in the past; the two most common are microvascular decompression of the trigeminal nerve root and percutaneous high frequency gangliolysis of the gasserian ganglion. The advantages of gangliolysis are that an intracranial approach to the trigeminal nerve is unnecessary and that 90% of patients obtain relief. Glycerol injections of the gasserian ganglion are also effective.

BRAIN TUMOR

Almost two-thirds of patients harboring a brain tumor complain of headache, with approximately 50% stating that their primary complaint is headache. A brain tumor headache is frequently a nonthrobbing, steady pain that is intermittent and frequently increased by activity and is often associated with nausea and/or vomiting. The patient with a brain tumor classically has a headache that awakens him or her from sleep. Although other conditions can lead to nocturnal headache (glaucoma, cluster), the presence of a headache that awakens the patient from sleep is a clue to the possible presence of a space-occupying lesion.

There are two distinctive headache patterns of brain tumor. *Paroxysmal headache* usually begins abruptly in a patient without a history of headache. The pain reaches its maximum intensity within a few seconds. It may persist for as long as a few hours, often disappearing as quickly as it began. The pain may be localized to bifrontal areas, but it is often generalized. Nausea, vomiting, transient visual loss, syncope, or "drop attacks" may also occur. Rapid head motion may precipitate a paroxysm, but changing the position of the head (down or supine) can dramatically relieve the head pain. This type of headache is usually caused by a midline mass that obstructs the ventricular system, causing episodic or continuous obstruction of CSF outflow and resulting in intermittent or constant increased intracranial pressure.

Exertional headache also may be associated with a brain tumor. It is characterized by transient pain induced by exertion, coughing, straining, sneezing, bending, or lifting. The headache is paroxysmal, lasting a few seconds to minutes. About 10% of patients with this type of pain have an intracranial lesion, usually in the posterior fossa. Arnold–Chiari malformation or basilar impression are the most common abnormalities, but any lesion in the posterior fossa can cause this type of pain. In common benign exertional headache, 30% of patients are symptom-free within five years, and the remaining 70% become symptom-free within ten years. In cases in which there is no structural lesion, indomethacin, 25 to 100 mg, often relieves the head pain.

Because supratentorial pain-sensitive structures are innervated by the trigeminal nerve, stimulation of these structures produces anterior head pain. Infratentorial pain structures are innervated by cranial nerves IX and X and the upper three cervical nerves. Stimulation of these structures results in pain localized to the posterior head areas. Thus, posterior fossa tumors usually result in occipital headache, whereas supratentorial tumors frequently produce anterior head pain. If obstructive hydrocephalus results, a bifrontal or generalized headache can occur. Headache is more likely to be the first symptom of a tumor located below the tentorium than one above it.

Brain tumors are discussed further in Chapter 21.

GIANT CELL ARTERITIS

Giant cell arteritis (temporal arteritis) is a systemic disease of the elderly in which headache can be a predominant symptom. It is not rare; incidence is 17 per 100,000. Women account for about 65% of the reported cases, and the average age of onset is 65 years. Onset before the age of 50 is extremely uncommon. The onset may be insidious or abrupt. Infrequently, the elderly patient notes a rapid development of severe proximal myalgia or headache with swollen temporal arteries. More often, the disease begins insidiously with fever, malaise, or weight loss. A low-grade fever may be present, and occasionally the patient presents as a case of fever of unknown origin. The most common initial symptoms are headache and polymyalgia rheumatica, but jaw claudication, weight loss, blindness, anemia, and limb claudication are other frequent presenting symptoms.

Headache is present in as many as 90% of patients with giant cell arteritis. The pain is usually sharp and boring, rarely throbbing, and it may be associated with occasional lancinating pains (ice pick-like). Most patients recognize that the pain is superficial, not deep. The head pain can be unilateral or bilateral and is commonly located temporally, but it may involve any area of the cranium. If headache is not localized in the temporal area, therefore, the diagnosis of giant cell arteritis should not be dismissed in the elderly patient with headache. Scalp tenderness may be present; brushing the hair may cause increased pain because of skin sensitivity. The headache is frequently worse at night and is often aggravated by exposure to cold. The patient may also complain of the feeling that his face is swollen, often on the side where the arteritic process is most active. The temporal artery on the involved side may be tender, nodular, and swollen, and pulsations may be diminished. Jaw claudication occurs in approximately two-thirds of patients with giant cell arteritis. It is associated with involvement of the facial artery by the arteritic process. It should be differentiated from pain in the temporomandibular joint that develops with simple opening or closing of the mandible.

Polymyalgia rheumatica, often associated with giant cell arteritis, is defined as aching and stiffness of the neck, shoulder, or hip girdle. It is associated with an elevated sedimentation rate. Polymyalgia rheumatica usually evolves insidiously, but in 40% of patients the onset is acute and resembles viremia. The symptoms characteristically disturb sleep, and pain and stiffness are worse in the morning. Localized muscle tenderness is not as marked as the pain elicited by movement.

Polyarticular involvement is not unusual; the knees and sternoclavicular joints may be swollen, and 25% of patients report swelling of the hands. Muscle enzyme levels, electromyographic examination, and muscle biopsy are normal.

Visual loss is the most common and most feared ocular symptom of giant cell arteritis. It is usually monocular initially and has an abrupt onset in 50% of patients. Transient visual blurring is common. Visual loss that is partial or incomplete is usually permanent, but approximately 10% of patients with visual symptoms describe recurrent amaurosis. About half of the patients with amaurosis caused by giant cell arteritis progress to permanent visual loss if untreated. When visual loss occurs unilaterally, the second eye is frequently affected in one to 21 days. Blindness rarely develops after a patient has been affected more than one year. The funduscopic picture of acute ischemic optic neuropathy is seen in most patients with blindness resulting from giant cell arteritis. It is characterized by pallor and swelling of the optic disc with associated hemorrhages and cotton-wool spots. Central retinal artery occlusion is observed in most of the remaining patients with visual loss; examination reveals retinal edema, a foveal cherry-red spot, and arteriolar "boxcars." Large-artery involvement is clinically detectable in approximately 10% of patients. Bruits have been reported over the carotid, subclavian, axillary, and temporal arteries when auscultation is performed carefully. Claudication of the upper and lower extremities may result. Involvement of the internal carotid artery and its branches is uncommon, so true cerebral ischemic symptoms in the carotid artery distribution are rare. Ischemic symptoms or infarction are more common in the vertebrobasilar system. Other uncommon manifestations of giant cell arteritis include glossitis, gangrene of the tongue, and scalp necrosis. Altered senses of taste and smell occur in as many as 50% of patients.

LABORATORY EVALUATION

The erythrocyte sedimentation rate (ESR) is the most helpful test for evaluating giant cell arteritis and is elevated in most cases. There are, however, well-documented cases of giant cell arteritis in which the ESR was normal even when corrected for the age of the patient. As age increases, so does the ESR (in general, the ESR for men should equal the age in years divided by 2; for women, it should equal the age in years plus 10, divided by 2), so that a normal, age-corrected ESR should not exclude the diagnosis of giant cell arteritis. A mild normochromic or hypochromic anemia is present in most patients (hemoglobin, 10 to 12 g/dL). The leukocyte count is often normal, but may be elevated in as many as 40% of patients. The platelet count may be markedly elevated, particularly in patients with visual or neurological symptoms. Liver function tests (SGOT, alkaline phosphatase) are elevated in many patients.

Biopsy of the temporal artery is the definitive test for the diagnosis of giant cell arteritis. A temporal artery biopsy should be obtained from all patients suspected of having giant cell arteritis. The arteritis can occur in a patchy distribution, often skipping segments of the involved artery. Thus a clinically involved portion of the artery should be biopsied, and a 5- to 6-cm segment should be obtained and examined at multiple levels. If the biopsied artery is normal, biopsy of the contralateral artery must be considered because giant cell arteritis is unilateral in only 5% of patients. Temporal artery angiography can be used either to establish the diagnosis or to identify abnormal segments of the vessel that should be biopsied, but it is by no means conclusive and has no advantage over temporal artery biopsy alone. Characteristic histologic findings of giant cell arteritis are a mononuclear inflammatory infiltrate throughout the vessel wall, disruption of the internal elastic lamina, and giant cells in the region of the internal elastic lamina.

MANAGEMENT

Giant cell arteritis is a self-limited disease that usually persists for one to two years. The mainstay of treatment is corticosteroids, instituted when the diagnosis is made. In patients in whom the clinical impression of giant cell arteritis is strong, steroids should be started *immediately*, usually prednisone, 60 to 80 mg per day. Treatment should not be delayed to allow for temporal artery biopsy. It takes at least three weeks of treatment with steroids to alter the pathological changes in the temporal artery; therefore, treatment must be started immediately. Biopsy can be scheduled for later. Small doses of steroids (10 to 20 mg per day) may improve symptoms for a few days, but larger doses are needed initially to prevent visual loss. There is no evidence that steroid therapy shortens the duration of giant cell arteritis, but it does prevent the complications, such as blindness, aortic rupture, and stroke.

The initial dose of prednisone (60 to 80 mg) should be continued daily for the first month (alternate-day therapy is not effective). Following that time, if the patient has improved and the ESR has returned to normal, the steroid dose can be tapered gradually. Most patients require lower doses of corticosteroids for several months. In one study, over half of the patients required treatment for less than a year. Steroids can be discontinued in most patients within a few years. As steroids are tapered, the ESR may become slightly elevated, but a relapse is unlikely if the patient remains asymptomatic.

Symptomatic relapses usually occur shortly after the steroid dose is reduced or stopped. After a patient has remained asymptomatic for one month or longer without steroids, further relapses are infrequent. Patients must be observed for complications of high-dose steroid therapy, including gastrointestinal bleeding, hyperglycemia, osteoporosis, cataracts, vertebral body collapse, aseptic necrosis of bone, and steroid myopathy.

CHILDHOOD HEADACHE

The principles of diagnosis and management of childhood headache are essentially the same as they are in the adult. As many as 25% of children will have experienced significant headache by the time they reach the age of 15. In one study, it was noted that by the age of fifteen 15.7% of children had experienced frequent nonmigraine headache; 5.3%, migraine, and 54%, infrequent nonmigraine headache. Four types of childhood headache have been classified on the basis of the temporal pattern of the head pain: (1) acute, (2) acute and recurrent, (3) chronic and progressive, and (4) chronic, nonprogressive.

A careful history should be obtained from the child and parents. The history should include information about pregnancy, labor, and delivery, as well as the child's developmental milestones and academic functions. The interaction of the child with the parents is an important observation to make; it may give clues to family discord. In certain cases, it is best to obtain the history from the child without the parents being present.

A severe headache without a prior history of headache, headache that awakens the child at night, localized head pain, changes in chronic headache pattern, and headache associated with specific neurological symptoms and signs all suggest an organic disorder.

A general physical examination should follow, with special attention paid to the height, weight, and blood pressure.The skin should be searched for cutaneous abnormalities, such as café-au-lait spots, hemangiomas, and adenoma sebaceum. A standard neurological examination should be performed. Head circumference should be measured and compared with normal values. The cranium should be auscultated because a bruit may indicate increased intracranial pressure or an underlying arteriovenous malformation. A visual field examination can be done easily in the cooperative child; a careful funduscopic examination must be performed to search for evidence of increased intracranial pressure.

The diagnostic tests to use depend on the differential diagnosis and the index of suspicion for an underlying intracranial lesion. Skull x-rays are of no real benefit for localizing abnormalities of the central nervous system. The EEG is of limited value because it is frequently abnormal in a nonspecific and unhelpful fashion. Epileptiform abnormalities occur with an increased incidence in children with migraine, but these changes are not specific. Computed tomography is the best method for evaluating the brain. It is safe, accurate, and usually well tolerated. If focal symptoms or signs are evident, it is mandatory that CT be performed to exclude an intracranial mass lesion. Lumbar puncture may be necessary to evaluate increased intracranial pressure (pseudotumor cerebri syndrome) or for intracranial infection (encephalitis, meningitis), but CT must be performed first, especially if there are focal signs. Angiography is necessary in selected cases (eg, evaluating the child for an intracranial aneurysm or arteriovenous malformation or for determining the vascular supply of a tumor).

Acute headache in a previously healthy child can have many causes, including systemic infection, CNS infection, toxic–metabolic disturbances, hypertension, and increased intracranial pressure. Associated symptoms and signs may yield a diagnosis, but focal signs or an altered level of consciousness must be evaluated rapidly. Acute localized headache may be the result of sinus infection, which is often associated with local tenderness of the sinuses and x-ray evidence of clouding of the sinuses. Refractive problems of the eyes are a rare cause of headache in children.

Acute recurrent headache is most commonly caused by migraine. In early childhood, boys are affected more frequently than girls, and there is a family history of migraine in more than 50% of cases. Classic migraine, usually associated with visual symptoms prior to the headache, occurs in 40% of children with migraine. Amnesia, confusion, and psychosis may also occur. Ophthalmoplegic migraine is uncommon overall, but occurs more frequently in childhood. Usually there is oculomotor nerve palsy at the time of the migraine that can persist for days or weeks.

Hemiplegic migraine occurs in patients with a family history of classic or complicated migraine, or in those with a family history of hemiplegic migraine. In children without a family history of hemiplegic migraine, episodes are briefer, not as severe, and tend not to recur frequently. In a child with a family history of hemiplegic migraine, attacks are usually recurrent, longer lasting, and quite severe. The face and arm tend to be involved more than the leg, and when the dominant hemisphere is affected, there is aphasia. Some patients with familial hemiplegic migraine have episodes of stupor, psychosis, or confusion during the attack; all the symptoms may last two or three days. When the attack is over, the neurological signs resolve completely, although some patients have residual neurological damage. Recurrent attacks may occur on either the same or the opposite side.

Basilar migraine, which is more common in childhood than in adulthood, is characterized by recurrent attacks of brain stem and cerebellar dysfunction. Symptoms can include an abrupt loss of consciousness, visual loss (at times cortical blindness), vertigo, tinnitus, and alternating hemiplegia and paresthesias, followed by severe occipital head pain (that is often throbbing), nausea, and vomiting.

Childhood migraine can present as an acute confusional state with an altered sensorium and agitation, often resembling an acute toxic psychosis. The duration of an attack is often a few hours, but it can be as long as 24 hours. Such confusional spells tend to occur over a relatively brief period of time, usually days to months, and they tend to evolve into typical migraine. Common migraine does not differ from that which affects the adult, although in the child episodes tend to be of briefer duration and nausea and vomiting may be more prominent than the headache. Unexplained paroxysmal and recurrent abdominal pain and cyclical vomiting may occur in childhood as manifestations of migraine. Usually there is a family history of migraine, and as the child gets older the spells of vomiting are replaced by, or associated with, more typical migraine symptoms.

TREATMENT

Analgesics and antiemetics are useful for treating the child with migraine. Unfortunately, non-narcotic analgesics do not provide adequate pain relief for most patients. Bed rest may be enough to treat the episode, but if headaches are recurrent, antimigraine medication is indicated. Ergotamine is used most often to treat the acute migraine attack. It must be used early, at the start of the headache or when vasoconstrictive symptoms (usually visual) are first noted. Sublingual ergotamine is better than the oral form, because it has a quicker onset of action and causes less gastric upset. The sublingual dose is 2 mg, and the second tablet may be taken 30 minutes after the first. No more than six tablets should be used weekly; the same complications discussed regarding ergotamine in the adult apply to the child.

Isometheptene mucate (Midrin) is a sympathomimetic agent that is more effective for the treatment of migraine than placebo. It causes less nausea and vomiting than ergotamine, but is no more effective for treating the headache. The usual dose is two tablets at the start of the attack, which may be repeated in 45 minutes.

If attacks occur more than once or twice a month, or if they are quite severe, a prophylactic agent should be considered. Propranolol, a beta-adrenergic blocking agent, is the only drug that demonstrates a consistent effect greater than that of placebo. The dosage for children is 2 mg per kg in three divided doses. It should be started at half the therapeutic dose and increased slowly. Even at low doses, adverse reactions can occur, including exacerbation of asthma, hypotension, and profound bradycardia. The drug is contraindicated in individuals with asthma, insulin-dependent diabetes, and heart failure.

Cyproheptadine (Periactin) a serotonin antagonist, has been reported to be effective for migraine prophylaxis. The usual dosage is 1 to 2 mg bid to tid. Sedation and weight gain are common side effects.

Methysergide maleate (Sansert), another serotonin antagonist, is effective for controlling migraine at a dosage of 2 mg tid after meals. Retroperitoneal or other fibrotic syndromes can occur with chronic use (longer than four to six months), and fear of these syndromes prevent methysergide from being utilized often.

Phenobarbital, 30 mg bid to tid, is occasionally effective in the child with chronic recurring migraine, especially if there are associated epileptiform abnormalities on an EEG. Amitriptyline may be effective in the selected older child. There are no convincing reports of the superiority of calcium-channel blockers in the treatment of migraine in the child, as there are in the adult.

Chronic progressive headache is uncommon in childhood, but when present it is usually caused by a brain tumor, increased intracranial pressure (hydrocephalus, pseudotumor cerebri), or subdural hematoma. Nonspecific signs of increased intracranial pressure include nausea and vomiting, personality changes, weakness, ataxia, seizures, and visual changes. The physical examination may be unrevealing, but in the presence of increased intracranial pressure papilledema should be present, and sixth cranial nerve palsies may be evident.

Headache caused by brain tumor is often progressive, but the patient may have pain-free intervals. Head pain is usually caused by the mass lesion or by obstruction of cerebrospinal fluid outflow. At least 70% of children with brain tumors have headache as a presenting symptom; in two-thirds it awakens them from sleep.

Subdural hematoma results from trauma; and it may be seen as part of the battered child syndrome. Symptoms and signs of increased intracranial pressure are often present, as are focal signs or seizures. A CT scan is diagnostic in most chronic progressive headache syndromes of children. Neurosurgical treatment of the offending lesion, whether it is a tumor, subdural hematoma, or hydrocephalus, often cures the headache.

Chronic nonprogressive headache is usually a result of muscle contraction-tension or depression, or it is post-traumatic. Functional headache in children tends to follow a clinical pattern similar to that in adults, and frequently there is a family history of a similar type of headache. It can be present for months to years. Secondary gain in children is quite common, occurring frequently in the form of frequent school absences. Headache may also be a sign of depression in the child; it is often associated with poor school performance, school phobia, withdrawal, or mood changes.

If the diagnosis of functional headache is suspected from the interview, it should be discussed with the parents and the child. Treatment modalities include individual counseling of the child, family counseling, and sometimes psychoanalysis. Drug treatment is often not helpful unless depression is a major factor. In such a case, amitriptyline, 25 to 75 mg at bedtime, is effective for the depression and the headache.

Bibliography

Appenzeller O, Raskin NH: *Headache.* Philadelphia, Saunders, 1980. (Overview of headache disorders, written for the generalist.)

Caniness VS Jr, O'Brien P: Headache. *N Engl J Med* 1980; 302:446-450. (Practical review of various headache disorders.)

Featherstone HJ: Clinical features of stroke in migraine: A Review. *Headache* 1986; 26:128-133. (Comprehensive review of stroke in migraine.)

Fenichel GM: Migraine in children. *Neurol Clin* 1985; 3:77-94. (Excellent overview of childhood migraine and its treatment; well referenced.)

Fisher CM: Late-life migraine accompaniments as a cause of unexplained transient ischemic attacks. *Can J Neurol Sci* 1980; 7:9-17. (Detailed case study of elderly patients with TIA likely caused by migraine.)

Fromm GH, Terrence CF, Chattha AS: Baclofen in the treatment of trigeminal neuralgia: Double-blind study and long-term follow-up. *Ann Neurol* 1984; 15:240-244. (Baclofen [Lioresal], an effective treatment for trigeminal neuralgia, is a useful adjunct in the patient who has not responded satisfactorily to carbamazepine.)

Huston KA, Hunder GG: Giant cell (cranial) arteritis: A clinical review. *Am Heart J* 1980; 100:99-107. (Comprehensive review of giant cell arteritis.)

Kaganov JA: The differential contribution of muscle contraction and migraine symptoms to problem headache in the general population. *Headache* 1981; 21:157-163. (Reviews the problem of muscle contraction headache and its relationship to migraine.)

Kunkel RS: Pharmacologic management of migraine—1985. *Cleve Clin Q* 1985; 52:95-101. (Current overview of pharmacologic treatment of migraine.)

Kunkel RS: Acephalic migraine. *Headache* 1986: 26:198-201. (Reviews "migraine equivalents" as they occur in all age groups.)

Lance JW: Headache. *Ann Neurol* 1981; 10:1-10. (Reviews current treatment and pathophysiology of various classes of headache.)

Leicht MJ: Non-traumatic headache in the emergency department. *Ann Emerg Med* 1980; 9:404-409. (Of 193 patients with headache evaluated by the author in 12 months, 54.5% had muscle contraction–tension or migraine headache.)

Packard RC (ed): Headache. *Neurol Clin* 1983; 1:359-569. (Monograph that comprehensively covers the diagnosis and management of major headache disorders.)

Piatt JH Jr, Wilkins RH: Treatment of tic doloreaux and hemifacial spasm by posterior fossa exploration: Therapeutic implications of various neurovascular relationships. *Neu-*

rosurgery 1984; 14:462-471. (Microvascular decompression is effective for the treatment of tic doloreaux.)

Porter M, Jankovic J: Benign coital cephalgia. Differential diagnosis and treatment. *Arch Neurol* 1981; 38:710-712. (Reviews a series of patients with benign sex headaches, a variant of migraine.)

Rothner AD: Diagnosis and treatment of headache syndromes in children. In, Moss AJ, Stiehm ER: *Pediatrics Update.* New York, Elsevier Biomedical, 1983, pp 55-77. (Good discussion of headache syndromes in childhood and their treatment.)

Solomon GD, Steel JG, Spaccavento LJ: Verapamil prophylaxis of migraine: A double blind, placebo-controlled study. *JAMA* 1983; 250:2500-2502. (Calcium channel blockers are effective in migraine prevention.)

Sweet WH: The treatment of trigeminal neuralgia. *N Engl J Med* 1986; 315:174-177. (Contemporary review of the treatment of trigeminal neuralgia; focuses on surgical therapies.)

Tyler GS, McNeely HE, Dick ML: Treatment of post-traumatic headache with amitriptyline. *Headache* 1980; 20:313-316. (Tricyclic antidepressant medications are effective in treatment of post-traumatic headache.)

Welch KMA, Ellis DJ, Keenan PJ: Successful migraine prophylaxis with naproxen sodium. *Neurology* 1985; 35:1304-1310. (Naproxen is effective and is the best nonsteroidal anti-inflammatory medication for migraine prophylaxis.)

Back and Neck Pain

LOW BACK PAIN

It has been estimated that 80% of persons will develop some type of back pain during their lifetime. By conservative estimate, each year 10% of Americans will suffer an episode of low back pain. Most patients recover from the episode of back pain within a month, but 4% have pain that persists for more than 6 months. More than 50% of those persons disabled for more than 6 months never return to work. It has been estimated that more than 10 million persons in the United States have functional limitations from low back pain, 3 million of whom have severe limitations, and more than 4 million are unable to work at all. When low back pain has persisted for more than two months, it is considered chronic.

A basic knowledge of the anatomy of the spine is necessary for the physician to diagnose and treat the patient with low back pain. The bony spine is divided into anterior and posterior parts. The anterior part consists of the vertebral bodies, which are articulated by the intervertebral discs and held together by the anterior and posterior longitudinal ligaments. In the lumbar area, the vertebrae are quite large because of their weight-bearing function. The posterior part of the vertebral bodies are less strong than the anterior sections and consist of the pedicles and laminae. The inferior portion of the pedicles from one vertebra, and the superior portion of the pedicle from below it, form the intervertebral foramen through which the spinal nerves pass. Within the foramen, the spinal nerves are vulnerable to compression by space-occupying lesions such as tumors, discs, or trauma. Any disruption of the normal anatomic configuration of the intervertebral foramen (spondylosis, stenosis) can cause nerve root entrapment.

The transverse and spinous processes project laterally and posteriorly and serve as the origins and insertions for the paravertebral muscles. The stability of the spine depends on the ligaments and attached muscles. The anterior longitudinal ligament runs anterior to the vertebral bodies and is attached to each of them. The posterior longitudinal ligament is weaker, and is located on the posterior surfaces of the vertebral bodies. The ligamentum flavum connects the lamina and extends laterally to the articular facets. Supraspinal ligaments join the spinous processes and the interspinal ligaments connect adjoining spinous processes.

The intervertebral disc consists of two compartments: the internal semifluid mass (nucleus pulposus) and its fibrous container, the annulus fibrosus. The vertebral and paravertebral structures, including the intraspinal ligaments, periosteum, outer annulus, and capsule of the articular facets, are innervated by the meningeal branches of the spinal nerves.

The alignment of the spinal nerve roots to the vertebra is of major clinical importance. There are eight cervical nerve roots, but only seven cervical vertebrae. The first cervical nerve root exits between the occiput and atlas; the eighth cervical nerve root exits between the seventh cervical and first thoracic vertebrae. Thus, cervical disc herniation affects the nerve root that is passing above the lower vertebra. A C5-C6 disc compresses the C6 nerve root as it passes above the C6 vertebral body. Because of the upward migration of the spinal cord that occurs during development, the lumbar nerve roots slant downward at an acute angle. In the lumbar area, lumbar disc herniation affects the nerve root corresponding to the lower vertebra, even though the exiting nerve root corresponds to the upper vertebra. Thus, an L4-L5 disc affects the L5 root, and an L5-S1 disc herniation affects the S1 root.

SYMPTOMS AND SIGNS

Back pain can arise from the bones, joints, ligaments, muscles, or nerve roots, and it can be referred to the back from elsewhere. Root pain (radicular) is caused by traction, compression, or irritation of the nerve root. It is usually intense, sharp, or knife-like, and radiates from an area in the spine to an extremity. Valsalva's maneuver increases pain, as does coughing or sneezing. The pain can usually be localized and is usually confined to a specific dermatomal area (Table 9-1). Pain from L3 irritation is usually felt in the anterior thigh; from L4, in the posterolateral thigh and medial calf; and from L5, in the posterior thigh and calf and dorsum of the foot. Soreness of the skin, tenderness, and paresthesias may accompany radicular pain.

Ligamentous and muscle pain may vary from a dull ache to a sharp, shooting pain and is occasionally "burning." This kind of pain is often difficult to localize, and it may radiate to the low back and legs in a nondermatomal pattern. The pain may lessen when the patient walks, and increase when he sits, lies in bed, or stands in one position for a long time.

Referred back pain is usually caused by a lesion of retroperitoneal or posterior peritoneal structures. This kind of pain is usually dull and aching, bilateral, constant, and not well localized. The severity of the referred pain depends on its cause. Movement or spinal percussion does not increase this kind of pain. Pain may also be referred from the back to the viscera. This discomfort is often deeply located, although a superficial component may also be present. Upper lumbar spine disease is usually referred to the flank, lumbar region, anterior thigh, and groin. Pain from the lower part of the lumbar spine is usually referred to the lower buttocks and posterior thighs. Local pain is usually ill-defined, steady, deep, and of

TABLE 9-1 DIFFERENTIAL DIAGNOSIS OF LOW BACK PAIN: CLINICAL FEATURES

	AFFECTED AREA		
	JOINT	MUSCLE	DISC
Onset	Sudden, during movement, with lock or snap	Sudden, with lifting, with tearing feeling	Sudden, with stressful move
Effect of rest	Relief	Stiffening	Relief
Effect of activity	Aggravating	Aggravating	Aggravating
Location	SI joint	Over muscle	Over interspace
Mobility	Localized reduction	Less well localized	Localized loss
Percussion	Brief sharp pain	—	Brief pain with radiation
Physical signs	One joint One level Referred pain No neurologic signs	No joint/area Unilateral Pain in muscle No neurological signs	One junction Same level joint bilateral radicular pain Mixed neurological signs
General observations	Patient lies still No systemic signs/ fever	Variable position No systemic signs/fever	Patient lies still No fever/systemic signs
X-ray	Negative	Negative	Negative, except for CT/myelogram/ MRI

Adapted from Cailliet R: *Low Back Pain Syndrome*, ed 3. Philadelphia, F.A. Davis, 1981, p 151. Used with permission.

a boring or aching nature. It can be caused by any process that impinges on or irritates sensory nerve endings.

DIAGNOSIS

A complete medical examination should be performed in the patient who complains of low back pain. Rectal and pelvic examinations are necessary because pathology in these areas can give rise to back pain. A neurological examination should also be performed with careful attention paid to the lower extremities. Inspection of the back must be done with the patient unclothed. Observation of standing posture allows determination of normal dorsal kyphosis and lumbar lordosis, or if there is scoliosis, lumbar spasm, or accentuation of lumbar lordosis.

Movements of the hips and spine can be observed when the patient walks. Difficulty with heel walking may indicate L5 root weakness, whereas defective toe walking may indicate an S1 root disturbance. Movements of the spine should be examined, including flexion, extension, and lateral motions, to determine if these maneuvers produce pain or limitation of movement. The patient should perform flexion by bending forward and attempting to touch the floor with his fingertips. If asymmetrical muscle spasm is evident, the patient may list to one side. To test hyperextension, the patient should bend backwards as far as possible while maintaining the normal position of the pelvis.

The spine should be palpated and percussed, beginning in the areas without pain. Exquisite tenderness of a spinous process may indicate inflammation or vertebral fracture. Tenderness over the costovertebral angle may indicate genitourinary tract disease or injury to the transverse processes of L1 or L2. With the patient supine, the lengths of the legs should be measured from the anterior—superior iliac spine to the top of the medial malleolus. Discrepancies of leg length can produce radiculopathy on the opposite side as a result of truncal tilt. The circumference of the calves and thighs should be measured to detect subtle atrophy.

Straight-leg raising (SLR, Lasègue's sign) should be tested. The patient should be supine and flex the extremity at the hip with slow extension of the knee. The degree of ability to extend the knee is noted, and the patient is instructed to notify the examiner if and when pain develops. During SLR, the first 15 to 30 degrees of elevation cause no movement of the nerve roots at the foraminal level; at 30 degrees there is traction of the sciatic nerve with the greatest degree of movement at L5. Because the L5 root has the greatest downward movement, a disc lesion at this level will produce a strongly positive SLR. If hysteria or malingering is possible, SLR can be tested when the patient is sitting; this should be performed prior to SLR when the patient is supine. As the patient extends the leg, the examiner looks for limitation of movement. If there is true nerve root entrapment, the patient will lean back and away from the side of involvement.

Occasionally, the performance of SLR on the unaffected leg will evoke pain on the involved side. This finding is known as Fajerstagn's crossed sciatic sign and indicates a ruptured disc. Patrick's test will show whether or not local hip pathology is the cause of low back pain. The test is also known as the "fabere" sign, an acronym that refers to the motions of the hip as the test is performed: **f,** flexion; **ab,** abduction; **er,** external rotation; **e,** extension. With the patient supine, the heel of the lower extremity being tested is placed on the opposite knee; the knee on the side being tested is pressed laterally and downward by the examiner as far as it will go. The procedure is positive if motion is restricted or if pain accompanies limitation of motion. With the patient in the prone position, reverse straight leg raising produces pain in the upper thigh if an L3 root lesion is present. In L1-L3 root lesions, the nerve roots do not migrate with conventional SLR, so Lasègue's sign is negative.

Motor function should be tested. The hip flexors are innervated by L2 and L3; the quadriceps (which maintains knee extension) by L4; the ankle dorsiflexors, by L4 and L5; the great toe extensor, by L5; and the plantar flexors of the foot, by S1. Deep tendon reflexes should be tested and plantar responses determined. Sensory examination is performed using pinpricks to determine dermatomal or other sensory abnormalities. Finally, an examination of the abdomen should be performed, including auscultation of the aortic area. Femoral, posterior tibial, and dorsal pedal pulses should be palpated because vascular disease of the lower extremities can cause low back and extremity pain.

Acute Low Back Pain

Acute low back pain has many causes. Most are benign, but sinister disturbances occasionally present in this fashion (Chapter 40). Low back pain of less than 2 months' duration is usually considered to be acute. Most cases of acute low back pain are a result of intervertebral disc disease or ligamentous/muscle injury.

Ruptured Intervertebral Disc

Herniation or rupture of an intervertebral disc can be caused by a bulging or protrusion of the nucleus pulposus into the annulus, which in turn protrudes into the spinal canal or intervertebral foramen. Because the anterior longitudinal ligament is much stronger than its posterior counterpart, disc herniation usually occurs in a posterior or posterolateral direction. Although disc material usually protrudes as a solid mass, free fragments of disc material may break off or protrude through the posterior longitudinal ligament and lie free in the spinal canal. The annulus degenerates with age as the nucleus pulposus shrinks. Many factors can lead to rupture of an intervertebral disc. Most cases are the result of trauma, either an acute flexion injury or related to chronic bending and lifting. Most lumbar disc herniations occur between the fourth and sixth decades of life; 80% occur in men.

SYMPTOMS AND SIGNS

Severe pain usually develops within a few hours of the injury. The initial complaint is often of a constant, dull, aching pain that is aggravated by activity. Pain is usually localized deep to the buttocks and lateral to and below the sacroiliac joint. Coughing, straining, sneezing, and flexion movement increase the pain. It is often relieved by lying on the unaffected side with the affected leg flexed. Pain may be associated with muscle spasm and flattening of the lumbar area. Often, the pain radiates into the lower extremity in a sciatic nerve distribution (buttocks and posterolateral aspect of the thigh and leg). As "sciatica" develops, the back pain may lessen as the leg pain increases. Extremity pain is increased by straining and activity; patients often have subjective paresthesias and numbness.

The pattern of radiation (radiculopathy) depends on the area of disc herniation (Table 9-2). Most (80% to 95%) of lumbar disc herniations occur at the L4-L5 or L5-S1 interspace, affecting the L5 and S1 nerve roots, respectively. If a fragment of disc material is free, it usually affects the root emerging above (rather than below) the herniated disc. Midline disc herniation is uncommon, but compression of the cauda equina may occur in the presence of a narrowed spinal canal, giving rise to paraparesis and sphincter disturbances. In some cases of lumbar disc herniation, back pain remains predominant, with little or no leg pain. In many cases, the back pain gradually subsides while leg pain and neurological deficits persist. Rarely, there is only leg pain.

DIAGNOSIS

Examination reveals reduced forward mobility, and in the acute stage almost all movements are restricted. The lumbar spine deviates away from the affected side because disc herniation is lateral to the nerve root. Range of motion is reduced

TABLE 9-2 CLINICAL FEATURES OF LUMBAR RADICULOPATHY

LEVEL	ROOT	PAIN	SENSORY LOSS	MOTOR LOSS	REFLEX LOSS
L3–L4	L4	Lower back, posterolateral thigh	Anteromedial thigh	Quadriceps	Patellar
L4–L5	L5	Over S1 joint and hip, lateral thigh and leg	Outer side of calf and great toe	Dorsiflexors of great toe and ankle	None
L5–S1	S1	Back of thigh outer calf to foot and lateral toes	Outer calf and foot and lesser toes	Plantar flexion (gastrocnemius)	Achilles

and the lumbar lordosis is lost. There is spasm of the paravertebral muscles. Tenderness may be present over the involved spinal area. Straight leg raising is often positive, but reverse SLR is positive if a lesion is located at L3 or L4. Motor signs are present in at least 90% of patients with lumbar radiculopathies; sensory findings are present in 80%.

An L5 root lesion produces pain in the groin, hip, posterolateral thigh, lateral calf (as far as the lateral malleolus), dorsal surfaces of the foot, and first to third toes. Tenderness is present in the lateral gluteal region and near the proximal femur. Extension of the big toe and ankle is weakened, and the Achilles reflex may be reduced.

An S1 root disturbance produces midgluteal pain, which is also felt in the posterior thigh and calf to the heel, and pain in the lateral surfaces of the foot and the fourth and fifth toes. Sensory changes also occur in these areas. Plantar flexion is weakened and the Achilles reflex is reduced or absent in most cases.

An L4 root lesion produces pain in the anterior thigh and the medial calf, with sensory abnormalities in a corresponding distribution. Weakness of hip flexion and knee extension and a decreased patellar reflex are also common clinical findings.

LABORATORY TESTS

X-ray examination of the lumbosacral spine (with oblique views) is necessary. A newly ruptured disc is usually not associated with disc-space narrowing, but an x-ray helps to exclude neoplasm, congenital diseases, or rheumatoid disease. A complete blood count, blood chemistry profile, and tests for calcium and phosphorus levels should be performed. In the selected patient, a test for the acid phosphatase level and serum protein electrophoresis is necessary. A CT scan of the L3-S1 spine will usually demonstrate disc herniation and will help exclude other lesions as the cause of the lumbar radiculopathy. The scan is best at determining the presence of a lesion at the L5-S1 interspace, where a myelogram can give a false-negative result.

If symptoms have been present for at least 14 to 21 days, then electromyography (EMG) and reflex studies can be performed, to help localize the site of the lesion based on the pattern of denervation. H-reflex abnormalities suggest an S1 root lesion and will become abnormal (delayed) sooner than the denervation potentials will develop. Myelography with water-soluble dye (metrizamide) is necessary if CT is not available, if results are equivocal, or if multiple lesions are suspected. The combination of high resolution CT and EMG will localize the lesion in over 95% of cases. MRI provides superb localization of spinal problems and has the advantage of being noninvasive. It will likely replace myelography in the future.

MANAGEMENT

Approximately 90% of first attacks subside with conservative therapy. Absolute bed rest is mandatory to remove weight-bearing from the disc. The hips and knees should be flexed to decrease the lordosis; 10 to 15 pounds of traction can be applied with a pelvic brace, although it is of questionable value. Heat can be applied to the low back. Analgesic (ibuprofen) and muscle relaxant (diazepam) medications are often indicated to reduce the degree of pain and muscle spasm. A corticosteroid (prednisone, 60 to 80 mg daily, with tapering over 10 to 14 days) has been used in the patient with acute lumbar radiculopathy to reduce pain and neurological deficit, in part by reducing edema of the inflamed–compressed nerve root. Within 10 to 14 days, ambulation can be started; a lumbar corset or brace will add stability to the spine. Lifting and bending should be forbidden. Exercises should be carried out daily to strengthen the spine extensors, glutei, and abdominal muscles.

Conservative therapy should not be abandoned until after a trial of strict bed rest for three to four weeks. Failure to respond to therapy is an indication for surgical intervention.. The best surgical results occur in the patient with objective neurological deficits and positive confirmatory tests (CT, EMG and/or myelography). Chemonucleolysis of the extruded disc material with chymopapain can be performed as an alternative to surgery. A variety of side effects may result from chymopapain, most notably an anaphylactoid reaction (a kit is available for screening for this sensitivity). Long-term results may not be as good as those obtained with surgery.

Lumbosacral Strain

The articulations of the spine, which are covered with cartilage and surrounded by ligaments, are subject to stretching and tearing. Degenerative changes, loss of the disc space, excessive weight, and chronic occupational strain all contribute to stress on these areas.

Repeated episodes of acute low back pain are caused by hyperextension injuries. Flexion movements decrease the pain, and hyperextension (eg, sleeping on the abdomen, sitting erect) tends to increase pain. When symptoms are acute, coughing, straining, or sneezing may increase symptoms. Although the pain is usually felt in the lower back and buttocks area, with time signs of nerve root irritation appear.

The patient with lumbosacral strain stands with a flexed posture. Tenderness is present at the lumbosacral junction, and in the acute stages, the paravertebral muscles may be in spasm. SLR may produce back pain, but usually there is no radiation into the legs. Strength may be reduced, but it is rarely focal, and probably is secondary to the pain. Likewise, deep tendon reflexes may be minimally and nonfocally reduced.

X-rays of the back with oblique views often demonstrate mild subluxation of the facet joints, with narrowing of the intervertebral foramina. In the acute stages, bed rest in a flexed position is mandatory, and hyperextension should be avoided. Pelvic or leg traction is often carried out, and heat, analgesics, and sedatives are often necessary to make the patient comfortable. An exercise program is necessary to strengthen the back muscles, and a lumbosacral corset may add stability to the lower lumbar spine. If pain is persistent and not responsive to conservative measures, spinal fusion will be necessary.

Chronic Low Back Pain

With advancing age, osteoporosis, osteoarthritis, and spondylosis are common causes of low back pain. Spondylosis begins with collapse of the dehydrated nucleus pulposus, with bulging and calcification of the annulus. Hypertrophic changes develop subsequently at the margins of the vertebral bodies, giving rise to osteophytic spurs. These bony spurs may encroach into the neural foramina, resulting in radiculopathy or narrowing of the spinal canal and causing cauda equina or spinal cord compression.

Lumbar Spinal Stenosis

Stenosis of the lumbar spine may result in symptoms of low back pain that radiates into the lower extremities. It usually occurs after the age of 50 and is the result of multiple levels of spondylotic narrowing that are sometimes superimposed upon congenital narrowing of the spinal column. This congenital narrowing of the spinal column may predispose the patient to symptomatic narrowing of the spinal canal in later years when hypertrophic changes develop. Severe lumbar spinal stenosis in the absence of marked degenerative disc or joint disease is uncommon. With extension of the spine (such as produced when walking or standing) the spinal canal narrows because of posterior bulging of the intervertebral discs, producing symptoms of pseudoclaudication. When the patient assumes a flexed posture, the canal widens and symptoms disappear. This condition is also known as intermittent claudication of the cauda equina.

SYMPTOMS AND SIGNS

The average patient with lumbar spinal stenosis is over 60 years of age and has had symptoms for an average of 24 months. Typical symptoms are those of pseudoclaudication: pain that develops in the buttocks, thighs, or legs when standing or walking. Most patients have pain, two-thirds have variable lower extremity numbness, and one-third a combination of numbness and pain. Pain is brought on by either prolonged standing or exercise when erect. Symptoms are relieved by lying flat, sitting, or adopting a flexed posture at the waist. These symptoms contrast with those of true vascular claudication, in which stopping an activity (such as walking) while the patient is standing relieves the symptoms. In 75% of patients the pain is above and below the knees; in two-thirds it is bilateral; and in two-thirds it also occurs in the lower back.

There is usually a paucity of findings on examination. Surprisingly few patients have sensory findings. One-third of patients have objective weakness of the lower extremities, usually unilateral and in the L5-S1 root distribution. More than one-third have reflex abnormalities in the lower extremities, usually depression of the Achilles reflex. If there is coexistent cervical spinal cord compression, corticospinal tract abnormalities may be evident in the legs, including spasticity or Babinski's reflex. Two-thirds of patients have decreased lumbosacral mobility on examination; 10% have positive SLR.

EMG usually demonstrates bilateral lumbosacral radiculopathies, often with involvement of the paraspinal areas; unilateral root abnormalities are rarely seen. Lumbosacral spine x-rays reveal degenerative disc disease in most patients, and almost two-thirds have radiographically demonstrable osteoarthritic changes of the facet joints. One-third of patients have evidence of spondylolisthesis. Myelography is abnormal in all patients, usually demonstrating total or subtotal obstruction at one or more levels in the lumbar region. Thirty percent of patients have multiple levels of obstruction to the flow of the myelographic dye. Most stenoses are at the L4 and L3 levels. A CT scan may demonstrate narrowing of the spinal canal, but it is much less sensitive than the myelogram for detecting true spinal stenosis. Almost 10% of patients have spinal stenosis *only* at the L1 or L2 levels, areas that are not routinely examined by lumbar CT. MRI is a sensitive procedure for determining the presence of spinal stenosis.

MANAGEMENT

Multiple-level laminectomy is often the treatment of choice for this condition. Common findings at surgery include ligamentous and facet-joint hypertrophy, degenerated discs, and multiple osteophytes. More than three-quarters of patients have a favorable surgical outcome. In a series of laminectomies reported by the Mayo Clinic, patients could walk only an average of 200 yards preoperatively before pseudoclaudication developed. After surgery, they could walk a mean of 1.5 miles. Back pain persisted after surgery in many patients.

NECK PAIN

The cervical spine is the most mobile part of the spinal column. With aging, degenerative changes occur within the intervertebral disc that lead to spondylosis. The differential diagnosis of conditions that affect the cervical spine is quite similar to those that affect the lumbar spine.

Intervertebral Disc Rupture

Acute rupture of a cervical disc rarely occurs in patients over 50 years of age. Many cases of cervical disc protrusion are caused by trauma that at times is seemingly trivial. Most acute cervical disc ruptures occur laterally, although midline herniations may occur. Thus, nerve root compression is more common than spinal cord compression. The C7 root is affected in 70% of cases; the C6 root in 20%; and the C5 or C8 root in the remaining 10%. The most common symptoms are pain in the neck and arm in a radicular pattern. Extension and rotation of the neck can exaggerate the arm and neck discomfort.

Symptoms and Signs

The clinical picture depends on the location of the laterally placed disc (Table 9-3). Involvement of the sixth cervical root produces pain in the ridge of the trapezius and the shoulder tip that radiates into the upper part of the arm and the radial forearm and that often extends into the thumb. Paresthesias and sensory loss can occur in the same area as the pain, with weakness of the biceps and brachioradialis muscles and depression of the biceps and brachioradialis reflexes.

Compression of the C7 nerve root produces pain in the shoulder blade, medial axilla, and pectoral areas, which radiates into the posterolateral upper arm, dorsal forearm, index and middle fingers. The area over the medial scapula adjacent to the third and fourth thoracic spinous processes is usually tender. Sensory loss is most evident in the hand, particularly in the second and third digits. Weakness is usually in the triceps and occasionally in the hand grip. The triceps reflex is reduced or absent.

Compression of the eighth cervical nerve root produces pain along the medial side of the forearm, with sensory loss in the medial forearm and in an ulnar-nerve pattern in the hand. The intrinsic hand muscles are weak and the finger flexor response may be diminished or absent, but the triceps reflex is usually preserved.

Limitation of neck movement develops in virtually all patients. Spurling's maneuver is of value in determining the presence of a laterally placed cervical disc. Downward pressure is applied to the top of the patient's head, with the neck hyperextended and laterally flexed toward the limb into which the pain extends. Aggravation of pain is a positive result. Neck traction relieves pain caused by compression of a cervical root. To determine this, the examiner grasps both sides of the patient's head and exerts strong traction upward, without inducing motion in the spinal column other than that of longitudinal stretching.

Large, centrally placed cervical discs can cause spinal cord compression which may be insidious and relatively painless. The myelopathy that results may be mistaken for a degenerative condition such as amyotrophic lateral sclerosis. (See the following section on cervical spondylosis.)

TABLE 9-3 CLINICAL FEATURES OF CERVICAL RADICULOPATHY

Level	Root	Pain	Sensory Loss	Motor Loss	Reflex Loss
C4–C5	C5	Neck, shoulder, upper arm	Shoulder and outer arm	Deltoid and biceps	Biceps
C5–C6	C6	Neck, shoulder lateral arm, and radial aspect of forearm to thumb and forefinger	Thumb, forefinger, radial forearm	Biceps	Biceps, brachioradialis
C6–C7	C7	Neck, lateral arm, ring and index fingers	Radial forearm, forefinger, middle finger	Triceps, extensor carpi ulnaris	Triceps
C7–T1	C8	Ulnar forearm, hand	Ulnar half of ring finger and little finger	Wrist extensors, intrinsic hand muscles	Finger flexor

DIAGNOSIS

The general evaluation of the patient with a cervical radiculopathy is similar to that of the patient with lumbar pain or radiculopathy. Cervical spine x-rays with oblique views are obtained. EMG may help to localize the involved nerve root and to exclude other causes of arm pain, such as carpal tunnel syndrome, ulnar neuropathy, or thoracic outlet syndrome (Chapter 11). A CT scan is of less value with cervical nerve root lesions than with lumbar nerve root lesions. Myelography is indicated to assess the cervical nerve roots and spinal cord. Cervical myelography with metrizamide (water-soluble) has more toxic side-effects than does lumbar myelography. Metrizamide should not be used for cervical myelography unless it can be injected into the cervical area (ie, not by the lumbar route). As with radiculopathies, MRI provides excellent visualization of the cervical spinal cord and adjacent structures.

MANAGEMENT

Cervical radiculopathy caused by disc disease is managed in much the same way as uncomplicated lumbar radiculopathy. Traction of the lumbar area is of questionable benefit, but cervical traction often produces considerable benefit. If pain does not respond to conservative treatment, or if the patient has a significant motor deficit, myelographic examination and surgical removal of the laterally placed disc is indicated. The patient with a cervical myelopathy caused by a centrally placed disc should not be treated conservatively; prompt surgical decompression is usually indicated. Chemonucleolysis is not performed on cervical discs.

Cervical Spondylosis

Abnormal stresses are placed on the anterior and posterior longitudinal ligaments because of their ball-bearing-type movement between the vertebrae. The C5-C6 joint is the most mobile joint and is thus the one most affected by spondylosis. Osteophytes that develop may form bars across the back of the vertebral bodies in the line of the intervertebral discs and may indent the spinal cord. This produces the clinical syndrome of cervical spondylotic myelopathy. The damage is the result of direct pressure of the osteophyte on the cord, and is sometimes associated with congenital narrowing of the spinal canal. Recurrent spinal cord trauma can occur, caused by narrowing of the spinal canal during neck extension and stretching of the tensed cord against osteophytes projecting from the posterior aspect of the vertebral bodies. Nerve root damage in cervical spondylosis is caused by compression of the roots by adjacent osteophytes as the roots pass through the intervertebral foramina. Clinically, neurological complications of cervical spondylosis manifest as radiculopathy or myelopathy.

Spondylotic radiculopathy

This condition is common, affecting both men and women over the age of 30. It is characterized by neck pain that radiates into one or both arms or hands. The pain is usually severe and aching and may start suddenly. It is often localized to one side of the neck and causes loss of neck mobility. Neck pain originates from both nerve roots and skeletal structures and produces secondary muscle spasm. Paresthesias and numbness arise in the distribution of the affected nerve root. During the acute stage, the patient's neck is stiff and tilted, and active and passive motion is restricted. Weakness and wasting of the muscles supplied by the compressed nerve root(s) is evident, as is suppression of the deep-tendon reflex supplied by the nerve root. The pain lasts four to six weeks and may recur. Abnormalities seen during examination usually persist between the bouts of pain.

Spondylotic myelopathy

This condition usually occurs in men over the age of 50. The patient's history extends over a few years, and his neurological deterioration may be intermittent or progressive. Trauma can cause sudden hyperextension of the spondylotic neck. Symptoms invariably involve the hands or legs; the hands may be numb or paresthetic, and these sensory complaints may extend to the elbows. Pain is uncommon, except in cases of associated radiculopathy. The patient's legs may feel weak and stiff, which is often the result of spasticity. He may have difficulty with fine movements of the hands, and his neck has a limited range of motion. Spasticity may be present in both arms, with wasting of hand or forearm muscles.

The weakness of spondylotic myelopathy is a mixed, upper-motor and lower-motor neuron type, with the lower-motor lesion corresponding to the area of maximum spinal cord compression. The legs are often spastic, with hyperreflexia and Babinski's responses, but isolated fasciculations have been reported. All sensory modalities in the hands are impaired, usually extending to the wrist or elbow. Proprioception and vibration sensation are often more reduced than pain and temperature sensation. Sensory signs in the legs also involve dorsal column (proprioception) functions predominantly. Sometimes radiculopathy and myelopathy combine and produce damage more on one side of the spinal cord than on the other, producing Brown–Séquard syndrome.

Both spondylotic radiculopathy and myelopathy must be differentiated from other conditions that affect the arms, including carpal tunnel syndrome, ulnar neuropathy, thoracic outlet syndrome, and brachial plexopathy. A lateral cervical disc protrusion usually cannot be differentiated clinically from spondylotic radiculopathy; spinal cord tumors can mimic spondylotic radiculopathy and myelopathy. Rheumatoid arthritis and ossification of the posterior longitudinal ligament are spinal diseases that can produce spinal cord compression. Primary or metastatic spinal cord tumors, subacute combined degeneration of the spinal cord, syphilis, and multiple sclerosis may also cause a cervical myelopathy. Motor neuron disease may mimic motor complaints, but sensory complaints are usually not present. High cervical cord or foramen magnum tumors may cause cervical myelopathy with tetraparesis and loss of sensation (primarily proprioception) in the hands. Any spinal cord lesion above C7 can produce the symptoms and signs of a cervical myelopathy.

Anterior-posterior, oblique, and lateral neck x-ray films should be taken, including flexion and extension views. Disc-space narrowing and osteophyte formation are often seen in persons more than 50 years of age. A test for vitamin B_{12}, a VDRL test, a complete blood count, and thyroid function studies should also be performed. Electromyographic examination and electroneurography help to localize the area of lower-motor neuron involvement in cases of spondylotic radiculopathy, but they are of little value in the patient with spondylotic myelopathy, except to exclude motor neuron disease. Myelography is the diagnostic procedure of choice; the entire cervical spinal cord should be visualized from C7 through the foramen magnum. The CSF should be examined with routine studies, VDRL, and in those cases where demyelination is possible, protein electrophoresis and an oligoclonal immunoglobulin assay. MRI imaging is a noninvasive way of looking at the cervical spinal cord and the caudal brain stem area. In the future it may obviate the need for invasive studies.

The pain of spondylotic myelopathy usually subsides spontaneously in four to six weeks. Immobilizing the neck with a soft cervical collar may relieve pain. Analgesic and anti-inflammatory medications help control the pain. Surgery should be considered if the root pain is severe, persistent, or unresponsive to conservative measures, but it is usually unnecessary in the patient with isolated neck pain. Eighty percent of patients with clinical radiculopathy improve after surgery. If cervical myelopathy is present, conservative therapy is usually of no major benefit because symptoms and signs are usually progressive. Decompressive laminectomy is necessary and is usually performed at multiple levels. Eighty percent of patients experience no further progression, and approximately one-third show improvement. These statistics underscore the need for early diagnosis and treatment.

Bibliography

Cailliet R: *Low Back Pain Syndrome*, ed 3. Philadelphia, F.A. Davis, 1981. (Monograph that covers all aspects of low back pain, with good discussion of biomechanics.)

Deyo RA: Conservative therapy for low back pain: Distinguishing useful from useless therapy. *JAMA* 1983; 250:1057-1062. (Discusses contemporary approaches to treatment of low back pain.)

Deyo RA, Diehl AK, Rosenthal M: How many days of bed rest for acute low back pain? A randomized clinical trial. *N Engl J Med* 1986; 315: 1064-1070. (Patients treated with only two days of bed rest missed 45% fewer days of work than patients treated with seven days of bed rest.)

Gregorius FK, Estrin T, Crandall PH: Cervical spondylotic radiculopathy and myelopathy. A long-term follow up study. *Arch Neurol* 1976; 33:618-625. (Excellent descriptions of signs, symptoms, and natural history.)

Hall S, Bartelson JD, Onofrio BM, et al: Lumbar spinal stenosis: Clinical features, diagnostic procedures, and results of surgical treatment in 68 patients. *Ann Intern Med* 1985; 103:271-275. (Best contemporary review of spinal stenosis.)

Junck L, Marshall WH: Neurotoxicity of radiological contrast agents. *Ann Neurol* 1983; 13:469-484. (Describes in detail the problem of metrizamide toxicity.)

Keim HA, Kirkaldy-Willis WH: Low back pain. *Clin Symp* 1980; 32(6):1-35. (Well-illustrated volume that describes causes and treatments of low back pain.)

Nakano KK, Schoene WC, Baker RA, et al: The cervical myelopathy associated with rheumatoid arthritis: Analysis of 32 patients, with 2 postmortem cases. *Ann Neurol* 1978; 3:144-151. (Good overview of rheumatoid myelopathy.)

Nurick S: The pathogenesis of the spinal cord disorder associated with cervical spondylosis. *Brain* 1972; 95:87-100. (Ischemia to the cord a likely factor.)

Parkinson D: Late results of treatment of intervertebral disc disease with chymopapain. *J Neurosurg* 1983; 59:990-993. (Of patients treated, 70% were cured or improved after chymopapain injection.)

Stanton-Hicks M, Boas RA: *Chronic Low Back Pain.* New York, Raven Press, 1982. (Good discussion of myofascial pain syndromes.)

10

Weakness

Weakness, one of the most common complaints in outpatient practice, is the condition in which a muscle cannot exert its normal force. Weakness can arise from dysfunction of any part of the motor system that governs voluntary muscle function. It may be subjective or objective, local or generalized, and of acute or gradual onset.

Patients may describe true weakness using other terms, such as stiffness, difficulty with fine hand coordination, or difficulty rising from the sitting position. Although weakness may be the cause of these complaints, the patient may not perceive them as due to a consequence of motor dysfunction. Patients often mention generalized "weakness" among the presenting symptoms of systemic and psychological disorders. True weakness must be differentiated from the lassitude and fatigue of depression or systemic disorders, in which there is lack of energy and loss of the sense of well-being; the patient is always tired, has no ambition, and lacks the pep to perform daily activities.

True weakness results from a lesion of the voluntary motor pathway, which is divided into the *upper motor neuron* (UMN) and the *lower motor neuron* (LMN) pathways. The UMN begins in the motor area of the cerebrum and extends along the corticospinal and corticobulbar tracts to end on the LMN in the spinal cord (anterior horn cell) and brain stem motor nuclei. The LMN arises within the gray matter of the spinal cord and brain stem motor nucleus, extends into the nerve, and terminates in the muscle. Muscle tone and movements are also influenced by the extrapyramidal system, the cerebellum, and proprioceptive systems. Involvement of the UMN or LMN can be caused by a wide variety of diseases (Table 10-1), and clinical findings depend on the area involved (Table 10-2).

A complete medical history must be obtained from the patient who complains of weakness. The nature of onset of weakness (gradual versus acute) should be determined, as well as the distribution and the pattern of progression of the weakness, including· any associated cranial nerve manifestations (eg, diplopia,

TABLE 10-1 COMMON CAUSES OF WEAKNESS BY ANATOMIC SITE

Area Involved	Etiologies
Upper Motor Neuron	Vascular; tumor; trauma; infection; degenerative; demyelinative; toxic/anoxic
Lower Motor Neuron Anterior horn cell	Infection (poliomyelitis); trauma; tumor; paraneoplastic; degenerative (ALS); disc (spondylotic myelopathy); radiation effect; vascular
Nerve roots	Intervertebral disc; neoplasm; trauma; infection; radiation; toxins
Peripheral nerve	Trauma; neoplasm; toxins (lead, alcohol); infections (diphtheria, Guillain–Barré); metabolic (porphyria, diabetes); vascular (arteritis); nutritional (vitamin B_{12} deficiency)
Neuromuscular junction	Toxins (botulinum, snake venom, tick bite); neoplastic (Eaton–Lambert syndrome); immunologic (myasthenia gravis); drugs (anticholinesterase toxicity)
Muscle	Congenital/hereditary (muscular dystrophy, congenital myopathies); infections (trichinosis); connective tissue disease-related (polymyositis, scleroderma, mixed connective tissue disease); endocrine (hypo-hyperthyroidism, hyperparathyroidism), neoplastic; drug-induced (clofibrate, corticosteroids)

Adapted from: Grob D: Weakness, in Barondess J (ed): *Diagnostic Approaches to Presenting Syndromes.* Baltimore, Williams & Wilkins, 1971, pp 197-300. Used with permission.

swallowing difficulties). As the patient provides information about the location and intensity of weakness, it may be possible to determine the location of motor system involvement (see Chapter 1 and Table 10-2). Knowing the time course of the weakness combined with the anatomic site of the involvement, helps in determining the nature of the illness. Provocative and palliative features of the weakness and the presence of pain should be ascertained as should the variability of symptoms according to the time of day. It is mandatory to know the patient's family history, occupation, drug exposure, and social history (including the amount of intake of alcohol). A brief psychiatric history should also be obtained to search for depression, hysteria or neurosis.

Weakness of particular muscle groups gives rise to characteristic symptoms. Weakness of extraocular muscles may give rise to diplopia or blurred vision; when the patient covers one eye, the vision usually returns to normal. Weakness of the muscles of mastication (temporalis and masseter muscles) may cause difficulty in chewing and may cause the jaw to sag. The patient with facial weakness may appear depressed because he lacks facial expression. The patient may additionally note that he is no longer able to drink liquids through a straw. Weakness of the vocal apparatus may cause dysphonia (from both palatal and vocal cord dysfunction) or dysarthria. Weakness of the pharyngeal muscles and of the palate invariably leads to episodes of choking, dysphagia, and nasal regurgitation of fluids.

TABLE 10-2 CLINICAL LOCALIZATION OF WEAKNESS

LOCATION	TONE	REFLEXES			ATROPHY	FASCICULATIONS
		DEEP-TENDON	SUPERFICIAL	BABINSKI		
Upper Motor Neuron	↑*	↑	−	+	no	no
Lower Motor Neuron						
Anterior Horn	↓	↓	−	−	yes	yes
Nerve	↓	↓ or −	+	−	yes	rarely
Neuromuscular junction	normal	normal	+	−	no	no
Muscle	normal	normal⁺	+	−	yes (late)	no

↑ = Increased.
↓ = Decreased.
+ = Present.
− = Absent.

*Hypotonia replaces hypertonia in infants.

+ Reflexes are absent with marked atrophy.

From Swanson PD: *Signs and Symptoms in Neurology.* Phialdelphia, Lippincott, 1984, p 134. Used with permission.

Weakness of neck flexors makes it difficult for a patient to sit up from a supine position. The patient with weak neck extensors usually supports his head by resting his chin on his hand. Proximal weakness of the arms is often recognized when tasks performed at the level of the shoulders are impaired such as reaching to place an object on a shelf or combing or washing the hair. Distal weakness of the arms and hands usually gives rise to difficulty in moving fingers, such as in writing or buttoning a shirt. Weakness of the proximal lower extremity muscles makes climbing stairs or rising from a chair or toilet seat difficult. Unilateral proximal weakness makes walking and running difficult. Quadriceps weakness can cause a patient's knees to intermittently buckle when he descends stairs. More severe weakness of the quadriceps can make it difficult for him to stand without assistance. Weakness of the distal lower extremity causes problems with walking. Foot drop can cause the patient to trip when he walks quickly; running can be difficult.

The patient may incorrectly interpret other physical conditions as weakness. Severe proprioceptive deficits can cause a feeling of weakness. Extrapyramidal dysfunction accompanied by rigidity and postural changes may also be interpreted by the patient as numbness or weakness. Limitation of joint motion by bone, tendon, or joint disorders are sometimes called weakness.

A complete medical evaluation should follow the history because systemic disease or occult endocrinopathies may give rise to weakness. A complete neurological examination should identify the distribution of weakness, allowing the examiner to determine the site of the lesion. The patient should be disrobed so that most muscles can be inspected. Muscle bulk should be determined and atrophy or hypertrophy noted. Posture, gait, and any limb or spinal deformities should be evaluated. Examination of the joints, including range of motion, is necessary; pain or limitation of motion is recorded.

The distribution of the weakness should be determined. Is it generalized or focal? Proximal or distal? Muscle power should be tested in all major muscle groups, including those muscles innervated by the cranial nerves as well as the axial muscles. If the patient complains of tiring easily, provocative maneuvers should be carried out to see if weakness can be reproduced. Tenderness should be determined by palpating muscles. Abnormal movements (at rest or during activity) should be noted; they should then be characterized as to whether they are increased or reduced by movement, rest, anxiety, or intention (Chapters 12 and 24). Deep-tendon and superficial reflexes and an extensor plantar response (Babinski's sign) should be tested. A careful sensory examination should be performed.

Table 10-2 lists characteristics of upper motor neuron and lower motor neuron lesions as they can be described on the basis of examination findings. Upper motor neuron lesions are associated with hyperactive deep-tendon reflexes, the loss of superficial cutaneous reflexes, the presence of Babinski's sign, and the lack of atrophy. Depending on the site of involvement, the patient may have sensory loss. A typical LMN lesion (neurogenic) is associated with hypoactive reflexes, muscle atrophy, and fasciculations. Diseases of the neuromuscular junction and of the muscles may have intact reflexes, however, and are not associated with sensory abnormalities or fasciculations.

Table 10-1 lists the many causes for weakness caused by disease of the UMN. Clinical manifestations depend on the abruptness of the insult and the anatomic location. Atrophy does not occur with UMN weakness unless the disease is chronic, in which case disuse results. Corticospinal tract weakness usually affects distal muscles more than proximal muscles. Groups of muscles (not individual muscles) are involved and not all muscles on one side are involved. Antigravity muscles are affected the most. In the upper extremities arm extensors are most involved; in the lower extremities leg flexors are weakest.

GENERALIZED WEAKNESS

The physician must first determine whether the patient is describing true weakness or fatigue and lassitude from depression. Causes of rapid, generalized weakness are listed in Table 10-3.

A slow progression without sensory loss may be caused by motor neuron disease (Chapter 25). Hypothyroidism, with resultant myopathy, may also cause slowly progressive weakness, in part as a result of slowed motor reaction times. Diffuse weakness that progresses over a few days can be caused by Guillain–Barré syndrome, polymyositis, or myasthenia gravis. Acute generalized weakness may result from periodic paralysis or myasthenia gravis. Causes of acute respiratory failure associated with diffuse weakness are listed in Table 10-4.

Weakness with pain may be a consequence of non-neurological as well as neurological conditions (Table 10-5). Localized fibrositis or fibromyositis may cause weakness that is usually more focal than generalized. Polymyalgia rheu-

TABLE 10-3 CAUSES OF ACUTE WEAKNESS BY TIME COURSE

Time	Cause
Minutes	Cerebrovascular diseases (infarct, hemorrhage)
	Trauma
	Postictal
	Peripheral nerve compression
	Drug related
	Spinal cord disease (vascular)
Hours	Myelitis
	Encephalitis
	Myasthenia gravis
	Periodic paralysis
	Botulism
	Poliomyelitis
	Toxins (eg, organophosphate poisoning)
	Spinal cord compression (eg, epidural hematoma)
Days	Guillain–Barré syndrome
	Myasthenia gravis
	Tick bite paralysis
	Polymyositis
	Trauma (subdural hematoma)
	Spinal cord compression

Adapted from Grob D: Weakness, in Barondess J (ed): *Diagnostic Approaches to Presenting Syndromes.* Baltimore, Williams & Wilkins, 1971; and from Pryse-Phillips W, Murray TJ: *Essential Neurology.* Garden City, NY, Medical Examination Publishing, 1986, p 339. Used with permission.

TABLE 10-4 WEAKNESS PRODUCING RESPIRATORY FAILURE

Upper Motor Neuron

Brain stem	Infarction or hemorrhage
Spinal cord	Trauma (above C4: phrenic nerve outflow)
	Infarction/hematoma (high cervical area)
	Motor neuron disease (combined with LMN dysfunction)

Lower Motor Neuron

Anterior Horn	Poliomyelitis
Nerve	Guillain–Barré syndrome
	Porphyria
	Diphtheria
NM junction	Myasthenia gravis
	Botulism
	Cholinergic drug toxicity
	Organophosphate poisoning
Muscle	Polymyositis*
	Myoglobinuria/rhabdomyolysis

* Rare.

Adapted from Pryse-Phillips W, Murray TJ: *Essential Neurology.* Garden City, NY, Medical Examination Publishing, 1986, p 343. Used with permission.

matica is associated with stiffness and pain in the muscles. Although patients complain of weakness, formal motor testing usually does not show objective abnormalities. Trichinosis can be associated with generalized weakness, with palpable muscle tenderness and severe pain.

Various connective tissue disorders can cause weakness with pain, the latter likely as a result of involvement of joint and connective tissue structures. Muscle tenderness may occur with various neuropathies, polyarteritis nodosa, and poliomyelitis. Local and severe pain of fibrositis, acute brachial or lumbosacral plexus neuritis, and radiculitis may also produce painful (often focal) weakness. Muscle pain occasionally occurs with myotonic muscular dystrophy. Some patients with extrapyramidal disturbances complain of local pain, possibly secondary to rigidity or drug-induced dystonia. Metabolic myopathies (myoglobinuria, McArdle syndrome) and viral myopathies can also be marked by weakness and pain. Drugs that occasionally cause painful myopathy are listed in Table 10-6.

LOCALIZED WEAKNESS
Monoplegia

Monoplegia is weakness confined to one extremity. This diagnosis should be a cautious one, however, when a patient complains of unilateral limb weakness, a careful examination often reveals that the weakness is caused by involvement of isolated muscles or that other limbs are involved.

TABLE 10-5 PAINFUL WEAKNESS

Upper Motor Neuron	
Brain	Thalamic syndrome
Spinal Cord	Acute compression (pain at site of compression or radicular)

Lower Motor Neuron	
Anterior Horn	Poliomyelitis
Nerve Roots	Disc
	Tumor
	Spondylosis
	Inflammatory
Nerve	Polyneuropathy
Muscle	Polymyositis
	Viral myositis
	Metabolic myopathy (with myoglobinuria)
	Alcoholic myopathy
	Drug-induced myopathy (see Table 10-6)
	Myotonic disorders
	Trichinosis
	Fibromyositis
Connective Tissue	Rheumatoid arthritis
	Mixed connective tissue disease
	Polymyalgia rheumatica
	Scleroderma
	Polyarteritis nodosa
	Lupus erythematosus
	Sjögren's syndrome
	Rheumatoid arthritis
	Fibrositis
Psychiatric	Depression
	Hysteria
	Malingering

Adapted from Grob D (1971) and from Adams RD, Victor M: *Principles of Neurology.* New York, McGraw-Hill, 1985. Used with permission.

TABLE 10-6 DRUG-INDUCED PAINFUL MYOPATHY

Necrotizing Myopathy
  Clofibrate
  Aminocaproic acid
  Heroin
  Emetine
  Alcohol

Hypokalemia-Producing
  Diuretics
  Purgatives
  Licorice
  Amphotericin B
  Depilatories

Rhabdomyolysis-Producing
  Heroin
  Aminocaproic acid
  Alcohol
  Amphetamine
  Phencyclidine (PCP)

Other
  Vincristine
  Danazol
  Allopurinol
  Cimetidine
  Lithium
  Cytotoxic drugs

Adapted from Mastaglia FL, Argov Z: Drug-induced neuromuscular disorders in man, in Walton JA: *Disorders of Voluntary Muscle,* ed 4. New York, Churchill Livingstone, 1981. Used with permission.

Monoplegia with Muscle Atrophy

This condition is more common than monoplegia without atrophy. Monoplegia is often the result of a lesion that affects the spinal cord or nerve roots. A patient may have muscle atrophy, depressed deep-tendon reflexes, and fasciculations. If atrophy is the result of disuse, reflexes are preserved longer. EMG and nerve conduction studies help determine the site of the lesion. Monoplegia of the arm can be caused by infection (poliomyelitis or other viral illnesses), syringomyelia, motor neuron disease, radiation therapy, or brachial plexus lesions, including trauma, neoplasm, and brachial plexus neuropathy. Monoplegia of the leg is more common than brachial monoplegia and is usually caused by trauma, ruptured disc, tumor, vascular disease, plexitis, or retroperitoneal neoplasm.

Monoplegia without Atrophy

Disease processes that interrupt the corticospinal pathways in the cerebral cortex, brain stem, or spinal cord are the usual causes of monoplegia without atrophy. Vascular lesions (infarcts, often lacunar) are the most common causes (Chapter 20), although tumor or infection may also cause isolated monoplegia. If there are contralateral cranial nerve signs, the lesion is most likely in the brain stem. Crural (leg) monoplegia may be caused by a spinal cord tumor or by demyelination (multiple sclerosis). A medial frontal lobe infarction in the distribution of the anterior cerebral artery also produces crural monoplegia, which is associated with aphasia and abulia if the dominant hemisphere is involved. Likewise, a neoplasm, hematoma, or abscess in this area may also produce crural paresis. In monoplegia without atrophy, the deep-tendon reflexes are increased and Babinski's sign is present.

Hemiplegia

Hemiplegia, weakness of the arm and leg on the same side, usually results from a lesion above the cervical spinal cord. Localization of the lesion may be determined by associated neurological findings. A cortical or subcortical lesion may cause contralateral hemiparesis with aphasia, neglect, visual symptoms, cortical sensory abnormalities, or seizures, depending on the site of brain involvement. Lack of associated cortical signs may place the lesion in the internal capsule or brain stem. If a cranial nerve palsy is present on the side opposite the hemiplegia (crossed hemiplegia), such as a third-nerve palsy with a contralateral hemiparesis (Weber's syndrome) the brain stem is the site of the lesion. With a cortical lesion, the face and arm tend to be affected more than the leg, but with a subcortical or brain stem lesion, the extremities and face are equally affected. The presence of facial weakness places the lesion above the spinal cord. Spinal cord lesions that produce hemiplegia (trauma, tumor) usually have associated loss of position and vibration sensation ipsilateral to the hemiplegia and the site of the lesion, associated with contralateral loss of pain and temperature sensation (Brown–Séquard syndrome; see Chapters 38 and 40).

Paraplegia

Paraplegia, paralysis of both lower extremities, may be caused by lesions of the UMN, LMN, or both. The acute and chronic causes of paraplegia are listed in Table 10-7. In acute paraplegia of spinal cord origin, there is loss of sensation below the site of involvement, pain, and bladder and bowel dysfunction. Peripheral nerve involvement usually does not cause paraplegia unless it is secondary to Guillain–Barré syndrome. A polyneuropathy produces a more distal pattern of weakness and sensory loss, and sphincter function is usually preserved. A cerebral lesion can also produce paraplegia with the pattern of involvement clinically that of a UMN weakness. The parasaggital area of the cerebral cortex gives rise to motor fibers that innervate the lower extremities and bladder/bowel areas. Neoplasms (glioma, meningioma), hematomas, or abscesses in this area can all produce paraplegia. Communicating hydrocephalus (Chapter 13) often presents with a gait disturbance, and although gait apraxia predominates, weakness may be evident.

The most common cause of acute paraplegia is spinal cord trauma (Chapter 38). Anterior spinal artery thrombosis and spontaneous spinal epidural hematoma (Chapter 40) may also cause acute spinal cord syndromes with paraplegia (or quadriplegia if trauma occurs in the cervical cord). Paraplegia from infection, neoplasm, demyelination, or paraneoplastic diseases (necrotizing myelopathy) usually develops over hours to days, but can occur acutely. In the adult, chronic

TABLE 10-7 CAUSES OF PARAPARESIS BY ANATOMIC SITE

Acute	
Spinal Cord	
Trauma	Laceration, fracture/dislocation, hematoma
Vascular	Anterior spinal artery thrombosis
	Epidural/subdural hematoma
Compressive	Hematomyelia/epidural hematoma
	Cervical or thoracic disc
	Vertebral collapse (neoplastic, degenerative, infectious)
Inflammatory	Viral or postinfectious myelitis
	Demyelinating disease
Lower Motor Neuron	Poliomyelitis
	Guillain–Barré
	Tick paralysis
	Porphyria
Chronic	
Intracranial	Bilateral lacunar strokes
	Parasagittal hematoma or neoplasm
	Communicating hydrocephalus
Spinal	Tumor
	Disc
	Spondylosis
	Abscess
	Syphilis
Degenerative	Multiple sclerosis
	Spinocerebellar degenerations
	Motor neuron disease
Metabolic	Vitamin B_{12} deficiency
	Hyperthyroidism

Adapted from Pryse-Phillips W, Murray TJ (1986, p 341). Used with permission.

paraplegia may be caused by vitamin B_{12} deficiency (Chapter 27), cervical spondylosis (Chapter 9), spinal cord tumor, motor neuron disease (Chapter 25), or a polyneuropathy (Chapter 28).

Quadriplegia

Weakness of all four limbs usually results from bilateral lesions of the corticospinal tracts, most often in the upper cervical spinal cord. If quadriplegia is associated with bifacial weakness, hyperreflexia, and bilateral Babinski's sign, the lesion is above the midpons. When a lesion is in the lower cervical cord (eg, spondylotic myelopathy) paralysis of the arms may be of the LMN type, but the legs will be spastic with hyperreflexia and Babinski's sign. Bilateral hemispheric or subcortical strokes (multi-infarct state) can also cause quadriplegia. Demyelinating disorders of the CNS, rheumatoid disorders and Down's syndrome (both producing C1-C2 subluxation), motor neuron disease, and primary lateral sclerosis can all cause a UMN-type of quadriplegia. LMN causes of paraplegia include Guillain–Barré syndrome, porphyric neuropathy, poliomyelitis, spinal muscular atrophy, and (rarely) polymyositis.

Proximal Weakness

Weakness of proximal muscles (limb-girdle weakness) is usually associated with LMN disorders. The patient notes an inability to raise his arms normally, or to arise from sitting or kneeling without support. Polymyositis and the muscular dystrophies (Chapter 29) are the most common causes. Periodic paralysis can also produce proximal weakness. A lesion that affects the C5-C6 or L2-L4 nerve roots or the brachial or lumbosacral plexus may produce proximal weakness. Diabetic amyotrophy is a common cause of painful asymmetrical proximal leg weakness. Occasionally motor neuron disease or Guillain–Barré syndrome is accompanied by weakness of proximal muscles.

Distal Weakness

Upper motor neuron or LMN lesions may cause distal weakness. Neuropathic diseases often produce distal weakness, whereas most myopathic processes produce proximal weakness (Chapters 28 and 29). Diabetes and alcohol are the most common causes of acquired neuropathy; Charcot–Marie–Tooth disease is the most common hereditary neuropathy. Corticospinal tract involvement produces more distal than proximal weakness, with reduced fine motions of the digits. A lower brachial plexus lesion (neoplastic, cervical rib) and lower cervical nerve root abnormalities (C7-C8) can cause progressive weakness and atrophy of hand muscles. An upper lumbosacral plexopathy or proximal (L2-L3) nerve root lesion causes weakness of proximal leg muscles. Atrophy, reflex loss, and fasciculations accompany these lesions. Syringomyelia and intramedullary spinal cord lesions (tumor, cyst) may cause distal weakness with lower motor neuron signs.

Myotonic muscular dystrophy may produce distal weakness, in contrast to the typical proximal involvement of the muscular dystrophies. Mononeuropathies (entrapment, arteritic, metabolic, traumatic) of the ulnar, radial sciatic, and peroneal nerves may also all cause distal focal weakness (Chapters 9, 11, and 29).

Ocular Palsy

Ocular palsies usually present with combinations of diplopia and bilateral ptosis that are often unaccompanied by pupillary abnormalities or exophthalmos. Myasthenia gravis, progressive external ophthalmoplegia (ophthalmoplegia plus) and thyroid ophthalmopathy may all cause isolated ophthalmoplegia. Other muscular diseases associated with ocular palsies include Kearns–Sayre syndrome, myotonic dystrophy, and Möbius' syndrome. Botulism and Fisher's syndrome (the ataxic–ophthalmoplegic variety of Guillain-Barré syndrome) are other LMN causes of ocular palsy. Granulomatous involvement of the cavernous sinus (Tolosa–Hunt syndrome), carotid cavernous fistulas, and tumors that invade the cavernous sinus (lymphoma, nasopharyngeal cancer) produce ophthalmoplegia, but often involve the pupils.

155

Bifacial Palsy

Bifacial palsy (facial diplegia) is usually associated with other neurological symptoms and signs. It is seen with myasthenia gravis, but in over 90% of cases facial diplegia is associated with ptosis and oculomotor abnormalities. Myotonic dystrophy can also produce bifacial palsy, but it has other signs, too. Other causes include the muscular dystrophies (fascioscapulohumeral, congenital myopathies), Möbius syndrome, and neuropathies (porphyria, Guillain–Barré syndrome). Sarcoidosis and other diseases that cause chronic basilar meningitis may produce facial diplegia.

Bulbar Palsy

The typical patient with bulbar palsy has a disorder of articulation (dysarthria, dysphonia) and dysphagia, often associated with weakness of facial and jaw muscles. Myasthenia gravis is the most common cause, but as is the case with bifacial palsy, bulbar palsy is usually associated with other cranial nerve abnormalities. If the patient has a droopy or hanging jaw, especially when fatigued, myasthenia gravis should be considered.

Myotonic dystrophy, botulism, and primary bulbar palsy (motor neuron disease) all can produce bulbar dysfunction. Bilateral involvement of the corticospinal pathways may produce a pseudobulbar palsy. Dysarthria and dysphonia have been reported with polymyositis. Poliomyelitis (rare today) and paraneoplastic disorders may also produce bulbar palsy, usually associated with other symptoms and signs.

Cervical Palsy

In cervical palsy, usually the patient cannot hold his head erect or lift it from a pillow. Inability to hold up the head is the result of weakness of the posterior neck muscles; difficulty in lifting the head from a pillow results from weakness of the sternocleidomastoids and anterior neck muscles. Weakness of the posterior neck muscles and of limb-girdle muscles is seen in polymyositis. In advanced forms of the disease, the head may hang so that the chin rests on the chest and must be supported by the patient's hand. Syphilitic meningoradiculitis, syringomyelia, and paraneoplastic disorders rarely cause cervical palsy.

Bibrachial Palsy

Restricted LMN involvement of both arms is unusual. Motor neuron disease is the most common cause of such involvement. Rarely, Guillain–Barré syndrome presents with proximal bilateral upper extremity weakness, but distal weakness soon follows. An extremely rare paraneoplastic disorder (encephalomyelitis) may produce bibrachial paralysis. Central cord syndrome (Chapter 38) is usually seen in the older patient who has cervical spinal cord trauma; it also produces weakness of both upper extremities (distal more than proximal), but there are associated corticospinal tract signs in the legs. Hypotension has been reported to cause bibrachial paralysis, producing the "man-in-a-barrel" syndrome, resulting from infarction in the anterior watershed areas of the cerebral cortex. Cervical spondylotic myelopathy in the C5-C6 area may produce bilateral upper extremity weakness that is associated with spasticity of the legs. Primary muscle disease almost never causes proximal weakness restricted to the arms.

Hysterical Weakness

The patient with hysterical paralysis usually has bizarre and nonanatomical weakness. The patient may be indifferent to his disability (*la belle indifférence*). Monoparesis or quadriparesis may be present. Tone is usually normal (but may be reduced or increased), deep-tendon reflexes are symmetrical and not hyperactive, and superficial reflexes are present. Sensory complaints may be bizarre and do not correspond to anatomical patterns. The cranial nerves are often not involved, but the patient may complain of blindness or deafness on the side of the paralysis. He may have total paralysis or have limited motion, often of the jerky, intermittent type.

Hoover's sign may be present with hysterical weakness of the leg. To elicit this response, the physician places both hands under the heels of the supine patient. The patient is then asked to press down his heels. If the leg weakness is organic, pressure should be felt only from the nonparalyzed leg. The examiner then places his hand on top of the normal foot (with the other hand still under the heel of the "weak" leg) and ask the patient to elevate the leg. With organic weakness, no downward pressure is exerted by the heel of the paralyzed leg on attempted elevation of the normal leg. If the weakness is hysterical, the heel of the "paralyzed" leg normally presses down against the examiner's hand. It is uncommon for hysterical weakness to persist for more than a few months, but if it does, disuse atrophy may result.

Subjective Weakness

Subjective weakness may be acute, recurrent, or chronic. The causes of acute or recurrent weakness are listed in Table 10-8. Subjective weakness is usually not associated with abnormalities on examination. Many acute or recurrent causes result from decreased blood flow to the brain (Chapter 7). Rarely, epilepsy, hyperventilation, and hypoglycemia are causes of weakness. Chronic subjective weakness may be associated with any chronic disease. Most patients have lassitude or fatigue. Emotional disorders, particularly depression, are also common causes of this type of weakness. Weakness of emotional origin may be superimposed on weakness from organic causes, so organic disease must be excluded in such patients.

TABLE 10-8 CAUSES OF SUBJECTIVE WEAKNESS

Transient Cerebral Ischemia
Arterial disease (atherosclerotic)
    Carotid
    Vertebrobasilar
    Extracranial vessels (eg, subclavian steal syndrome)
Decreased Cardiac Output
    Postural hypotension (decreased venous return)
        Decreased blood volume
            Blood loss
            Dehydration (diarrhea, vomiting)
        Diminished sympathetic vasoconstrictor tone
            Drugs (antihypertensives, beta-blockers, tricyclics)
            Vasovagal reaction
            Heat
            Peripheral nerve diseases (polyneuropathies; amyloid, alcohol, diabetes,
              Guillain–Barré; porphyria)
            Central nervous system (posterior fossa tumors, demyelination)
            Spinal cord (trauma, vascular)
Cardiac Failure
    Myocardial infarction or ischemia
    Brady or tachyarrhythmias
    Carotid sinus hypersensitivity
    Glossopharyngeal neuralgia
    Mechanical cardiac obstruction (valvular disease, myxoma, pericardial effusion)
    Myocarditis

Other
    Hyperventilation
    Seizures (akinetic)
    Cerebrovascular (drop-attacks)
    Narcolepsy/cataplexy
    Hysrterical
    Metabolic
        Periodic paralysis
        Hypoglycemia
        McArdle's disease

Adapted from Grob D (1971). Used with permission.

Bibliography

Adams RD, Victor M: Principles of clinical myology: Diagnosis and classification of muscle diseases, in *Principles of Neurology,* ed 3. New York, McGraw-Hill, 1985, pp 1020-1031. (Discusses the approach to the patient with weakness caused by muscle disease.)

Grob D: Weakness, in Barondess J (ed): *Diagnostic Approaches to Presenting Syndromes,* Baltimore, Williams & Wilkins, 1971, pp 197-300. (A most comprehensive review covering the entire clinical spectrum of weakness.)

Lane RJM, Mastaglia FL: Drug-induced myopathies in man. *Lancet* 1978; 2:562-566. (Reviews major drug-induced myopathies, including those that produce painful weakness.)

McHardy KC: Weakness. *Br Med J* 1984; 288:1591-1594. (Presents a clinical algorithm for evaluating the weak patient.)

Pryse-Phillips W, Murray TJ: Weakness, in *Essential Neurology,* ed 2. Garden City, NY, Medical Examination Publishing, 1982, pp 328-335. (Presents a brief approach to the patient with weakness.)

Schneider S, Rice DR: Neurologic manifestations of childhood hysteria. *Pediatrics* 1979; 94:153-156. (Hysteria in childhood is not rare. This article reviews the neurological manifestations of a group of hysterical children.)

Weintraub MJ: Hysteria: A clinical guide to diagnosis. *Ciba Clinical Symposia* 1977; 29(6):1-31. (Well-illustrated overview of the clinical signs associated with hysteria.)

11 Hand Numbness

Numbness of the hands is a common complaint. The correct diagnosis usually can be made with a careful history and examination (Chapter 1). Cervical nerve roots C6 to C8 all contribute to the formation of mixed motor and sensory nerves that supply the hands. From a dermatomal standpoint, the C6 root supplies sensation to the thumb and forefinger and occasionally to the middle finger; C7 supplies the middle finger and at times part of the index finger; and C8 supplies the fourth and fifth digits.

Lesions of the brachial plexus may also result in numbness of the hand, but such lesions tend to be distal or to involve the lower segments of the plexus. The radial three digits on the palm side, and distally on the dorsum, are invariably supplied by the median nerve. The ulnar nerve supplies the fourth and fifth digits, both palmar and dorsal areas, although the radial half of the fourth digit is often innervated by the median nerve. The dorsal surface of the hand on the radial side is innervated by the superficial radial nerve. The ulnar nerve innervates the majority of the intrinsic hand muscles, so that many of the lesions involving that nerve can also cause weakness of the hand. The median nerve supplies the abductor pollicis brevis and opponens pollicis. The superficial radial nerve does not supply any muscles in the hand as it is purely sensory.

The patient who feels that his whole hand is numb or "asleep" more likely has a median nerve lesion than an ulnar nerve lesion, and the patient who complains of weakness more than numbness often has a lesion of the ulnar nerve. In this chapter, common causes of hand numbness are discussed. They are divided into lesions that affect (1) the peripheral nerves, (2) the brachial plexus, and (3) the cervical nerve roots and spinal cord. It is from pathology affecting these three main areas that the vast majority of cases of hand numbness arise.

Entrapment neuropathies are lesions of peripheral nerves that result from injury at vulnerable anatomic sites, typically occurring where a nerve passes through an opening in fibrous tissue or an osseofibrous canal. Their onset is gradual and the clinician must consider factors that can precipitate the compression neuropathy. Entrapment neuropathy of the median nerve is one of the most common causes of hand numbness and can occur at two different sites.

MEDIAN NEUROPATHY
Carpal Tunnel Syndrome

Carpal tunnel syndrome (CTS), caused by median nerve compression at the wrist, is the most common entrapment neuropathy affecting the upper extremities, and is the most common cause of hand numbness. The carpal tunnel is the anatomic space on the palmar aspect of the wrist bounded below by the carpal bones and above by the flexor retinaculum (transverse carpal ligament) through which pass the long finger flexor tendons. Compression of the median nerve at this site leads to a characteristic group of symptoms and physical findings that have come to be known as CTS.

The causes of CTS are varied. Any condition that causes an increase in the mass of the carpal tunnel can cause compression of the median nerve. Most patients with CTS have nonspecific tenosynovitis, and they often have other evidence of tenosynovitis. Tenosynovitis may be induced occupationally from repeated flexion and extension of the hand or fingers. CTS is the most frequent rheumatoid compression neuropathy, affecting about 25% of patients with rheumatoid arthritis. Acute or chronic CTS can be associated with trauma. Acute CTS may be associated with Colles' fracture, fracture of both bones of the forearm, or dislocation or fracture of the carpus. CTS is one of the symptoms of Volkmann's ischemic contracture. Acute CTS has been reported from bleeding into the median nerve, occurring spontaneously or caused by anticoagulants. Chronic CTS may result from prior bony injury at the wrist. Tumors within the carpal canal or various flexor tendon anomalies can also lead to the CTS. There is also a syndrome of familial liability to pressure palsies, in which numerous entrapment neuropathies may occur. CTS frequently accompanies pregnancy, typically with onset in the sixth month; the cause is not clear. It may also occur with systemic amyloidosis and with myxedema or acromegaly.

CTS occurs five times more often in women than in men and often begins in middle life. Paresthesias in the finger and pain in the hand, often radiating as high as the shoulder, are the most common and most troublesome complaints. The thumb, index finger, middle finger, and radial half of the ring finger are common areas of numbness, but many patients claim numbness of the entire hand. If isolated numbness occurs, it is most often in the middle finger. Patients with CTS often shake their hand to decrease pain and restore sensation. Nocturnal acroparesthesias, common with CTS, will awaken the patient from sleep; shaking the arm or hanging it down over the side of the bed will help relieve symptoms. As the condition progresses, symptoms may also occur during the day and may be precipitated by any motion of the hand and wrist, such as sewing, knitting, holding a book, or driving a car.

Pain and paresthesias can occur without any abnormal neurological signs in the hand. When sensory symptoms have been present for longer than several months, thenar atrophy and weakness may begin. Early cases may occur without evidence of sensory impairment. As CTS advances, there may be slight hypo-esthesia to point location, primarily in the middle finger. These sensory changes may spread to the entire distribution of the distal median nerve. Tinel's sign occurs at the wrist over the median nerve in about 50% of cases. It is elicited by tapping over the volar wrist area, and a positive sign is an electric shock-like sensation that radiates distally into the median nerve-innervated digits. The wrist flexion test (Phalen's sign) is carried out by placing the wrist in unforced flexion for 30 to 60 seconds. If positive, the symptoms of CTS will be exacerbated. This test is helpful, but many patients with documented CTS have negative responses. Atrophy of the thenar eminence may be prominent, involving the opponens pollicis and abductor pollicis brevis. In most patients, CTS occurs in the dominant hand; 10% to 25% of cases are bilateral.

DIAGNOSIS

Diagnosis is in part based on the history and physical examination but should be confirmed by electrophysiological testing. Both electromyography (EMG) and nerve conduction studies are of benefit in diagnosing CTS. Sensory nerve conduction slowing is the most sensitive abnormality seen; prolongation of the median motor and sensory distal latencies are also common. There is poor correlation between the severity of the symptoms and the electrophysiological changes. Electromyographic examination may show denervation confined to the thenar eminence when there is advanced compression with secondary axonal degeneration. However, it is not uncommon to see abnormalities of sensory or motor nerve distal latencies without electromyographic abnormalities. The degree of abnormalities on electrophysiologic testing may predict a response to treatment. When axonal degeneration has started, as shown by the denervation in the abductor pollis brevis muscle, the prognosis for complete recovery is not as good as when the patient has only sensory symptoms or loss of sensation.

The differential diagnosis of CTS includes other entrapment neuropathies and more proximal lesions. CTS must be differentiated from the pronator teres syndrome (see below). CTS can be associated with the "double crush" syndrome, in which there is cervical radiculopathy at the C6 or C7 level associated with distal CTS. Likewise, a generalized peripheral neuropathy or thoracic outlet syndrome may also cause symptoms that may mimic CTS. Focal seizures, transient vascular episodes, or atypical migraine may present with episodic unilateral hand numbness, at times in an ostensibly median nerve distribution, but usually not associated with pain. One of the values of electrophysiological testing is differential diagnosis from these other conditions.

TREATMENT

Treatment is both nonsurgical and surgical. If there is electrophysiologic evidence of very mild nerve entrapment associated with minimal symptoms, steroids (usually injected into the carpal tunnel) and splinting of the hand at night may help. This treatment is advised for patients with mild symptoms or those who have an acute flare. Precipitating factors should be avoided, and the wrist should be splinted; a single, short course of nonsteroidal anti-inflammatory drugs or oral steroids may be of benefit. The night splint should be worn for a few weeks, with the wrist in a neutral position. Local steroid injection usually helps a patient who has intermittent or mild symptoms. It is contraindicated in the presence of muscle wasting or severe sensory loss. Injections usually afford only temporary relief, but complete relief occurs in 30% to 40% of patients, lasting from a few weeks to as long as six months. Correction of associated metabolic conditions may also revert CTS; those associated with pregnancy spontaneously abate, usually soon after delivery. Correction of hypothyroidism also causes the symptoms of CTS to abate. The same is true of treatment of acromegaly.

Surgery is indicated in cases in which there is failure of nonsurgical treatment, progressive muscle wasting, sensory loss, or recurrence of symptoms. Division of the flexor retinaculum is the common surgical approach. Pain and paresthesias are relieved almost immediately, but recovery of power and sensation may take as long as a year. Surgical results depend on surgical skill and on the degree of motor and sensory loss. Patients with a long history of symptoms do not fare as well as those with a shorter history.

Pronator Teres Syndrome

The pronator teres syndrome is caused by entrapment of the median nerve at the level of the pronator teres muscle. It produces pain and tenderness of the proximal forearm as well as paresthesias of the hand. This is a relatively uncommon syndrome, often caused by trauma from repeated pronation and finger flexion or from tight casts. Occasionally, tumors, tenosynovitis, or fibrous bands are the cause. Patients with a pronator teres syndrome demonstrate weakness of the flexor pollicis longus and of the abductor pollicis brevis, although pronation of the forearm remains normal. Sensory abnormalities are usually poorly defined, but correspond anatomically to the distribution of the median nerve. Tinel's sign may be present over the median nerve in the forearm.

DIAGNOSIS
The differential diagnosis includes carpal tunnel syndrome, which is much more common, and thoracic outlet syndrome. Signs and symptoms of carpal tunnel syndrome may overlap, and electrophysiologic tests are necessary to establish the diagnosis. Many symptoms of thoracic outlet syndrome are similar to those of pronator syndrome. There may be nonspecific pain and weakness of the forearm and shoulder, although there tends to be more shoulder pain in thoracic outlet syndrome. Furthermore, thoracic outlet syndrome sensory involvement tends to occur on the ulnar side of the hand, as opposed to the radial side in pronator teres syndrome. In addition, intense pain on palpation over the pronator teres muscle associated with Tinel's sign is quite specific. Patients with cervical spine disease affecting the C6 or C7 nerve roots may have sensory involvement in an area similar to that of the pronator teres syndrome, but neck pain with radicular features and weakness in more proximal muscles is more suggestive of a cervical nerve root disturbance.

Unfortunately, abnormalities on EMG and nerve conduction studies are only present in a minority of cases. Because some cases show evidence of median nerve injury below the elbow but above the wrist, the value of the electrical studies is primarily to exclude other nerve and nerve root compression syndromes.

TREATMENT

In cases caused by occupational trauma (repeated elbow flexion and pronation), avoiding these activities may alleviate symptoms. For persistent or progressive symptoms, surgical exploration of the forearm is necessary to release the offending compressive band. Making the correct diagnosis results in favorable prognosis after surgery, but proper diagnosis is not always easy.

ULNAR NEUROPATHY

Although entrapment can occur anywhere along the course of the ulnar nerve, major sites of entrapment are at the *elbow* and more distally in the *wrist* or *palm*. The second most common upper extremity entrapment neuropathy involves the ulnar nerve at the elbow.

Elbow Neuropathy

The initial symptoms of ulnar neuropathy at the elbow are intermittent hyperesthesias in an ulnar nerve distribution, often induced by elbow flexion. Use of the arms, especially elbow flexion and extension, exacerbates these sensory complaints. The patient may be awakened at night with pain in the elbow, or the pain may radiate into the fourth and fifth fingers. Most patients seek medical attention because of sensory dysfunction, but occasionally the initial complaint is weakness of the hand.

Acute and chronic compression of the nerve in the cubital tunnel (a result of local scarring or impingement) can lead to chronic compression of the ulnar nerve. In one-third of cases, there is no identifiable cause; 8% to 20% of patients have bilateral ulnar nerve involvement. Neuropathy may follow elbow trauma, and may occur because of improper positioning of the arm during periods of unconsciousness, in bedridden patients, and during anesthesia. Ulnar nerve compressions can complicate elbow pathology, including osteophytes or rheumatoid arthritis.

Physical examination discloses decreased sensation at the ulnar aspect of the palm, including the volar surface of the fifth digit and the ulnar half of the fourth digit. The dorsal sensory branch of the ulnar nerve supplies the ulnar aspect of the hand and the fourth and fifth fingers. Two-point, light-touch, pinprick, or thermal sensation may be diminished. There are anatomical variations in the sensory supply to the hand, so that in about 20% of the patients the ulnar nerve supplies the entire ring finger and the ulnar half of the middle finger.

Weakness of ulnar-innervated muscles of the hand is common; so is weakness of pinch. Grip is diminished because of the involvement of the interosseous muscles and the flexor digitorum profundus of the fourth and fifth digits. Atrophy of the first dorsal interosseous muscle and hypothenar eminence develops.

DIAGNOSIS

Diagnosis is based on clinical findings and electrophysiological examination. Nerve conduction studies disclose slowing of the nerve conduction across the elbow segment of the ulnar nerve. EMG often shows evidence of denervation of the ulnar-innervated hand muscles.

Differential diagnosis includes other sites of ulnar nerve compression, particularly at the wrist. A C8 nerve-root lesion or a brachial plexopathy may also present as fourth- and fifth-finger numbness. If motor signs predominate, then distinction from evolving motor neuron disease may be difficult. Syringomyelia can present as ulnar-type sensory and motor complaints. Brachial plexus involvement caused by the thoracic outlet syndrome may cause more C8 nerve-root-like involvement; at times, sensory loss may be more medial. Tumors of the superior pulmonary sulcus (Pancoast tumor) may involve the medial cord of the brachial plexus and may give rise to hand numbness and weakness in addition to hoarseness.

THERAPY

Nonsurgical treatment is advised initially for most patients. Flexion and extension at the elbow should be minimized in patients with intermittent symptoms or with acute or chronic mild compression. Splinting the elbow in an extended posture may help; this may be necessary for two to three months. Foam rubber elbow pads can help reduce external trauma. Surgical treatment is usually indicated when there is definite evidence of denervation on EMG or when the patient is unresponsive to medical treatment. The nerve can be decompressed or can be transplanted to an anterior position. Patients with intermittent symptoms or those produced by elbow flexion have good results if symptoms and signs are not marked. Patients with severe symptoms or marked sensory loss and weakness have less favorable results.

Wrist or Palm Neuropathy

The ulnar nerve can be compressed at several sites below the elbow, most often at the palm or wrist. Many distal ulnar nerve lesions occur at the base of the palm where the nerve enters the hand through Guyon's canal (ulnar tunnel); these lesions tend to produce motor and sensory symptoms. Lesions that are more distal in the palm tend to spare all sensory branches and produce a purely motor syndrome. Compression at the wrist level is caused by disorders similar to those that cause carpal tunnel syndrome. Ganglion of the wrist, certain occupations, and laceration of the wrist area may predispose to ulnar neuropathy. Fractures of the wrist, especially of the hook of the hamate, may also produce ulnar neuropathy. Bicyclists may develop bilateral ulnar neuropathies as a result of compression at the wrist caused by pressure when holding the handlebars. Any mass in the area of the distal ulnar nerve, such as a ganglion, lipoma, or aberrant muscle, can also cause distal ulnar neuropathy.

A lesion of the deep palmar branch of the ulnar nerve is the most common site of distal ulnar nerve compression near the wrist. Symptoms are usually those of painless weakness of the hand without definite sensory loss. If compression occurs within Guyon's canal (distal to the wrist), there is isolated involvement of the intrinsic hand muscles, including the hypothenar muscles. Such compression within Guyon's canal may be purely sensory, with loss of sensation occurring over the volar aspect of the digits but normal sensation over the dorsum of the hand (dorsal sensory branch territory).

Electrophysiological testing reveals denervation in the intrinsic hand muscles; distal latency of the ulnar motor nerve at the wrist is characteristically prolonged. Other electrophysiological changes are determined by the site of the ulnar nerve compression.

Differential diagnosis is similar to that of ulnar nerve compression at other sites. Dorsal sensation is normal because the dorsal branch arises from the ulnar nerve about 6 to 8 cm proximal to the wrist, and this helps differentiate distal and more proximal compression. The major diagnoses to consider are C8 or T1 cervical radiculopathy, brachial plexus lesion, and motor neuron disease, especially when there is atrophy of the intrinsic hand muscles without sensory loss. The examination, and more importantly the electrophysiological studies, help determine the primary cause of the hand numbness or weakness.

TREATMENT

If symptoms are mild, therapy is initially conservative. Wrist trauma should be avoided, and a night splint may be of benefit. Avoidance of precipitating factors is crucial. For patients who have significant denervation or who are unresponsive to conservative treatment, exploration and decompression is indicated. Results are similar to those of surgical treatment of carpal tunnel syndrome.

THORACIC OUTLET SYNDROME

The thoracic outlet is a channel through which nerves and blood vessels of the arm leave the neck and thorax. The apex of the thoracic outlet is formed anteriorly by the scalenus anticus muscle, inferiorly by the first rib, and posteriorly by the scalenus medius muscle. Through this triangular space run the subclavian artery and the brachial plexus. Enlargement of the scalenus anticus muscle can compress the neurovascular supply of the arm; anomalous cervical ribs or bands can cause compression posteriorly. True thoracic outlet syndrome (TOS) is overdiagnosed: it is far less common than carpal tunnel syndrome, ulnar nerve entrapment, or cervical spondylosis. Symptoms of neurovascular compression at the thoracic outlet may be of purely vascular or neural origin or a combination of the two.

SYMPTOMS AND SIGNS

Paresthesias are usually the first symptoms; they tend to precede overt pain or weakness. Usually the ulnar nerve distribution is affected, as well as the medial forearm area because of lower brachial plexus involvement. Pain may then develop, which may be localized in the shoulder, chest, arm, or hand. The pain is usually aching and may be produced by carrying heavy objects with the involved limb. Elevating the affected limb also characteristically produces pain and paresthesias. When a patient carries or lifts objects, the thoracic outlet becomes narrowed and exacerbates neurovascular compression. Some patients complain of nocturnal numbness. Playing certain musical instruments or typing may also bring on the symptoms.

Motor loss is uncommon, although fatigability is common. Weakness, if present, usually involves those hand muscles innervated by the lower brachial plexus. Atrophy is uncommon unless there is a congenital band or cervical rib. In such cases, atrophy affects all the intrinsic muscles of the hand.

Vascular symptoms occur in 5% to 10% of patients with TOS. The complaints caused by vascular compression are quite different from those caused by neural compression. Coldness, muscle aching, and diminished strength are typical and are usually noticed with continued use. The hand may become pale or cyanotic; often it feels cold to the touch. Vascular compression usually results from a large cervical rib or compressive band.

Various maneuvers may reproduce the symptoms of TOS. Radial pulse obliteration may be detected by performing Adson's maneuver. In this test the seated patient takes a deep breath with his head extended and rotated to the affected side, while the ipsilateral arm rests on the knee. A positive test occurs when the ipsilateral radial pulse is obliterated when the breath is taken. Obliteration of the ipsilateral radial pulse, however, occurs in many normal people, so this test is nonspecific. Reproducing the patient's symptoms with an elevated posture of the arm suggests TOS, whether or not the radial pulse changes. A bruit over the clavicle, particularly when the arm is hyperabducted, is a common finding in normal individuals without arm symptoms. In most cases, compression of the thoracic outlet results from a fibrous band. Cervical ribs or elongated transverse processes of C7 are less common causes.

DIAGNOSTIC TESTS

Cervical spine films may demonstrate true or rudimentary cervical ribs in 30% of patients with TOS. The syndrome can be simulated by a Pancoast tumor, which can be identified on apical lordotic chest x-rays. Arteriography is often normal, but angiographic demonstration of subclavian artery compression, which occurs only with the arm or head in the position that reproduces the patients symptoms, suggests the diagnosis of TOS, and predicts a favorable surgical result.

Electrophysiologic tests may be helpful but often are not. Nerve conduction studies are most helpful for excluding other causes of symptoms, such as ulnar nerve or median nerve compressions. Nerve conduction latency of the ulnar nerve across the thoracic outlet can be performed, but the technique is difficult and results are often not clear. Anatomical differences that determine the points of stimulation, as well as difficulties in measuring the true distance of proximal stimulation (Erb's point) to the arm, make it difficult to determine abnormal values for proximal conduction. EMG of the arm and hand may be useful if there is objective wasting of muscles: denervation potentials may be seen in a pattern that suggests brachial plexus involvement instead of a compressive neuropathy or cervical radiculopathy. F-wave studies, in which conduction in the proximal nerve routes is determined, may be of benefit in helping to diagnose TOS; however, it has been shown (as with other nerve conduction tests) that F-wave prolongation is not a sensitive measurement for TOS. Somatosensory-evoked responses may be of value in diagnosing TOS; abnormalities occur when the involved arm is abducted and rotated externally.

DIFFERENTIAL DIAGNOSIS

Many diseases (low cervical spinal cord abnormalities, such as tumors, syringomyelia, spondylosis, or vascular cord disease) can produce symptoms that seem to resemble those of TOS. Brachial plexus involvement by tumor can simulate TOS and is much more common than true TOS. Radiation therapy to the chest may cause radiation-induced brachial plexopathy, but this condition usually is relatively painless and involves the upper plexus. Brachial neuritis, whether compressive (caused by carrying a knapsack) or idiopathic, may also produce a thoracic outlet-like symptom complex. Entrapment neuropathy that affects the median and ulnar nerves may also be misdiagnosed as TOS. Sensory loss is not in the C8-T1 (or ulnar nerve) distribution, and thenar atrophy (median nerve) does not occur with ulnar nerve entrapment. Cervical radiculopathy that affects the C8 nerve root may cause hand numbness, but usually other roots are involved. Neck pain is a helpful clue in the diagnosis.

TREATMENT

The easiest initial therapy is restraint of the arms while the patient sleeps; an attempt should be made to prevent sleeping positions in which the arms are elevated or the hands are placed behind the head. Prevention of elbow flexion during sleep, if there is a coincidental ulnar nerve entrapment, is of benefit. During the day, avoiding positions in which symptoms develop—such as elevating the arms or carrying objects—is also helpful.

Exercises designed to strengthen the neck and shoulder muscles and to prevent droopy shoulders lead to improvement in most patients. Such exercises consist of range-of-motion movements of the shoulder girdle, lateral rotational movements of the neck, and exercises to induce erect posture. Regular exercise relieves symptoms in as many as 80% of cases. Nonsurgical therapy should be continued for a minimum of a few months. Conservative therapy is considered a failure when pain becomes incapacitating, when paresthesias are replaced by sensory loss, or when muscle wasting appears.

The thoracic outlet can be exposed surgically via a supraclavicular approach. With this technique, resection of the anterior scalene muscle can be performed and the brachial plexus can be thoroughly explored; if an offending cervical rib or band is found, it can be removed. The first rib can also be resected with this technique. Good results with the supraclavicular approach have been reported in as many as 80% of cases. The disadvantages of this approach are that the surgical scar is more pronounced, and there may be temporary damage to the phrenic nerve or to the long thoracic nerve. Transaxillary first rib resection has also been used with good results in treating TOS. Neurological symptoms appear to respond better to first rib resection than do vascular symptoms, although a satisfactory result is achieved in about 90% of patients. The recurrence rate is 15%.

Bibliography

Cherington M: Proximal pain in carpal tunnel syndrome. *Arch Surg* 1974; 108:69. (Documentation of occurrence of predominant proximal—and thus confusing—complaints in CTS.)

Dawson DM, Hallett M, Millender LH: *Entrapment Neuropathies.* Boston, Little Brown, 1983. (A comprehensive and easy to read monograph on all aspects of entrapment neuropathies. Has excellent current chapters on all subjects discussed in this chapter; highly recommended.)

Hirsh LF, Thanki A: The thoracic outlet syndrome: Meeting the diagnostic challenge. *Postgrad Med* 1985; 77:197-207. (Excellent and accessible review of TOS, written for the primary care physician.)

Lascelles RG, Mohr PD, Neary D, et al: The thoracic outlet syndrome. *Brain* 1977; 100:601-612. (British review of 31 patients with TOS, with comments on diagnosis and treatment.)

Miller RG: The cubital tunnel syndrome: Diagnosis and precise localization. *Ann Neurol* 1979; 6:56-59. (Review of the clinical and electrophysiologic features of ulnar nerve compression at the elbow.)

Miller RG, Camp PE: Postoperative ulnar palsy. *JAMA* 1979; 242:1636-1639. (Warns that improper positioning of the arm during surgery may lead to this neuropathy; the situation can be a cause of litigation against the physician.)

Morris HH, Peters BH: Pronator syndrome: Clinical and electrophysiological features in 7 cases. *J Neurol Neurosurg Psychiatry* 1976; 39:461-464. (A good clinical overview of the uncommonly encountered pronator syndrome.)

Phalen GS: The carpal tunnel syndrome: Seventeen years experience in diagnosis and treatment of 654 hands. *J Bone Joint Surg* 1966; 48A:211-228. (A large clinical and surgical review of this common problem.)

Roos DB: Congenital anomalies associated with thoracic outlet syndrome: Anatomy, symptoms, diagnosis, and treatment. *Am J Surg* 1976; 132:771-778. (Comprehensive review of this syndrome by a physician who has examined over 2,300 patients with alleged thoracic outlet syndrome.)

12

Tremor

As both a symptom and a sign, tremor is frequently encountered in clinical practice. Tremors span a broad spectrum from innocuous to serious and from asymptomatic to disabling. The classification by appearance and pathophysiology is useful because specific treatments are effective for specific classes of tremors.

DEFINITION AND CLASSIFICATION

Formally, tremor is defined as an involuntary rhythmic oscillatory movement produced by alternating or synchronous contractions of repircrocally innervated antagonist muscles. Tremor is differentiated from other involuntary adventitious movements (described in Chapter 1) chiefly by its rhythmic nature. All tremors disappear during sleep, which helps to differentiate them from myokymia and palatal myoclonus, two rhythmic disorders that persist during sleep.

Descriptively, tremors are first classified as (1) those that occur at rest (static tremors); and (2) those that occur during voluntary muscle movement (action tremors). Action tremors are further classified into three groups: (a) those that are most prominent on maintenance of sustained antigravity posture (postural or "sustention" tremors); (b) those that are most prominent with tonic muscle contraction (contraction tremors); and (c) those that are worst on dynamic goal-directed limb movements (intention or kinetic tremors).

Pathophysiologically, tremors are classified as physiologic, essential, cerebellar, parkinsonian, and polyneuropathic types as listed in Table 12-1.

EXAMINATION

The patient is examined for static tremor by observing his or her muscles at rest. The examiner then asks him to extend his arms in an outstretched position with the fingers spread apart. Postural tremor is most apparent in this position. The patient is then asked to make a fist and is observed for contraction tremor. Then he is asked to perform the finger-to-nose test and is observed for evidence of intention tremor. A similar assessment for leg tremor follows. The patient is also observed for head tremors which may be flexion-extension ("yes-yes"), rotation ("no-no"), or lateral flexion types. The examination of handwriting should always be part of tremor assessment.

An effective method of amplifying an intention tremor is to affix a large rubber band around the patient's wrist and ask him to perform the finger-to-nose test. The examiner maintains tension on the rubber band, which requires the patient to overcome resistance in the finger-to-nose movement. The addition of resistance to the system amplifies the tremor.

PHYSIOLOGICAL TREMOR

Normally, there exists a low-amplitude action tremor of the limbs, head and tongue, which is not ordinarily noticeable. This physiological tremor may become noticeable when it is amplified by anxiety, stress, fatigue, the effects of certain drugs, certain endocrinopathies, or alcohol withdrawal (Tables 12-1 and 12-2). The frequency of physiological tremor varies with age. It is about 6 Hz in children under 9 years and gradually increases in frequency to 10 Hz at 16 years of age. At age 40, the tremor begins to slow down and again reaches the childhood frequency of 6 Hz at 70 years of age. The mechanism of physiological tremor is uncertain, but its blockade by intra-arterial propranolol strongly suggests the action of peripheral beta-adrenergic receptors.

The physiological tremor may be demonstrated by amplification techniques. When a sheet of paper is placed on the dorsum of the outstretched pronated hand, the edges of the paper can be seen to rhythmically shake if observed carefully. Similarly, the physiological tremor can be appreciated if the subject is asked to extend his arm and hold a point light source (eg, lecture pointer) so that the light shines on a wall 30 feet away. The rhythmic oscillations of the light on the wall can then be seen.

An independent body tremor is passively induced by ballistocardiac forces. This ballistocardiac tremor, which has the frequency of the pulse, is increased in patients with a wide pulse pressure. It can be particularly prominent in patients with aortic regurgitation.

ESSENTIAL TREMOR

Essential tremor is the most common action tremor seen in clinical practice. Prevalence rates from 4/1000 to 60/1000, without gender predominance, have been reported. The wide variation probably reflects inconstant diagnostic criteria among studies.

The tremor usually begins in young adulthood and worsens with age. By the sixth decade, patients have marked tremor. With advancing age, the tremor amplitude increases and the frequency decreases, and the tremor may spread to other parts of the body. When the tremor begins in old age it may be called "senile tremor."

TABLE 12-1   CLASSIFICATION OF TREMORS

Physiologic
  Normal
  Actentuated
    Anxiety, stress, fatigue
    Endocrinopathy (pheochromocytoma, hypoglycemia, hyperthyroidism)
    Drug-induced (Table 12-2)
    Alcohol withdrawal

Essential
  Sporadic
  Hereditary
  Senile

Cerebellar
  Cerebellar degeneration
  Multiple sclerosis
  Midbrain damage
  Drug-induced (Table 12-2)

Parkinsonian
  Idiopathic
  Secondary
    Postencephalitic
    Drug-induced (Table 12-2)
    Chronic hepatocerebral degeneration

Multisystem disorders
    Progressive supranuclear palsy
    Shy-Drager syndrome
    Olivopontocerebellar atrophy
    Joseph disease
    Huntington's disease
    Wilson's disease

Polyneuropathic
  Acute postinfectious polyneuropathy
  Hereditary motor-sensory neuropathies, Types 1-4
  Metabolic polyneuropathies
    Diabetes
    Uremia
    Alcohol-induced and nutritional
    Acute intermittent porphyria
    Amyloidosis

Miscellaneous
  Writing
  Spasmus nutans
  Psychogenic

Adapted from Jankovic J, Fahn S: Physiologic and pathologic tremors. *Ann Intern Med* 1980; 93:461. Used with permission.

Essential tremor is an action tremor that is worse during sustained posture. It often has a mild intentional worsening and when severe can also be present at rest. Affected limbs show a characteristic flexion–extension movement unlike the primarily pronation–supination movement of parkinsonism. The tremor usually occurs at a frequency of 7 to 11 Hz.

Essential tremor has been called "familial" and "benign," but not all cases fit either description. When familial, there is usually an autosomal dominant mode of

TABLE 12-2 DRUGS AND POISONS THAT ACCENTUATE TREMOR

ACCENTUATION OF PHYSIOLOGIC TREMOR

Sympathomimetic Agents
Amphetamines
Epinephrine
Isoproterenol
Metaproterenol
Terbutaline
Dopamine
Levodopa

Psychotropic Agents
Neuroleptics
Lithium
Tricyclic antidepressants

Xanthines
Caffeine
Theophylline

Heavy Metals and Poisons
Mercury
Lead
Arsenic
Bismuth
Carbon monoxide
Methyl bromide

Other Agents
Sodium valproate
Monosodium glutamate
Oral hypoglycemic agents
Corticosteroids
Thyroid hormone

ACCENTUATION OF CEREBELLAR TREMOR
Phenytoin
Barbiturates
Lithium
Alcohol
Mercury
5-Fluorouracil

ACCENTUATION OF PARKINSONIAN TREMOR
Phenothiazines
Butyrophenones
Reserpine
Carbon monoxide
Carbon disulfide
Manganese

inheritance with incomplete penetration. Many cases are sporadic. Mild cases may be benign, but the tremor can produce occupational and social disability when severe.

The tremor usually affects the distal upper extremities out of proportion to other body parts and is somewhat asymmetric. In the typical case, the patient notes fine distal hand shaking when holding an object. The more the patient tries to hold the object without shaking, the greater the amplitude of the tremor. Holding a cup of coffee is one of the most difficult tasks for such a patient.

Handwriting becomes impossible in advanced cases. Some patients can hold an object more steadily if they grasp it with both hands.

The tremor may affect the legs, head, and voice in particular cases. Usually, these are later events, but more patients have an early involvement of head tremor. Head tremor is not specific for essential tremor, nor is the direction of head tremor useful for making a differential diagnosis.

Essential tremor is exacerbated by the conditions listed in Table 12-1, of which anxiety is the most important clinically. These conditions also exacerbate physiological tremor. Embarrassment experienced by the patient in social interactions tends to amplify the tremor. The tremor is diminished by any sedating medication, particularly alcohol. The patient soon learns that an alcoholic drink will temporarily reduce the tremor and allow an hour or two of improved functioning. Some studies have shown an increased rate of subsequent alcoholism among patients with essential tremor.

Electrophysiological studies of essential tremor have shown 7 to 11 Hz periodic paroxysms of motor unit potentials from affected muscles, with simultaneous agonist and antagonist contractions. Only in a small percentage of cases are there true alternating contractions of agonist and antagonist muscles.

Neuropharmacological studies have shown a central mechanism for essential tremor. Intra-arterial beta blockade with propranolol blocks physiological tremor but does not block essential tremor, although intravenously administered propranolol does. The tremor cannot be blocked by limb ischemia or by local procaine anesthesia but is ablated by contralateral ventrolateral thalamotomy. Thus, current evidence suggests that essential tremor is not an exaggeration of physiological tremor.

MANAGEMENT

The mainstay of treatment for essential tremor is beta blockade. Most studies showing the efficacy of beta blockade have used propranolol. Treatment with propranolol has been estimated to improve 50% to 75% of patients with essential tremor but has certain difficulties in practice. Although there is a correlation between plasma propranolol levels and tremor suppression, there is a great patient-to-patient variation in the plasma propranolol levels resulting from a given oral dosage. Patients are usually begun on low dosages (20 mg tid) that are increased as tolerated until improvement occurs or side effects limit further dosage increases. Most patients require 120 to 240 mg/day in divided doses, but some require 320 to 480 mg/day.

Propranolol is contraindicated in bronchospastic pulmonary disease, congestive heart failure, and second- or third-degree heart block, all of which are worsened by the drug. It should not be used in diabetics who use insulin because it can block symptoms of early hypoglycemia. Reduction of pulse rate is common and dose-related. The pulse should not be allowed to fall below 55 beats a minute. Fatigue and exercise intolerance are common side effects of high-dose propranolol.

Propranolol reportedly reduces tremor by 50% to 60%. It is thought to improve hand tremors more than those of the legs, trunk, head, or voice. In addition, propranolol is useful in blocking stress/anxiety exacerbation of essential tremor. It has been used to reduce symptomatic physiologic tremor, particularly in performers with stage fright.

Recent reports have shown the efficacy of several other beta-blockers in essential tremor, including metoprolol, nadolol, and timolol. Because of its beta-one receptor selectivity, metoprolol has been assumed to be safe for use in asthmatic patients. In higher dosages, it blocks beta-two receptors, so metoprolol should not be used at dosages of more than 100 mg/day in patients with bronchospastic lung disease. Nadolol has the advantage of being used in a single daily dose because of its long half-life. Atenolol has poor penetration of the brain and does not improve essential tremor.

Benzodiazepines help suppress essential tremor, but produce sedation in the effective dosage range for tremor improvement. Nevertheless, a small dose before a social engagement may be beneficial. Because alcoholic beverages similarly provide dose-related tremor suppression, many patients have a few drinks before dinner or a social engagement. Primidone (Mysoline) has been reported to improve essential tremor in some patients who are refractory to beta-blockers. Phenobarbital is helpful occasionally.

Only in very severe cases should ventrolateral thalamotomy be considered. In experienced hands, the procedure is relatively safe and effective. Complications include hemiplegia and hemianesthesia. Even in patients with bilateral tremor, thalamotomy should be performed on only one side.

CEREBELLAR TREMOR

Whereas the features of essential tremor are principally postural and contractional, those of cerebellar tremor are mostly postural and intentional. The tremor is inconspicuous at rest, present during sustained postures, and worst during intentional movements. It is seen most often in cerebellar degeneration, in multiple sclerosis, and as a side effect of medications listed in Table 12-2. The frequency of cerebellar tremor is usually 3 to 5 Hz.

The major cerebellar outflow tract, the superior cerebellar peduncle, is usually the site of cerebellar damage in cases of tremor. Lesions of the red nucleus in the brain stem produce a similar disorder (rubral tremor). Cerebellar dysfunction also may produce ataxia, which can be distinguished from tremor by its irregularity and the decomposition of movements it produces. Cerebellar tremor and ataxia frequently coexist, particularly in multiple sclerosis. Electromyographic (EMG) recordings reveal regular 3 to 5 Hz bursts of motor unit discharges alternating between agonist and antagonist muscles.

The finger-to-nose and heel-to-shin tests are the most sensitive methods for revealing cerebellar tremor. The amplitude of the tremor is greatest at the end points of movement at which the greatest amount of fine-tuning of motor feedback data is required. Performing either test more slowly also accentuates the tremor. Patients with cerebellar tremor should be observed for other signs of cerebellar dysfunction, including ataxia, dysdiadochokinesia, loss of checking, and hypotonia.

Treatment of cerebellar tremor is not effective. Some have advocated isoniazid (because of its gamma aminobutyric acid agonist action) and propranolol, but

TABLE 12-3 DIFFERENTIAL DIAGNOSIS OF TREMOR

	Physiologic	Essential	Cerebellar	Parkinsonian
Resting tremor	+	+	+	+ + + +
Postural tremor (against gravity)	+ + + +	+ + +	+ + +	+ +
Contraction tremor (independent of gravity)	+ +	+ + + +	+ +	+
Intention tremor	+ +	+ +	+ + + +	+ +
Frequency (Hz)	6-12	6-11	3-5	3-7 (rest) 7-12 (action)

    + = Mild, rare.
  + + = Moderate, occasional.
 + + + = Prominent, frequent.
+ + + + = Severe, characteristic.

Adapted from Jankovic J, Fahn S: *Ann Intern Med* 1980; 93:462.

these agents have not successfully withstood controlled trials. Stereotactic thalamotomy occasionally helps reduce the tremor but has no effect on the accompanying ataxia.

PARKINSONIAN TREMOR

Tremor is the most conspicuous feature of Parkinson's disease, but bradykinesia and rigidity are more disabling symptoms. Parkinsonian tremor is classified as a resting or "static" tremor. It is of maximal intensity when the patient is not actively moving but is diminished in states of deep relaxation and is absent during sleep. As is true with all tremors, it is exacerbated by anxiety, fatigue, and hypervigilance.

The incidence of parkinsonism is about 1/1000 in the United States. About 70% of parkinsonian patients have tremor as a prominent sign. The patient who has tremor as the predominant sign has a better prognosis than the patient who has severe bradykinesia or rigidity on presentation. Usually reversible, drug-induced parkinsonism is present in over half of patients on high-dose neuroleptic drugs.

The appearance of parkinsonian tremor is so characteristic that it is difficult to confuse it with other tremors. When the patient sits or stands, he has a coarse 3 to 7 Hz rhythmic pronation–supination movement of the wrist with an adduction–abduction movement of the thumb tip across the index finger tip (pill-rolling). The tremor is usually bilateral but asymmetric. The diagnosis of parkinsonism is made easily by observing the characteristic tremor in the patient who walks with small shuffling steps, head and trunk flexed, arms slightly flexed at the elbows, no associated arm swinging movements, fingers and thumb adducted, and fingers extended at the proximal interphalangeal joints and flexed at the metacarpophalangeal joints (see Chapter 24).

Tremor in parkinsonism also may affect the head, producing tremors resembling essential head tremors. The lips, tongue, and voice are frequently tremulous, but symptomatic leg tremors are unusual. In addition to the resting tremor, many parkinsonian patients have an action tremor, usually present at 7 to 12 Hz, which has both postural and intentional components.

Electromyographic studies show the resting tremor to be caused by motor unit discharges from rhythmically alternating antagonist muscle groups. The tremor reflects impairment of basal ganglia motor control mechanisms that results from the dropout of dopaminergic neurons arising in the substantia nigra and projecting to the corpus striatum. A correlation has been shown between tremor severity and the concentration of homovanillic acid (a catecholamine metabolite) in the globus pallidus.

Examination of the patient for parkinsonian tremor includes observing him at rest when stressed with mental status memory and cognitive questions. If the tremor is present at rest and becomes worse with anxiety, the patient is asked to outstretch his arms to see if the tremor lessens. Finally, finger-to-nose testing is performed, which should not disclose tremor unless the patient also has an action tremor. The clinician should assess gait, muscle tone, facial appearance, presence of associated movements, and bradykinesia, and should look for other features of parkinsonism as discussed in Chapter 24. Handwriting in parkinsonism reveals micrographia that is specific for parkinsonian tremor.

Table 12-1 lists the disorders other than idiopathic parkinsonism in which the parkinsonian tremor is seen. The multisystem disorders are discussed in Chapter 24; chronic hepatocerebral degeneration is discussed in Chapter 32. The most common disorder in this group is drug-induced parkinsonism. The patient on phenothiazines, butyrophenones, or related neuroleptic drugs often develops a dose-related parkinsonian syndrome in which tremor may be present but in which bradykinesia, rigidity, and loss of associated movements are more conspicuous. This disorder responds to anticholinergic drugs but not to levodopa. The parkinsonian features may persist for several weeks or months after the neuroleptic drug is discontinued.

Management

Treatment of tremor in idiopathic parkinsonism is usually successful. Levodopa and levodopa–carbidopa combinations (Sinemet) generally improve bradykinesia and rigidity more effectively than they suppress tremor, but tremor is improved in 70% of treated patients. Anticholinergic agents are particularly useful for suppressing tremor, and the combination of anticholinergic drugs and levodopa is the most effective treatment of all. The action tremor of parkinsonism is usually exacerbated by anticholinergic and levodopa therapy but may respond to treatment with propranolol. As in essential tremor, stereotactic ventrolateral thalamotomy is effective for suppressing tremor. Stereotactic thalamotomy for parkinsonian tremor reached its pinnacle in the 1960s; it is performed infrequently today because of the uniform success of medical therapy.

POLYNEUROPATHIC AND MISCELLANEOUS TREMORS

The polyneuropathic syndromes listed in Table 12-1 have been associated with tremor. Usually, the tremor has all the features of an essential tremor except that it is refractory to treatment with propranolol. The mechanism causing the tremor is unknown but is usually explained as resulting from impaired proprioceptive input caused by damage to the peripheral nerves.

Writing tremor is an otherwise unclassified disorder in which a tremor appears only when the patient attempts to write. The tremor is brought out by pronation of the writing hand and is not seen with other postural or intentional activities. It is often classified with writer's cramp under the rubric "occupational neuroses" but is distinct from this focal dystonia. Anticholinergics may help writing tremor, but propranolol is of no therapeutic value. Local anesthesia at the motor point of the pronator teres muscle may be helpful.

Spasmus nutans is a self-limited and reversible syndrome affecting infants 4 to 18 months old in which pendular nystagmus is seen with a rhythmical head tremor. The tremor is worst when the infant is supported in a sitting position. Newer tremor classifications exclude spasmus nutans as a true tremor.

Numerous cases have been reported of a variety of psychogenic tremors. Patients who have conversion or true malingering can manifest static, action, postural, and intentional tremors, usually of the arms. The clinician must exercise his usual degree of caution in assigning this diagnosis.

Bibliography

Desmedt JE (ed): Physiological tremor, pathological tremor, and clonus. *Prog Clin Neurophysiol* 1978; 5:1-218. (Several chapters discuss tremor pathophysiology.)

Fahn S: Differential diagnosis of tremors. *Med Clin North Am* 1972; 56:1363-1375. (Somewhat dated, but still a very useful discussion of the differential diagnosis of tremors.)

Jankovic J, Fahn S: Physiologic and pathologic tremors. Diagnosis, mechanism, and management. *Ann Intern Med* 1980; 93:460-465. (The best short reference, from which Tables 12-1 and 12-3 were adapted.)

Koller WC: Diagnosis and treatment of tremors. *Neurol Clin* 1984; 2:499-514. (The most current source; includes good references on recent treatment trials.)

Young RR, Shanhani BT: Pharmacology of tremor, in: Klawans HL (ed): *Clinical Neuropharmacology.* New York, Raven Press, 1979, pp 39-156. (Useful discussions of tremor pharmacology and treatment.)

13

Dementia

CLINICAL SIGNIFICANCE

Dementia is a global decline of mental function, primarily involving thought and memory and, to a lesser degree, behavior and emotion. Its incidence is unknown; the incidence of severe dementia is 4% to 5% of the population over the age of 65 and that of mild to moderate dementia is approximately 10%. Using these estimates, today there are approximately 1.3 million severe cases of dementia in the United States with an additional 2.8 million patients in the mild to moderate category. It has been estimated that over two-thirds of the approximately 1.5 million elderly individuals in nursing homes are demented, but one-third to one-half of patients with dementia are cared for at home.

In 1900 persons over the age of 65 represented only 3% of the population of the United States; by the 1970s they constituted over 11% (23 million). By the year 2000 to 2030 they will represent over 20% of the population. The fastest growing segment of the U.S. population is the group over age 85, and their mortality has fallen 20% in the last decade. Thus, over the next few decades dementia will become one of the major health care problems in this country.

ETIOLOGY

Dementia has no single cause; it may result from a wide range of disturbances. Because dementia is a clinical syndrome, there are a cluster of symptoms and signs that should lead the physician to search for an underlying cause. Most demented patients have a diagnosable condition, although the number varies from series to series. The accepted common diagnoses in patients with dementia syndrome are listed in Table 13-1. Approximately 70% of patients have Alzheimer's-type dementia, with a lower percentage having other irreversible causes. The physician should attempt to diagnose the patient with dementia because some cases are reversible and treatable. If unrecognized, however, they may progress to irreversible–untreatable types (Table 13-2).

The dementias are classified clinically as cortical (Alzheimer's, Pick's) and subcortical (normal pressure hydrocephalus, multi-infarct dementia, Bin-

TABLE 13-1   COMMON TYPES OF DEMENTIA

Illness	Frequency (% of all dementias)
Alzheimer's disease	50-70
Multi-infarct dementia	10-25
Alcoholic dementia	5-10
Brain tumors	5
Normal pressure hydrocephalus	5
Drug intoxications	3-5*
Miscellaneous (metabolic, degenerative)	7-10
Undiagnosed	3
Pseudodementia (including psychiatric causes)	7

*Low estimate.

TABLE 13-2   CAUSES OF TREATABLE (REVERSIBLE) DEMENTIA

Medications

Sedative-hypnotics
Chloral hydrate
Barbiturates
Benzodiazepines (diazepam, lorazepam, chlorodiazepoxide, flurazepam)
Antihistamines (diphenhydramine)

Antihypertensives
Beta-blockers (propranolol, timolol)
Methyldopa
Reserpine
Clonidine
Guanethidine

Cardiac drugs
Digitalis
Procainamide
Quinidine
Beta-blockers
Atropine

Antidepressants
Tricyclics (amitriptyline, imipramine, desipramine)
Tetracyclics (maprotoline)
Lithium carbonate
Monoamine oxidase (MAO) inhibitors

Antipsychotics
Phenothiazines (chlorpromazine, thioridazine, trifluoperazine)
Butyrophenones (haloperidol)
Lithium carbonate

Anticonvulsants
Phenobarbital
Phenytoin
Primidone
Carbamazepine

Toxins and Heavy Metals
Carbon disulfide
Organophosphates
Alcohol
Carbon monoxide
Arsenic
Thallium
Lead
Copper (Wilson's disease)

TABLE 13-2 *continued*

Vitamin Deficiency States
Vitamin B$_{12}$ deficiency
Pellagra
Folate deficiency

Infections
Neurosyphilis
Whipple's disease
Chronic meningitis (eg, tuberculosis, cryptococcosis)
Cysticercosis
Brain abscess
AIDS encephalopathy (HIV)

Intracranial Diseases
Chronic subdural hematoma
Meningioma
Hydrocephalus
Multiple sclerosis
Epilepsy

Endocrine Diseases
Hypothyroidism
Hyperthyroidism
Addison's disease
Hypoparathyroidism
Hyperparathyroidism
Cushing's disease

Systemic Diseases
Porphyria
Portosystemic encephalopathy
Uremia
Hyponatremia
Pulmonary insufficiency
Anemia-polycythemia
Hypertension
Sarcoidosis

Vascular (Including Collagen-Vascular Diseases)
Systemic lupus erythematosus
Giant cell arteritis
Buerger's disease
Behçet's syndrome
Bilateral carotid artery stenosis

swanger's dementia). The former have prominent cortical signs (aphasia, apraxia, agnosia) without pyramidal signs; the latter have prominent pyramidal signs without cortical signs. This chapter considers the more common types of dementia, emphasizing Alzheimer's disease and the treatable dementias.

SYMPTOMS AND SIGNS

Patients with dementia have significant defects of orientation, memory, intellectual function, judgment, and affect. Memory loss is often the most persistent and earliest symptom. However, the patient who persistently complains of memory loss is unlikely to have organic brain disease; such a complaint correlates better with depression than with brain damage. Memory impairment tends to be minimized by patients with dementia but emphasized by their family or others in contact with them.

Early on, family or friends note that the patient with dementia is "not himself"; this is somewhat nonspecific, but they have seen the onset of the dementia syndrome. Such early, minimal manifestations may be alterations of mood, drive, and enthusiasm for living or projects. The patient may complain of decreased enthusiasm and energy. He or she may lose interest in daily activities and become more anxious. Creativity is diminished, and subsequent goals and achievements are reduced. Any frustration or failure at this point tends to upset the patient more than would normally be expected, and recovery to the baseline state may not occur. As the disease progresses the patient becomes less concerned with social and personal responsibilities and ambitions and is less sensitive to the feelings of others.

Anxiety and frustration increase, producing irritability. Depression may develop, and at this time the patient may begin to complain of memory loss. Complaints of memory loss are worse with recent memory; there may be preservation of remote events (Ribot's law of regression). In practice, Ribot's law is often not at play; the majority of patients have concomitant problems with past memory.

The patient has trouble making decisions and has poor judgment. There is difficulty in dealing with new situations and in initiating and making plans. The patient becomes more intolerant and frustrated and ignores personal hygiene. Affect becomes more flattened; concern for others is diminished. At this time defective recent memory is most obvious, and problems arise in time and space orientation. The patient has difficulty understanding, is easily lost, and often loses his train of thought.

At this stage motor and sensory signs of brain dysfunction may appear. How rapidly the disease progresses, coupled with the site and extent of the brain damage, are the major factors in the development of neurological abnormalities. If the disease is rapidly progressive, signs and symptoms of motor and sensory dysfunction may predominate, whereas in cases with a slow onset, the neurological examination may remain normal for a long period of time.

As the disease worsens, drive and ambition are lost; the patient no longer has his "personality" because emotional responses and feelings are blunted. Gross disorientation is present, recent and remote memory are defective, and the patient is unaware of situations or people. Changes in the level of consciousness are usually not noted until the disease is advanced. The signs and symptoms of early dementia are psychological and are appreciated best on psychological testing or psychiatric examination. As the disease progresses, neurological deterioration is added to the psychological dysfunction. At the time of the early symptoms, a progressive dementia should be recognized and an attempt made at diagnosis and therapy.

ALZHEIMER'S DISEASE

CLINICAL SIGNIFICANCE

Alzheimer's disease is one of the most common degenerative diseases of the brain. Alois Alzheimer first described the characteristic pathological changes. In both the presenile and senile patient, approximately 50% to 70% of all cases of dementia are caused by Alzheimer's disease (Table 13-1). It is estimated that the disease afflicts 1.5 to 2 million Americans and that at least 100,000 of them die every year. Ten billion of the 21 billion dollars spent on nursing care in the United States in 1982 was for the care of patients with this disorder. With the longer survival of the elderly, billions of dollars will be spent in the future for the care of patients with Alzheimer's disease.

ETIOLOGY

The cause of Alzheimer's disease is unknown. Acetylcholine has been found to be substantially reduced in the brains of patients with Alzheimer's type dementia. So is choline acetyltransferase, the enzyme that synthesizes acetylcholine in the brain—much more so than in age-matched controls. The most marked reduction of choline acetyltransferase is in the temporal lobes, less so than in the frontal lobes, hippocampus, and amygdala. These areas are vital to cognition, memory, and emotional control. The degree of cognitive deficit during life is proportional to the loss of choline acetyltransferase. Not all cholinergic neurons are equally affected in Alzheimer's disease, however. Cortical degeneration of the basal forebrain (nucleus basalis of Meynert) is a common finding. Younger patients, who have a more rapid progression of dementia, have a greater degree of loss of choline acetyltransferase activity than do elderly patients. Muscarinic (acetyl-choline) receptors in the brain do not seem to be decreased. By the time Alzheimer's disease is recognized clinically, irreversible structural damage has already occurred.

There is a familial or genetic predisposition in some cases of Alzheimer's disease. Approximately 5% to 10% of patients have a positive family history for this condition with what appear to be an autosomal-dominant mode of inheritance. Most cases occur sporadically, but the risk of developing the disease at any given age is increased to four- to fivefold among first degree relatives of Alzheimer probands.

Alzheimer's disease occurs with great regularity in individuals with Down's syndrome (trisomy 21). The brains of these patients who survive past their fourth decade show characteristic features of Alzheimer's disease as well as a decrease in acetylcholine. Recently, a gene has been located on chromosome 21 that is likely responsible for the development of Alzheimer's disease. The finding of elevated levels of aluminum in the brains of Alzheimer's disease has not been corroborated, nor has the disease been transmitted to experimental animals or from human to human. A decline in cholinergic activity in the brain correlates with symptoms of Alzheimer's disease, but the reason for the decline in cholinergic activity is not known.

SYMPTOMS AND SIGNS

Alzheimer's disease is the quintessential dementing illness. It usually begins in the sixth or seventh decade and is associated with defects of higher cognitive functioning and global intellectual decline. Thought processes are slowed and memory is impaired. Judgment is impaired as is the ability to concentrate. Personality changes occur and language disturbances frequently develop (aphasia, anomia). Depression occurs in 25% of patients. Motor signs are uncommon early, but, as the disease develops, reflex changes may develop and parkinsonian signs appear in 25% of patients. Seizures occur in 10%, and myoclonus may also be present. In the seventh decade of life or later, a progressive decline of global intellectual functions may develop, at times similar to the more standard presentation. The patient with Down's syndrome who lives past the age of 30 may demonstrate further decline in cognitive functions, resulting from Alzheimer's disease. Approximately 50% of patients with Alzheimer's disease die within five years of diagnosis; only 18% are alive ten years later.

LABORATORY TESTS

Table 13-3 outlines the medical workup of the demented patient. Because the diagnosis of Alzheimer's is ultimately made at postmortem examination, evaluation is directed toward determining whether a reversible–treatable process is responsible for the dementia. There is no specific diagnostic test for Alzheimer's disease. A CT scan frequently demonstrates cerebral atrophy, but it cannot differentiate atrophy from normal aging. Mental status testing is quite important; more formal neuropsychiatric tests can document the presence of higher cortical dysfunction, although a premorbid baseline will not be known. Serial testing helps to quantify intellectual deterioration. The EEG often shows generalized, nonspecific slowing. Examination of CSF usually is not necessary, but increased CSF protein levels are occasionally noted. Drug screens and heavy metal analysis may also be necessary in selected cases to rule out treatable causes (see section "Treatable Dementia"). Brain biopsy is not indicated for the elderly patient whose clinical course seems to be compatible with Alzheimer's disease and who does not have evidence of other treatable diseases.

At autopsy there is evidence of cerebral atrophy, usually diffuse, and most severe in the frontal and temporal lobes. Senile plaques and neurofibrillary tangles are characteristic pathologic changes. Neurofibrillary tangles are composed of paired helical filaments; they occur in a high proportion of demented patients, although their presence is not specific for Alzheimer's disease. The number of senile plaques present correlates with the severity of the dementia.

TABLE 13-3 BASIC EVALUATION OF THE DEMENTIA PATIENT

Medical history and examination (including neurological examination)
Mental status examination
Psychometric examination
Laboratory tests
  -CBC, blood chemistry profile (including electrolytes, calcium, glucose, liver function tests)
  -VDRL, ESR, T_4, vitamin B_{12} level
  -CT of head
  -EEG
  -Chest x-ray
Additional tests for selected cases
  -Drug screen
  -Heavy metal analysis of urine and blood
  -EMG
  -Evoked potentials
  -CSF examination with studies for fungal or neoplastic disease
  -Neuropsychiatric tests

Widespread axonal degeneration in the optic nerves is another common (albeit only recently recognized) pathological finding. It may be an indication of a sensory system degeneration that occurs in Alzheiner's disease (and not other dementias).

DIAGNOSIS

The diagnosis of Alzheimer's disease is based on the development of a progressive dementia without focal changes when other diagnoses have been excluded. The list of other possible diseases is long and will be covered in a subsequent section of this chapter. The major differential diagnosis includes alcoholic dementia, pseudodementia, and communicating hydrocephalus. Table 13-4 lists the proposed National Institutes of Health criteria for the clinical diagnosis of Alzheimer's disease.

MANAGEMENT

After the diagnosis has been established, there are a number of management goals. The patient's personal safety should be maintained and safety issues discussed with the patient's family. Because the patient may be disoriented and confused, he or she is vulnerable to accidents. Poor judgment and slowed motor reaction times often make it best to restrict driving privileges. The patient's health must be monitored closely because he may not complain of, or recognize potentially life threatening illnesses.

Calendars and memory aids can help maintain the patient's orientation. A well-established daily routine will help reduce confusion. Catastrophic reactions should be avoided (for example, moving the patient out of a structured environment). Family members need to be supported and advised about how they can find an appropriate nursing home when it becomes necessary. Appropriate reading material (see "Suggested Reading for Caregivers") can be given to the family, and they can be referred to their local Alzheimer's disease chapter or to another formal support group.

There is no specific treatment for Alzheimer's disease. Many pharmacologic agents have been used, but none has reversed the dementia significantly. Because of the known brain cholinergic defect in the brain, attempts have been made to increase central acetylcholine levels. The use of oral choline and lecithin has been unrewarding. The inhibition of central acetylcholinesterase with physostigmine, coupled with oral lecithin, has resulted in improvements in neuropsychological testing, but there are no long-term clinical benefits. Chelation therapy is of *absolutely no benefit*. The use of various vasodilators (papaverine, hydergine) may be comforting to the physician and to the family but they are not of proven efficacy. Because some patients seem to improve modestly on hydergine, it may be used as long as it does not cause significant side effects. Vasodilator drugs, such as papaverine, should be avoided in the elderly patient because of possible hypotension.

Because physostigmine has been shown to temporarily improve memory (correlated with its concentration in the spinal fluid) studies are in progress to constantly infuse bethanecol chloride into the ventricular CSF. The subjective response to this form of therapy has been encouraging, with reports of improved cognitive and social functions during the drug infusion and few side effects.

TABLE 13-4 CLINICAL CRITERIA FOR THE DIAGNOSIS OF ALZHEIMER'S DISEASE

Criteria for clinical diagnosis of PROBABLE Alzheimer's disease include:
- Dementia established by clinical examination and documented by the Mini-Mental Test, Blessed Dementia Scale, or similar examination, and confirmed by neuropsychological tests;
- Deficits in two or more areas of cognition;
- Progressive worsening of memory and other cognitive functions;
- No disturbance of consciousness;
- Onset between ages 40 and 90, most often after age 65; and
- Absence of systemic disorders or other brain diseases that alone could account for progressive deficits in memory and cognition.

The diagnosis of PROBABLE Alzheimer's disease is supported by:
- Progressive deterioration of specific cognitive functions such as language (aphasia), motor skills (apraxia), and perception (agnosia);
- Impaired activities of daily living and altered patterns of behavior;
- Family history of similar disorders, particularly if confirmed neuropathologically;
- Laboratory results of:
  Normal lumbar puncture as evaluated by standard techniques;
  Normal pattern or nonspecific changes in EEG, eg, increased slow-wave activity; and
  Evidence of cerebral atrophy on CT with progression documented by serial observation.

Other clinical features consistent with the diagnosis of PROBABLE Alzheimer's disease, after exclusion of causes of dementia other than Alzheimer's disease, include:
- Plateaus in the course of progression of the illness;
- Associated symptoms of depression, insomnia, incontinence, delusions, illusions, hallucinations, catastrophic verbal, emotional, or physical outbursts, sexual disorders, and weight loss;
- Other neurologic abnormalities in some patients, especially with more advanced disease and including motor signs such as increased muscle tone, myoclonus, or gait disorder;
- Seizures in advanced disease; and
- CT normal for age.

Features that make the diagnosis of PROBABLE Alzheimer's disease uncertain or unlikely include:
- Sudden, apoplectic onset;
- Focal neurologic findings such as hemiparesis, sensory loss, visual field deficits, and incoordination early in the course of the illness; and
- Seizures or gait disturbances at the onset or very early in the course of the illness.

Clinical diagnosis of POSSIBLE Alzheimer's disease:
- May be made on the basis of the dementia syndrome, in the absence of other neurologic, psychiatric, or systemic disorders sufficient to cause dementia, and in the presence of variations in onset, presentation, or clinical course;
- May be made in the presence of a second systemic or brain disorder sufficient to produce dementia but that is not considered to be the cause of the dementia; and
- Should be used in research studies when a single, gradually progressive severe cognitive deficit is identified in the absence of other identifiable cause.

Criteria for diagnosis of DEFINITE Alzheimer's disease are:
- The clinical criteria for probable Alzheimer's disease; and
- Histopathologic evidence from a biopsy or autopsy.

Classification of Alzheimer's disease for research purposes should specify features that may differentiate subtypes of the disorder, such as:
- Familial occurrence;
- Onset before age 65;
- Presence of trisomy 21; and
- Coexistence of other relevant conditions, such as Parkinson's disease.

Criteria are those of the NIH–Alzheimer's Disease and Related Disorder Association (NINCDS–ADRDA group). See McKhann et al, Bibliography.

Formal neuropsychiatric testing of these patients did not document significant improvement, however. Research in this area is being carried out at several centers, and its true efficacy remains to be shown. Tetrahydroaminoacridine (THA), a centrally active anticholinesterase, has recently been shown to produce significant improvement in memory functions of a group of patients in the middle and late stages of suspected Alzheimer's disease. Although further clinical studies will be required before a clear assessment can be made of the role of THA in the treatment of the disease, these initial results are most encouraging.

Naloxone, an opiate antagonist, has been reported to produce transient improvement in memory of patients with Alzheimer's disease, but the results are only transient and large amounts of medication are required. This method of treatment has no clinical applicability at the present time.

About 25% of Alzheimer's disease patients become depressed. Tricyclic antidepressants may be of benefit, especially if vegetative symptoms are present. Drugs have anticholinergic activity, however, so they may increase the degree of confusion. Neuroleptic agents such as haloperidol or chlorpromazine may help control agitation, but they may overly sedate the patient or produce extrapyramidal signs.

WHEN TO CONSULT

When the patient first develops symptoms of dementia, a neurologist should be consulted. A follow-up examination can be scheduled for neuropsychiatric testing to assess the patient's rate of intellectual decline. The neurologist can help determine the type of dementia process and help direct a cost-efficient evaluation.

PATIENT EDUCATION

There are numerous family support groups for demented patients and their families. There are both local and national chapters of the Alzheimer's Disease Association (see Appendix). See the end of the chapter for a list of self-help books suggested by the Alzheimer's Disease Society.

PICK'S DISEASE

Pick's disease is a rare degenerative disease that usually occurs in the presenium. It's incidence is less than 2% that of Alzheimer's disease. It is transmitted as an autosomal dominant and is slightly more common in females. The clinical presentation is similar to Alzheimer's disease and is often impossible to differentiate premortem. Language disturbances (echolalia, dysphasia) may be the first symptoms of Pick's disease; they have a late onset in Alzheimer's disease. Throughout the course of Pick's disease, the language disturbance predominates; significant memory loss and dyspraxia are uncommon. Focal atrophy of the brain (frontal and temporal lobes, sparing the parietal lobes) may be seen on CT and can help in differentiating Pick's from Alzheimer's disease. At autopsy, the neurofibrillary tangles and neuritic plaques typical of Alzheimer's disease are absent. Swollen neurons with silver-staining inclusions (Pick bodies) are evident and diagnostic. There is no effective therapy for Pick's disease. The clinical approach is the same as that of Alzheimer's disease.

NORMAL PRESSURE HYDROCEPHALUS

CLINICAL SIGNIFICANCE

Normal pressure hydrocephalus (NPH) is a symptom complex associated with panventricular dilatation and normal CSF pressure. The clinical triad in adults consists of dementia, apraxic gait (or other gait disturbances) and urinary urge incontinence. NPH is clinically significant because it is one of the most treatable dementias. Because there is no intraventricular block, NPH is also known as communicating hydrocephalus.

ETIOLOGY

Normal pressure hydrocephalus frequently occurs on an idiopathic basis. Infrequently, it is associated with subarachnoid hemorrhage, head trauma, meningitis (as a sequela), or surgical procedures on the posterior fossa. Scarring or fibrosis of the meninges, intermittent blockage of the aqueduct of Sylvius, edema, and clogging of the arachnoid granulations blocking CSF resorption have all been implicated as possible mechanisms for the development of NPH.

SYMPTOMS AND SIGNS

The disease is characterized by the insidious onset of the triad of dementia, apraxia of gait, and urinary urge incontinence. Headache and signs of increased intracranial pressure do not occur. The dementia may be global and mild but is rarely an isolated abnormality. The gait disturbance, characteristically described as apraxia or "glue-footed," occurs, and episodes of falling are common. The gait may be wide-based, shuffling, and slow. In the most severe form of the disorder, attempts at self ambulation are inhibited. Incontinence, initially sporadic, usually follows the mental and gait disturbances. The patient frequently complains of urinary urgency that progresses to urge incontinence and, rarely, to overflow incontinence. Rectal incontinence is rare. The course of NPH is associated with increasing neurological symptoms, although short periods of remission sometimes occur. In general, the gait disturbance is the earliest and most severe disturbance.

LABORATORY TESTS

A CT scan demonstrates panventricular dilation, usually without evidence of cortical atrophy, although the latter may occur. The injection of a radioactive isotope into the CSF provides a measure of CSF flow dynamics. In NPH, the classical cisternogram shows retention of the isotope in the ventricles for 48 hours, with delayed or absent flow over the convexities. Intrathecal injection of metrizamide, with sequential CT scans at 24 and 48 hours, also can be used to follow the CSF circulation. Because leptomeningeal carcinomatosis or occult chronic meningitis may initially present as NPH, careful CSF analysis should be performed. Neuropsychological testing can quantitate the degree of dementia, and a cystometrogram can test for the presence of a neurogenic bladder. The EEG findings may be nonspecific, at times showing high voltage slow waves directed more frontally.

DIAGNOSIS

The diagnosis of NPH is made when the triad of symptoms are associated with CT changes. Gait disturbance is usually the initial presentation, before dementia develops. The pattern of primary panventricular dilatation without significant cortical atrophy is the opposite of that seen in Alzheimer's disease, in which the ventricles enlarge to fill the void left by the atrophic brain (hydrocephalus *ex vacuo*). Some neurologists believe that NPH will transiently improve following the removal of 30 mL of CSF, and that this response predicts the success of a CSF shunt.

MANAGEMENT

The treatment of NPH is neurosurgical. Shunting is usually performed from the ventricle into the peritoneum, although lumboperitoneal shunts have also been used. The results of surgical shunting vary widely. Some patients respond quickly and dramatically to shunting, whereas others do not improve. Usually the gait disturbance and incontinence respond more quickly than does the dementia. In one series of patients with NPH, 74% with the full triad of symptoms and signs responded to shunting. A recent review from the Mayo Clinic shows that the typical patient has a 75% chance of some improvement after shunting and a 40% chance of satisfactory enduring results (median duration 24 months). In their experience, however, patients had a 31% likelihood of complications from the procedure itself. Patients who had symptoms for less than two years were most likely to improve. Although CT played an important role in diagnosis and follow-up, ventricular size or degree of atrophy did not correlate with response.

WHEN TO CONSULT

The generalist should consult the neurologist to evaluate the diagnosis and the likelihood of improvement with shunting in any patient with clinical or CT evidence of NPH.

ARTERIOSCLEROTIC MULTI-INFARCT DEMENTIA

CLINICAL SIGNIFICANCE AND ETIOLOGY

Of dementia cases, 20% to 25% have a vascular cause. The most common vascular etiology is multiple strokes, producing the syndrome called multi-infarct dementia. These strokes may be embolic, thrombotic, or hemorrhagic. Cognitive impairment usually becomes evident when 50 to 100 grams of the cerebral hemisphere has been destroyed. Multiple small subcortical infarcts (lacunae) can also give rise to dementia, but the most common cause of multi-infarct dementia is thromboembolism. Dementia has been reported to be caused by multiple stenoses or occlusions of the extracranial arteries leading to the brain, primarily of both carotid arteries. In these rare patients, the etiology seems to be reduced cerebral blood flow. Following carotid endarterectomy, improvement has been noted and has been documented on neuropsychiatric testing. Both systemic lupus erythematosus and thrombangitis obliterans may involve small vessels. Binswanger's dementia, characterized by subcortical demyelination, usually occurs in the hypertensive patient and may present with progressive dementia and disturbances of gait. Once considered to be rare, it is now believed that this disease is common in hypertensive patients.

SYMPTOMS AND SIGNS

When it occurs as a primary disorder, multi-infarct dementia can be identified by its sudden onset associated with focal neurological signs in hypertensive patients who have a stepwise decline in intellectual function. Binswanger's disease (subcortical arteriosclerotic encephalopathy) tends to be progressive; the dementia is coupled with signs of focal cerebral disease, such as hemiparesis or aphasia. Progression of this disease is slow, usually over five to ten years, and convulsive episodes may develop. Clinical similarities exist between Binswanger's disease and multi-infarct dementia, although there are pathological differences.

In general, symptoms and signs associated with arteriosclerotic or multi-infarct dementia states are those of progressive decline of higher cortical function associated with focal or multifocal signs, especially sensory, motor, and visual. These may initially be transient, but fixed deficits soon develop. Multi-infarct dementia and Binswanger's disease are subcortical dementias with prominent pyramidal signs.

LABORATORY TESTS

Neurodiagnostic tests, including CT and neuropsychiatric testing, can help determine vascular causes of dementia. The basic screening tests for dementia (Table 13-3) should be performed. The erythrocyte sedimentation rate should always be measured; it will be elevated in the majority of patients with collagen–vascular disease as a cause of their multiple small-vessel occlusions. Holter monitoring should also be obtained in the patient with suspected vascular dementia, especially if multiple embolic episodes are possible.

In the patient with global decline in functions associated with carotid artery bruits, noninvasive vascular studies may be performed to determine if blood flow is reduced. If so, cerebral angiography can be performed on the selected patient; if multiple extracranial stenoses are evident, cognitive function may improve following endarterectomy. Only rare patients improve with this approach.

MANAGEMENT

Control of blood pressure is necessary in most patients who have vascular dementia. It is important that the antihypertensive drug being utilized does not contribute to the dementia (Table 13-2). Other than antihypertensive medications, no other drugs seem to be beneficial. The cessation of cigarette smoking in normotensive patients with multi-infarct dementia is associated with improvement of cognition. Overall, although control of risk factors may produce some improvement, multi-infarct dementia is often irreversible.

WHEN TO CONSULT

In the patient with an abrupt loss of cognitive functions or with multiple episodes of neurological deterioration associated with memory impairment it is best to obtain neurological consultation to help determine the cause and to reassure the primary care physician and the family.

TREATABLE DEMENTIA

CLINICAL SIGNIFICANCE

Dementia is often assumed to be a chronic, irreversible condition. It is true that most patients with dementia have an irreversible illness, but 10% of those with apparent dementia have a potentially treatable disorder. Another 10% are not really demented, but have significant depression or transient confusional states. The clinician must first determine whether the patient is demented. An error rate has been reported of from 10% to 50% of the diagnosis of dementia on first evaluation.

Some patients who show transient improvement following treatment do not have reversible dementia. In one recent report of patients with possible reversible dementia, only 3 of 92 returned to their normal mental status. Most of the patients in the series with reversible dementia also had coexistent irreversible dementia. However, many of these patients had improved cognitive functions after treatment of coexistent previously undiagnosed or untreated medical illnesses.

ETIOLOGY

Many of the causes of potentially reversible dementia are listed in Table 13-2. The most common cause is medication, either single drugs or polypharmacy. In general, patients with reversible dementia have a shorter duration of symptoms, are less demented, and tend to receive more prescription drugs (usually sedative-hypnotic or antihypertensive drugs). A discussion of the more common categories of treatable dementia follows.

Depression

Of patients labeled demented, 8% to 15% are in fact depressed. Depression in the elderly often mimics dementia, producing the syndrome of pseudodementia. Depression and dementia may coexist: 20% to 30% of demented patients have an associated depressive reaction. Depression can be mistaken for dementia because of an inadequate mental status examination. Such patients often have a history of significant depressive illnesses and only a modest degree of memory loss. Treatment with antidepressant medications is required.

Patients with the following psychiatric disorders may be occasionally misdiagnosed as having dementia: manic-depressive state, atypical psychosis, anxiety, hysterical conversion reaction, post-traumatic neurosis, malingering, and personality disorder. Individuals with benign senescent forgetfulness have transiently impaired recall of unimportant past experiences, but (unlike the demented patient) they can remember and relate the essentials of their experience. Those who forget where they put their eyeglasses probably have benign senescent forgetfulness, whereas those who forget that they wear glasses are more likely to have dementia.

Drugs and Toxins

In the elderly, polypharmacy is, unfortunately, widespread. Furthermore, there are age-related changes in the pharmacokinetics of drugs. Almost any drug taken in large quantities will cause mental status impairment in the elderly. Many drugs listed in Table 13-2 can cause apparent dementia when taken in excessive dosages. The major groups of drugs reported to cause "dementia" are 1) psychotropics 2) antihypertensives, 3) anticonvulsants, 4) anticholinergics and 5) sedative-hypnotics.

Metabolic Disorders

Thyroid disorders are the most common endocrinopathies that cause reversible impairment of mental status. Either hypothyroidism or apathetic hyperthyroidism may cause reversible dementia. Frequent episodes of hypoglycemia can also cause a progressive dementia. Confusion and lethargy may result from hyperthyroidism or hypercalcemia. Hepatic insufficiency may cause global cognitive impairment; Cushing's syndrome may cause reversible dementia. Treatment of Wilson's disease with penicillamine improves the mental status of some patients.

Intracranial Disorders

Any space-occupying intracranial lesion may produce memory loss or dementia. Lesions producing dementia without localizing signs include: meningioma (especially if located frontally), subdural hematoma and hydrocephalus. The frontal lobe is one area where tumors often cause a dementia syndrome. Chronic subdural hematoma may be overlooked in the elderly patient when a history of trauma is not prominent. Occasionally, progressive deterioration in a patient with a subdural hematoma is caused by a nonconvulsive seizure that can be reversed when the seizures are treated. In patients with multiple sclerosis, dementia is seen occasionally. It may exacerbate and remit just as the primary illness does.

Vitamin Deficiency States

Vitamin B_{12} deficiency may cause memory deficits that predate abnormalities in the bone marrow and peripheral blood. The dementia of vitamin B_{12} deficiency and folate deficiency may reverse after replacement therapy, but if the duration of deficiency is long, dementia may not reverse. Vitamin B_1 (thiamine) deficiency can lead to Korsakoff's psychosis, with specific impairment of recent memory. Last, general malnutrition is linked to cognitive impairment.

Metals and Toxins

Toxic exposure to certain heavy metals (lead, mercury, thallium, arsenic) can cause a dementing illness that is reversible with chelation therapy. Long-term exposure to organic agents such as carbon disulfide, trichlorethylene, toluene, carbon monoxide, and organophosphates can also lead to abnormalities of mental status that reverse when the offending substance is eliminated. Alcohol and other drugs of abuse can produce dementia that may remit with abstinence.

Cardiovascular Problems

Dementia has been noted in patients with myocardial infarction, atrial myxoma, and bilateral carotid artery disease. Some cases of dementia in patients with heart block improve with cardiac pacing. Multi-infarct dementia often is treatable (eg, with antihypertensive drugs) but is not reversible.

Infectious Diseases

Chronic meningitis (due to cryptococcosis, tuberculosis, and blastomycosis) may cause primary changes in mental status that may resemble dementia. The underlying dementia of neurosyphilis (uncommon but rising in incidence) can be partially reversed with therapy. Progressive multifocal leukoencephalopathy, Whipple's disease, and acquired immune deficiency syndrome (AIDS) may be marked by dementia, but treatment is unsatisfactory in reversing the condition.

Collagen Vascular Diseases

Some collagen-vascular disorders, including systemic lupus erythematosus, Buerger's, sarcoid, and Behçet's disease may cause a reversible dementia, usually on the basis of small vessel inflammatory disease.

LABORATORY TESTS AND DIAGNOSIS
The basic medical evaluation for the patient with dementia is listed in Table 13-3. If the dementia is mild and has come on rather suddenly, a reversible condition is more likely to be present. A careful evaluation of the patient's medications is mandatory because of the high incidence of polypharmacy as a cause of mental impairment in the elderly. The EEG may show changes caused by toxic or metabolic disturbances, or may show evidence of frequent temporal lobe seizures. If chronic or occult meningitis is considered, CSF analysis should be performed. A CT scan should be performed in all patients with dementia. It can give evidence as to the degree of cortical atrophy, the presence of ventriculomegaly, and the presence of occult, space-occupying lesions. More specific investigations for particular etiologies should be ordered by the neurologist.

MANAGEMENT
A wide variety of conditions, both psychiatric and nonpsychiatric, can produce a reversible dementia syndrome. An attempt should be made to find any treatable causes of the dementia, although many patients with a "reversible" dementia do not reverse to normal and may continue to show progressive dementia. If polypharmacy and social and sensory deprivation are avoided, the patient may be able to use his remaining intellectual functions to the maximum extent.

Suggested Reading for Caregivers of Alzheimer's Patients

Brown, DS: *Handle With Care: A Question of Alzheimer's*. Buffalo, NY, Prometheus Books, 1985.

Heston, LL, White, JA: *Dementia: A Practical Guide to Alzheimer's Disease and Related Illness*. New York, W.H. Freeman, 1983.

Mace, NL, Rabins, PV: *The 36-Hour Day*. Baltimore, Johns Hopkins University Press, 1981.

Powell, LS, Courtice, K: *Alzheimer's Disease: A Guide for Families*. Reading, PA, Addison-Wesley, 1983.

Reisberg, B: *A Guide to Alzheimer's Disease*. New York, Free Press, 1981.

Roach, M: *Another Name for Madness.* Boston, Houghton Mifflin, 1985.

Zarit, SH, Orr, NK, Zarit, JM: *Caring for the Patient with Alzheimer's Disease: Families under Stress.* New York, New York University Press, 1985.

Bibliography

Adams RD, Fisher CM, Hakim S, et al: Symptomatic occult hydrocephalus with "normal" cerebrospinal fluid pressure: a treatable syndrome. *N Engl J Med* 1965; 273:117-126. (The classic article, first describing the syndrome of NPH in English literature).

Cummings J, Benson DF, LoVerme S: Reversible dementia. Illustrative cases, definition, and review. *JAMA* 1980; 243:2434-2439. (Comprehensive review of treatable dementias.)

Hachinski V: Multi-infarct dementia. *Neurol Clin* 1983; 1:27-36. (Best review of multi-infarct dementia.)

Hollister LE: Alzheimer's disease. Is it worth treating? *Drugs* 1985; 29:483-488. (Reviews drug treatment for Alzheimer's disease.)

Khachaturian ZS: Diagnosis of Alzheimer's disease. *Arch Neurol* 1985; 42:1097-1106. (Results of a joint conference on Alzheimer's disease; provides much more factual information than the McKhann reference, but both should be read.)

Kokmen E: Dementia-Alzheimer type. *Mayo Clin Proc* 1984; 59:35-42. (Concise overview of all aspects of Alzheimer's disease.)

Larson EB, Reifler BV, Featherstone HJ: Dementia in elderly outpatients: A prospective study. *Ann Intern Med* 1984; 100:417-423. (Reviews outpatient study of dementia victims; emphasizes that all treatable cases may not be reversible.)

Mace NL, Rabins PV: *The 36-Hour Day: A Family Guide to Caring for Persons with Alzheimer's Disease, Related Dementing Illnesses, and Memory Loss in Later Life.* Baltimore, Johns Hopkins U. Press, 1981. (Excellent guide for family members and professionals who deal with dementia victims.)

McKhann G, Drachman D, Folstein M: Clinical diagnosis of Alzheimer's disease: Report of the NINCDS-ADRDA Work Group under the auspices of Department of Health and Human Services Task Force on Alzheimer's Disease. *Neurology* 1984; 34:939-944. (Reviews criteria for clinical diagnosis of Alzheimer's disease.)

Meyer JS, Judd BW, Tawakinat T, et al: Improved cognition after control of risk factors for multi-infarct dementia. *JAMA* 1986;256:2203-2209. (Improvement of risk factors does produce improvement in cognition in patients with multi-infarct dementia).

Peterson RC, Mokri B, Laws ER Jr: Surgical treatment of idiopathic hydrocephalus in elderly patients. *Neurology* 1985; 35:307-311. (Reviews surgical results with long-term follow-up of 45 patients with NPH.)

Roca RP, Klein LE, Kirby SM, et al: Recognition of dementia among medical patients. *Arch Intern Med* 1984; 144:73-75. (Johns Hopkins Medical School study of how often dementia is misdiagnosed.)

Rossor MN: Dementia. *Lancet* 1982; 2:1200-1204. (Reviews the role of neurotransmitters in dementia syndromes.)

Small GW, Jarvik LF: The dementia syndrome. *Lancet* 1982; 2:1443-1446. (Gives a synopsis of the major types of dementia.)

Summers WK Majorski LV, Marsh GM, et al: Oral tetrahydroaminoacridine in long-term treatment of senile dementia, Alzheimer type. *N Engl J Med* 1986;315: 1241-1245. (First study to show dramatic improvement in memory function of a group of Alzheimer's patients given an oral medication [THA, a central anticholinesterase].)

Terry RD, Katzman R: Senile dementia of the Alzheimer type. *Ann Neurol* 1983; 14:497-506. (Good clinical and pathophysiologic review.)

Wells CE: *Dementia*. Philadelphia, FA Davis, 1977. (Comprehensive monograph covering all aspects of the dementia syndrome.)

14

Delirium

The diagnosis and management of the acutely confused patient is one of the more challenging activities in medicine. The clinician must be both thorough in considering a large number of etiologic factors, and efficient in rapidly reducing the patient's agitation and the family's anxiety.

A number of terms have been used to describe the acutely confused patient: acute confusional state, toxic psychosis, acute brain syndrome, delirium, beclouded dementia, and primary mental confusion. Although there may be subtle characteristics distinguishing each of these syndromes, clinically it is more useful to lump them all under the rubric delirium. According to Lipowski (1967), delirium has the following characteristics:

"(1) The individual is awake and usually capable of responding verbally;

"(2) There is evidence of impairment of thinking, memory, perception, and attention. This impairment tends to fluctuate irregularly over time;

"(3) There is impaired ability to comprehend the environment and internal perceptions in accordance with the individual's past experience and knowledge (as a result of item 2), i.e., defective reality testing;

"(4) There is usually a concomitant change in the frequency of the EEG pattern, which tends to vary pari passu with the level of cognition."

ETIOLOGY

Delirium is best regarded as the behavioral manifestation of an acute, diffuse, and potentially reversible dysfunction of brain neuronal metabolism. As such, any disorder capable of producing such an insult can provoke delirium. When the insult is stopped and brain neuronal metabolism returns to normal, the delirium will clear. If the insult becomes more severe, the patient will drift into stupor, then coma (Chapter 36). Several of the most common causes of delirium are described here.

1. *Drug intoxication.* The elderly or chronically ill patient is highly susceptible to delirium due to intoxication from ostensibly therapeutic doses of many

prescription drugs. The intoxication is the result of decreased clearance and increased sensitivity to these agents. Psychotropic drugs are the most obvious offenders, but delirium can also be produced by digitalis, beta-blockers, calcium-channel blockers, cimetidine, and anticholinergics. Occult alcohol intoxication is a very common cause of episodic confusion.

2. *Drug withdrawal.* Reduction in dosage or absolute abstinence from alcohol or any other central nervous system depressant drug that has been taken over a long period can provoke drug withdrawal delirium. Delirium tremens is the best known syndrome in this regard (Chapter 33). Such a patient may become acutely confused shortly after a hospital admission or just into the course of a viral gastroenteritis, when he or she cannot eat or drink and, hence, must stop consuming alcohol.

3. *Metabolic disturbances.* Delirium can herald major organ system failure, including portosystemic encephalopathy (Chapter 33), uremic encephalopathy, pulmonary failure, and congestive heart failure. In instances of portosystemic and uremic encephalopathy, the brain is assaulted by blood-borne toxins. In pulmonary failure, neuronal metabolism is impaired by hypoxemia and hypercapnia. In congestive heart failure, cardiac output falls and cerebral perfusion pressure drops. Myocardial infarction and pulmonary embolism may present as delirium as a result of hypoxemia and impaired cardiac output. Fluid and electrolyte imbalances, particularly of sodium and calcium, can provoke delirium. Hypoglycemia should always be considered in the acutely delirious patient.

4. *Infections.* Systemic infections and fever from any source can provoke delirium, particularly in the elderly and in children. An acute confusional syndrome may be the most conspicuous sign of pneumococcal pneumonia in the octogenarian. Patients with meningitis and encephalitis usually develop a confusional state before coma ensues.

5. *Seizures.* In the patient with an unwitnessed seizure, a postictal confusional state may be reported. In the rare patient with complex partial status epilepticus, confusion lasting several days can be caused by persistent ictal activity.

6. *Focal and multifocal structural brain lesions.* Strokes, tumors, and other focal brain lesions can produce a confusional state if bilateral hemispheric function is impaired or if right parietal function is suddenly affected. Generally, focal neurologic signs are elicited in such cases. Subarachnoid hemorrhage can produce headache and confusion, but few other signs, in its early stage.

7. *Systemic disease.* Systemic disorders, including connective tissue diseases, bacterial endocarditis, widely metastatic carcinoma, and acute intermittent porphyria, often produce delirium.

8. *Head injury.* Diffuse closed-head injury with concussions or cerebral contusions often features a confusional state.

9. *Predisposing factors.* Delirium is often multifactorial and usually has predisposing factors. The patient with dementia has a greatly diminished "cerebral reserve" so that seemingly minor insults may provoke delirium. Minor electrolyte and hematologic abnormalities, such as borderline hyponatremia and anemia, may be additive in predisposing the patient with fever or drug intoxication to develop delirium. Old age alone is a predisposing factor.

Symptoms and Signs

The onset of delirium can be gradual, as in portosystemic encephalopathy, or sudden, as in acute hypoglycemia. In delirium of gradual onset, the floridly delirious state has a prodrome of more mild global cognitive impairment, usually most pronounced for attention and concentration. Such a patient may be easily distracted, tired, restless, and irritable. The prodrome is not conspicuous and is very transient in cases of delirium of sudden onset.

The severity of delirium fluctuates throughout the day, often from minute to minute. There may be brief intervals of relative lucidity between more floridly delirious episodes. Many patients reach the peak of delirium at night (sundowning) when visual, auditory, and other sensory cues are minimal.

Although there is global impairment of all mental functions in such a patient, the major defect is in selective attention. The patient is incapable of focusing his complete attention on the task at hand because of his being constantly distracted by irrelevant competing stimuli. For example, the clinician may find, while attempting to interview a delirious patient, that any noise or movement in the room will command the attention and interrupt the train of thought of the patient. He will then not be able to return to his previous task and to continue a coherent conversation. This type of distraction may occur several times per minute.

There is diminished alertness and awareness of the environment, producing disorientation for place and time. Temporal disorientation is the earliest impairment, followed by spatial disorientation. It is rare for delirium to be so severe that personal identity is forgotten. The patient usually believes he is at home or in some other familiar environment. Date disorientation often places the patient several or many years earlier in his life. The degree of disorientation is directly proportional to the severity of the delirium.

The train of thought becomes impaired early in delirium. The patient may be aware that his thinking is confused or muddled and that he "can't concentrate or think straight." Perseveration of thought is evident, and those thoughts that are expressed show an incoherence in order and logic. Frustration, angry outbursts, evasiveness, and facetiousness are evident. As a result, behavior is erratic and disorganized.

In delirium, memory is impaired for registration, retention and recall tasks. Recent memory is most affected, so anterograde amnesia is more profound than retrograde amnesia. With clearing of the delirium, there is usually permanent amnesia for the delirious episode.

Perceptual abnormalities include misperceptions, hallucinations, and delusions. Misperceptions, or illusions, are common; they result from disordered integration of sensory input. The telephone cord in the patient's room may be mistaken for a snake, or a picture on the wall for an animal. A hallucination may be visual, auditory, tactile, or olfactory. Rarely does a hallucination have a neutral emotional tone; it is usually frightening. Similarly, delusions (incorrect beliefs) exhibited by delirious patients tend to have a paranoid flavor as best exemplified by the patient with delirium tremens who believes that the nursing staff is trying to kill him. Even in the patient with a "quiet delirium," who displays no agitation, the clinician should inquire about misperception, hallucinations, and delusions.

The degree of psychomotor activity in delirium varies greatly. In the hyperactive delirious patient there are signs of autonomic arousal, gross agitation, restlessness, and acute anxiety and screams for help. Such a patient must be restrained to avoid injury to himself or others. Other delirious patients are hypoactive and sit or lie quietly. Yet they may have the same degree of attentional, cognitive, and perceptual deficits as the hyperactive patient. Whether a particular delirium is hyperactive or hypoactive may be an indication of its cause. Depressant drug-withdrawal syndromes and anticholinergic intoxications produce hyperactivity; portosystemic encephalopathy and Wernicke–Korsakoff syndrome usually produce hypoactivity.

Disturbances of sleep–wake cycles and circadian rhythms are common in delirium. The patient sleeps intermittently for only brief periods through the day or night. Slow-wave and rapid eye movement (REM) sleep (Chapter 30) is reduced so that the little sleep that occurs is not refreshing. REM and slow-wave sleep deprivation probably contributes to the severity of the delirium.

Disturbances of emotion are seen, including anxiety, fear, depression, or apathy. The particular emotional state of the delirious patient depends on several factors, including the premorbid personality structure, the nature of the brain insult, the effect on the limbic system, cultural factors, and the psychological stresses of the underlying illness.

LABORATORY TESTS

Laboratory tests are performed to assist both in the diagnosis and in the management of the delirious patient. The electroencephalogram (EEG) aids the diagnosis by confirming the clinical syndrome as delirium and by assessing its severity. A series of blood tests and other investigations are undertaken to identify the precise causes of the delirium.

The EEG is a sensitive indicator of delirium of any cause but is not specific for a particular etiology. In portosystemic, uremic, hypoxemic and hypoglycemic metabolic encephalopathies, there is slowing of the background EEG rhythms that becomes worse in direct proportion to the clinical severity. In mild cases, there is an excess of theta activity over both hemispheres. With greater severity, bifrontal delta activity appears and background theta activity is slower. In depressant drug withdrawal states and some toxic encephalopathies, there is increased fast-wave activity and increased slow-wave activity.

The EEG also aids in differential diagnosis. Uncomplicated cortical dementias such as Alzheimer's disease do not produce striking EEG abnormalities in the early stages. A normal EEG in a very confused patient suggests the diagnosis of dementia rather than delirium. Functional psychiatric illnesses with which the delirium may be confused usually are marked by normal EEGs or mild, nonspecific abnormalities.

The choice of laboratory investigations to identify the etiology of delirium will be directed by the clinical setting and by the findings of a thorough physical examination. Most patients need a series of blood tests—CBC, glucose, electrolytes, calcium, BUN, creatinine, AST (SGOT), alkaline phosphatase, and arterial blood gases. An electrocardiogram, chest x-ray, and urinalysis are usually necessary. Full body fluid cultures will be necessary in the febrile patient. Cerebrospinal fluid examination may become necessary in the confused, febrile patient if no other source of fever is found and the neurological examination discloses no focal signs or signs of raised intracranial pressure. Should either of the latter be present, a CT scan of the brain should be performed first to assure the safety of lumbar puncture (Chapter 5).

DIAGNOSIS

Delirium is a clinical diagnosis made in the acutely confused patient with the characteristics previously described. A history should be elicited from those caring for the patient to include the premorbid mental state, complete medication history, the events leading to the delirium, and the rapidity of its onset. A complete physical examination is performed to search for infection, organ dysfunction, and states of intoxication and withdrawal. Laboratory tests are then performed.

The differential diagnosis of delirium includes dementia, aphasia, and several psychiatric disorders. Dementia may be excluded because it has a more gradual onset, does not affect alertness, and in early cases may produce a relatively normal EEG. Both disorders may coexist, however, and the demented patient may become delirious after a seemingly minor insult.

Aphasia is occasionally confused with delirium by the unwary physician. A complete language examination as described in Chapter 16 differentiates the two. The aphasic patient makes characteristic errors in naming, repetition, reading, writing, comprehension, and spontaneous speech that are not fully mimicked by other states.

Psychiatric disorders, including schizophrenia, mania, and agitated depression, can mimic delirium. A proper history and psychiatric examination usually differentiates the two diagnoses, but an EEG is often necessary in difficult cases.

MANAGEMENT

The goals of management of the delirious patient are to correct the underlying cause of diffuse neuronal dysfunction and to protect and calm the patient. Specific underlying causes (eg, hypovolemia, infection, hyponatremia, drug withdrawal, congestive heart failure) are treated appropriately to produce optimal conditions for neuronal metabolic functioning. Exact treatment protocols for underlying illnesses are found in textbooks of internal medicine.

All medications taken by the patient should be scrutinized because unintentional overdosage is a very common cause of delirium, particularly in the elderly. All medications that are not absolutely necessary should be stopped; serum levels of necessary medications (eg, digoxin, aminophylline) should be tested to guarantee therapeutic not toxic concentrations.

Humane measures should be provided to calm the confused patient. Because multisensory deprivation is a major cause of delirium in the elderly, the patient should receive adequate sensory stimulation. In the ideal circumstance, a family member or friend should stay with the patient (particularly at night) to provide reality cues and reassurance to calm him. In the absence of an attendant, radio or television may help provide sensory stimulation. In the hospitalized patient, familiar objects from home in the room will help him relax.

Sedation of the delirious patient is complicated. The goals should be to insure a proper amount of sleep for the patient and to reduce states of agitation. Chloral hydrate, 500 to 1000 mg, is the safest hypnotic medication and should be tried first to aid sleep. Rapid-acting benzodiazepines such as triazolam (Halcion), 0.125 to 0.25 mg, or temazepam (Restoril), 15 to 30 mg, may be beneficial to aid sleep if chloral hydrate fails. Using tranquilizing drugs to reduce agitation runs the risk of further reducing sensory input and worsening the delirium. Haloperidol (Haldol), 0.5 to 2.0 mg, is probably the most useful agent for reducing agitation because it does not produce drowsiness or hypotension in therapeutic dosages. Larger dosages may be necessary in younger patients or in those with severe agitation. Dosage requirements change frequently in delirium, so the physician should frequently re-evaluate the patient and write new orders.

Restraints for the delirious patient should be avoided unless necessary because they tend to increase agitation. They are necessary for the agitated patient who tries to climb out of his chair or bed, or who removes vital parenteral lines and tubes. Restraints should be applied by a skilled nurse or physician and repositioned every two hours to improve comfort, prevent decubitus ulcers, and optimize pulmonary function.

The family of the delirious patient should be reassured that the patient is not insane, and that the frightening state is caused by a temporary imbalance in brain metabolism. Knowing that the disturbance is temporary helps them cope with the patient's illness and enables them to provide a better therapeutic environment.

In the patient suspected of alcoholism, thiamine, 100 mg, should be given intramuscularly and daily vitamin therapy instituted. The management of specific alcohol withdrawal syndromes is discussed in Chapter 33.

Prevention of delirium depends first on identification of the patient at risk. The patient with dementia, alcoholism, chronic illnesses, or advanced age can develop delirium with relatively minor metabolic or toxic stimuli. Such a patient should be carefully monitored during systemic illnesses, the initiation of new drug regimens, and the postoperative period. The family should be alerted to the symptoms of early delirium so that the patient can be treated in the early stages.

Bibliography

Brenner RP: The electroencephalogram in altered states of consciousness. *Neurol Clin* 1985; 3:615-631. (A discussion of the value of EEG in delirium and coma.)

Caplan LR, Kelly M. Kase CS, et al: Infarcts of the inferior division of the right middle cerebral artery: Mirror image of Wernicke's aphasia. *Neurology* 1986; 36: 1015-1020. (Provides anatomical basis for delirium following right hemispheric strokes.)

Engel GL, Romano J: Delirium, a syndrome of cerebral insufficiency. *J Chronic Dis* 1959; 9:260-277. (The classic paper that introduced the concepts later reiterated by others.)

Lipowski ZJ: Delirium, clouding of consciousness and confusion. *J Nerv Ment Dis* 1967; 145:227-255. (Another classic paper worth reviewing.)

Lipowski ZJ: *Delirium: Acute Brain Failure in Man.* Springfield, Ill, Charles C Thomas, 1980. (An expansion of the 1967 paper, including the results of a large prospective study of delirious patients.)

Massie MJ, Holland J, Glass E: Delirium in terminally ill cancer patients. *Am J Psychiatry* 1983; 140:1048-1050. (Outlines strategies for the management of delirium in terminal cancer patients.)

Mesulam M-M, Geschwind N: Disordered mental states in the postoperative period. *Urol Clin North Am* 1976; 3:199-215. (Discusses postoperative delirium in detail.)

Obrecht R, Okhomina FOA, Scott DF: Value of EEG in acute confusional states. *J Neurol Neurosurg Psychiatry* 1979; 42:75-77. (Points out the usefulness and limitation of EEG in delirium.)

Strub RL: Acute confusional state, in Benson DF, Blumer D (eds): *Psychiatric Aspects of Neurologic Disease.* New York, Grune & Stratton, 1982, vol 2, ch 1. (An excellent summary of practical information useful in the diagnosis and management of delirious patients.)

15

Seizure Disorders

CLINICAL SIGNIFICANCE

Epileptic seizures are the most common serious neurological disorder seen in outpatient practice. In the United States (population 236 million), about 4 million persons have suffered at least one seizure; 2 million have suffered two or more seizures; and 200,000 (0.1%) suffer more than one seizure per month despite treatment.

Seizures have no geographic or gender predominance and can begin at any age. The most common ages of onset are before age 2 and during adolescence. In general, the higher the age at onset, the higher the percentage of seizures that are symptomatic of an identifiable, underlying structural or metabolic brain abnormality.

It is desirable for physicians to use the term "seizure disorder" rather than "epilepsy" when talking to patients. For many patients, the word epilepsy conjures up frightening images of deformed and retarded people consigned to institutional life. Since most patients with seizure disorders are treated successfully and thus live more or less normal lives, such connotations are misleading and harmful.

ETIOLOGY

The causes of seizure disorders as a function of age are presented in Table 15-1. Idiopathic (primary, essential) epilepsy occurs at all ages. Heredity has a role in this disorder, but it does not follow a simple Mendelian inheritance pattern. About 3% of first-degree relatives of affected patients have seizure disorders, a rate three times that of the general population. A much higher percentage of relatives have electroencephalographic (EEG) abnormalities without seizures.

Perinatal injuries, intracerebral hemorrhages, hypoglycemia, pyridoxine deficiency, anoxia, and infections are the causative factors for seizures in the neonate. Hereditary or acquired defects in metabolism of amino acids, carbohydrates, or lipids can produce seizures that begin in infancy or childhood. Congenital anomalies such as the phakomatoses (tuberous sclerosis, Sturge–Weber syndrome) produce seizures that begin in infancy or early childhood.

TABLE 15-1 ETIOLOGY AND TIME OF ONSET OF SEIZURE DISORDERS

	NEWBORN	INFANCY	CHILDHOOD	ADOLESCENCE	ADULTHOOD
Perinatal injury	X	X			
Metabolic defect	X	X			
Congenital malformation		X	X	X	X
Genetic disease		X	X	X	
Myoclonic syndromes	X	X	X	X	
Head trauma		X	X	X	X
Brain tumor			X	X	X
Cerebrovascular	X				X
Idiopathic			X	X	X
Metabolic encephalopathy	X	X	X	X	X

Head trauma can produce seizures at any age, but it is a particularly common cause in young adults. The onset of seizures in the middle-aged or elderly patient should immediately suggest five possible etiologies: stroke, brain tumor (primary or metastatic), metabolic encephalopathy (particularly hypoglycemia, hyponatremia, hypocalcemia, hypomagnesemia, and hypoxemia), meningoencephalitis, or withdrawal from a depressant drug (including alcohol).

SYMPTOMS AND SIGNS

The classification of seizure types is not synonomous with the classification of seizure disorders (epilepsies). A particular seizure disorder may feature one, two, or several types of seizures. Seizure disorders can be classified in several ways: by seizure type, EEG, etiology, seizure magnitude, seizure severity, and affected body part. Clinically, the most useful classification scheme uses observed seizure type and EEG findings; it is presented in Table 15-2. These criteria also separate seizure disorders by their response to anticonvulsant drugs.

Absence Seizures

A common form of minor motor generalized seizure of childhood and young adulthood is absence. The best known type of absence is classical petit mal, a highly stereotyped disorder of children with characteristic EEG findings. The seizure begins abruptly with a stare and unresponsiveness. Most children are not entirely motionless during petit mal, although major tonic or clonic muscle contraction does not occur. There are often minor movements, including eyelid fluttering, lip smacking or chewing, minor limb movements, and motor automatisms. The frequency of automatism increases with the duration of the seizure.

Petit mal attacks usually last six to ten seconds and end abruptly with immediate resumption of normal consciousness and no postictal confusional state. There is no falling to the ground or loss of continence, although an object held in the hand may be dropped. If the child is talking, speech is arrested. Attacks are often unnoticed by the patient (and also often by observers) and may occur 10 to 20 times or more per day. They are regularly precipitated by hyperventilation.

The EEG reveals characteristic 3-Hz spike-and-wave discharges, recorded from all electrodes, which begin and end abruptly and synchronously. Non-petit mal absence seizures also occur with slightly different clinical features (eg, myoclonic

TABLE 15-2 CLASSIFICATION OF SEIZURE DISORDERS

Primary generalized epilepsies

Absence
  Classical absence of childhood, with diffuse 3-Hz spike-and-wave complexes*
  Absence of juvenile myoclonic epilepsy; staring, with diffuse 3- to 6-Hz multispike-and-wave complexes during adolescence
  Juvenile absence with diffuse 8- to 12-Hz rhythms
  Myoclonic absence with diffuse 3- to 6-Hz multispike-and-wave complexes
  Myoclonus absence: staring, fragmentary myoclonus, automatisms, and diffuse 12-Hz rhythms
Myoclonic
  Myoclonic seizures of early childhood, with 3- to 6-Hz multispike-and-wave complexes, without mental retardation (Doose syndrome)
  Juvenile myoclonic seizures of Janz or benign myoclonic seizures of adolescence and late childhood, with diffuse 4- to 6-Hz multispike-and-wave complexes
Clonic–tonic–clonic (grand mal)
Tonic–clonic (grand mal)*

Partial epilepsies

Simple partial*
  Focal motor
  Somatosensory
  Auditory
  Visual
  Uncinate
  Rolandic
Complex partial*
  Simple partial at onset, followed by impairment of consciousness and automatisms
  Impairment of consciousness at onset
      Motionless stare and impaired consciousness, followed by automatisms (temporal lobe epilepsy)
      Complex motor automatisms at start of impaired consciousness (frontal lobe, somatosensory, or occipital lobe epilepsy)
      Drop attack with impaired consciousness and automatisms (temporal lobe syncope)

Secondary generalized epilepsies

  Simple partial evolving to tonic–clonic (secondary tonic–clonic)*
  Infantile spasms (propulsive petit mal, infantile myoclonic encephalopathy with dysarrhythmia or West syndrome)
  Myoclonic astatic or atonic epilepsies (epileptic drop attacks of Lennox–Gastaut in children with mental retardation)
  Progressive myoclonic epilepsies in adolescents and adults with dementia (myoclonic epilepsies of Lafora, Lundborg, Hartung, Hunt, or Kuf)

Reflex epilepsies

Unclassified epilepsies

*Common.

Adapted from Delgado-Escueta AV, Treiman DN, Walsh GO: The treatable epilepsies. *N Engl J Med* 1983; 308:1508-1514, 1576-1584.

jerks), and EEGs reveal findings of "petit mal variant," including atypical spike-wave discharges of 2.5 to 3.5 Hz.

Family members of affected children and teenagers with petit mal have a high incidence of 3-Hz spike-wave EEG discharges. They also have a higher incidence of seizure disorders (about 10%) occurring at some time during their lives. About one-third of petit mal patients develop tonic–clonic seizures in adult life.

The most common diagnostic error in seizure disorders is to confuse absence seizures with partial complex seizures. Both have unresponsiveness and automatisms without tonic–clonic phases. The major points of differentiation are (1) partial complex seizures have a phase of postictal confusion or stupor, but absence attacks have no postictal phase whatsoever; and (2) absence seizures usually last less than 10 seconds, whereas partial complex seizures last more than 10 seconds. The EEG findings of the two disorders also differ, but EEG is helpful only if a seizure discharge can be captured.

Myoclonic seizures

Children and young adults can also develop myoclonic attacks without unconsciousness. In such patients, attacks of irregular arm and/or leg myoclonic jerking lasting many seconds suddenly occur, often within an hour after awakening in the morning. Such patients also often report absence attacks and generalized tonic–clonic seizures.

During such a seizure, EEG abnormalities include 16- to 24-Hz spikes; interictal abnormalities include 4- to 6-Hz polyspike-wave complexes. As with absence, there is a marked increase in first-degree relatives with seizure disorders and EEG abnormalities. The prognosis for patients with most myoclonic seizure disorders is good because valproate is very effective. More serious myoclonic seizure disorders are rare; see Porter RJ (1984) and Delgado-Escueta AV, et al (1983).

Tonic–Clonic Seizures

Generalized tonic–clonic (grand mal) seizures are the best known variety and the type most often referred to when the term epilepsy is used. Generalized tonic–clonic seizures are best regarded as the most extreme form of maximal epileptic neuronal discharges. Only a small percentage of patients (usually children) have primary generalized tonic–clonic seizures. In most adults and many children with this seizure type, tonic–clonic seizures occur secondarily to a partial seizure disorder that has generalized to induce maximal neuronal involvement. Drug therapy is different for primary and secondarily generalized tonic–clonic seizures, so it is important to differentiate primary and secondary causes.

Tonic, clonic, and postictal phases are recognized. The tonic phase lasts 10 to 20 seconds, and begins with a brief flexion movement during which all muscles contract, the eyelids remain open, and the eyes look up. The arms are elevated, abducted, and externally rotated with flexed elbows; and the legs may be flexed but tend to be less involved than the arms. The extension portion of the tonic phase immediately follows the brief flexion. Here, the epileptic cry is heard, a bird-like sound lasting 2 to 12 seconds. Then the back and neck are arched and hyperextended into an opisthotonic position, and the arms and legs are extended. The tremor next begins at 8 Hz, gradually slowing to 4 Hz. It consists of intermittent relaxation of the tonic contraction of the muscles and graduates into the clonic phase. Cyanosis occurs in the tonic phase because of paralysis of respiratory muscles and apnea.

The clonic phase lasts 30 seconds or so (longer in young children) and consists of violent flexor spasms of all muscle groups that alternate with regular periods of relaxation. The patient bites his tongue, and limb injuries are common. Cyanosis persists in the clonic phase and is accompanied by marked hypertension, tachycardia, hyperhydrosis, mydriasis, and increased salivation.

The postictal phase begins when the clonic phase ends. All muscle activity ceases and a deep coma ensues. The level of consciousness gradually increases until wakefulness occurs about 15 minutes later. Normal consciousness may not occur for one to two hours after the seizure. Patients awaken with fatigue, muscle soreness, and headache.

The EEG discloses typical findings during a tonic–clonic seizure. The tonic phase begins with desynchronization of all EEG rhythms, which lasts a few seconds. The tonic muscle contractions correlate with a 10-Hz spike discharge recorded over all electrodes. During the clonic phase, there is a polyspike and wave pattern, the polyspikes corresponding to the clonic muscle contractions and the waves corresponding to the brief relaxations between contractions. During the postictal phase, the EEG is initially isoelectric (flat) corresponding to the deeply comatose state. With lightening, high-voltage slow waves appear, and the EEG normalizes over the next few hours as the patient's consciousness returns to normal.

Simple Partial Seizures

The largest group of seizure disorders are those in which only a portion of the cortical neurons develop epileptic discharges. These partial seizures can be further classified into those in which consciousness is not impaired (simple or elementary) and those in which consciousness is impaired (complex).

Signs and symptoms of simple partial seizures depend on the location of the seizure focus. Thus, several subtypes are identified:

1. *Focal motor seizures.* Tonic or clonic muscle contractions of one limb or one side of the body occur with the patient remaining fully conscious. There may be a proximal-to-distal march as the seizure focus spreads over one hemisphere. These attacks usually occur from frontal lobe lesions. If clonic movements persist for long periods, the term "epilepsia partialis continua" is applied.

2. *Somatosensory seizures.* Paresthesias or dysesthesias occur unilaterally with a march. These seizures are usually from a parietal lobe focus.

3. *Auditory seizures.* This uncommon type, usually of temporal lobe origin, produces auditory hallucinations of poorly formed sounds and noises.

4. *Visual seizures.* Another uncommon type, these are caused by epileptic discharges in the occipital lobe, which produce poorly formed visual hallucinations of light flashes or sparkles.

5. *Uncinate seizures.* This type is caused by a discharge in the mesial temporal lobe. It features an olfactory hallucination of a noxious, but very hard to characterize, odor. It correlates highly with pathology in the uncus of the temporal lobe, particularly neoplasm.

6. *Rolandic seizures.* Rolandic, or benign focal, epilepsy of childhood occurs in children 5 to 9 years of age. It consists of unilateral arm and facial contractions with speech arrest. EEG findings include high-voltage spikes and slow waves in the

rolandic region. Patients with this disorder have a good prognosis with or without treatment. The disorder usually disappears by the teenage years.

EEG findings in partial epilepsies are focal paroxysmal spike, spike-wave, or slow-wave discharges. Postictal states after motor partial seizures include Todd's paralysis, a transient hemiparesis previously thought to be caused by neuronal exhaustion but more recently believed to be the result of active inhibition.

Complex Partial Seizures

The complex partial seizure is the most difficult to control of the common adult seizure types. It lasts about two minutes (11 seconds to 8 minutes) and begins with an absence-like stare and unresponsiveness. Automatisms then begin, with fumbling of the hands, lip-smacking, chewing movements, and foot shuffling. Automatisms can continue into the postictal phase. Consciousness is clearly abnormal, with no evidence of cognition or appropriate interaction with the environment but not full unconsciousness.

Complex psychological phenomena are common and may include the following: peculiar dream-like states; fear; feelings of depersonalization; feelings of peculiar familiarity (*déjàs vu*); feelings of peculiar unfamiliarity (*jamais vu*); formed visual, auditory, or olfactory hallucinations; illusions; and distortions of body image.

Autonomic phenomena are occasionally present. A sensation of the epigastrium rising to the throat is often noted. Patients may be able to correctly execute complex acts, such as driving a car. Violence has been reported, but it is exceedingly rare. There is subsequent amnesia for the total ictal episode and for part of the postictal state as well. The length of the seizure and the presence of postictal confusion distinguish the complex partial seizure from the absence seizure. Many patients have interictal behavioral abnormalities including hypersexuality, hyperreligiosity, hypergraphia, and paranoid ideations.

Secondary Generalized Seizures

Seizures that have partial onset may generalize to tonic–clonic convulsions. Most adult tonic–clonic seizures have a focal onset, but it may not be conspicuous. The patient may note an aura of focal motor activity preceding the tonic phase which points to the focal onset. In the "jacksonian march," a seizure of partial onset gradually spreads to generalized seizure activity and loss of consciousness. The patient notices clonic activity beginning in one hand, spreading to that arm, and then to the face and leg, until consciousness is lost in a generalized seizure. After the second or third decade of life, a jacksonian march suggests the presence of an underlying, identifiable structural lesion.

Infantile spasms, a syndrome of seizures in children under 1 year of age, has characteristic findings of hypsarrhythmia on EEG. Other early childhood seizure forms include atonic and astatic types. See Porter RJ (1984) for further discussion.

Reflex Seizures

Reflex epilepsies are an unusual but fascinating group of related disorders in which partial or generalized seizures are induced by a certain highly stereotyped stimulus. Seizures in individual patients may be reported after one of the following activities: eating, reading, seeing flashing lights, hearing music, touching a certain body part, or sensing heat—to name the more common types. The particular stimulus somehow lowers the seizure threshold. Treatment is directed toward biofeedback and avoidance of the stimuli.

LABORATORY TESTS

Laboratory evaluation of the patient with a newly diagnosed seizure disorder depends primarily on his age and the type of seizure. Many neurologists would not order any laboratory tests other than an EEG for the well-controlled patient with childhood idiopathic epilepsy. In such patients, the EEG reveals interictal paroxysmal abnormalities about 70% of the time. The EEG in patients with symptomatic epilepsy (eg, as a result of stroke, head trauma, alcohol withdrawal) is marked by interictal paroxysmal EEG abnormalities much less often.

For the patient with adult-onset seizures a laboratory screening battery should be performed to investigate structural causes that may be medically or surgically remediable as well as metabolic causes. Such patients should have CBC, serum chemistry screen with electrolytes, lumbar puncture, brain CT scan, and EEG. The child with poorly controlled seizures should undergo a CT scan to investigate a structural cause.

Closed-circuit video EEG recordings in inpatient epilepsy centers are reserved for the patient with medically intractable seizures or to help differentiate organic from psychogenic seizures. Intracerebral depth electrode studies to determine the precise location of seizure foci are reserved for the medically intractable epileptic in whom surgical resection is planned.

DIAGNOSIS

Epilepsy is primarily a diagnosis of history. A detailed account of the seizure episode is vital and should include the setting, aura, initial and subsequent ictal events, postictal events, and sequelae. Eyewitnesses to the seizure should be identified and interviewed.

The physical exam is useful to search for focal neurologic signs that suggest a focal cerebral lesion. In childhood-onset seizures, examination for cutaneous manifestations of phakomatoses should be performed (see Chapter 25). The value of the EEG and other tests was discussed previously. Utilizing clinical and EEG findings, the diagnosis and the identification of the type of seizure disorder is possible.

Several syndromes that resemble epilepsy are part of the differential diagnosis. Syncope and how it is differentiated from seizure are discussed in Chapter 7. Migraine (Chapter 8) can have a march of sensory dysfunction caused by spreading cerebral depression, which resembles a sensory seizure. Distinguishing features of migraine include a slower march, a subsequent headache, and a history of migraine.

TABLE 15-3 FEATURES OF PSEUDOSEIZURES

Bizarre actions during seizure
EEG is normal during and after seizure
Anticonvulsant medication not helpful
No postictal confusion
May recall events during attack
Primary and secondary gain are present
Usually no incontinence, tongue-biting, or injury
Pupillary reflexes and plantar signs are normal during seizure
Serum prolactin concentration remains normal.

Conversional epilepsy or pseudoseizures are seen occasionally. Even experienced epileptologists may have difficulty in distinguishing pseudoseizures from real ones. Table 15-3 lists some of the features of pseudoseizures. The patient suspected of having pseudoseizures should be referred to a neurologist. Occasionally, transient ischemic attacks (TIA) can have a few clonic movements just before or during the attack. A TIA (Chapter 20) should be considered when the paralysis is more notable than the clonic activity.

MANAGEMENT

The overwhelming majority of patients with seizure disorders can be managed with anticonvulsant medications. The clinician should understand the principles of anticonvulsant drug use, the drugs of choice for different seizure types, and the basic pharmacology of major anticonvulsant drugs.

General Principles

1. *Make the correct diagnosis*. Patients with syncope, dizzy spells, and other nonepileptic disorders do not respond to anticonvulsant drugs. In adults, failure to respond to several of the major drugs itself argues against the diagnosis of epilepsy.

TABLE 15-4 ANTICONVULSANT DRUGS OF CHOICE FOR SEIZURE DISORDERS

	FIRST-LINE DRUGS	SECOND-LINE DRUGS
Primary generalized epilepsies		
Absence (petit mal)	Ethosuximide	Valproic acid
Myoclonic	Valproic acid or clonazepam	Ethosuximide
Tonic–clonic (some childhood grand mal)	Valproic acid	Clonazepam
Partial Epilepsies		
Simple	Phenytoin or carbamazepine	Primidone or phenobarbital
Complex	Phenytoin or carbamazepine	Primidone or phenobarbital
Secondary generalized epilepsies		
Tonic–clonic (most adult grand mal)	Phenytoin or carbamazepine	Primidone or phenobarbital
Infantile spasms	ACTH or nitrazepam	
Astatic, atonic	Valproic acid or clonazepam	Ethosuximide
Reflex epilepsies	Phenytoin or carbamazepine	Primidone or phenobarbital

2. *There is a drug of choice for each type of seizure disorder.* Table 15-4 lists first-line and second-line drugs for each type of seizure disorder. The two major clinical distinctions that must be made are absence versus complex partial, and primary tonic–clonic versus secondary tonic–clonic. Valproic acid, ethosuximide, and clonazepam are valuable in absence and primary tonic–clonic cases, whereas phenytoin and carbamazepine are valuable in complex partial and secondary tonic–clonic cases.

3. *Begin with a single drug, not a combination.* Despite the past custom of beginning adults on phenytoin and phenobarbital, there is now excellent evidence that single-drug treatment (monotherapy) is optimal for most patients. The beginning drug is chosen from Table 15-4. The pharmacologic properties of each drug are listed in Table 15-5.

4. *Adjust dosage to bring the serum drug level within the therapeutic range.* Therapeutic ranges have been established for each anticonvulsant drug. The important issue is not how many tablets or capsules are taken daily, but what serum level of drug is achieved. Serum for measuring drug levels should be obtained in the early morning before the first dose. This trough level should be higher than the effective level listed in Table 15-6. In the patient with suspected

TABLE 15-5 DOSAGES AND INDICATIONS OF MAJOR ANTICONVULSANT DRUGS

GENERIC (TRADE NAME)	INDICATIONS	AVERAGE DAILY MAINTENANCE DOSE (MG/KG)		SERUM HALF-LIFE (HR)	
		ADULTS	CHILDREN	ADULTS	CHILDREN
Phenytoin (Dilantin)	Generalized tonic–clonic seizures; all forms of partial seizures	3-5	4-7	24 ± 12	20 ± 2
Carbamazepine (Tegretol)	All forms of partial seizures; generalized tonic–clonic seizures	10-20	20-30	17 ± 7	14 ± 5
Valproic acid (Depakene)	Absence seizures; photosensitive seizures; atonic seizures; akinetic seizures; myoclonic seizures; generalized tonic–clonic seizures	30-60	30-60	12 ± 6	12 ± 6
Ethosuximide (Zarontin)	Absence seizures	20-40	20-30	55 ± 5	30 ± 6
Clonazepam (Clonopin)	Myoclonic seizures; infantile spasm; atonic seizures; absence and akinetic seizures	0.05-0.2	0.01-0.2	32 ± 13	23 ± 10
Primidone (Mysoline)	Generalized tonic–clonic seizures; all forms of partial seizures	10-25	10-25	12 ± 6	†
Phenobarbital (Luminal)	Generalized tonic–clonic seizures; all forms of partial seizures	2-3	3-5*	96 ± 12	55 ± 15

*Infants, 8 mg/kg.
†Data not available.
Adapted from: So EL, Penry JK: Epilepsy in adults. *Ann Neurol* 1981; 9:3-16

TABLE 15-6 BLOOD LEVELS AND SIDE EFFECTS OF MAJOR ANTICONVULSANT DRUGS

Generic (Trade Name)	Blood Levels* Effective	Blood Levels* Toxic	Most Common Side Effects	Most Common Toxic Signs and Symptoms
Phenytoin (Dilantin)	>10µg/mL	>20µg/mL	Skin eruptions, hypertrichosis, gingival hyperplasia, coarsening of facial features, decreased blood folate level, hypocalcemia, osteomalacia, lymphadenopathy, hepatitis, systemic lupus erythematosus, fever	Nystagmus, ataxia, slurred speech, drowsiness, diplopia, blurred vision
Carbamazepine (Tegretol)	>4µg/mL	>8µg/mL	Nausea, vomiting, anorexia, blood dyscrasias	Vertigo, drowsiness, nystagmus, diplopia, unsteadiness
Valproic acid (Depakene)	>50µg/mL	>100µg/mL	Nausea, vomiting, drowsiness, weight gain, transient alopecia, hypersalivation, diarrhea, thrombocytopenia, hepatic toxicity	Ataxia, sedation
Ethosuximide (Zarontin)	>40µg/mL	>100µg/mL	Nausea, skin rash, blood dyscrasias, drowsiness, hiccups	Nausea, vomiting, anorexia, lethargy, headache, hiccups
Clonazepam (Clonopin)	>20ng/mL	>80ng/mL	Sedation, drowsiness, ataxia, behavioral problems, anorexia	Somnolence, confusion, coma, hypotension
Primidone (Mysoline)	>5µg/mL	>12µg/mL	Sedation, paradoxical excitement, rash, irritability and hyperactivity, especially in children	Drowsiness, ataxia, nystagmus, slurred speech
Phenobarbital (Luminal)	>15µg/mL	>40µg/mL	Same as primidone	Same as primidone

*Total blood levels, free and protein-bound.

Adapted from So EL, Penry JK: Epilepsy in adults. *Ann Neurol* 1981; 9: 3-16.

drug toxicity, serum drug levels should be obtained several hours after a dose, and should be compared to the toxic level listed in Table 15-6.

5. *Don't administer drugs less frequently than one drug half-life between doses.* The clinician attempts to achieve a relatively constant serum level of anticonvulsant drugs. A drug with a short half-life, such as valproate or carbamazepine, must be given several times daily, whereas a drug with a long half-life, such as phenytoin or ethosuximide, usually can be given once daily.

6. *If partial improvement occurs, add a second drug.* In the patient on monotherapy whose seizures improve but do not stop, when serum drug levels have been documented to be within the high therapeutic range, the addition of a second drug is indicated. It may raise or lower the serum level of the first drug, so both levels should be followed. The second drug can be selected from Table 15-4.

7. *If improvement does not occur, change drugs.* When the seizure frequency does not fall with monotherapy, the clinician should reassess his seizure diagnosis. Another drug should be chosen from Table 15-4, and the first drug discontinued.

8. *Avoid sedative side effects whenever possible.* Patients do not like to take medications with sedative effects. Of the drugs listed in Tables 15-4 and 15-5, those that are most sedating are primidone, phenobarbital, and clonazepam. They should be avoided, if possible, because patient compliance is likely to be poor.

9. *Give drugs at bedtime and after meals to reduce toxicity.* When large doses of anticonvulsant medication must be taken, prescribing a substantial portion of the dosage for just before bedtime reduces the awareness of bothersome side effects. When drugs are mixed with food at mealtime, they are absorbed more slowly and provide a more constant serum level.

10. *Rapidity of administration depends upon the particular clinical situation.* The rapid induction of anticonvulsant medications in status epilepticus is discussed in Chapter 39. With phenobarbital and phenytoin, loading doses are customarily given to boost the serum level into the therapeutic range quickly. By giving only maintenance-level doses, the serum drug level slowly reaches a steady-state therapeutic level in about five or six half-lives.

11. *The major cause of uncontrolled seizures is noncompliance.* Patients may skip doses of medications because of forgetfulness, illness, apathy, or intent. Patients should be counseled carefully as to the importance of taking the medications. The physician should try to deal with any problem induced by the medication. When forgetfulness is common, the patient should be instructed to remove a full day's dosage of each drug and place it in a receptacle in a prominent place (eg, on the kitchen table). All dosages for that day should be taken from the receptacle. The patient should inspect the receptacle each night to ascertain that it is empty.

Specific Syndromes

1. *Seizure disorders in pregnancy.* When managing the pregnant epileptic, the physician should consider the effect of pregnancy on the course of maternal epilepsy, the effect of epilepsy on the course and outcome of the pregnancy, the effect of anticonvulsant drugs on fetal development, and the effect of anticonvulsant drugs on the health of the neonate. These are discussed further in Chapter 34.

Pregnancy is associated with declining seizure control in about 40% of patients. This decline is caused by two factors: poorer compliance, perhaps from fear of teratogenic fetal effects, and changes in the maternal metabolism of anticonvulsant drugs, which produces drops in serum levels. Seizures in about 10% of patients are controlled better during pregnancy.

The effect of a seizure disorder on the outcome of pregnancy is not clear. Early studies showed a twofold increase of microcephaly, stillbirth, and mental retardation, but these were conducted in the era before measurement of serum anticonvulsant levels when seizure control was not optimal. There is not an increased incidence of toxemia, abruptio placentae, or hyperemesis gravidarum.

Anticonvulsant drugs do produce a twofold-to-threefold increase in the incidence of fetal abnormalities, from 2% of births to 4.6%. Trimethadione, a third-line drug, causes serious fetal anomalies in more than 75% of cases, so it should be avoided. Valproic acid also should be avoided because it is associated with a high rate of teratogenic effects. Phenytoin can produce the fetal hydantoin syndrome of hypertelorism, short, low-bridged nose, low-set ears, nail and distal phalangeal hypoplasia, microcephaly, growth disturbance, and mental retardation. No anticonvulsant agent is free of teratogenic effects, although the data on carbamazepine are incomplete.

The newborn of a mother who takes anticonvulsant drugs may develop a bleeding diathesis because of vitamin K deficiency. The management of this and other complications of the pregnant epileptic is described in Table 15-7.

2. *Neonatal seizures.* Seizures in the neonatal period can be caused by hypocalcemia, intracranial hemorrhage, other birth injury, perinatal hypoxemia, infection, congenital malformation, hypoglycemia, and pyridoxine deficiency. Neonatal seizures are managed by controlling hypocalcemia and hypoglycemia, treating infection, administering pyridoxine, and treating the patient with loading doses of phenytoin and/or phenobarbital.

3. *Febrile seizures.* Probably because of a genetic mechanism, 2% to 5% of children 3 months to 5 years of age experience one or more febrile seizures. Such seizures are usually self-limited and are associated with high fevers from a viral exanthem, bacterial otitis or pharyngitis, or other non-central nervous system

---

TABLE 15-7 MANAGEMENT OF SEIZURE DISORDERS IN PREGNANCY

- Before a planned pregnancy, control seizures, stabilize drug doses, and simplify drug regimens.
- Discontinue anticonvulsants if the mother has been free of seizures for many years.
- Advise prospective mothers taking anticonvulsants that they have a twofold to threefold increased risk of fetal malformation.
- Women on trimethadione or other oxazolidinediones should not become pregnant; if pregnant, they should be given the option of abortion. Valproic acid should also be avoided.
- Have more frequent prenatal checkups and fetal monitoring than normal.
- Follow monthly serum anticonvulsant levels.
- Newborns should receive prophylactic vitamin K and have coagulation studies performed every 4 hours for the first 2 days of life.
- Breast feeding is generally all right, but barbiturates in milk can produce neonatal drowsiness.

infection. Mortality is about 0.1%; febrile seizures recur in 34%, and nonfebrile epilepsy develops in 2% to 4%.

Anticonvulsant drugs probably do more harm than good in most children with febrile seizures. A subgroup of about 6% of children with febrile seizures should receive daily phenobarbital until the age of 5. This group is composed of children who have two or more of the following risk factors: (1) family history of nonfebrile epilepsy; (2) abnormal neurological status or development; (3) prolonged or focal febrile seizures. See Wolf (1979) for further discussion.

4. *Status epilepticus.* Management of this emergency condition is discussed in Chapter 39.

COMPLICATIONS

The incidence of sudden death is increased in epilepsy. It can be caused by asphyxia or cardiac arrhythmia, but a frequent cause is drowning while swimming. Porter (1984) suggests that although an epileptic should be encouraged to lead a normal life, swimming must be carefully regulated. The epileptic patient should never swim without a companion who can swim well; he should always wear a lifejacket designed to keep the head above water should a seizure occur.

Psychosocial issues are a major concern for the epileptic patient and his family. The physician has an important role to play in educating them about how to cope with the limitations placed on the patient by society with respect to employment, driving, recreation, and insurance.

Employers are reluctant to hire a patient with a seizure disorder because of the fear that the employee will have a higher risk of injury and that the employer's workman's compensation payments will increase. Neither fear is justified by the data. The physician can intervene to educate employers, to recommend a safer job (eg, not working on or near heavy machines), and to state the level of control of the seizures.

Physicians should educate the patient and family about state laws pertaining to driving automobiles. Most states require that before an epileptic patient can obtain a driver's license, he must be under a physician's care, on anticonvulsant medications, and seizure-free for 6 to 12 months. Whether physicians are permitted or obligated to notify state motor vehicle bureaus that a patient has suffered a seizure varies from state to state.

The patient with a seizure disorder should be encouraged to participate in a full range of recreational activities, except those involving water and heights. Participation in contact sports is not prohibited.

Epileptic patients are rated as uninsurable by almost all commercial carriers of health and life insurance. Patients should be told they can obtain group life and health insurance through the Epilepsy Foundation of America (see address below).

WHEN TO CONSULT

The neurologist should evaluate the newly symptomatic patient with a seizure disorder, but the generalist can follow and manage most cases. The patient with difficult seizure control should be followed up by the neurologist. The patient with an intractable seizure disorder should be referred to a regional epilepsy center for intensive inpatient management and consideration for a neurosurgical palliative procedure (temporal lobectomy, corpus callosotomy).

PATIENT EDUCATION

Patients with seizure disorders should be referred to their local chapter of the Epilepsy Foundation. Numerous helpful educational, counseling, and clinical services are available through the Foundation. For the address of the local chapter, write to: Epilepsy Foundation of America, 4351 Garden City Drive, Landover, MD 20785, or to The American Epilepsy Society, 179 Allyn Street, Suite 304, Hartford, CT 06013. Patients can also purchase one of three good self-help books.

Suggested Reading for Patients

Lechtenberg R: *Epilepsy and the Family.* Cambridge, Mass., Harvard University Press, 1984, 223 pp ($16.50).

Laidlaw MV, Laidlaw J: *People with Epilepsy: How They Can Be Helped.* New York, Churchill-Livingstone, 1984, 177 pp ($9).

Middleton AH, Attwell AA, Walsh GO: *Epilepsy. A Handbook for Patients, Parents, Families, Teachers, Health and Social Workers.* Boston, Little Brown, 1981, 295 pp ($14.95).

Bibliography

Aird RB, Masland RL, Woodbury DM: *The Epilepsies: A Critical Review.* New York, Raven Press, 1984. (A very good and current review of basic mechanisms and clinical features of epilepsy.)

Bergman I, Painter MJ, Hirsch RP, et al: Outcome in neonates with convulsions treated in an intensive care unit. *Ann Neurol* 1983; 14:642-647. (Shows that poor outcome was related to seizures of late onset, tonic seizures, and seizures lasting many days.)

Dalessio DJ: Seizure disorders and pregnancy. *N Engl J Med* 1985; 312:559-563. (A recent review with recommendations.)

Delgado-Escueta AV, Treiman DN, Walsh GO: The treatable epilepsies. *N Engl J Med* 1983; 308:1508-1514, 1576-1584. (Current and authoritative review. Does a better job reviewing the literature and presenting the UCLA approach than providing clinically useful tips.)

Dreifuss F, Farwell J. Holmes G, et al: Infantile spasms: Comparative trial of nitrazepam and corticotropin. *Arch Neurol* 1986;43:1107-1110. (Multicenter study showing equivalent efficacy of nitrazepam and ACTH, with fewer complications from the former.)

Engel J, Jr, Troupin AS, Crandall PH, et al: Recent developments in the diagnosis and therapy of epilepsy. *Ann Intern Med* 1982; 97:584-598. (Discusses PET scans, new drugs, biofeedback, and surgical approaches.)

Gates JR, Ramani V, Whalen S, et al: Ictal characteristics of pseudoseizures. *Arch Neurol* 1985; 42:1183-867. (Describes differential diagnosis of true seizures and pseudoseizures.)

Mattson RH, Cramer JA, Collins JF, et al: Comparison of carbamazepine, phenytoin, and primidone in partial and secondarily generalized tonic–clonic seizures. *N Engl J Med* 1985; 313:145-151. (Shows that phenytoin and carbamazepine are first-line drugs and that phenobarbital and primidone are second-line drugs.)

Penry JK, Newmark ME: The use of antiepileptic drugs. *Ann Intern Med* 1979; 90:207-218. (Excellent review of the clinical pharmacology of anticonvulsant drugs.)

Porter RJ: *Epilepsy: 100 Elementary Principles.* Philadelphia, Saunders, 1984. (A gem of a book, packed with clinical pearls and the wisdom gained from the sensitive management of thousands of epileptic patients. Highly recommended.)

So EL, Penry JK: Epilepsy in adults. *Ann Neurol* 1981; 9:3-16. (Strong on new diagnostic techniques and the clinical pharmacology of anticonvulsant drugs.)

Wolf SM: Controversies in the treatment of febrile convulsions. *Neurology* 1979; 29:287-290. (Discusses the subgroup that needs daily treatment, and provides recommendations.)

16

Aphasia

Behavioral neurology is largely concerned with the study of syndromes of communicative and perceptual dysfunction arising from focal hemispheric lesions. The three major groups of these syndromes are the aphasias (language dysfunction), apraxias (disconnection of language from movement), and agnosias (perceptual dysfunction). Aphasia is the most conspicuous and the most frequently encountered. This chapter, considers aphasia and the related syndromes of apraxia, agnosia, and neglect.

Aphasia is an acquired impairment of previously intact language function. It is distinguished from dysarthria and dysphonia, which refer specifically to mechanical disturbances in the articulation and phonation of speech. In aphasia, the symbolic interpretive and generative language centers are damaged, resulting in impairment in numerous areas of communication including speech production and comprehension, word finding, repetition, reading ability and comprehension, and writing. A dysarthric or dysphonic patient at a typewriter can produce prose with normal sentence structure, syntax, and grammar. An aphasic patient at a typewriter can produce only aphasic sentences with impairment in sentence structure, syntax, and grammar. Aphasia also must be distinguished from developmental dyslexia, which is discussed in Chapter 19.

DOMINANCE

The paired cerebral hemispheres are ostensibly exact mirror images, but are neither structurally nor functionally homologous. In development that begins prenatally, one hemisphere becomes specialized for language functions and the other for nonlanguage, mostly perceptual, functions. The "language hemisphere" also becomes the "dominant" hemisphere for handedness by subserving the contralateral hand and leg, preferred for fine and coarse motor activities such as handwriting and throwing and kicking a ball. Anatomic studies show that the perisylvian language center, particularly the planum temporale, is grossly larger in the dominant than in the nondominant hemisphere. This asymmetry is present at birth and can be seen by computed tomographic (CT) scan.

More than 99% of right-handed people and about 50% of left-handed people have left-hemisphere dominance. Most other left handers have codominance; only about 10% have right-hemisphere dominance. Plasticity of dominance is maintained until about age 10 to 12. Children who sustain severe injuries to their dominant hemispheres can change dominant sides successfully before that age and usually suffer no permanent aphasia.

Hemisphere dominance can be inferred from answers to detailed surveys of handedness. Subjects are asked to answer questions, such as with which hand they prefer to write, eat, thread a needle, button a button, and throw a ball. Handedness is not an all-or-none phenomenon; it may be present in degrees. Many patients born left-handed, especially elderly ones, were forced to convert to right-handedness in childhood. The only way to establish hemisphere dominance with certainty is to perform the Wada test, in which a rapid-acting barbiturate is injected sequentially into each carotid artery and the patient undergoes a neurological examination. Transient global aphasia will accompany hemiplegia when the carotid artery that perfuses the dominant hemisphere is injected.

CLASSIFICATION OF APHASIA

Table 16-1 outlines the currently accepted classification of aphasia and the essential features of each type. The classification is based on the location of the underlying lesion and the findings of the aphasia examination.

TABLE 16-1   CLASSIFICATION OF APHASIA

With impaired repetition
Broca's
Wernicke's
Conduction
Global

With intact repetition
Anomic
Transcortical aphasias
    Motor transcortical
    Sensory transcortical
    Isolation of the speech area
Single modality aphasias
    Aphemia
    Pure word deafness

Related disturbances
Aprosodia
Alexia
Agraphia
Acalculia
Apraxia
Agnosia
Neglect

EXAMINATION FOR APHASIA

The aphasia examination must include tests for spontaneous speech, repetition, naming, comprehension of written and spoken words, reading, writing, and praxis. Each phase of language function is tested first with common, easy tasks. If the patient completes them successfully, he is given more difficult language tasks until the threshold of error for each task is reached. When all subtests are completed, the responses are compared to those in Table 16-2 to identify the type of aphasia and the presumed location of the underlying lesion.

Spontaneous Speech

The separation of aphasias into fluent and nonfluent types carries the greatest anatomic significance: nonfluent aphasias suggest an anterior lesion and fluent aphasias, a posterior lesion. Benson and Geschwind (1986) identified eight characteristics of spontaneous speech that can be assessed in the aphasic patient: (1) rate of output; (2) rhythm, inflection, and prosody (emotional expression); (3) pronunciation; (4) effort; (5) press of speech; (6) phrase length; (7) paraphasias; and (8) word content. Nonfluent aphasias are characterized by sparse output (fewer than 50 words per minute), much effort, poor articulation, dysprosody, short phrase length, and use of substantive words. Fluent aphasias, by contrast, feature normal or increased word output (100 to 200 words per minute), often with press of speech, normal pronunciation, prosody, and phrase length, but with paraphasias.

A paraphasia is an idiosyncratic, newly created word substituted for the intended word by the aphasic patient. Benson and Geschwind identify three classes of paraphasias: phonemic, semantic, and neologistic. The phonemic or literal paraphasia sounds like the intended word. The semantic or verbal paraphasia substitutes a semantically similar, but not synonomous, word. The neologistic paraphasia bears no recognizable phonemic or semantic similarity to the intended word. For example, when a fluently aphasic patient wants to say, "Place your book upon the table," a phonemic paraphasic substitution might be, "Place your book upon the teeble." A semantic paraphasia might be "Place your book upon the drawer." A neologistic paraphasia might be "Place your book upon the glossfarnel."

Repetition

The ability to correctly repeat spoken phrases is impaired in most aphasias (but not in transcortical aphasias). Patients are asked to repeat phrases of increasing difficulty, beginning with "hello," "good-bye," "today is Tuesday," and "down to earth." They are then challenged with more improbable phrases, such as "the fox slept on the bush" or "the pale yellow dress with green checks." Finally, they are given the most difficult phrase of all: "no ifs, ands, or buts." Mildly aphasic patients may correctly repeat the simple, high-probability phrases but fail to repeat the low-probability phrases. "No ifs, ands, or buts" is very difficult for aphasic patients

TABLE 16-2 CHARACTERISTICS OF APHASIA

	SPONTANEOUS SPEECH	COMPREHENSION	NAMING	REPETITION	SELF-MONITORING	RESPONSE TO CUING	PARAPHASIAS	PRAXIS
Broca's aphasia	Nonfluent	Good	Poor	Poor	Good	Good	Rare	Left hemi-apraxia
Wernicke's aphasia	Very fluent	Poor	Poor	Poor	Poor	Poor	Common	Cannot follow instructions
Conduction aphasia	Fluent	Good	Poor	Poor	Good	Poor	Common	Apraxia
Global aphasia	Nonfluent	Poor	Poor	Poor	Poor	Poor	Occasional	Left hemi-apraxia
Anomic aphasia	Fluent	Good	Poor	Good	Good	Good	Absent	Normal

to repeat because it makes nouns of three words ordinarily used as conjunctions. Most aphasics cannot perform this linguistic maneuver.

Naming

The ability to name common objects (word-finding) is almost universally impaired in aphasia. Patients are asked to name common articles of clothing worn by the examiner, body parts, common objects, and so forth. If a patient can name common objects, the examiner asks him to name less probable objects, such as the parts of a wristwatch (crystal, face, stem). The ability to name fingers and colors can also be tested. The inability to name (dysnomia) is occasionally seen in nonaphasic disorders, particularly in acute delirium.

Comprehension

Posterior aphasias impair the comprehension of spoken or written words to varying degrees. Comprehension is difficult to test in the aphasic patient because verbal and performance measures of successful comprehension may be impaired even when comprehension is intact. The nonfluently aphasic patient with intact comprehension cannot respond verbally to the examiner's questions, leading the unwary examiner to suspect a comprehension disturbance. The apraxic aphasic patient with intact comprehension may not be able to follow the examiner's commands, producing similar conclusions in the unwary.

Spoken comprehension is properly tested by having the patient respond to the question with a nonverbal, simple gesture. He can be asked to point to the object named by the examiner in a group of assembled common objects (safety pin, rubber band, paper clip, key, thumb tack, penny, nickle, dime, quarter) or asked to point to objects in the room (window, door, ceiling, floor).

Written comprehension can be tested by telling the patient to follow a command that the examiner has written on a card—without reading it aloud first. The examiner can write "close your eyes," "raise your hands," "open your mouth," and so forth.

Reading

The patient is asked to read aloud sentences in a magazine or newspaper after the examiner ascertains that he can see the letters with proper refraction. If the patient can read the sentences aloud, he can then be asked to explain their meaning. Inability to read (alexia) is discussed later in this chapter.

Writing

Agraphia, the inability to write, is just as common in aphasia as is the inability to speak. In fact, written output usually follows speech output. Verbally nonfluent patients with anterior lesions write with poorly formed letters, reduced output, and retained substantive words, in short, graphic nonfluency. Similarly, verbally fluent patients are also graphically fluent, with lengthy, wordy sentences and frequent paraphasias. The examiner should dictate simple sentences for the patient to print or write, allowing for clumsiness if the nondominant hand is used because of paresis of the dominant hand. Patients should not be asked to sign their name because this overlearned act frequently survives the aphasic insult and is not diagnostically useful. Agraphia is considered later in this chapter.

Praxis

Left hemiapraxia frequently complicates anterior aphasias. The patient is asked to use his left hand to "show me how you brush your teeth,...comb your hair,...salute,...wave goodbye." Inability to perform these learned acts properly despite intact hearing, comprehension, strength, and coordination is termed apraxia, which is considered later in this chapter.

Formal Aphasia Assessment

The two standardized and validated aphasia assessment batteries in general use are the Boston Diagnostic Aphasia Examination (BDAE) and the Porch Index of Communicative Ability (PICA). They have been tested extensively and use scores that classify aphasias into types that have implications for lesion localization. The PICA takes about one hour; the BDAE, about eight hours.

TYPES OF APHASIA

Principally as the result of the writings of the late Norman Geschwind (1965, 1986), the pioneering works of Broca, Wernicke, Dejerine, Liepmann, and others have been resuscitated and incorporated into an anatomic schema representing the organization of language in the brain (Figure 16-1). This schema is based on studies of naturally occurring ablative hemispheric lesions, usually caused by stroke, and on the characteristics of the aphasias that result. The extent and types

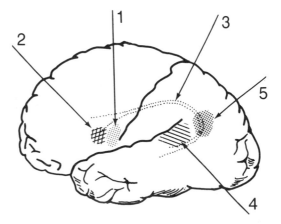

Figure 16-1. Anatomy of the language areas of the dominant hemisphere. Lateral surface of the left hemisphere. (1) Face area of motor cortex; (2) Broca's area; (3) lesion involving arcuate fasciculus (dotted lines); (4) Wernicke's area; (5) angular gyrus. (Reproduced, with permission, from Geschwind N: *Selected Papers on Language and the Brain. Vol XVI: Boston Studies in the Philosophy of Science.* Dordrecht, The Netherlands, D. Reidel, 1974, p 435.)

of aphasia are a continuum because lesions may be large or small, discrete or diffuse, and located in any part or in more than one part of the language hemisphere. Nevertheless, it is a useful clinical simplification to reduce the types of aphasias seen by the clinician into those listed in Table 16-1.

Broca's Aphasia

The patient with Broca's aphasia is nonfluent. His speech is poorly articulated, filler words (conjunctions, prepositions) are absent, and the remaining few words are substantive (telegraphic speech). Comprehension remains essentially intact, and the monitoring of impaired language output that results produces severe frustration. Naming and repetition are impaired; reading aloud is not possible, but reading comprehension is present. Writing with the left hand is analogous to speech: sparse, messy, and nonfluent.

The lesion that produces Broca's aphasia includes Broca's area and the cortex just posterior to it. Because of concomitant involvement of the precentral gyrus (motor strip) of the posterior frontal lobe, the patient has a right hemiparesis affecting the face and hand more than the leg. He cannot protrude the tongue on command or whistle. The typical patient has had a stroke involving frontal branches of the left middle cerebral artery. The unusual patient with a discrete lesion only of Broca's area that spares the surrounding cortex does not develop Broca's aphasia, but has a peculiar form of mutism called aphemia, discussed later.

Wernicke's Aphasia

The patient with Wernicke's aphasia is fluent—often to a fault. Whole sentences are produced effortlessly, but the sentences lack substance and bear little relation to what the patient is apparently trying to express. Comprehension is severely impaired, and the patient is unable to monitor his disordered language output. There is no frustration except that produced when the patient senses the inability of others to decipher his speech. Paraphasias are prominent, with many semantic substitutions and often very humorous neologisms. Naming, repetition, writing, and reading aloud are severely contaminated with paraphasias. Spontaneous speech may become utterly incomprehensible ("jargon aphasia").

The lesion that produces Wernicke's aphasia includes the posterior portion of the superficial temporal gyrus (Heschl's gyrus) just inferior to the most posterior extent of the Sylvian fissure. Patients frequently have no hemiparesis, but have a contralateral homonymous hemianopia or superior quadrantanopia. Often, patients with acute Wernicke's aphasia from posterior temporal branch occlusions of the left middle cerebral artery are admitted to psychiatric wards because of their bizarre jargon aphasia and no other obvious signs of neurologic dysfunction.

Conduction Aphasia

The patient with conduction aphasia shows a disturbance of repetition out of proportion to other language deficits. Spontaneous speech is reasonably fluent, with frequent paraphasic substitutions, but neither are as pronounced as in

Wernicke's aphasia. Unlike Wernicke's aphasia, comprehension is quite intact. Naming, writing, and reading aloud are impaired. Written comprehension is usually excellent. Apraxia for limb movements is often present.

Conduction aphasia is usually produced by a lesion of the arcuate fasciculus, the white matter tract connecting Broca's and Wernicke's areas. This lesion is usually in the posterior left perisylvian region and often underlying the supramarginal gyrus. Parietal branch occlusions of the left middle cerebral artery are the most common cause. Affected patients have variable degrees of right hemiparesis, but usually show loss of cortical sensory modalities on the right side and often have right-sided visual field defects.

Global Aphasia

Many unfortunate patients suffer damage to the entire language area, including Broca's area, Wernicke's area, and the arcuate fasciculus. When the entire perisylvian language area is dysfunctional, the result is the most profound possible aphasia, known as global aphasia. These patients are totally nonfluent. They may be mute initially, but they invariably recover a vocabulary of one or a few stock words, often profanities. They are severely impaired in all spheres of language function, including naming, repetition, reading, writing, and spoken and written comprehension.

Complete left middle cerebral artery infarction caused by left middle cerebral artery stem occlusion or left internal carotid artery occlusion is the common underlying pathology. Patients with global aphasia also have a dense right hemiplegia, right hemihypesthesia, right homonymous hemianopia, and some degree of right voluntary gaze paresis.

Transcortical Aphasias

Transcortical aphasias differ in two respects from those described previously. Whereas, other aphasias feature a repetition disturbance, repetition is normal in transcortical aphasias. Other aphasias are usually the result of a dominant hemispheric focal lesion, usually an infarction in a single arterial territory. Transcortical aphasias are caused by a diffuse border-zone lesion in the watershed region between the distribution of the middle cerebral artery and the anterior and posterior cerebral arteries. Transcortical aphasias usually result from diffuse cerebral insults, such as hypotension or hypoxemia, in which the watershed areas of the brain are most severely affected because of their marginal blood supply.

Transcortical aphasias are motor, sensory, or global. In the motor type, patients are nonfluent and have intact verbal and written comprehension, and intact repetition. Naming is impaired. The lesion is in the border zone between the anterior cerebral artery and the frontal branches of the middle cerebral artery. In the less-common sensory transcortical aphasia, patients are fluent with paraphasias and impaired comprehension and naming. The lesion is in the border zone between the posterior cerebral artery and posterior parietal and temporal branches of the middle cerebral artery. In the unusual instance of combined motor and sensory transcortical aphasias (isolation of the speech area), no language function except repetition remains. Echolalia, the mindless repetition of heard phrases, is present more often in isolation of the speech area than in either motor or sensory transcortical aphasia.

Anomic Aphasia

Anomic aphasia is characterized by difficulty in word-finding of varying severity. Repetition, spontaneous speech, reading, writing, and comprehension are normal. Paraphasias are not present, but patients may substitute synonymous words or phrases for words they cannot find, a process known as circumlocution. Their otherwise normal syntax is interrupted by pauses as they search for words.

The lesion of anomic aphasia can be localized with less certainty than that of any of the aphasias. While it is classically said to result from a lesion of the angular gyrus, the most clear-cut cases are seen in lesions of the basal aspect of the posterior temporal lobe. Anomic aphasia is also seen in cases of metabolic encephalopathy and from other focal lesions scattered throughout either hemisphere.

Single-Modality Aphasias

Rare cases of single language modality impairment have been reported. Damage to the primary auditory cortex in the superior temporal gyrus (Heschl's gyrus) produces the syndrome of pure word deafness. Here, despite normal language output and intact hearing, the patient has total incomprehension of spoken language. Written comprehension remains normal. The neurological exam is usually normal.

Aphemia is an analogous motor impairment. Here, muteness recovers to hypophonia with normal syntax, comprehension, reading, writing, naming, and repetition. A discrete lesion only in Broca's area is usually present. The neurological exam is normal. Because aphemia and pure word deafness affect only speech, some have classified them as nonaphasic speech disorders. But because they affect the higher language centers, they are better classified as aphasias.

PROGNOSIS AND THERAPY FOR APHASIA PATIENTS

The signs of aphasia from stroke evolve with time as gradual, spontaneous recovery occurs. The best predictor for return of fluency in Broca's aphasia is the CT scan appearance of the infarct six weeks after the stroke. If the volume of the infarct is less than 25 cm^3, the prognosis for recovery of fluency is good; if the infarct is greater than 100 cm^3, location becomes a factor in prognosis. If the infarct includes the precentral or postcentral gyrus, prognosis for recovery is poor; otherwise, recovery is satisfactory (Knopman et al, 1983). Other prognostic variables include age and handedness. Young patients recover better than do old patients. Left-handed patients recover better than right-handed ones—probably because they have a higher likelihood of codominance.

The role of speech therapy in aphasia rehabilitation is controversial. Although it is customarily performed, several studies have shown it is ineffective. Clearly, attention, encouragement, and motivation conveyed to an aphasic person is instrumental in speeding his recovery. Recent evidence shows that volunteers talking regularly with aphasic patients are as effective in producing improvement as trained speech therapists are.

Aphasias vary in their amenability to therapy. Those in which the patient's intact comprehension permits self-monitoring of language output (Broca's, conduction, anomic) are more likely to improve with therapy than those with poor self-monitoring (Wernicke's, global). Experimental therapies using musical notes and sign language have had mixed success and are not widely used.

RELATED HEMISPHERIC SYNDROMES
Aprosodia

The use of facial expression, word inflection and emphasis, and gesticulation to convey emotional feelings—in short, the emotional expression of speech—is called prosody. While the functions of language content, syntax, word choice, and word comprehension reside in the dominant hemisphere, language prosody is believed to be a nondominant hemispheric function.

In states of nondominant (usually right) hemispheric dysfunction, aprosodia may occur. The patient's speech may be normal in content but may be devoid of emotional expression. When the patient is tested by asking him to repeat a phrase such as "I am going to the circus" in a voice conveying happiness, then anger, then sadness, he is incapable of expressing an emotional vocabulary (motor aprosodia). Some patients lose the ability to comprehend emotional statements of others (sensory aprosodia). Conduction and transcortical aprosodias, analogous to aphasias, also occur. Ross (1981) believes the nondominant hemisphere lesions responsible for the aprosodias to be the exact homologues of the dominant hemisphere lesions responsible for the aphasias.

Alexia and Agraphia

Alexia is the acquired inability to comprehend written language. In addition to alexias that result from aphasias, there are two specific alexic syndromes: alexia without agraphia and alexia with agraphia.

The patient with alexia without agraphia can write but cannot read what he has just written. Aphasia, per se, is not present, although the patient may have a mild dysnomia, particularly for colors, and acalculia. A dense right homonymous hemianopia is present, but there is no hemiparesis.

The lesion that most often gives rise to alexia without agraphia is a left posterior cerebral artery occlusion producing infarction of the left occipital cortex and the splenium of the corpus callosum. Vision from the intact right occipital cortex is disconnected from the left hemispheric language centers by the callosal lesion, producing alexia. Handwriting and language are otherwise intact because the left hemispheric language center in the middle cerebral artery territory is spared.

Less often, alexia with agraphia occurs. Here, a severe disturbance of writing accompanies alexia, often with apraxia and acalculia. Occasionally the full

Gerstmann's syndrome manifests with the tetrad of agraphia, acalculia, right–left disorientation, and finger agnosia. In practice, formes frustes of Gerstmann's syndrome are seen more often than the full tetrad. A lesion of the dominant (left) angular gyrus lesion is responsible for alexia with agraphia; Gerstmann's syndrome only localizes the lesion to the dominant parietal lobe.

Apraxia

Apraxia is the inability to execute learned skilled movements despite normal motor and sensory systems, comprehension, attention, and cooperation. Apraxia is best regarded as a disconnection syndrome in which the language centers in the left hemisphere are disconnected from the motor centers in either hemisphere.

Apraxia is tested in several ways. By pantomime, the patient is asked to "show me how you brush your teeth...comb your hair," etc. By imitation of pantomime he is told "watch how I brush my teeth...now show me how you do it." Finally, to test the ability to use a real object, the patient is given a fingernail clipper and asked to show the examiner how it is used.

When told to pantomime or to imitate, an apraxic patient makes a clumsy movement of the affected arm and hand, but cannot correctly perform the act. When asked to pantomime brushing his teeth, he may slowly raise his arm, regard it quizzically, and crudely place it near his face. Similarly, he will operate a fingernail clipper clumsily and improperly when asked to demonstrate its use.

In callosal apraxia, a lesion of the corpus callosum separates the left hemispheric language center from the right hemispheric motor centers, which produces apraxia of the left hand only. Patients do not have aphasia, right hemiparesis, or right-sided apraxia. In ideomotor apraxia, concomitant aphasia damages the motor engrams for movement in the dominant hemisphere, which in turn disconnects the homologous motor engrams in the nondominant hemisphere that require dominant hemisphere activation. These patients have aphasia, right hemiparesis, and left hemiapraxia. Right hemiparesis makes apraxia testing impossible, but these patients also have right hemiapraxia.

Agnosia and Neglect

Agnosia is a modality-specific, but spatially nonspecific, failure of recognition, whereas neglect is a modality-nonspecific but spatially-specific failure of recognition. In visual agnosia, for example, the patient does not recognize and respond appropriately to items seen in every visual field, despite normal visual acuity and processing. In left hemineglect, there are lack of attention and visual, auditory, and somasthetic nonrecognition of any item placed in left hemispace. The syndromes of agnosia and neglect are listed in Table 16-3.

Agnosia is examined by asking the patient to name common objects, colors, and forms by sight and touch. Prosopagnosia can be assessed by asking the patient to name pictures of well-known faces. Neglect is tested by asking the patient to draw a clock, copy a picture, or bisect a line. In cases of left hemineglect, the left side of the figure is left incomplete and the line is bisected far to the right of midline.

TABLE 16-3 AGNOSIA AND NEGLECT SYNDROMES

Name	Characteristics	Lesion
Apperceptive visual agnosia	Failure of visual recognition of objects; cannot draw or trace outline of object	Bilateral occipital cortex
Associative visual agnosia	Cannot name objects on visual presentation; alexia without agraphia	Left occipital lobe and splenium of the corpus callosum
Color agnosia	Cannot name colors or point to a named color; seen with syndrome of alexia without agraphia	Left occipital lobe and splenium of the corpus callosum
Prosopagnosia	Inability to recognize faces; inability to recognize types of animals, trees, etc; left superior quadrantanopia	Right occipitotemporal
Tactile agnosia	Inability to recognize objects by touch	Anterior middle ⅓ of the contralateral postcentral gyrus
Auditory agnosia	Inability to recognize nonspeech sounds; may include the inability to appreciate the characteristics of music (amusia)	Right superior temporal gyrus and angular gyrus
Hemispatial neglect	Inattention to all objects in left visual hemispace	Right parietal lobe
Anosognosia	Denial by patient of accompanying left hemiparesis; when severe, denial that the left side of the body belongs to him	Acute large right parietal lobe

Bibliography

Benson DF: *Aphasia, Alexia, and Agraphia.* New York, Churchill Livingstone, 1979. (A complete summary of the principles of the Benson–Geschwind school of aphasia.)

Benson DF, Geschwind N: The aphasias and related disturbances. In Baker AB, Joynt RJ (eds): *Clinical Neurology.* Philadelphia, Harper & Row, 1986, Chapter 10. (The best short work on the clinical aspects of aphasia. Recommended as the first source to consult.)

Brown JW: *Aphasia, Apraxia, and Agnosia.* Springfield, Ill, Charles C Thomas, 1972. (Difficult to read but presents a counterpoint to the Benson–Geschwind approach.)

Geschwind N: Disconnexion syndromes in animals and man. *Brain* 1965; 88:237-294, 585-644. (The single most important original work on aphasia and apraxia in this generation.)

Goodglass H, Kaplan E: *The Assessment of Aphasia and Related Disorders,* ed 2. Philadelphia, Lea & Febiger, 1983. (An excellent treatise by the developers of the Boston Diagnostic Aphasia Examination; includes the entire BDAE, its scoring, and its interpretation.)

Heilman KM, Valenstein E (eds): *Clinical Neuropsychology,* ed 2. New York, Oxford University Press, 1985. (The single best reference source, with excellent critiques of past research studies; well referenced.)

Knopman DS, Selnes OA, Niccum N, et al: A longitudinal study of speech fluency in aphasia: CT correlates of recovery and persistent nonfluency. *Neurology* 1983: 33: 1170-1178. (Shows how language recovery in aphasia is related to lesion size and location.)

Rose FC (ed): *Progress in Aphasiology Advances in Neurology* Ser, vol 42. New York, Raven Press, 1984. (Up-to-date comprehensive account from the British perspective.)

Ross ED: The aprosodias. Functional–anatomic organization of the affective components of language in the right hemisphere. *Arch Neurol* 1981; 38:561-569. (The best work on aprosodias, with complete descriptions of each type.)

Sarno MT: *Acquired Aphasia.* New York, Academic Press, 1981. (A series of papers on aphasia, many from the linguistic viewpoint; particularly strong on rehabilitative aspects.)

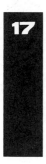

17

Bladder, Bowel, and Sexual Dysfunction

NEUROGENIC BLADDER DYSFUNCTION

CLINICAL SIGNIFICANCE

Impairment of bladder innervation at any level can produce the syndrome of neurogenic bladder. Neurogenic bladder dysfunction can therefore complicate a wide variety of nervous system diseases. In outpatient practice, neurogenic bladder is most commonly seen in patients with myelopathies and peripheral autonomic neuropathies.

Normal bladder emptying consists of a complex reflex action of several steps:

1. There is appreciation of bladder fullness at bladder volumes of 100 to 200 mL, provided by sensory impulses originating from the stretched bladder wall and projecting to the parasagittal frontal lobe cortex.

2. Tonic contraction of the external urinary sphincter is first inhibited; the induced state of sphincter relaxation persists throughout the act of micturition, although several brief contractions may occur.

3. Several seconds after relaxation of the external sphincter, there is sustained contraction of the detrusor muscle of the bladder wall. When intravesical pressure exceeds urethral pressure, urine is voided.

4. The pulse rate and systolic and diastolic blood pressure often rise during voiding.

5. As the bladder volume returns to normal, detrusor contraction subsides and the external urinary sphincter tone returns to normal.

ETIOLOGY

Abnormal bladder emptying of neurogenic origin can be simply classified into three major groups.

1. *Detrussor hyperreflexia (spastic bladder).* Detrussor hyperactivity is the result of impaired higher spinal cord and brain micturition inhibitory centers. Detrussor hyperreflexia can be produced by hydrocephalus or parasagittal meningiomas that interfere with higher urinary control centers in the parasagittal

frontal cortex. Similarly, interference with descending inhibitory pathways at the level of the cervical or thoracic spinal cord can result from spinal cord compression, injury, or multiple sclerosis.

2. *Detrussor hyporeflexia (flaccid bladder).* Detrussor hypoactivity is the result of impaired direct sacral segmental bladder innervation by lesions of the sacral spinal cord, cauda equina, or peripheral nerves to the bladder. Commonly, his type of neurogenic bladder results from compressive lesions of the sacral spinal cord (conus medullaris) and cauda equina, and from peripheral autonomic neuropathies such as those produced by diabetes mellitus.

3. *Detrussor-urethral sphincter dyssynergia.* This disorder may accompany both aformentioned types of neurogenic bladder. Dyssynergia refers to loss of coordination between muscular contraction of the detrussor and relaxation of the external sphincter. The sphincter may fail to reflex during detrussor contraction, or there may be inappropriate sphincter relaxation without detrussor contraction. Table 17-1 lists the specific causes of detrussor hyperreflexia and hyporeflexia.

SYMPTOMS AND SIGNS

Although patients with neurogenic bladders may complain of hesitancy, frequency, urgency, and retention, it is urinary incontinence that most often causes them to seek medical attention. This complaint is divided into five types:

1. *Urge incontinence.* The patient suddenly feels the need to void, but cannot

---

TABLE 17-1 ETIOLOGY OF DETRUSSOR HYPOREFLEXIA AND HYPERREFLEXIA

Detrussor hyperreflexia

Interruption of pathways to and from the detrussor part of the frontal cortex to the brain stem
    Stroke
    Brain tumor
    Head injury
    Parkinsonism
    Motor neuron diseases
    Multiple sclerosis
    Dementia

Interruption of pathways from the brain stem to the detrussor motor centers in the sacral spinal cord
    Spinal cord trauma
    Syringomyelia
    Multiple sclerosis
    Spinal cord tumor
    Adhesive arachnoiditis

Detrussor hyporeflexia

Interruption of peripheral nerve to spinal cord bladder motor and sensory fibers
    Cauda equina or conus medullaris injury
    Adhesive arachnoiditis
    Central disc herniation
    Spinal cord birth defects

Interruption of peripheral nerve to spinal cord bladder sensory fibers
    Diabetes mellitus

Interruption of spinal cord innervation of detrussor nuclei
    "Spinal shock" following acute spinal cord injury
    Multiple sclerosis

Adapted from Bradley WE: Cystometry and sphincter electromyography. *Mayo Clin Proc* 1976; 51:331. Used with permission.

reach the bathroom quickly enough. This pattern is characteristic of, but not specific for, detrussor hyperreflexia.

2. *Overflow incontinence*. There is steady dribbling of urine from a large, overfilled bladder under low pressure. This pattern is common in detrussor hyporeflexia.

3. *Reflex incontinence*. There is neither the sensation of bladder filling nor the urge to void, but the bladder spontaneously and frequently voids small amounts of urine. This pattern is common with total suprasacral bladder denervation by spinal cord lesions.

4. *Stress incontinence*. Sudden increases in intraabdominal pressure during coughing or laughing induce involuntary voiding of small amounts of urine. Stress incontinence is not usually caused by a neurogenic bladder, but by an anatomic disruption of the urethral angle or length. It is most common in women following childbirth and in men following prostatectomy.

5. *Total incontinence*. The sphincter is totally incompetent so that any urine in the bladder automatically leaks out. Incontinence is worse when standing than when lying. Total incontinence is the "endpoint" of stress incontinence and is produced by the same disorders.

LABORATORY TESTS

Urinalysis should be performed on all patients with neurogenic bladder. If pyuria or bacteriuria is present, a clean-catch urine specimen should be submitted for culture and sensitivity testing. Urinary catheterization is also indicated to measure postvoiding residual urine volume. A neurogenic bladder with more than 50 mL of postvoid residual urine puts the patient at high risk for urinary tract infection.

Cystometry and sphincter electromyography (EMG) are the best techniques for classifying the type of neurogenic bladder. Cystometry can be performed with water, saline, or carbon dioxide. The cystometrogram is a pressure versus volume tracing obtained by filling the bladder at a constant rate through a urinary catheter. Pressure transducers and surface EMG electrodes can simultaneously record intraurethral pressure, sphincter motor activity, and intravesical pressure.

In the normal person, there is only a slight rise in intravesical pressure when the bladder is filled with 200 mL. The first sensation of filling occurs at 100 to 150 mL, and the desire to void, at 200 to 250 mL. Intravesical pressure rises with voluntary contractions.

In detrussor hyperreflexia, there are uninhibited bladder contractions that induce voiding at very low bladder volumes. The patient may or may not be aware of the contractions. In detrussor hyporeflexia, a large bladder volume is required before intravesical pressure rises; the patient may not have the urge to void. In detrussor–urethral sphincter dyssynergia, EMG reveals inappropriate sphincter contractions during detrussor contraction. Administration of anticholinergic, cholinergic, or alpha-sympatholytic agents at the time of cystometry can guide subsequent therapy.

DIAGNOSIS

Historical data should include any history of enuresis, urinary tract surgery, urinary tract infection, and past patterns of voiding. Present illness history should include assessment of current medications, nocturia, frequency, urgency, burning, hesitancy, retention, weak stream, intermittency, dribbling, incontinence, back or neck pain, weakness or numbness in the legs, and associated symptoms of bowel or sexual dysfunction.

Physical examination should include a careful neurological examination and an inspection of the external urethral apparatus. Rectal examinations in men'and pelvic examinations in women are necessary to assess prostate size and uterine and bladder suspension.

In the patient with suspected neurogenic bladder, two major complicating or coexisting factors must be excluded: urinary obstruction and infection. Both can produce symptoms of urgency, dribbling, burning, nocturia, and hesitancy. A clinical diagnosis of neurogenic bladder is made only when infection and obstruction have been excluded. Cystometric testing is necessary to define the type of neurogenic bladder.

MANAGEMENT

Therapeutic modalities for urinary incontinence include pharmacotherapy, catheterization, physical measures, and surgery. An indwelling Foley catheter should be avoided if possible because it has a propensity for producing chronic urinary tract infection, bladder calculi, bladder spasm, hematuria, and urethral strictures, fistulas, and abscesses. An indwelling Foley catheter may be indicated in several situations: (1) seriously ill or debilitated patients with incontinence or retention; (2) patients too ill to undergo a corrective urologic or gynecologic procedure to relieve obstruction or combat incontinence; and (3) patients with hydronephrosis or vesicoureteral reflux. Condom catheters are acceptable for patients with overflow or total incontinence.

Clean, intermittent self-catheterization is recommended for the patient with chronic neurogenic bladder who has the muscular control to perform the procedure. Paraplegics with spastic bladders from multiple sclerosis or spinal cord injury are particularly good subjects to learn to catheterize themselves. With self-catheterization four times daily, bladder volumes can be optimized and residual urine evacuated. This results in a greatly reduced risk of urinary tract infection and incontinence.

Physical measures useful in some patients include trigger voiding, Credé's method, and Kegel exercises. Trigger voiding may be successful in patients with detrusor hyperreflexia. Stroking the thigh, pulling pubic hairs, tapping the suprapubic region, or stroking the glans penis may incite reflex voiding. Each patient can discover his or her own trigger point and optimum body position to reflexively induce voiding.

Credé's method may aid patients with detrussor hyporeflexia. Here, the bladder must be manually compressed to empty. The patient sits erect and pushes one or both open hands deep into the suprapubic area while performing a Valsalva maneuver. Intravesical pressure thus is made to exceed urethral pressure.

Kegel exercises alleviate stress incontinence in women by strengthening the pubococcygeus muscle. These exercises include: (1) squeezing the muscles of the vaginal introitus and wall upon the inserted finger; (2) drawing the perineum up and in; (3) constricting the anal sphincter as if to interrupt a bowel movement; and (4) contracting the external urethral sphincter as if to interrupt voiding.

Several surgical measures may be useful to aid voiding in patients with neurogenic bladders. They include transurethral external sphincthotomy, pudendal neurectomy, transurethral resection of the bladder neck, enterocystoplasty, and sacral rhizotomy. See Krane RJ, Sinoky MB (1979) for further discussion of these procedures.

Pharmacotherapy remains the mainstay of neurogenic bladder treatment. It is selected on the basis of findings on cystometry and urethral EMG. Some empirical manipulation of drugs and dosages is usually also necessary because of individual variation in response.

Detrussor hyperreflexia is treated with anticholinergic drugs and those that directly relax smooth muscle. Propantheline bromide (Pro-Banthine), 15 to 30 mg two to four times daily, can be prescribed. Its anticholinergic effect opposes detrussor hyperreflexia and reduces bladder resting tone. It is contraindicated in glaucoma and in urinary obstruction. Oxybutynin chloride (Ditropan) is the most useful agent for treating detrussor hyperreflexia because, in addition to its anticholinergic effects, it directly relaxes bladder smooth muscle. It is given in a dosage of 5 mg two to three times daily. It is contraindicated in glaucoma, urinary tract obstruction, and pregnancy.

Detrussor hyporeflexia is treated with cholinergic drugs to increase bladder smooth muscle tone. Bethanechol (Urecholine), 40 to 150 mg daily in divided doses, is the drug of choice. It is contraindicated in pregnancy, peptic ulcer, asthma, hyperthyroidism, and parkinsonism.

Detrussor-urethral sphincter dyssynergia is treated with cholinergic or anticholinergic agents, depending on whether it complicates detrussor hyporeflexia or hyperreflexia. If inappropriate sphincter contraction is of the bladder neck and proximal urethra, the alpha-adrenergic blocker phenoxybenzamine (Dibenzyline), 10 to 40 mg daily in divided doses is prescribed. This drug is contraindicated in severe cardiac or pulmonary disease. It can induce hypotension and ejaculatory failure.

If inappropriate sphincter contraction is from the external sphincter, baclofen (Lioresal) is the drug of choice. It is usually prescribed as two 10 mg tablets three times daily. Side effects include gastric irritation and drowsiness.

WHEN TO CONSULT

Patients with neurogenic bladders should undergo urodynamic studies (cystometry, sphincter EMG) by a urologist trained in these techniques, because urodynamic studies direct pharmacotherapy. The urologist should also assess the presence of any surgically remediable mechanical factors.

NEUROGENIC BOWEL DYSFUNCTION

CLINICAL SIGNIFICANCE

Impairment of bowel and rectal innervation by disorders of motor or sensory neurons can produce constipation, diarrhea, or fecal incontinence. There is a high degree of concordance between neurogenic bladder and neurogenic bowel disorders because their innervation is analogous and they are subject to the same set of neurological disorders.

ETIOLOGY, SYMPTOMS, AND SIGNS

The causes of fecal incontinence are listed in Table 17-2. Diabetes mellitus, multiple sclerosis, and parkinsonism (constipation) are the most common neurogenic bowel disorders seen in outpatient practice.

Denervation of the external anal sphincter is most often a mechanical disturbance resulting from weakness of the pelvic floor musculature. Pudendal nerves may be compressed or damaged by straining at bowel movements or during childbirth. Pudendal neuropathy produces weakness and incompetence of the external rectal sphincter.

Internal anal sphincter incompetence is most often caused by peripheral neuropathies (particularly diabetes) interfering with reflex tonic contraction. Similar dysfunction is also produced by spinal cord diseases and lesions of the parasagittal cerebral hemispheres. Internal sphincteropathy induces diarrhea, which magnifies the incontinence.

Mechanical factors must also be considered. Previous anal surgery can produce fecal incontinence. Hemorrhoidectomy produces fecal soilage in 25% of patients. Anal dilation and sphincterotomy produce incontinence in 5% of patients.

Diarrhea induces incontinence in patients with marginal competence of the anal sphincter. A common clinical scenario is to find new diarrhea as the basis for recently developed fecal incontinence. This is particularly common in the elderly patient with reduced baseline anal sphincter pressure.

LABORATORY TESTS AND DIAGNOSIS

Mechanical factors, diarrhea, previous surgery, hemorrhoids, and nervous system disease are ascertained by history, rectal examination, and neurological examination. Appropriate investigations of the nervous system and gastrointestinal tract may be ordered. Diarrhea is evaluated according to usual protocols.

MANAGEMENT

The treatment of neurogenic constipation embraces the following general principles:

1. *Ensure adequate fluid intake.* The patient should take at least 2 liters of fluids by mouth daily as juice, coffee, tea, or any other beverage.

TABLE 17-2 ETIOLOGY OF FECAL INCONTINENCE

External sphincter dysfunction
　Denervation caused by pelvic floor descent
　Damage from prior anal surgery
　Spinal cord injuries
Internal sphincter dysfunction
　Autonomic neuropathies
　Diabetes mellitus
　Damage from prior anal surgery
　Parasagittal brain lesions
Diarrhea
Fecal impaction
Partial obstruction in malignancy
Hemorrhoids (fecal soilage)

Adapted from Lieberman DA: Common anorectal disorders. *Ann Intern Med* 1984; 101:843. Used with permission.

2. *Ensure adequate fiber intake.* A diet of foods high in fiber (bran cereals, fruits, some vegetables, whole wheat bread) should be encouraged. Fiber increases stool bulk and water-retaining capability and facilitates normal bowel movements.

3. *Schedule regular physical activity.* Contraction of abdominal muscles and aerobic elevation of resting heart rate help produce regular bowel movements.

4. *Schedule regular bowel movements.* Utilizing the gastrocolic reflex, patients should attempt evacuation 20 to 30 minutes after meals at the same time each day. The voiding environment should be quiet and relaxed. Hot beverages are particularly likely to stimulate the gastrocolic reflex.

For the more severe cases of neurogenic constipation, additional measures can be undertaken:

1. *Stool softeners.* Docusate sodium (Colace), 100 mg daily, can increase the water content of stool through surface action.

2. *Bulk supplements.* Psyllium hydrophilic mucilloid (Metamucil) adds bland fiber to the stools and promotes normal elimination.

3. *Glycerine suppositories.* These can be inserted 30 minutes prior to planned evacuation to aid the passage of dry, hard stools.

In severe instances of constipation, laxatives and enemas may be necessary. Frequent use of laxatives or enemas is potentially harmful because constant irritant stimuli produce bowel desensitization and tolerance to medications. Spontaneous evacuation becomes impossible and progressively stronger irritant stimuli become necessary. A reasonable approach follows:

1. Mild laxatives, such as milk of magnesia, should be tried first.

2. Bisacodyl (Dulcolax), 5 mg tablets or 10 mg suppositories, can be tried next.

3. Tap-water enemas twice weekly can be added if the above regimen fails. Soap suds or oil enemas should be avoided if possible.

4. Manual rectal disimpaction may be necessary for the obstipated patient.

Management of neurogenic diarrhea and incontinence is difficult. General measures previously listed should be instituted. Chronic neurogenic diarrhea may be reduced by the judicious use of diphenoxylate hydrochloride with atropine sulfate (Lomotil) or a paregoric, pectin, and kaolin mixture (Parapectolin). Neurogenic fecal incontinence can be treated with exercises to improve rectal sphincter tone and by biofeedback conditioning. Surgical procedures to improve fecal incontinence have uneven results.

NEUROGENIC SEXUAL DYSFUNCTION

CLINICAL SIGNIFICANCE

Neurogenic disturbances of sexual function are common in patients with neurogenic bladder and bowel dysfunction. Both the parasympathetic and sympathetic nervous systems are required for normal sexual functioning. Although separating sexual functions by these pathways is an oversimplification, penile and clitoral tumescence and erection primarily are parasympathetically innervated. The series of muscular contractions of the seminal vesicles, prostate, vas deferens, and ampulla that constitute ejaculation in the man and of the uterus, fallopian tubes, and vagina during orgasm in the woman are primarily sympathetically innervated.

Etiology

Table 17-3 lists the causes of sexual dysfunction associated with diseases of the nervous system. Anatomic, vascular, psychogenic, and endocrine causes may be present as well, and must be considered.

Symptoms and Signs

Neurogenic complaints of sexual dysfunction fall into one of several categories: (1) loss of libido, (2) failure to achieve or maintain erection or arousal, or (3) failure to achieve orgasm and ejaculation.

Some studies report that as many as 90% of cases of male erectile failure are psychogenic, but a more reasonable current figure is 25%. The following questions help separate psychogenic from organic erectile failure. If any are answered in the affirmative, impotence is probably psychogenic.

1. Do you have erections when you awake in the morning? (Morning erections are normally present because erection occurs during REM sleep and REM sleep cycles are frequent in the early morning. If impotence is totally organic, there should be no morning erection.)

TABLE 17-3 CLASSIFICATION OF SEXUAL DISORDERS ARISING FROM DISEASES OF THE NERVOUS SYSTEM

Disorders of libido

Decreased
  Due to effects of chronic disease (pain, disability, depression, leg spasticity)
  Specific disorders: secondary hypogonadism from pituitary disorders, frontal lobe disorders
Increased
  Temporal lobe epilepsy
  Frontal lobe disorders
  Delirium

Disorders of tumescence

Impaired erection caused by lesions of:
  Parasagittal region of brain
  Spinal cord
  Peripheral nerves
  Autonomic nervous system
Drug effects
Impaired detumescence (priapism)
  Spinal cord lesion

Disorders of emission and ejaculation

Lesions of sympathetic nervous system
Drug effects
Metabolic/endocrine disorders
Postoperative: sympathectomy, aortic aneurysm resection, abdominal-perineal resection

---

Adapted from Seiden MR: *Practical Management of Chronic Neurologic Problems.* New York, Appleton-Century-Crofts, 1981, p 144. Used with permission.

2. Do you have erections with dreams? (The same explanation holds: dreams occur during REM sleep.)

3. Do you have erections during masturbation, sexual daydreams, or fantasies?

4. Do you have erections when performing with sexual partners other than your wife?

5. Have you lost sexual interest (libido)?

6. Have you been depressed?

A careful history of current medication use is mandatory. Impotence can be produced by several classes of drugs, including anticholinergics, tricyclic antidepressants, phenothiazines, alcohol, benzodiazepines, narcotic analgesics, and sympatholytic antihypertensives (beta-blockers, alpha-methyldopa, guanethidine, reserpine).

LABORATORY TESTS AND DIAGNOSIS.
If the patient's impotence does not have an obvious neurological basis, several laboratory tests are indicated.

A fasting blood glucose test or two-hour postprandial glucose test should be done to exclude diabetes mellitus, which predisposes to vascular impotence. A serum testosterone test can be used to screen for hypogonadism. Thyroid function and prolactin tests should also be performed because impotence can be produced by hyperthyroidism, hypothyroidism, and hyperprolactinemia. If the diagnosis of organic impotence is in question, a sleep laboratory study with measurement of penile tumescence can be performed (Chapter 30). A psychologic screening interview should be conducted to search for signs of depression, including anorexia, weight loss, loss of interest, anhedonia, and morbid thoughts.

MANAGEMENT
Therapy for neurogenic sexual dysfunction begins with the identification and treatment of reversible causes. Thus, impotence-producing drugs should be stopped, depression treated, and underlying medical conditions treated.

Patients should be questioned about the importance of sexuality in their day-to-day lives and about the impact of sexual dysfunction on them and their partners. They should be counseled that the goal of therapy is a satisfying sexual outlet for them and their partners. The range of sexual activity can include any activity that is pleasurable, harmless, and inoffensive to both partners. Masturbation and anogenital and orogenital activities should be presented as acceptable options to the neurologically disabled patient. Nongenital erogenous zones (nipples, lips, earlobes, etc.) should be identified by experiment. *Sexual Options for Paraplegics and Quadriplegics* by Mooney TO, Cole TM, Chilgren RA (1975) provides more detailed information.

Penile erection in the impotent patient may be produced reflexively by stroking the glans penis or the inside of the thigh. Placing a rubber band at the base of the penis to create a constriction pressure greater than venous pressure but less than arterial pressure safely produces partial erection. The band should not be kept in place for more than 20 minutes, however.

Penile prostheses should be offered as an option. There are two types: the semirigid rod and the inflatable type. The semirigid rod keeps the penis in a state of perpetual partial erection. When pointed downwards it can be concealed in the pants; when pointed upward it can be used to function sexually. The inflatable prosthesis contains a pump that is placed in the scrotum and that will inflate the prosthesis. This prosthesis allows the penis to appear relatively normal when noninflated, but it produces a full erection when inflated. It is more expensive, however, and has more complications, including phimosis, penile irritation, and plastic tube migration.

Female sexual dysfunction includes vaginal dryness, dyspareunia, and failure to achieve orgasm. A water-soluble, sterile jelly (K-Y) can be used as a vaginal lubricant. Vaseline is not recommended because it is not water-soluble and can produce urinary tract infection. Women must experiment to find locations and techniques that they find pleasurable and to teach their partners how to please them. A relationship of open communication, caring, and love is necessary.

Bibliography

Bradley WE: Cystometry and sphincter electromyography. *Mayo Clin Proc* 1976; 51:329-335. (Good description of urodynamic studies and their interpretation.)

Bradley WE, Rockswold GL, Timm GW, et al: Neurology of micturition. *J Urol* 1976; 115:481-486. (Readable review that is still current.)

Brocklehurst JC: Management of anal incontinence. *Clin Gastroenterol* 1975; 4:479-487. (Practical tips for therapy.)

Krane RJ, Siroky MB (eds): *Clinical Neuro-Urology.* Boston, Little, Brown, 1979. (Contains much detailed information, particularly on surgical options in treatment.)

Lieberman DA: Common anorectal disorders. *Ann Intern Med* 1984; 101:837-846. (Contains useful section on fecal incontinence, particularly the causative roles of diabetes, hemorrhoids, and diarrhea.)

Mooney TO, Cole TM, Chilgren RA: *Sexual Options for Paraplegics and Quadriplegics.* Boston, Little, Brown, 1975. (Provides information on positions and techniques; to be read by patient.)

Morley JE: Impotence. *Am J Med* 1986; 897-905. (A recent reveiw of the anatomy, etiology, and management of the impotent patient.)

Resnick NM, Yalla SV: Management of urinary incontinence in the elderly. *N Engl J Med* 1985; 313:800-805. (Classifies urinary incontinence and discusses management.)

Scheinberg LC (ed): *Multiple Sclerosis: A Guide for Patients and Their Families.* New York, Raven Press, 1983. (Contains excellent chapters on bladder and bowel management and sexuality. Most of the information presented is applicable to other neurological diseases in addition to MS.)

Seiden MR: *Practical Management of Chronic Neurologic Problems.* New York, Appleton-Century-Crofts, 1981. (Useful and well-described tips for the management of bowel, bladder, and sexual disorders that complicate specific diseases of the nervous system.)

Slag MF, Morley JE, Elson MK, et al: Impotence in medical clinic outpatients. *JAMA* 1983; 249:1736-1740. (Discusses the etiologies of impotence in 401 cases of male impotence screened from an outpatient population. Unlike previous studies, this one found that 14% of cases were psychogenic, 83% had an identifiable organic cause, and only 7% were of unknown cause.)

18

The Floppy Infant

Not uncommonly, the generalist is faced with the evaluation of a hypotonic or "floppy" infant. Hypotonia refers to decreased resistance of the limbs with passive motion. The features of floppy infant syndrome include (1) bizarre or unusual postures; (2) decreased resistance of the joints to passive motion; and (3) increased range of motion of the joints. Hypotonia usually accompanies weakness, but it may occur in isolation.

Hypotonia, a common problem in infancy, may be associated with a wide variety of conditions that affect either the upper motor neuron or the lower motor neuron. The associated clinical features of diseases affecting these neurons are listed in Table 18-1.

A careful neurological history must be obtained when evaluating the floppy infant. Depending on the age of the infant, various symptoms and signs may be evident that suggest neuromuscular disease. An inadequate cry, weak sucking, or a paucity of body movements in the newborn may be a clue that he or she is affected by a neurological disease. In the case of weakness producing floppiness (Table 18-2) the temporal profile of the development of the weakness is important to ascertain. Did the infant move normally in utero, or did movements decrease as the pregnancy progressed? Did the weakness have an abrupt onset, or did it develop slowly or insidiously? Abrupt weakness is usually associated with vascular disease or trauma, whereas insidious weakness is suggestive of degenerative or metabolic disease. Is the process progressive, episodic, or static? A complete developmental history must be obtained (Chapter 2). Because the infant is less than a year old, crawling, walking, and vocalization are important milestones to assess. Based on the history, it should be determined whether the disease process is diffuse or focal. The family history should be investigated thoroughly, because many diseases that cause floppy infant syndrome are hereditary.

The classical posture of the floppy infant is the "frog posture," with the hips abducted and externally rotated, and the limbs in contact with the surface that the infant is lying upon, because of poor postural tone. (The normal position is that of

TABLE 18-1 LOCALIZATION OF WEAKNESS/HYPOTONIA

LOCATION	TONE	DEEP-TENDON	SUPERFICIAL	BABINSKI'S	ATROPHY	FASCICULATIONS
			REFLEXES			
Upper motor neuron	↑ *	↑	−	+	No	No
Lower motor neuron Anterior horn	↓	↓	−	−	Yes	Yes
Nerve	↓	↓	+	−	Yes	Rarely
Neuromuscular junction	Normal	Normal	+	−	No	No
Muscle	Normal	Normal†	+	−	Yes	No

↓ = Decreased.

↑ = Increased.

+ = Present.

− = Absent.

*Hypotonia replaces hypertonia in infants.

†Reflexes are absent with marked atrophy.

Adapted from Wright FS: Weakness, fatigue, hypotonia, in Swaiman KF, Wright FB (eds): *The Practice of Pediatric Neurology* (ed2). St Louis, McGraw-Hill, 1982, pp 278-286.

flexion and adduction of the hips.) The spontaneous movements of the infant should be observed.

Ventral suspension and traction of the hands (when supine) are two positions that are most helpful in assessing hypotonia (Chapter 2). In ventral suspension, when the infant is supported prone by a hand under the chest, the normal infant holds his head at 45° angle or less to the horizontal. The back is straight or slightly flexed, with the arms flexed at the elbows and extended (partially) at the shoulders, and the knees partially flexed. In contrast, the floppy infant's head and limbs hang limply, like a "rag doll." When the normal infant is supine, traction on the hands to raise the shoulders off the couch results in some flexion of the head in full-term and immature infants. Most full-term infants can keep their head in the same plane as the body, whereas the floppy infant shows a marked head lag.

The neurological examination should help determine whether hypotonia is the result of upper motor neuron or lower motor neuron disease (Table 18-1). If the infant can move its limbs against gravity or spontaneously following a stimulus to the soles or hands, or can maintain a posture of a passively elevated limb, then weakness cannot be significant. Infants, in contrast to older children or adults, have hypotonia as a manifestation of upper motor neuron disease. Upper motor neuron dysfunction, caused by involvement of the pyramidal and extrapyramidal pathways from the cerebral cortex to the spinal cord, classically produces weakness that is distal more than proximal and that is not associated with atrophy or fasciculations. Deep-tendon reflexes are exaggerated, superficial reflexes are lost, and an extensor plantar response (Babinski's sign) is present. In the older child and adult, spasticity also accompanies upper motor neuron disorders.

Involvement of the lower motor neuron produces segmental weakness, atrophy, depressed or normal reflexes (depending on the level of lower motor neuron involvement), and fasciculations (if the anterior horn cell or peripheral nerve are involved). The range of motion of the joints should be tested. The floppy

TABLE 18-2 DISORDERS THAT PRODUCE HYPOTONIA

Nonparalytic conditions (hypotonia without significant weakness)

Central nervous system diseases

Hypotonic cerebral palsy
Birth trauma
    Cerebral
    Spinal cord
Perinatal asphyxia
Intracranial hemorrhage
Dysgenetic syndromes, eg, trisomy 21 (Down's syndrome)
Metabolic disorders
    Leukodystrophies
    Sphingolipidoses
    Aminoacidurias
    Mucopolysaccharidoses
Failure-to-thrive syndromes
Prader–Willi syndrome (hypotonia–obesity)
Benign congenital hypotonia
Metabolic and endocrine diseases
    Organic acidemia
    Hypothyroidism
    Hypercalcemia or hypocalcemia
    Leigh's syndrome

Connective tissue disorders

Congenital laxity of ligaments
Ehlers–Danlos syndrome
Marfan's syndrome
Mucopolysaccharidoses
Osteogenesis imperfecta

Paralytic conditions (weakness prominent; hypotonia incidental)

Anterior horn cell disorders

Infantile spinal muscular atrophy (Werdnig-Hoffman Disease)
    "Benign" variants
Poliomyelitis

Peripheral nerve disorders

Guillain–Barré syndrome
Neuroaxonal dystrophy
Metachromatic leukodystrophy
Globoid cell leukodystrophy
Hereditary neuropathies

Neuromuscular junction disorders

Neonatal and congenital myasthenia gravis
Infant botulism

Muscle diseases

Congenital myotonic dystrophy
Congenital muscular dystrophy
Congenital myopathies
    Metabolic
        Lipid storage myopathy
        Glycogen storage disease: types II (Pompe's disease) and III
        Periodic paralysis
    Structural
        Myotubular myopathy
        Nemaline (rod) myopathy
        Central core disease
        Congenital fiber-type disproportion
        Other morphological myopathies

Adapted from Dubowitz V: *The Floppy Infant. Clinics in Developmental Medicine No. 76*, ed 2. Philadelphia, Spastics International and Lippincott, 1980; and Dubowitz V: The floppy infant syndrome, in *Muscle Disorders of Childhood*. Philadelphia, Saunders, 1978.

infant is able to be placed in bizarre postures. Placement of the foot to the chin or head and adduction of the elbow past the midline toward the opposite side of the body are possible only in the hypotonic infant.

Upon examination of the cranial nerves, the presence of ptosis or weakness of extraocular movements may indicate lower motor neuron disease, either of the neuromuscular junction or muscle. Symmetry of the facial muscles should be present when the infant is crying. The gag reflex should be assessed, and the presence of abnormal tongue movements (fasciculations) should be determined.

Deep-tendon reflexes are normally obtainable in the infant, although the triceps reflex is usually more difficult to elicit because of the predominant flexor tone in the upper extremities. When all reflexes are brisk, the possibility of upper motor neuron disease must be considered. Eight to ten beats of clonus is normal in infants, but unilateral ankle clonus is abnormal.

Moro and Landau reflexes and tonic neck response should be tested (Chapter 2). Although all muscles should be inspected visually, muscle atrophy is usually not visible because of the presence of subcutaneous fat. The muscle should be tapped (percussed) to look for contraction. No response occurs in normal patients or those with muscle disease, but a positive response is likely with neurogenic lesions. Sensory examination is difficult to perform, but the infant's response to noxious stimulation (pinprick) should be tested in the limbs, trunk, and face. By the end of the examination, the physician should be able to determine whether the infant has true weakness with incidental hypotonia (usually arising in the lower motor neuron), or whether the infant is truly hypotonic without weakness.

Diagnostic categories in Table 18-2 can be based on the age of the infant, and on whether there is weakness or just hypotonia (without weakness). Three-fourths of the cases of hypotonia are caused by perinatal insult to the spinal cord or the brain, spinal muscular atrophy, and dysgenetic syndromes. A spinal cord injury usually follows a uterine malposition or a traumatic birth. Focal hypotonia may be of developmental origin or the result of trauma. Upper brachial plexus injury is often accompanied by paralysis of the diaphragm. Lower plexus injuries (Klumpke's paralysis) are often accompanied by Horner's syndrome.

The anatomical approach to the infant with hypotonia begins with diseases that affect the cerebral cortex and associated corticospinal tract projections to the spinal cord. Anterior horn cell dysfunction, peripheral nerves, and neuromuscular structures are then considered, followed by muscle and tendon (connective tissue) diseases. A list of common causes of floppy infant syndrome based on this classification is presented in Table 18-2.

Hypotonia may be associated with mental deficiency or can be caused by other disorders such as cerebral palsy (Chapter 26). Nonparalytic conditions that produce hypotonia without weakness are usually caused by connective tissue disorders. Metabolic disease may also produce this syndrome, but usually there are other symptoms and signs. Most upper motor neuron diseases are non-paralytic, and most lower motor neuron diseases are paralytic.

A brief discussion of common diseases that produce hypotonia with or without weakness follows. Related topics are discussed further in Chapters 10, 25, 26, 28, and 29. For a complete discussion of these diseases the reader is referred to Dubowitz (1978 and 1980).

PARALYTIC DISORDERS
(WITH INCIDENTAL HYPOTONIA)
Severe Infantile Spinal Muscular Atrophy

Also known as Werdnig–Hoffman disease, infantile spinal muscular atrophy (SMA) is the most common cause of hypotonia with weakness. Inherited as an autosomal recessive trait, infantile SMA has an early onset—possibly in utero (noticed as diminished fetal movements by the mother)—or during the first three months of life. Paralysis can occur acutely, but it is usually more insidious in onset. The infant usually demonstrates marked weakness and hypotonia, and when supine assumes a frog-leg posture. The legs tend to be more severely affected than the arms; the infant is often able to raise the arms against gravity.

Marked head lag is present, with ventral suspension and with traction. These infants cannot raise their heads or roll over, but usually appear quite alert and responsive. Bulbar and respiratory muscles are affected, so swallowing is difficult and there is respiratory distress. Breathing is often diaphragmatic; a bell shape to the chest results. The cry is weak and high-pitched. Muscle atrophy or fasciculations are not evident on examination, and deep-tendon reflexes are always absent. Severe cases with early onset rarely survive the first year of life. The main variable that determines survival is the extent of the bulbar and respiratory involvement.

Nerve-conduction velocities may be normal or slowed, and electromyography (EMG) reveals fibrillations and a reduced interference pattern. Muscle biopsy is the only way to confirm the diagnosis. At autopsy, there are degenerative changes in the anterior horns of the spinal cord and the motor nuclei of the cranial nerves.

The child should be treated symptomatically. Tube feedings may be necessary because of bulbar involvement. The child should not be placed on a ventilator when respiratory insufficiency develops: once on the ventilator, he can never be weaned from it.

Intermediate Infantile Spinal Muscular Atrophy

Intermediate SMA has an insidious onset. The child develops normally during the first six months of life, but then is noted to have lower extremity weakness. This is first noticed when the infant has difficulty placing weight on his legs and cannot stand or walk. The child can sit, however, without much difficulty. Weakness is symmetrical in the legs, and mild weakness may develop in the arms. Weakness affects proximal muscles more than distal muscles. There are no bulbar symptoms, but atrophy and fasciculations of the tongue are common. The face is not affected; intercostal weakness is insignificant. Although generalized fasciculations are absent, there is often a coarse tremor of the hands. This type of SMA has a relatively benign course, with survival possible into adolescence and adult life. Ultimately, the prognosis depends on the severity of respiratory dysfunction.

The creatine kinase level is often normal, but may be elevated. Motor nerve conduction velocities are normal; EMG demonstrates fibrillations, with a reduced voluntary interference pattern. Muscle biopsy is diagnostic and reveals large-fiber atrophy with type 1 fiber hypertrophy.

NONPARALYTIC DISORDERS (HYPOTONIA WITHOUT SIGNIFICANT WEAKNESS)

A large percentage of children with hypotonia are in this category. Many present with hypotonia as the major symptom or have delayed motor milestones. Most have associated mental retardation; many children with hypotonia associated with delay in motor milestones and mental retardation have no specific identifiable cause for their disease. Hypotonic cerebral palsy is a cause of floppy infant syndrome (Chapter 26).

Birth trauma and other perinatal insults are common causes of infantile hypotonia. Hypotonia is often seen after difficult labor or in the infant with severe asphyxia. In both cases, hypotonia tends to be short-lived, and as the child improves neurologically, so does the hypotonia. Maternal diazepam exposure (usually given during labor) produces severe hypotonia in the neonate that is characteristically out of proportion to other neurological signs, and that may take up to two weeks to disappear.

Hypotonia is often present from birth in the child with Down's syndrome, in contrast to most other trisomy (dysgenetic) syndromes, in which there is increased tone. Various metabolic disorders (Table 18-2) are associated with hypotonia (and mental retardation), including abnormalities of amino acid metabolism and the organic acidemias. Lipid-storage diseases (sphingolipidoses) are associated with hypotonia, but usually intellectual deterioration is severe and is associated with visceromegaly and other neurological signs. The hypotonia is only an incidental feature of the illness.

CONNECTIVE TISSUE DISORDERS

Disorders of connective tissue involve fibrous elements or are disorders of mucopolysaccharide degradation. Many disorders of connective tissue are associated with hypotonia and delays in reaching motor milestones.

Congenital Laxity of Ligaments

Laxity of ligaments, often familial, is the most common connective tissue disorder that produces a floppy infant. Most cases are inherited in a dominant pattern. There is usually no associated intellectual impairment, and strength and deep tendon reflexes are normal. Many affected infants are asymptomatic. Children with laxity of joints and joint hypermobility may have hypotonia in infancy, delayed motor milestones, or congenital dislocations of the hip.

The following joint abnormalities are present in the child with joint laxity and hypermobility: (1) increased mobility of the thumb and wrist, with the thumb capable of being approximated to the anterior aspect of the forearm; (2) hyperextension of the metacarpophalangeal joints of the fingers—the wrist can be extended to 90°; (3) hyperextension of knees and elbows beyond 180°; (4) dorsiflexion of the ankles beyond 45° from the neutral position; and (5) increased range of abduction of the hips (often to 90°).

Ehlers–Danlos Syndrome

There are several varieties of this syndrome, which is characterized by excessively stretchable, easily bruised, fragile skin and hyperextensible joints. Classical forms are inherited in an autosomal dominant fashion; other subtypes (seven in all) are autosomal recessive, although type V Ehlers–Danlos is X-linked

Marfan's Syndrome

Marfan's syndrome is an autosomal recessive trait. It features the triad of ectopia lentis, long thin extremities, and aortic aneurysm. It has many clinical features of homocystinuria. There are at least four varieties of Marfan's syndrome; in the variety associated with joint hypermobility it has associated features of Ehlers–Danlos syndrome.

Bibliography

Brooke MH, Carroll JE, Ringel SP: Congenital hypotonia revisited. *Muscle Nerve* 1979; 2:84-100. (Excellent review of congenital hypotonia.)

Dubowitz V: *The Floppy Infant. Clinics in Developmental Medicine No. 76,* ed 2. Philadelphia, Spastics International and Lippincott, 1980. (Classic monograph that covers in detail all aspects of the floppy infant syndrome.)

Dubowitz V: The floppy infant syndrome, in *Muscle Disorders of Childhood* (*Major Problems in Clinical Pediatrics* Ser, vol 16). Philadelphia, Saunders, 1978, pp 223-231. (Concise review of the floppy infant syndrome; the rest of the book covers all aspects of pediatric muscle diseases.)

Wright FS: Weakness, fatigue, hypotonia, in Swaiman KF, Wright FB (eds): *The Practice of Pediatric Neurology,* ed 2. St Louis, McGraw Hill, 1982, vol 1, pp 278-286. (Reviews the clinical approach to the floppy or weak infant.)

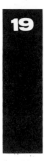

Failure in School

Learning disabilities are a group of related disorders that result in motor and behavior disturbances. Because children with learning disabilities are distracted very easily, they have difficulty performing tasks that require selective attention and discrimination. Approximately 10% of school-aged children have some degree of learning disability. Most of them have normal intelligence, are properly motivated, and are free of physical handicaps—yet they cannot, by conventional methods of education, make scholastic progress commensurate with their measured intelligence.

Childhood learning disorders have many causes. Such terms as hyperactivity, impulsivity, and minimal brain dysfunction (MBD) have been applied to learning disabilities. MBD is a term that was previously used synonymously with learning disorder and indicated that an observed behavioral disorder was based on brain abnormalities that could not be demonstrated by neurological examination. But MBD is a vague term, and many pediatric neurologists believe it is not a true clinical entity. Attention deficit disorder, also known as hyperactivity, is the major nonprogressive disorder that affects learning. This chapter focuses on attention deficit disorders, the common causes of school failure.

MINIMAL BRAIN DYSFUNCTION

As defined by the National Institute of Neurological and Communicative Disorders and Stroke (NINCDS) Task Force 1, minimal brain dysfunction refers to children "of near average, average or above average general intelligence with learning and behavioral disabilities ranging from mild to severe, which are associated with deviations of function of the nervous system. These deviations manifest themselves by various combinations of impairment of perception, conceptualization, language, memory, control of attention, impulse or motor function."

Clinical Significance
Abnormalities of nervous system function that can lead to MBD are caused by genetic changes, biochemical abnormalities, prenatal and perinatal insults,

trauma, or other diseases of the nervous system. Children with MBD may have learning difficulties, hyperactivity, discoordination, or combinations of these.

Some children with primary learning disabilities suffer from dyslexia. Developmental dyslexia is a language learning disability in which the child is unable to learn to read adequately in school in spite of normal intelligence. Reading, writing, and spelling are all involved to some degree. Word substitution, inversion of words or letters, and reversals of letter sequences are often seen in dyslexia. The letters most often reversed are "B," "D," "P," and "Q." A number of neurological abnormalities may have a direct relationship with dyslexia including lack of cerebral dominance, confused laterality, incoordination, and abnormal eye movements.

Dysnomia, the difficulty in finding and naming words, also may be present; it often precedes stuttering. Dyscalculia (difficulty in utilizing and comprehending numerical concepts) and dysgraphia (inability to copy or write letters, words, or numbers) may also develop.

Both learning-disabled and hyperactive children perform tasks that demand sustained attention less successfully than groups of normal "control" children do. Learning-disabled children have difficulty performing tasks that require selective attention and discrimination, too.

DIAGNOSIS

The child is often brought to the physician's office because of a learning or behavior problem or because of a motor disability. First, a detailed history must be obtained, including the perinatal and postnatal periods. The age at which the child reached major motor and developmental milestones should be noted. A psychosocial history is important; the family history, including the parents' relationship with each other, should be explored. A history of exposure to drugs or toxins by the child or mother must be obtained. A focused neurological history is required. The physician must determine whether the present problem is acute or chronic, slowly progressive or static.

Based on the history, the physician must determine if the problem is the result of a neurological disease, a learning disorder, visual or auditory defect, or emotional or psychiatric disease. A complete medical examination is necessary. Although the medical examination of such a patient is usually normal, the physician must carefully examine the child looking for cutaneous stigmata of inherited disease (Chapter 26). A complete neurological examination should be performed (as detailed in Chapter 2) including a brief mental status examination. The child should be observed, and his interaction with his parents noted. An older child may be easier to communicate with than a younger one. The spontaneous speech that the child produces before he is questioned formally probably represents an accurate sample of the child's language abilities. Clues to possible auditory dysfunction may be noted at this time and can be evaluated later in the examination.

An examination of the cranial nerves should follow. Visual acuity should be tested; a more detailed examination of hearing can be made if indicated. Gross motor skills should be assessed. Distal versus proximal muscle areas should be tested; fine distal movements, such as buttoning clothes or tying shoestrings, should be tested. Truncal and appendicular cerebellar functions must be assessed by walking (looking for maintenance of balance with symmetrical arm swing); finger-to-nose testing can be performed (looking for ipsilateral cerebellar or corticospinal pathology). The hands and arms must be observed for unilateral pronation, downward drift, or abnormal posture when the upper extremities are held extended in front of the body. Deep-tendon reflexes are examined and plantar response is tested. Gross sensory testing can be performed at this time to look for major sensory functions.

Hard or soft neurological signs should be noted. Hard findings are those that are abnormal at any age (eg, Babinski's reflex). Soft neurological signs are those that are normal in early ages but, when present after early childhood, are abnormal and represent a maturation delay in neuromuscular development. Table 19-1 lists major soft signs.

Fine motor incoordination (demonstrated by finger tapping or rapid alternating movements) is one of the more frequently observed soft signs. Mirror movements are involuntary movements in the fingers and hand opposite to that with which a task is being performed. They are best demonstrated by having the child rapidly move one hand while attempting to keep the other still. Mirror movements are seen in 14% of normal 9- to 10-year old children, however, and they can be considered normal up to the age of 11 or 12. Involuntary choreiform movements when the arms are outstretched occur in children with learning disabilities, but they also occur in normal children. Backwards tandem gait can be performed normally by 70% of 6-year-old children and by 90% of those age 7.

Cortical sensory abnormalities are often listed as soft neurological signs in children. Right-left confusion may be seen; 75% to 80% of 7-year-olds and 100% of 8-year-olds should normally be able to distinguish their right from left sides. Finger gnosis, the ability to recognize, identify, and differentiate the fingers, is tested by saying, "Show me your thumb," "Which finger is this?" and so forth. More than 50% of children have finger gnosis by the age of 5 or 6 years; more than 90%, by the age 7½. Children with learning disabilities have greater difficulty identifying fingers than controls do.

Soft neurological signs have a debatable significance. Isolated soft signs are not diagnostic of brain damage. They may identify a child at risk for developing a

TABLE 19-1 "SOFT" NEUROLOGICAL SIGNS

Clumsiness with tasks that require fine motor coordination
Mirror movements
Choreiform movements
Tremor
Reflex asymmetries
Awkward (clumsy) gait
Finger agnosia
Dysdiadochokinesia
Graphesthesia
Extinction to double simultaneous stimulation
Mixed laterality

Adapted from Schain R: *Neurology of Childhood Learning Disorders*, ed 2. Baltimore, Williams & Wilkins, 1977, p 54; and Shaywitz S, Grossman HJ, Shaywitz B: Symposium on learning disorders. *Pediatric Clin NA* 1984; 31:305. Used with permission.

learning disability, however, and can be followed as the child is treated with medication. Soft neurological signs often improve with treatment. Most normal "control" patients have no soft signs or only one, whereas 90% to 95% of learning-disabled children have two or more soft signs.

LABORATORY TESTS

There are no specific laboratory tests to confirm the diagnosis of a learning disability. Computed tomography (CT) and auditory evoked potentials are normal, so are routine blood studies and chromosomal analysis. The electroencephalogram is usually normal, although it is not uncommon to see minor abnormalities of doubtful significance (Table 19-2). Rarely, a learning disability is caused by a seizure disorder, usually of the petit mal or complex-partial type.

Numerous psychological tests can be performed on the child with a suspected learning disability (Table 19-3). The Denver Developmental Screening Test can be performed at the initial evaluation. It measures personal and social skills, fine and gross motor skills, and language skills in children through the age of 6 years. It is primarily used to identify lags in developmental milestones, but it does not identify mildly retarded or neurologically impaired children.

The intelligence test used most often is the Wechsler Intelligence Scale for Children—Revised (WISC-R). This, and other intelligence tests, are fairly good predictors of school performance. The WISC-R is designed for children 6 to 16 years of age; a preschool test is available for children 4 to 6½ years of age. The

---

TABLE 19-2   EEG VARIATIONS IN SCHOOL-AGE CHILDREN

Definite Abnormality

Paroxysmal polyspike complexes
Paroxysmal spike-wave discharges
Amplitude asymmetries > 50%
Repetitive focal spiking or slowing

Questionable Abnormality

14 Hz and 6 Hz positive spike waves
Occipital or posterior temporal slow waves
Nonfocal sharp waves
Excessive slowing or amplitude potentiation with hyperventilation

Adapted from Schain R (1977, p 56). Used with permission.

TABLE 19-3   TESTS FOR THE CHILD WITH A SUSPECTED LEARNING DISABILITY

Screening
  Denver Developmental Screening Test (DDST)
  Gesell Developmental Screening Inventory
Intelligence
  Wechsler Intelligence Scale for Children—Revised (WISC-R)
  Stanford-Binet
Academic
  Peabody Individual Achievement Test
  Wide Range Achievement Test
Adaptive Behavior
  Adams Behavior Scale
  Vineland Adaptive Behavior Scale

Stanford–Binet test, developed in 1905, is the oldest intelligence test. It tests language, memory, motor skills, and reasoning skills. Tests of academic strengths and weaknesses include the Peabody Individual Achievement Test and the Wide Range Achievement Test. These tests should be tailored to the individual child with a known learning disability, but they are also helpful for evaluating the child with a suspected learning disability.

ATTENTION DEFICIT DISORDERS

Behavioral disorders all have in common deficits in attention. These attention deficit disorders (ADD) are characterized by impulsivity, distractability, short attention span, and (occasionally) hyperactivity. Their prevalence is 4% to 6%; they are the most frequently observed neurobehavioral problems in children. Major subgroups are: (1) attention deficit disorder with hyperactivity (ADDH); (2) attention deficit disorder without hyperactivity; and (3) attention deficit disorder, residual type. Criteria for making the diagnosis of ADD are listed in Table 19-4.

CLINICAL SIGNIFICANCE

ADDH is marked by inattention, impulsivity, and hyperactivity. Cardinal features of ADD without hyperactivity are inattention and impulsivity. ADD, residual type, occurs in adolescents and adults who at younger ages satisfied criteria for ADDH, but who are no longer hyperactive. Characteristics of the attention deficit disorders appear in Table 19-4.

ADDH occurs in younger children, and has double the prevalence of ADD with

TABLE 19-4 DIAGNOSTIC CRITERIA FOR ATTENTION DEFICIT DISORDERS

Inattention (when at least 4 of the following characterize the child)
Often asks to have things repeated
Needs a calm and quiet atmosphere to work (if this is not provided, cannot complete assignments)
Easily distracted
Does not finish what he starts
Confuses details
Hears but does not seem to listen
Difficulty concentrating except in a one-to-one environment

Impulsivity (when at least 3 of the following are present)
Is extremely excitable
Calls out or makes noise in class
Talks excessively
Has trouble waiting his turn
Disrupts other children

Hyperactivity (when at least 3 of the following are present)
Always on the go; runs rather than walks
Fidgets or squirms
Climbs onto furniture and cabinets
Does things in a noisy way
Fidgets unless doing something

Other criteria
Onset before 7 years of age
Duration of at least 6 months

Adapted from Shaywitz S, Grossman HJ, Shaywitz B: *Pediatr Clin NA* 1984; 31:437.

no hyperactivity. As children grow up, hyperactivity tends to abate, and the prevalence of ADDH declines. Boys are affected four times as often as girls.

ETIOLOGY

The etiology of ADD is not clear, but popular conception is that it is a result of structural brain damage. Most children, however, do not have a history of birth injury or associated neurological illness. Occasionally, damage to the CNS is followed by behavioral disturbances that satisfy the criteria for ADD. Survivors of Reye's syndrome have a high incidence of ADD, for example. ADD can develop as the result of exogenous toxins, evidenced by its increased incidence in the offspring of alcoholic women. Elevated levels of lead (without clinical encephalopathy) can also be associated with cognitive and behavioral difficulties. Genetic factors probably play an important role in most cases of ADD. The incidence of ADD is increased in the siblings of girls with ADD and when the mother or both parents had ADD.

DIAGNOSIS

Diagnostic evaluation begins with information obtained from the history and from a personal data inventory of the child, which is a comprehensive computer-indexed program. This inventory includes demographic information, genetic background, prenatal and perinatal events, developmental and social history, educational experiences, recent life stresses, and current areas of difficulty. A Teacher's Behavior Rating Scale should be performed to evaluate the child's school performance. This questionnaire tests the activity, attention, social and emotional qualities, and the acquisition of learning skills.

Physical examination of the child with ADD is usually normal. A complete neurological examination is necessary. The visual and auditory systems get special attention, for a child with impaired vision or hearing may appear restless and inattentive. Although "soft" neurological signs (Table 19-1), are more common in learning-disabled children, they can be present in ADD. Children with ADD do not have a higher incidence of left-handedness, mixed dominance, or choreiform movements.

LABORATORY TESTS

Psychometric tests, including the WISC-R and the Stanford-Binet tests, are useful. Routine laboratory tests and chromosomal studies are not helpful, and the EEG shows nonspecific changes in 50% of patients. True petit mal epilepsy or other forms of seizures are rarely the cause of ADD. A CT scan is usually normal. The diagnosis is based on findings listed in Table 19-4. Exclusionary criteria are listed in Table 19-5. The presence of a psychiatric disturbance or mental retardation makes the diagnosis of ADD unlikely.

TABLE 19-5 EXCLUSION CRITERIA FOR ATTENTION DEFICIT DISORDERS

Disorders of the sensory organs, particularly hearing or vision
Severe or profound mental retardation
Progressive developmental disorders
   Autism
   Childhood schizophrenia
Seizure disorders (petit mal)

MANAGEMENT

Conventional therapy for ADD is both nonpharmacological and pharmacological (Table 19-6). An optimal educational plan must be decided upon with the cooperation of the child and the parents. A self-contained classroom or a structured classroom environment works best. It is often necessary to remove the child from distracting stimuli at school. Behavior modification can be used, but there is doubt as to whether it is superior to pharmacotherapy. Individual psychotherapy may be important for some children with ADD, but it does not produce satisfactory results overall.

A number of nonconventional therapies have been used (Table 19-7). *Dietary modification* has been popularized in the lay press. There does appear to be a small subgroup of affected children who are sensitive to ingested food colorings. Placing them on an additive-free diet may help, but more standard therapies should not be ignored. The Feingold diet is nonstandard and controversial. It's basic hypothesis is that certain food additives and colorings produce the syndrome of learning disability and hyperactivity in susceptible children. Feingold reports that as many as half of affected children show dramatic improvement in their learning and behavior when these substances are removed from their diet. However, when such studies were repeated by other researchers, the majority of children did not improve on the Feingold diet. There is no inherent danger in an additive-free diet as long as attention is paid to basic nutritional principles. The National Institutes of Health Consensus Development Conference on Defined Diets and Hyperactivity concluded that "initiation of a trial of dietary treatment or continuation of a diet in patients whose families and physicians perceived benefits may be warranted."

Megavitamin therapy. The use of "orthomolecular" or megavitamin therapy is based on the concept of genetotrophic disease introduced in 1950. This theory holds that some individuals have a genetic abnormality that produces a requirement for a specific nutrient greater than that required by the general population. The failure to provide adequate amounts of the required substance produces a

---

TABLE 19-6 THERAPY FOR ATTENTION DEFICIT DISORDERS

Nonpharmacologic

Educational
    Structured classroom environment
    Removal from disturbing influences
    Curriculum modification
Behavioral modifications

Pharmacologic

Stimulants
    Methylphenidate (MPH)
    Dextroamphetamine
    Pemoline
Clonidine
Tricyclic antidepressants
    Imipramine
Phenothiazines
    Thioridazine
    Chlorpromazine

TABLE 19-7 CONTROVERSIAL THERAPIES FOR ATTENTION DEFICIT DISORDERS

Feingold diet
Megavitamin therapy
Orthomolecular mineral therapy
Hypoglycemia diets
Patterning (Doman–Delacato technique)
Optometric training
Vestibular stimulation

All are without proven scientific value.

disease state. Most studies that report benefits from this kind of therapy are flawed. There is no evidence that megavitamin therapy is of any use in the treatment of developmental disabilities. Megadoses of vitamins may produce toxicity; the risk of toxicity from taking large doses for long periods of time is unknown. The use of orthomolecular mineral supplements in treating brain disturbances has been made possible by the availability of accurate methods of measuring minerals in body tissues, eg, hair and nails. However, these analyses are nonspecific and do not take into account unknown environmental factors. Overall, the evidence for body deficiencies of certain minerals in children with learning disabilities is weak, and there is no support for the treatment with supplementary minerals.

Hypoglycemia diets. There are two differing opinions regarding the efficacy of hypoglycemia diets in the treatment of learning disabilities and ADD. Some physicians believe that hypoglycemia is a problem and that frequent feedings are necessary with diets low in carbohydrate and high in protein. There is also the excessive sugar theory, which holds that an excessive intake of sugar leads to an increase in hyperactive behavior. Few clinical studies have been performed to test this theory. There is no scientific support for either hypothesis.

A number of other nonmedical therapies have been advocated. These include *optometric training,* based on the assumption that learning disabilities are due to abnormal visual perception and abnormalities in the coordination of eye movements and binocular fixation. No controlled studies support this view. Sensory motor integration is said to be improved by vestibular stimulation produced by spinning or rocking the child. No studies prove its effectiveness.

Stimulants. Amphetamine, the first effective drug for treating the disruptive behavior of hyperactive children, was introduced in 1937. Stimulants have been shown to be the most effective, least toxic agents for treating hyperactive children: 70% to 80% of children demonstrate sustained improvement. Stimulants improve attention span, reduce impulsivity, improve the performance of fine motor tasks, and reduce motor activity levels. However, the effect of stimulants on cognition is controversial. The WISC-R scores have improved in some children following administration of stimulants, but, it remains questionable as to whether stimulants produce a sustained effect on learning. When stimulants are combined with supportive therapies, including modification of school programs, sustained benefits in learning may result.

When should therapy with stimulant drugs be started? Ideally, the child should be placed in the proper class with attention paid to target symptoms; this requires that the child be properly evaluated so that school placement is appropriate.

255

Target symptoms must be identified so that the effects of any therapy can be easily identified. Stimulants are most useful in the management of attention difficulties; hyperactivity alone is usually not a sufficient reason for the initiation of pharmacotherapy.

Ideally, it is best to start therapy only after the child has had the opportunity to adjust to changes in the school environment. This means that medicine usually should not be given at the start of the school year. However, if prior experience suggests that medication will likely be necessary at the start of the school year, then it is best to give it early, rather than producing a negative effect at school or at home. Amphetamines and methylphenidate (MPH) (Ritalin) are the most widely used drugs. MPH has fewer side effects and is the drug of choice (Table 19-8).

MPH should be taken in the morning before the child leaves for school. The initial dose is 0.3 mg/kg. Pharmacokinetics and behavioral effects of the drug are no different whether it is given 30 minutes before breakfast or with breakfast. By the time school starts, MPH should be absorbed; peak levels occur within three to four hours. Academic activities should be scheduled in the morning so that in the afternoon, when levels of medication are falling, medication will not be as necessary for nonacademic activities (eg, physical education). Weekly feedback is needed from the parents and the teacher. If the child does not seem to be responding after two weeks of treatment, the dosage should be raised by 0.1 mg/ kg. It can be increased every two weeks, if necessary, until a dosage of 0.6 mg/kg is reached.

If the child does not respond favorably to the maximum dosage, plasma drug levels should be obtained two and three hours after a dose. If the level is in the therapeutic range (15 to 20 ng/mL) at the maximum dosage of the medication, it may be necessary to switch to another medication. If the plasma level is low, the dosage should be increased every two weeks by 0.1 mg/kg increments, to a maximum of 0.8 mg/kg or to a blood level of 10 to 20 ng/mL.

If the child does well in the morning on the 0.3 mg/kg dosage but the effects of the drug seem to wear off by early afternoon, an identical second dose at lunch time should be added. A sustained-release MPH can be used in such a case, but there have been no studies showing that the behavioral effects from this preparation are of longer duration than those of MPH tablets.

Dextroamphetamine is as effective as MPH but has greater side effects. The initial dosage is usually 0.2 mg/kg/day, with a maximum dosage of 0.5 mg/kg/day.

Pemoline, a CNS stimulant that is structurally different from the amphetamines and MPH, is as effective as both amphetamines and MPH at a dosage of 2 mg/kg/ day. Hypersensitivity reactions occur in 1% to 2% of patients, usually involving the liver. Thus, liver function should be monitored. The advantage of pemoline is its

TABLE 19-8 DOSAGES OF DRUGS OFTEN USED TO TREAT HYPERACTIVITY

Drug	Daily dosage
Methylphenidate	0.3 to 0.8 mg/kg
Dextroamphetamine	0.2 to 0.5 mg/kg
Pemoline	2.25 mg/kg
Imipramine	2.5 to 5.0 mg/kg
Thioridazine	0.5 to 1.0 mg/kg

long duration of action, which requires the child to take medication only before school.

The side effects of stimulants include insomnia, sleep disturbances, depressed appetite, and, occasionally, nausea and vomiting. Growth retardation occurs, and, in certain children, Gilles de la Tourette's syndrome may be precipitated by the use of amphetamine or other stimulants. The effects of MPH are dose-related. Higher dosages administered for a longer time produce the greatest decrement in height. These drugs should probably be discontinued during the summer, and they should not be given if the child or the family has a history of tics.

The tricyclic antidepressants exert beneficial behavioral effects in hyperactive behavioral disorders. The preferred drug is imipramine, 2.5 mg to 5.0 mg/kg, in divided doses. The total daily dosage ranges from 10 to 150 mg. An advantage of imipramine is that its effect persists throughout the day.

Both behavioral and attentional difficulties are improved with clonidine; its side effects tend to be minimal. Other drugs—haloperidol, phenothiazines (chlorpromazine and thioridazine), and anticonvulsants—have been used. Their role is limited because they are not as effective and their potential for side effects is somewhat greater than that of stimulants. Phenobarbital is contraindicated because it can exacerbate hyperactivity.

PROGNOSIS

ADD has a fairly good outcome. Only a minority of children do not do well in school or later in life. Attention deficits in adolescents are widespread, however, and hyperactivity is not limited to young school children. Hyperactivity diminishes at adolescence, but associated traits may become worse, including restlessness, task and persistence distractability, and problems with planning and organization. These children also have a tendency to tire easily during sustained cognitive effort.

Management of adolescent learning disabilities usually involves special education services such as tutoring and speech and language therapy. An individual therapist may be able to help the child with motor and interpersonal skills; likewise, counseling with a social worker, guidance counselor, or psychologist is important. An appropriate teacher and careful course selection is also important. The child should be encouraged to pursue his strengths, and vocational services should be enlisted. An occasional adolescent responds to stimulant medication such as dextroamphetamine or MPH, but usually drug therapy is not necessary.

Bibliography

Huessy HR, Cohen AJ: Hyperkinetic behaviors and learning disabilities followed over seven years. *Pediatrics* 1976; 57:4-10. (MBD is not always a benign disorder; many children have continued social or school problems.)

Ottenbacher KJ, Cooper HM: Drug treatment of hyperactivity. *Dev Med Child Neurol* 1983; 25:358-366. (Reviews current drug therapies for ADD.)

Schain RJ: *Neurology of Childhood Learning Disorders,* ed 2. Baltimore, Williams & Wilkins, 1977. (Relatively short book (156 pages) that covers all practical areas of learning disabilities.)

Shaywitz S, Grossman HJ, Shaywitz B (eds): Symposium on learning disorders. *Pediatr Clin North Am* 1984; 31:279-518. (Current review of all aspects of attention deficit disorders; well referenced.)

Silver LB: Controversal approaches to treating learning disabilities and attention deficit disorder. *AM J Dis Child* 1986; 140: 1045-1052. (Current review of acceptable and controversial treatment for the child with a learning disability or an attention deficit disorder.)

Wright FS, Schain RJ, Weinberg WA, et al: Learning disabilities and associated conditions, in Swaiman KF, Wright FS: *The Practice of Pediatric Neurology,* ed 2. St. Louis, C.V. Mosby, 1982, vol 1, pp 1083-1132. (Accessible overview of childhood learning disorders.)

THREE

Diseases

Cerebrovascular Diseases

CLINICAL SIGNIFICANCE

Each year in the United States at least 120,000 people die of cerebrovascular disease, and about 1 million suffer a nonfatal stroke. After cancer and heart disease, stroke is the third most common cause of death in the U.S.; the incidence is approximately 200/100,000/year. For example, in July 1976 there were 1.7 million survivors of stroke in the United States, a prevalence of 794/100,000. Prevalence rates are 66/100,000 in persons under 45 years of age; 998/100,000 in those ages 45 to 64; and 5063/100,000 in those 65 and over. The American Heart Association has estimated that 170,400 persons died from stroke and 1,830,000 survived stroke in 1980. Approximately 50% of patients hospitalized for acute neurological disease are suffering from a stroke; the estimated annual cost for care of stroke victims in the United States in 1976 was more than 3 billion dollars. Each year in the United States, 400,000 patients with stroke are discharged from acute care hospitals; three-quarters after suffering their first stroke, and the remainder for recurrent stroke.

In men, the age-adjusted annual incidence myocardial infarction is 8.5/1000, in contrast to the incidence of atherothrombotic brain infarction of 2.7/1000. For women, the annual incidence of myocardial infarction and atherothrombotic brain infarction were almost the same: 2.4/1000 and 2.1/1000. The frequency of stroke by type is listed in Table 20-1. Over two-thirds of strokes are caused by ischemia and infarction.

TABLE 20-1 TYPES AND FREQUENCY OF CEREBROVASCULAR DISEASE

Thrombosis	32
Embolism	32
Lacunes	18
Hypertensive hemorrhage	11
Subarachnoid	7
aneurysmal, AVM	
hemorrhages	

Adapted from Adams RD, Victor M: Cerebrovascular diseases, in *Principles of Neurology.* New York, McGraw-Hill, 1985, ed 3. Used with permission.

The rate of stroke mortality has clearly declined; the age-adjusted cardiovascular mortality has declined approximately 32% over the past 30 years. This decline has accelerated during the past decade, accounting for two-thirds of the 30-year decline. In the 1940s and 1950s stroke mortality declined at a rate of 1% per year; since 1972 the rate of decline has been 5% per year. Preventive measures, particularly control of hypertension and better medical care, are major contributing factors to this decline in stroke mortality.

This chapter discusses major classes of nonhemorrhagic stroke: transient ischemic attack (TIA) and cerebral infarction. Hemorrhagic stroke and its management are addressed in Chapter 37.

RISK FACTORS FOR STROKE

Hypertension is the dominant precursor of stroke. The incidence of atherothrombotic brain infarction rises as the systolic or diastolic blood pressure rises. The elderly person has a twofold increased risk of brain infarction when the systolic pressure is greater than 160 mmHg accompanied by a diastolic pressure of less than 95 mmHg. Increasing age is itself a risk factor for stroke.

Cardiac impairment ranks third among risk factors for stroke after age and hypertension. Persons with cardiac disease have more than twice the average risk of stroke. Atrial fibrillation is a powerful precursor of stroke, specifically embolic stroke. Patients with nonrheumatic atrial fibrillation develop strokes at more than five times the rate of those without atrial fibrillation.

The association of total cholesterol content or of lipoprotein cholesterol fractions with stroke is less clear than it is with coronary artery disease. The serum level of total cholesterol in persons older than 65 years is inversely related to the general incidence of stroke and the risk of atherothrombotic brain infarction. In contrast to coronary artery disease, high-density lipoprotein has no significant protective effect on stroke.

Atherothrombotic brain infarction often occurs in diabetics, particularly women; diabetics have at least a three-fold increased risk of stroke. Above blood glucose levels of 160 mg/dL, the risk of atherosclerotic brain infarction is doubled.

Women who take oral contraceptives have an increased risk of fatal stroke, but it is more often a result of subarachnoid hemorrhage than ischemic stroke. The stroke risk is increased four-fold for those women who are over the age of 35, especially if they smoke cigarettes.

Cigarette smoking is more strongly related to the incidence of peripheral vascular disease and coronary artery disease than to stroke in men. Smoking is a slight risk factor for atherothrombotic brain infarction only in men under the age of 65.

ETIOLOGY

The characteristics of a stroke depend on the collateral vascular supply to the affected area. The more proximal the lesion the greater the collateral flow. Of asymptomatic elderly adults, 7% to 10% have an occluded or severely stenotic carotid artery without evidence of brain infarction. Artery-to-artery emboli are a common cause of cerebrovascular ischemia. If an atherosclerotic plaque on an arterial wall ulcerates, the associated necrotic material may dislodge and embolize. Platelets also adhere to this necrotic area and may form a platelet mass that dislodges and embolizes distally.

Cardiogenic emboli usually associated with atrial fibrillation or mitral valve prolapse, or that occur after myocardial infarction, are common causes of cerebral emboli and subsequent ischemic stroke. Systemic hypotension usually produces global CNS symptoms; focal symptoms are quite rare. Stenosis or occlusion of a cerebral artery can lead to hemodynamic impairment, usually when the diameter of the lumen is reduced by at least 75%. Systemic hypotension, however, can produce focal neurological symptoms and signs when there is associated carotid artery stenosis, especially if the patient is also hypertensive.

Most episodes of cerebrovascular ischemia occur suddenly, are focal, and can be isolated to dysfunction in a specific arterial distribution. Approximately 95% of abrupt focal cerebral defects are of vascular nature. Common nonvascular causes are seizures with resulting postictal paralysis, tumor producing a seizure or spontaneous hemorrhage, demyelination, and psychogenic.

CLINICAL SYNDROMES

Clinical manifestations of cerebral ischemia are defined best in terms of the arterial distribution involved (anatomical profile) and the time course of the resulting symptoms and signs (temporal profile).

CAROTID ARTERY SYNDROMES
Common Carotid Artery

Occlusion of the common carotid occurs in fewer than 1% of carotid artery syndromes. Occlusion of this vessel may not produce symptoms because of the extensive anastomosis between the carotid and vertebral arteries at the circle of Willis and because of extracranial branch anastomoses.

Internal Carotid Artery

The internal carotid artery (ICA) supplies the ipsilateral eye by way of the ipsilateral ophthalmic artery, and by way of the intracranial branches (middle cerebral artery, anterior cerebral artery) it supplies the entire frontal lobe and almost all of the temporal lobe and parietal lobe. Atherosclerosis often involves the origin of the ICA at the bifurcation. In autopsied white persons over 60 years of age, atherosclerotic ICA occlusion occurred in 6% to 15% of cases, with stenosis and roughening of intimal surfaces, in about 10%. A fibrous plaque with ulceration occurs commonly in the posterior wall of the carotid sinus; atheromas also occur in the adjacent external carotid (ECA) and common carotid arteries. A mural thrombus can form at the plaque.

In 95% of patients with ICA occlusion, the greatest degree of stenosis is found in the carotid sinus; other locations for stenosis are uncommon. Blood flow tends to decrease only when the lumen of the vessel is decreased by 90%. Most symptoms of ICA disease are of cerebral hemispheric origin, with contralateral motor and sensory abnormalities most common. Symptoms of retinal or optic nerve ischemia may also occur, resulting in amaurosis fugax (transient monocular blindness). Symptoms occur with ICA disease because there is limited collateral blood flow both extracranially and intracranially.

Middle Cerebral Artery

The arterial distribution of the brain supplied by the middle cerebral artery (MCA) is the site of most strokes. It is occluded more often by emboli than by thrombi. The MCA has a number of important branches. Small lenticulostriate arteries penetrate deep into the brain to supply a portion of the basal ganglia and the internal capsule. The superior division of the MCA supplies most of the frontal lobe and almost all of the anterior parietal lobe. The inferior division supplies the posterior parietal lobe, most of the temporal lobe, and the lateral occipital region.

Occlusion of the proximal portion of the MCA usually produces a contralateral hemiplegia, hemianesthesia, and hemianopia. If the dominant hemisphere is involved, aphasia will be present. Ischemia of the superior division produces contralateral weakness of the face and arm more than the leg, with contralateral hemisensory loss. If the dominant hemisphere is involved, Broca's (nonfluent) aphasia will be present. Neglect (impaired awareness) of the opposite side will be present in nondominant hemispheric involvement. In involvement of the inferior division, weakness is usually absent, but apraxia of opposite limbs and conduction aphasia are seen. With involvement of the nondominant hemisphere, left-sided neglect, apraxia, and hemianopia will be present.

Anterior Cerebral Artery

The anterior cerebral artery (ACA) gives rise to branches that supply the anterior limb of the internal capsule, the caudate nucleus, and the putamen. Cortical surfaces supplied by the ACA include the medial frontal lobe and the anterior parietal lobe. Collateral flow from the anterior communicating artery and branches of the MCA is usually adequate, so the extent of brain damage resulting from occlusion of this vessel is variable.

Ischemia in the territory of the ACA produces paralysis of the opposite leg and foot, with minimal weakness of the arm, and sparing of the face. Sensory loss may also occur in the same distribution as the weakness. Involvement of the dominant hemisphere can produce a transcortical motor aphasia (nonfluent, with intact repetition and comprehension). Behavioral changes, including abulia or akinetic mutism and urinary incontinence, may also develop.

Anterior Choroidal Artery

The anterior choroidal artery arises from the ICA or the MCA. This vessel supplies the posterior limb of the internal capsule, the medial temporal lobe, and the optic radiations. Ischemia in the distribution of this artery produces contralateral hemiplegia, sensory loss, and hemianopia.

VERTEBROBASILAR ARTERY SYNDROMES
Posterior Cerebral Artery

Both posterior cerebral arteries (PCAs) arise from the basilar artery in 70% of persons; one or both PCA's are supplied by the ICA by way of the posterior communicating artery in 25%. A number of small penetrating arteries originate from the proximal PCA, supplying the midbrain and the thalamus. Branches to the cortical surfaces supply the inferior temporal regions and the parietal and occipital cortex.

Ischemia of the main trunk of the PCA produces a syndrome that mimics occlusion of the inferior branch of the MCA. When there is ischemia of the cortical branches of the PCA, a contralateral homonymous hemianopia develops. When collateral flow is adequate from the anterior cerebral artery, ischemia may result only in the inferior occipital lobe area, with signs of a contralateral superior quadrantanopsia. With ischemia of the dominant occipital lobe, reading disturbances (dyslexia) and difficulties in naming and discriminating colors may result. A state of agitated delirium has been reported following occipital lobe ischemia.

If the smaller penetrating vessels are involved, a variety of clinical manifestations can result. Infarction of the thalamus (usually lacunar) produces a contralateral pure sensory syndrome. Involvement of the midbrain and thalamic areas may produce a number of signs, including ipsilateral oculomotor nerve palsy with contralateral hemiparesis (Weber's syndrome), ataxia, hemiballismus-hemichorea, and tremor.

Basilar Artery

The basilar artery is formed by the two vertebral arteries at the pontomedullary junction. It supplies the pons, midbrain, and cerebellum, and it bifurcates into the PCAs. Multiple branches of the basilar artery supply the brain stem and surrounding areas; the wide spectrum of neurological syndromes that result from basilar arterial disease depends on the anatomical areas involved. The paramedian branches, seven to ten in number, supply a wedge of the pons on either side of the midline. The short circumferential branches, numbering five to seven, supply the lateral two-thirds of the pons and the middle and superior cerebellar peduncles. The long circumferential branches (the anterior inferior and superior cerebellar arteries) supply the cerebellar hemispheres and several paramedian branches at the bifurcation ("top") of the basilar supply the subthalamic and midbrain areas.

Rostral basilar artery involvement by atherosclerosis can produce ischemia to the midbrain, subthalamus, thalamus, and a portion of the temporal–occipital lobe. The resulting infarction is known as the "top" of the basilar syndrome; it features visual-field defects, pupillary defects, gaze abnormalities (primarily in the vertical plane), ataxia, weakness, sensory loss, and visual hallucinations.

Involvement of the paramedian vessels usually results in paresis of the contralateral arm or leg, associated with ipsilateral cranial nerve signs. Most paramedian syndromes involve the pons. Ocular abnormalities are frequent and include nystagmus, ocular bobbing, gaze paresis, convergence spasm, internuclear ophthalmoplegia, and abducens nerve palsy. The combination of unilateral abducens nerve weakness with ipsilateral peripheral facial nerve weakness and contralateral hemiparesis is known as Millard–Gubler syndrome. When the reticular formation is involved, somnolence or coma may result. Although weakness may be unilateral, any pattern of abnormalities is possible, including monoplegia or tetraplegia. Nausea, vomiting, and vertigo result from ischemia of the vestibular nucleus; ataxia results from involvement of the cerebellar peduncles.

Involvement of the dorsolateral areas of the brain stem and cerebellum produce a characteristic group of syndromes. Occlusion of the major vessels to these areas (superior cerebellar artery, anterior inferior cerebellar artery) causes abnormalities of cerebellar and sensory function, as well as abnormalities of the sympathetic nervous system. Ischemia of the superior cerebellar artery produces ipsilateral cerebellar dysfunction with palatal myoclonus and contralateral hypesthesia. Infarction of the anterior inferior cerebellar artery (AICA) that supplies the lower quarter of the pons, cranial nerves VII and VIII, the cochlear and lateral vestibular nuclei, and the inferior one-third of the middle cerebellar peduncle produces severe vertigo, unilateral deafness, vertical diplopia, facial weakness, dystaxia, dysarthria, Horner's syndrome, ipsilateral loss of touch sensation in the face, and contralateral loss of pain and temperature sensation of the body.

Manifestations of basilar artery ischemia may be varied because of the compactness of the brain stem and the branching of the basilar artery. When symptoms and signs can be attributed to a single vessel, branch occlusion is likely. Rostral disease of the proximal basilar artery is likely when there are bilateral signs.

Vertebral Artery

The paired vertebral arteries (VA) nourish the spinal cord and the posterior inferior cerebellum; they are the major arteries that supply the medulla. Many congenital abnormalities of the vertebral artery exist. In approximately 10% of them, one vessel is so small that the other is the only artery that supplies the brain stem. Ischemia or occlusion of the VA may be asymptomatic, but if one VA is hypoplastic and if collateral flow from the circle of Willis is unavailable, occlusion of the vertebral artery will produce brain stem infarction. Occlusion of a VA at its origin is usually asymptomatic because collateral circulation develops through the ipsilateral external carotid artery branches. Intracranial occlusion usually results in infarction of the lateral medulla because of occlusion of the posterior inferior cerebellar artery (PICA) branch that supplies this area; however, 80% of lateral medullary infarctions are caused by vertebral artery occlusion alone.

Lateral medullary ischemia or infarction (Wallenberg's syndrome), is the most common brain stem stroke. The classic syndrome consists of the following features: (1) contralateral impairment of pain and temperature sensation over half of the body because of spinothalamic tract involvement; (2) ipsilateral Horner's syndrome caused by involvement of the descending sympathetic tract; (3)

dysphagia, hoarseness, hiccups, palatal and vocal cord weakness caused by involvement of cranial nerves IX and X; (4) ipsilateral ataxia caused by involvement of the inferior cerebellar peduncle–spinocerebellar tract; and (5) pain, numbness or hypesthesia on the ipsilateral half of the face that is the result of involvement of the descending tract of cranial nerve V.

Occlusion of the distal PICA produces infarction in the posterior medullary area and the inferior cerebellum. Symptoms mimic acute labyrinthitis, with the sudden onset of vertigo, nausea, vomiting, ataxia, and nystagmus. Brain stem compression by the infarcted cerebellum may occur, and death occasionally results.

TRANSIENT ISCHEMIC ATTACK

Clinical Significance

The TIA is an episode of ischemic focal neurological dysfunction that lasts for less than 24 hours. About 50% of strokes caused by cerebrovascular disease are preceded by a TIA. Because the best treatment of stroke is prevention, recognition of a TIA makes preventive treatment possible.

The annual incidence of TIAs ranges from 2.2 to 8/1000 persons. Thirty-five percent of untreated TIA patients will develop a completed stroke within five years (approximately 5% to 7% per year); the greatest risk for stroke is in the first few weeks following the TIA. Approximately 20% of strokes will occur within the first month following the TIA, and approximately 50%, within the first year. Most patients who develop strokes have fewer than four preceding TIAs.

Most TIA's last less than 20 minutes. Those that last longer than 60 minutes are usually caused by an embolus. Short-duration TIAs correlate with tight stenosis of the ipsilateral carotid artery. The reversible ischemic neurological deficit (RIND) is a focal ischemic event that lasts longer than 24 hours, but that completely resolves within three weeks. The following discussion of TIA also applies to RIND.

Etiology

Men are affected twice as frequently as women, with onset usually between the ages of 50 and 70. Approximately 90% of TIAs occur in the carotid artery distribution, 7% occur in the vertebrobasilar distribution, and 3% occur in both arterial distributions. Forty percent of patients are hypertensive, 50% have ischemic heart disease, and 20% have diabetes mellitus. The incidence of myocardial infarction following a TIA is approximately 21%.

The precise mechanism of a TIA is not understood. In one study of patients with TIAs that exceeded one hour, 87% had abnormal cervical angiograms, whereas 37% of those with TIAs of shorter duration had carotid stenosis. Embolization of fibrin–platelet material from atheromatous plaques is a cause of many TIA's. It is unclear why each successive embolus in patients with multiple TIAs follows the same arterial distribution, but laminar intravascular flow has been proposed to explain this fact. Cerebral vascular hypotension and vasospasm have also been proposed as mechanisms for TIA, but they are uncommon. Disorders of the red blood cells can cause TIAs secondary to sludging of blood flow in the cerebral microcirculation. Thrombocytosis may cause micro-occlusions, particularly when the platelet count is above 500,000/μL. A single episode that lasts more than one hour and multiple episodes in a different arterial distribution suggest embolism as a cause of the TIA. Brief recurrent attacks in the same pattern suggest thrombosis or atherosclerosis.

SYMPTOMS AND SIGNS

Clinical manifestations depend on the vascular territory involved. Typical manifestations are listed in Table 20-2, and were discussed earlier in the chapter. Anatomical classification of TIA by the carotid or vertebrobasilar arterial distribution is important. Usually the patient is not examined during the TIA, and the history is anecdotal. For this reason, from 10% to 20% of patients admitted to the hospital with possible TIAs will not have had a true TIA. Symptoms that occur in isolation and cannot be considered to indicate a TIA are listed in Table 20-3. They include isolated loss of consciousness, dizziness, falling spells, dysarthria, and headache.

Transient hemispheric attacks are a common variety of carotid-artery TIA; the symptoms are those of middle cerebral artery distribution dysfunction. Usually, there is a combination of motor and sensory deficits involving mostly the arm and hand. If the dominant hemisphere is involved, transient disturbances of language may occur. Episodic dyskinesias may have been reported rarely, but the limbs are usually motionless. A TIA usually begins suddenly and subsides slowly over a few minutes.

Transient monocular blindness (amaurosis fugax) is a common carotid-artery TIA. The patient usually describes this visual disturbance as a dark shade being drawn over one eye, developing in a few seconds, and spreading from the periphery to the center of vision. Amaurosis fugax is painless, the "shade" often lifts within a few minutes, and vision returns to normal. The entire episode usually lasts 5 to 15 minutes. The patient with critical carotid or ophthalmic-artery

---

TABLE 20-2 SYMPTOMS OF TRANSIENT ISCHEMIC ATTACKS

Carotid Artery
Contralateral weakness (usually hemiparesis)
Contralateral sensory complaints (numbness, paresthesias)
Aphasia (motor or sensory if dominant hemisphere is involved)
Confusion (nonspecific, usually with nondominant hemisphere ischemia)
Transient monocular visual blurring or blindness (amaurosis fugax)
Transient dyskinesias

Vertebrobasilar Arterial System
Weakness (may be unilateral, bilateral, or of all 4 limbs)
Sensory complaints (may be unilateral, bilateral, or generalized)
Ataxia
Dysarthria
Diplopia
Dysphagia
Vertigo
Deafness
Visual deficits (usually binocular, occasionally cortical blindness)
Drop attacks
Confusion, agitation, or coma

Adapted from Easton JD, Hart RG, Sherman DG, et al: Diagnosis and management of ischemic stroke. *Curr Probl Cardiol* 1983; 7(5):13. Used with permission.

TABLE 20-3 SYMPTOMS OFTEN NOT CAUSED BY TIA IF OCCURRING ALONE

Vertigo
Dizziness (nonspecific, lightheadedness)
Syncope (often cardiac)
Confusion
Falling spells
Headache
Dysarthria

stenosis may complain of ipsilateral monocular visual blurring or loss on exposure to bright sunlight. There is inability to resaturate visual pigments because of compromise of the ocular circulation; it is brought out by increased metabolic demand resulting from exposure to the bright sunlight.

Vertebrobasilar TIAs can be characterized by blindness of both eyes, diplopia, oscillopsia, vertigo, dysarthria, dystaxia, deafness, or drop attacks (Table 20-2).

The neurological examination should be normal in the patient with a true TIA because the episode has been completed. If symptoms persist for longer than 24 hours, abnormalities should be found on neurological examination, and they will depend on the arterial system involved. Although the presence of a carotid-artery bruit is helpful in possibly localizing the cause of a carotid-system TIA, its absence does not exclude the presence of localized carotid-artery disease. More than 80% of cerebral infarctions occur in patients without cervical bruits, and the presence of a bruit does not necessarily mean that it arises from the carotid artery or that it is related to the TIA.

LABORATORY TESTS

Clinical and laboratory investigations may help differentiate the cause of the TIA. Because there are many causes of a TIA, a directed laboratory examination should be performed that is based on the age and health of the patient and the number and location of the TIAs.

Carotid Artery Distribution TIAs
Single Hemispheric or Retinal TIA

Basic laboratory studies that should be performed on all patients include erythrocyte sedimentation rate (ESR), complete blood count (CBC), platelet count, blood chemistry profile, coagulation profile, and VDRL test. In the younger patient, a serum protein electrophoresis, antinuclear antibody (ANA) determination, a plasma fibrinogen test, and cerebrospinal fluid (CSF) analysis should be considered. Because cardiogenic embolism is a common cause of TIA, a 12-lead electrocardiogram (ECG) should be performed on each patient, looking for evidence of atrial fibrillation or recent myocardial infarction. Chest x-rays should be taken, looking for evidence of neoplastic disease, pulmonary arteriovenous fistulae, congestive heart failure, and congenital heart disease. The use of two-dimensional echocardiography is more controversial; it should be performed in patients under the age of 50 and in those in whom a specific cardiac diagnosis is suspected (eg, atrial myxoma or mitral valve prolapse). It is also indicated in patients with normal carotid angiograms, and in those with evidence of systemic embolization. The yield in these selected groups is 10% to 20%, compared to 2% in the group overall. Holter monitoring usually is not of benefit in patients with focal TIAs unless there might be a cardiac arrhythmia that can predispose to stroke (eg, intermittent atrial fibrillation).

A variety of noninvasive vascular tests are available to investigate carotid artery disease. Noninvasive tests can identify clinically relevant structural and hemodynamic changes at the bifurcation and distal hemodynamic alterations with 90% accuracy. The optimal set of noninvasive vascular studies includes direct assessment of the carotid bifurcation by duplex Doppler examination, combined with quantitative phonoangiography when a bruit is present. Transcranial Doppler studies are now available; they can demonstrate stenosis of major intracranial arteries with good accuracy. Oculoplethysmography indirectly measures the pressure in the ICA and assesses the hemodynamic importance of the lesion. Noninvasive tests assess a stroke or TIA of major consequence in the territory fed by the ICA and permit the physician to follow the progress of a known carotid bruit. They may be of use for evaluating the patient with an asymptomatic bruit. These tests tend primarily to monitor physiology rather than anatomy, however, and they are preliminary, usually used to select patients for contrast studies.

Computed tomography (CT) with and without contrast should be performed in all patients with a TIA to help exclude nonischemic causes of TIA, including hemorrhage and neoplasm. A CT scan of the neck can be performed to look at the carotid bifurcation; areas of stenosis and intraplaque hemorrhage can be identified occasionally with this technique.

Cerebral angiography is the definitive, most reliable technique for evaluating the patient with a TIA. In most patients, it carries a 1% risk of stroke and aortic dissection. Contrast agent reactions also occur. The prevention of hypotension and dehydration are important safeguards in the patient who is undergoing cerebral angiography. If these conditions are not corrected, toxic reactions can occur involving the CNS and kidneys (contrast-induced acute renal failure).

Angiography can detect ulcerative lesions, severe stenosis, mural thrombus formation, and carotid artery dissection. Transfemoral angiography is the technique of choice. Views of the aortic arch and the clinically diseased artery should be obtained, including intracranial views.

Digital subtraction angiography is available in many communities. It allows intravenous or intra-arterial injection of contrast. When given intravenously, the bolus of contrast must be large, which increases the possibility of contrast-induced complications. The aortic arch is usually well visualized, but views of the intracranial circulation are usually suboptimal. When performed intra-arterially, the computer-reconstructed images are of excellent quality, and the volume of contrast used is less than that used with conventional angiography. If the patient is not an endarterectomy candidate, there is usually no reason to perform angiography unless other uncommon causes are suspected clinically (eg, arteritis, aneurysms that have embolized and extracranial or intracranial arterial dissections).

The electroencephalogram (EEG) usually offers little information in evaluation of the patient with a TIA. Slowing of brain rhythms can occur over the involved hemisphere when there is a hemodynamically significant arterial stenosis. Epileptiform discharges may be identified in the patient who has a TIA resulting from a postictal state (Todd's paralysis).

Multiple Carotid TIAs in the Same Distribution

If the patient has multiple TIAs in the same circulation, there is a high probability that he has an atherosclerotic lesion of the involved vessel. Embolism is a less common cause of such stereotyped multiple TIAs. Angiography should be performed sooner in this kind of patient. If angiography is negative, an alternative diagnosis must be considered; cardiac evaluation still should be performed, but the yield will be low.

Multiple Carotid TIA's in Two Circulations

When TIAs are recurrent and occur in two different arterial circulations, then either embolic disease or a systemic disease is present. Cardiac evaluation should be performed early, including a 12-lead ECG, two-dimensional echocardiography, and Holter monitoring. Tests of ESR, ANA, and partial thromboplastin time (PTT) and a platelet count should be performed to look for occult arteritis or a circulating lupus anticoagulant. If these tests are negative, cerebral angiography can be performed to look primarily for small-vessel disease or multiple-vessel occlusions.

Vertebrobasilar TIA
Single

The diagnostic tests discussed for carotid artery disease must be performed in the patient with a single vertebrobasilar (VB) TIA. Noninvasive vascular tests cannot be used to assess the VB system as well as the carotid system. Cerebral angiography is performed less often because the number of surgical procedures available for the treatment of posterior circulation arterial disease is very limited. Cardiac or other hemodynamic diseases must be considered, as is the case in anterior circulation disease.

Multiple

As with carotid-artery disease, multiple episodes of VB TIAs in the *same* circulation usually indicate focal arterial disease. Angiography can be performed to distinguish between extracranial (eg, subclavian steal syndrome) and intracranial stenoses. The carotid circulation should also be investigated because lesions of both carotid arteries, combined with occlusive disease of the VB system, can result in decreased posterior circulation through the circle of Willis. If there are multiple TIAs in multiple arterial distributions, emboli are a less common cause and multiple levels of VB stenosis are likely. If the patient also has carotid artery symptoms, a systemic illness or multiple cardiac emboli must be considered. In addition to cerebral angiography, CSF examination is indicated to look for infection, demyelination, or leptomeningeal carcinomatosis.

MANAGEMENT

Because a TIA may be followed by a completed stroke within a few days, it must be considered a medical emergency and treatment must be started immediately. Treatment of TIA is medical, surgical, or both.

Medical Therapy

Any risk factors that contribute to the development of cerebrovascular disease should be treated immediately, particularly hypertension and hyperglycemia. Overtreatment of hypertension, however, can induce cerebral infarction, particularly if carotid-artery stenosis coexists.

The TIA is a predictor of myocardial infarction as well as stroke. The patient should undergo a workup for and treatment of coronary artery disease as well as for cerebrovascular disease.

Anticoagulant Therapy

There have been few well-performed studies of the role of anticoagulant (heparin or warfarin) therapy for TIA. In a few studies anticoagulants reduced the number of recurrent TIAs, subsequent stroke, and death. Contraindications to the use of anticoagulants include bleeding ulcer, malignant hypertension, hepatic failure, poor patient compliance, advanced age, systolic blood pressure greater than 190 mmHg, or bleeding diathesis. It is mandatory that a CT scan be performed prior to starting anticoagulant therapy; if there is no evidence of hemorrhage and if the clinical presentation does not suggest a subarachnoid hemorrhage, then therapy can be started. Lumbar puncture is not necessary if the CT scan is negative. If CT is not available, lumbar puncture should be performed; if there are no red blood cells in CSF anticoagulant therapy can be started, but it should be delayed for two to four hours to reduce the likelihood of a spinal hematoma.

Hemorrhagic complications of anticoagulant therapy increase with the duration of therapy. To help minimize bleeding complications, the prothrombin time should not exceed 1.8 times the control value. A rebound hypercoagulable state can occur in five to seven days after warfarin is stopped.

Heparin infusion with a bolus of 5000 units, followed by 1000 units every hour, can be given as soon as the patient is evaluated and the decision to anticoagulate is made. It should be continued for seven to ten days, at which time warfarin is introduced. Careful attention must be paid to ensuring that the PTT is not excessively prolonged; the platelet count should be monitored because heparin may produce thrombocytopenia, which can lead to hemorrhagic complications in the absence of an excessively prolonged PTT.

For the patient who is not a surgical candidate, short-term therapy for three to four months is usually safe during this high-risk period. Patients with carotid stenosis who refuse surgery, who are not surgical candidates, who remain symptomatic on antiplatelet drugs, or who have VB TIAs are candidates for short-term therapy with warfarin. The relative efficacy of warfarin and aspirin in this regard are not known.

Antiplatelet Drugs

Aspirin is an effective antiplatelet drug that inhibits intra-arterial thrombus formation in vivo, an effect that lasts for the life of the platelet. Aspirin exerts its antiplatelet effect by inhibiting cyclo-oxygenase, the enzyme involved in the synthesis of thromboxane A_2 in platelets and of prostacyclin in the vascular endothelium. Thromboxane A_2 is a potent vasoconstrictor and platelet-aggregating agent, whereas prostacyclin is a powerful vasodilator and platelet antiaggregating drug. The optimal dose of aspirin for the treatment of TIA is not yet known. Too much aspirin inhibits both thromboxane A_2 and prostacyclin; however, aspirin in low dosages (5 grains daily) inhibits production of thromboxane A_2 (a beneficial effect) more so than it does prostacyclin. Most neurologists prescribe aspirin 300 mg daily for the treatment of TIA.

The two largest studies have shown that aspirin is beneficial in preventing subsequent TIA, stroke, retinal infarction, and death. In these studies, aspirin, 1200 mg daily reduced the risk of stroke in three years from 19% to 12%. Some studies have shown a greater efficacy in men than in women. Most neurologists have abandoned the use of coumadin in favor of aspirin in all TIA patients except those with a clear cardiac source of emboli.

Other antiplatelet drugs have been used to treat TIA. Sulfinpyrazone (Anturane) was shown in the Canadian Cooperative Study (1978) not to be of benefit in reducing the incidence of stroke or death after a TIA. Dipyridamole (Persantine), a drug released for the treatment of angina pectoris, acts by inhibiting platelet phosphodiesterase, with a resulting increase in the platelet level of cyclic adenosine monophosphate, which produces platelet antiaggregation. Dipyridamole, widely used to treat TIA, is expensive; however, two recent studies have shown that in a dose of 225 mg daily in combination with aspirin it does *not* exert any benefit in decreasing the stroke rate following a TIA.

Surgical

Carotid endarterectomy is the most widespread surgical therapy for TIA caused by carotid stenosis. The frequency of this procedure has increased at a remarkable rate: from 7.4/100,000 cases to more than 24/100,000 in the past decade. It is widely believed to be effective in preventing additional TIAs and stroke. The morbidity of the procedure is lowest when the surgeon and anesthesiologist are experienced. As long as the combined complication rate of surgery and angiography is less than 3%, surgery is more effective than medical therapy. Relatively few centers can boast of such a low complication rate, and those that cannot should treat the TIA patient medically rather than surgically or refer the patient to a center where the surgical complication rate is low.

Stenosis of the ICA at the bifurcation ipsilateral to the site of the TIA is a widely used indication for endarterectomy. The degree of critical stenosis is unclear; 40% to 60% is likely when symptoms begin. The ideal surgical candidate is the patient who is symptomatic, who has no deficit, who has carotid stenosis of greater than 50%, and who has minimal generalized vascular disease. Neurologically unstable patients, those with chronic obstructive pulmonary disease or severe angina, those over 70 years of age, and those with a recent (within six months) myocardial infarction are at increased risk from the procedure (7% morbidity/mortality). Such patients should be treated medically. Recurrent stenosis occurs in 4% to 5% of patients, usually within 24 months of the first endarterectomy; surgery in this setting is more difficult to perform.

The role of bypass procedures in the treatment of TIA or incomplete stroke caused by carotid artery occlusion was reported recently by the EC/IC Bypass Study Group (1985). Bypassing an occluded carotid artery by using a branch of the external carotid artery (usually the superficial temporal artery) anastomosed to the middle cerebral artery has many theoretical benefits. The result of the comprehensive multicenter study, however, was that there was no benefit from this risky and expensive procedure and that it should be abandoned.

Therapy for Vertebrobasilar TIA

TIAs in the VB circulation can be caused by atherosclerotic disease of the small penetrating branches of the basilar and vertebral arteries or by the major arteries themselves. Small-vessel disease occurs with great regularity and is less threatening than disease of the basilar trunk. Thus, it is important to try to determine clinically if the basilar artery itself or one of the penetrating vessels is stenotic or occluded.

Basilar arterial disease usually produces bilateral symptoms, whereas involvement of penetrating vessels usually produces unilateral symptoms. If neurological fluctuation occurs, a seven- to ten-day course of heparin is indicated after CT or lumbar puncture has excluded an intracranial hemorrhage. Angiography then should be considered if the patient is stable. If basilar stenosis is associated with an improving or partial (minor) stroke, long-term (at least one year) anticoagulation with warfarin is indicated. The value of long-term antiplatelet therapy is not known, but aspirin is a reasonable alternative medication.

Surgical revascularization or reconstruction now can be performed on the VB arterial system. Vertebral artery endarterectomy, transposition, or transluminal angioplasty have all been performed, but their indications are not established and these techniques are practiced safely by few surgeons. Likewise, bypass procedures can be performed on the posterior circulation, but their indications are poorly defined and they carry a high surgical mortality rate.

STROKE-IN-EVOLUTION

The progressing stroke is characterized by a gradually accumulating neurologic deficit that occurs within the span of a few hours to 48 hours. Progression tends to be stepwise. The patient stabilizes for as little as a few minutes or as long as several hours before further progression occurs. Stroke-in-evolution occurs in approximately 20% of carotid-artery distribution strokes and in 40% of VB strokes. Several mechanisms exist for this neurological deterioration. Brain edema may occur but usually develops after 48 hours. There may be recurrent embolization or extension of a thrombus. The primary brain lesion may be an expanding hematoma and not an ischemic infarction.

The symptoms and signs depend on the brain region involved. Severe vomiting and headache may indicate intracranial hemorrhage, although severe head pain occurs in as many as 25% of patients with ischemic stroke. A CT scan should be performed on an emergency basis in the acutely deteriorating patient to exclude a focal mass lesion. Angiography usually is not performed in this acute setting. If there is no CT evidence of intracranial hemorrhage, therapy should be started immediately with intravenous heparin if there are no contraindications. Heparin infusion should be continued for at least seven to ten days, until the deficit has stabilized. Hemorrhagic complications of anticoagulant therapy in this setting are discussed under management of embolism.

THROMBOTIC STROKE

ETIOLOGY
Approximately 32% of strokes are the result of cerebral thrombosis (Table 20-1). Progressive atherosclerosis of the carotid artery or other extracranial or intracranial arteries may stenose the lumen and predispose the patient to vessel occlusion by thrombosis. Thrombosis of the vessel may occur even in the absence of severe atherosclerotic involvement because of platelet adhesion at the area of the vessel irregularity. If the lumen of the artery has become occluded, the thrombus can propagate distally and block the next-encountered vessel or its branch.

SYMPTOMS AND SIGNS
In at least three-quarters of patients with thrombotic infarction, the major stroke will have been preceded by TIAs. Usually the stroke episode evolves over a period of a few hours. A stuttering course may develop, with intermittent progression of the disorder over several hours to as long as a day. Multiple episodes can occur over several days, leading to a fixed deficit; or a partial deficit can occur and be followed later by a more complete process. Almost 60% of thrombotic strokes occur during sleep. Rarely, the patient with a thrombotic stroke may have evolution of the neurological syndrome over one to two weeks. This protracted course is more suggestive of a tumor or subdural hematoma.

Headache can occur localized to the side of the stroke. It is most common frontally in the case of carotid disease, in the back of the head with basilar occlusion, and behind the ear in vertebral occlusion. The headache is usually not severe, does not have a sudden onset, and may precede the stroke by a week or so. Other symptoms and signs depend on the anatomic distribution of the stroke.

LABORATORY TESTS
A CT scan demonstrates evidence of cerebral infarction in most cases within a few days of the onset of symptoms. The EEG is of limited value when CT is available. Asymmetrical slow waves often are seen over the involved hemisphere. The CSF is usually not sampled unless there is concern about subarachnoid hemorrhage. The CSF protein level may be elevated and a few white blood cells may be present in CSF at first, occasionally rising to several hundred per mm^3 by the third or fourth day. A pure cerebral thrombosis does not cause red blood cells to enter the CSF. A

VDRL test should also be performed on the CSF. In the case of a completed stroke, cerebral angiography is usually not necessary.

The patient with a mild completed stroke and minimal residual neurological deficits needs the same basic evaluation as the patient with a TIA. The risk of further completed stroke in this group of patients is approximately 7% per year. The patient with a moderate stroke who is ambulatory and independent in the activities of daily living is also at higher risk for another infarction. A search for systemic and cardiac diseases should be carried out. If the patient is an acceptable angiographic and surgical risk, then angiography can be performed to look for a surgically correctable lesion. In the patient with a major stroke, there is usually no reason to perform an invasive evaluation because the risk of losing any more functioning tissue on the side of the stroke is slight. Some studies have shown an unacceptably high risk of complications with endarterectomy in patients with completed strokes.

MANAGEMENT

In the patient who has a nonprogressive stroke, there is no benefit from anticoagulation therapy. Most physicians use antiplatelet drugs in this setting to decrease platelet aggregation. Aspirin, 300 to 650 mg/day, may be of benefit, but other antiplatelet drugs, including dipyridamole and sulfinpyrazone, have been shown to be of no benefit. Because hyperglycemia potentiates ischemic damage, a blood glucose level above 140 mg/dL should be lowered. Vasodilators such as papaverine or pentoxyfylline have no role in the treatment of cerebrovascular disease. They can exacerbate the neurological deficit because they steal blood from the infarct site.

Experimental therapies that have shown some benefit in the treatment of stroke include large doses of IV naloxone, infusion of prostacyclin, and hypervolemic hemodilution. In the patient with an uncomplicated infarct, there is no need to give osmotic diuretics such as mannitol. Corticosteroids have *no proven efficacy* in the treatment of ischemic stroke; they can exacerbate the deficit.

With massive infarcts, swelling of infarcted tissue can lead to tentorial herniation and death. In most large infarcts, swelling that results in increased intracranial pressure occurs after 24 to 48 hours; it can cause progression of the neurological deficit over the next 48 to 72 hours but most are not fatal. For large infarcts, a 20% mannitol infusion combined with IV furosemide and fluid restriction reduce swelling and lower intracranial pressure. A cerebellar infarction may acutely raise posterior fossa pressure in the way a cerebellar hemorrhage can (Chapter 37) and can cause sudden death as a result of herniation of the caudal brain stem. Dehydrating therapy should be given to all patients with documented cerebellar infarcts. In cases of progression, surgical removal of the infarcted hemisphere may be lifesaving.

Within a few days after stabilization of deficits, the patient who has suffered a stroke should begin physical therapy and rehabilitation therapy. If language functions have been affected, speech therapy is necessary. Transfer to a rehabilitation unit facilitates the patient's attempts to regain his independent functions. Depression can complicate cortical infarcts, especially those that involve the left hemisphere. These patients may not reach anticipated levels of recovery; some may have vegetative symptoms. Treatment with antidepressant medication (usually nortriptyline) often produces a dramatic change in their affect and recovery.

Recovery depends in part on the extent of the lesion and the age of the patient. The longer the beginning of recovery is delayed, the poorer the prognosis. If early recovery has not begun by two to three weeks after the stroke, the outlook is not good. Patients with mild deficits or those caused by small lesions may begin to improve within a few days and may be totally recovered in a few weeks. More than 90% of recovery occurs within six months of the stroke.

EMBOLIC STROKE

CLINICAL SIGNIFICANCE AND ETIOLOGY

About 30% to 50% of brain infarctions are caused by a cerebral embolus (Table 20-1). Most are of cardiac origin. Less commonly, the source is intra-arterial, arising from damaged endothelium or an ulcerated plaque. The resultant infarction may be pale, hemorrhagic, or have both features. Hemorrhagic infarction almost always indicates cerebral embolism. Any region of the brain may be affected, but the MCA territory is involved most frequently. Because the embolic occlusion occurs rapidly and is usually distal, there is little time for the development of collateral flow.

Causes of cardiogenic emboli are listed in Table 20-4. The most common cause is chronic atrial fibrillation resulting from rheumatic or atherosclerotic disease. Atrial fibrillation produces left atrial thrombi. In the patient with rheumatic mitral valvular disease, there is a 17-fold increase in stroke as compared to age-matched patients without rheumatic heart disease. Systemic emboli occur in approximately 15% to 20% of patients. In nonrheumatic atrial fibrillation, there is a fivefold to sixfold increase in the incidence of cerebral emboli. Myocardial infarction can cause ventricular thrombi to form, which may embolize into the arterial circulation. If the myocardial infarct is transmural, anteroseptal in location, and associated with congestive heart failure, thrombus formation is more likely to occur. The incidence of clinically significant peripheral emboli that follow acute myocardial infarction is 2% to 3%. Patients with cardiomyopathy also are at risk for systemic embolization, particularly if congestive heart failure is present.

TABLE 20-4 CARDIAC CAUSES OF CEREBRAL EMBOLISM

Atrial fibrillation (rheumatic and atherosclerotic)
Myocardial infarction with mural thrombus
Bacterial endocarditis
Nonbacterial thrombotic endocarditis (marantic endocarditis)
Prolapsed mitral valve
Prosthetic cardiac valves
Cardiomyopathy
Paradoxical Embolism
Cardiac tumors (myxoma)
Complications of heart surgery
Valvular disease (aortic stenosis, mitral stenosis)
Congenital heart disease

Adapted from Adams RD, Victor M: Cardiovascular diseases in *Principles of Neurology,* ed 3. New York, McGraw-Hill, 1985. Used with permission.

Mitral valve prolapse (MVP) is a cause of embolic stroke, particularly in the patient less than 45 years old. In young patients with cerebral ischemic events, there is a twofold to tenfold increase in the prevalence of MVP. Embolization of valvular thrombi is the most common mechanism of cerebral ischemia in MVP. The incidence of stroke in asymptomatic young adults with MVP is low, approximately 1 per 6000 persons/year.

SYMPTOMS AND SIGNS

The typical embolic stroke develops suddenly and without warning; it reaches maximal deficit in a few seconds or minutes (rarely, hours). The signs depend on the location of the embolus, as described under the discussion of stroke syndromes. Although the embolus can occlude a major vessel, such as the carotid artery, more commonly the embolus is small and occludes a branch of the MCA, producing a focal disorder such as fluent aphasia. Although VB emboli are uncommon, they can reach the top of the basilar artery to produce coma and paralysis. More often, the embolus enters the posterior cerebral artery and produces homonymous hemianopia. The embolus can cause a severe initial neurological deficit that rapidly improves as the embolus breaks up and passes distally. Seizures may occur, with postictal paralysis.

LABORATORY TESTS

The tests discussed in the section on thrombotic disease and TIA apply here. A CT scan should be performed; often, it demonstrates a hemorrhagic infarction. Hemorrhagic infarction occurs in one-third of patients, but in only 5% does hemorrhagic infarction become evident on initial CT. Red blood cells may be present in CSF, but lumbar puncture is not necessary. Cerebral angiography may reveal single or multiple arterial branch occlusions. Because emboli can lyse rapidly, a delayed angiogram may be normal. Routine blood studies should be performed, including a clotting profile, ANA, CBC, ESR, and VDRL. Blood cultures may be necessary in the patient with bacterial endocarditis. Cardiac evaluation is important in the patient with suspected cerebral emboli from a cardiac source. Two-dimensional echocardiography is indicated in all patients, and Holter monitoring for 24 to 48 hours may be necessary. Two-dimensional echocardiography will identify MVP and mural thrombi in a high percentage of patients with these conditions.

MANAGEMENT

The measures outlined in the section on thrombotic stroke in this chapter apply to the patient with an embolic infarction. General medical management, with attention to cardiorespiratory functions and fluid balance, is important. The major additional therapeutic issue is whether to anticoagulate to prevent recurrent embolus. Recurrent brain embolism occurs within a few days in approximately 13% of patients with embolic stroke from all cardiac sources. Hemorrhage into the infarction occurs in one-third of all patients with embolic stroke, but usually it is not evident for two to four days. Early anticoagulation reduces the incidence of recurrent stroke but carries the risk of exacerbating the cerebral hemorrhage. If the infarct is hemorrhagic on a CT scan, anticoagulation should be delayed. If the infarct is massive or associated with depressed levels of consciousness anticoagulant therapy should be withheld.

In the patients who have nonhemorrhagic infarcts, immediate anticoagulation with intravenous heparin can be started. Many neurologists, however, prefer to delay anticoagulation for three to four days and repeat the CT scan to exclude late hemorrhage. In the patient with a hemorrhagic infarct on CT, anticoagulation should be withheld for five to ten days, CT repeated, and, if the hemorrhage has cleared, heparin started. Cardiogenic embolism is an indication for long-term anticoagulation with warfarin. There is no consensus on whether to preventively anticoagulate the patient with atrial fibrillation or recent myocardial infarction who has not embolized.

LACUNAR INFARCTION

CLINICAL SIGNIFICANCE AND ETIOLOGY
Ten to thirty percent of all strokes are caused by occlusions of penetrating branches of large cerebral arteries. The lacuna is small: it ranges from 0.2 mm^3 to 15 mm^3, with most about 2 mm^3, depending on the size of the occluded penetrating vessel. Lacunae are located in the deep regions of the brain, primarily in the basal ganglia, internal capsule, brain stem, and thalamus. Lacunae are not found in the white matter of the cerebral hemispheres or in the superficial grey matter of the cortex. Most lacunae occur in the territory of the lenticulostriate branches of the anterior and middle cerebral arteries, the thalamoperforant branches of the posterior cerebral artery, and the paramedian branches of the basilar artery.

Lacunar disease is a microvasculopathy. Hypertension and diabetes are present in most patients. Most larger lacunae are caused by microatheroma that involves the wall of the penetrating artery, leading to stenosis and occlusion. Lipohyalinosis is an arteriopathy responsible for most smaller lacunes, many which are clinically asymptomatic. Microembolism is a rare cause of lacunae. Basilar artery atheroma may lead to branch occlusion producing the brainstem lacunar syndromes.

SYMPTOMS AND SIGNS
The onset of symptoms is usually gradual. Almost one-third of lacunae develop over 36 hours. TIAs had occured previously in 20% of patients. Several distinct lacunar syndromes have been described, and the list is growing.

Pure Motor Stroke

The pure motor stroke is the most common lacunar syndrome, accounting for 60% of cases. The lacuna is most often in the internal capsule (the most common site documented by CT), although sites in the corona radiata, cerebral peduncles, pons and the medulla have also been reported. The initial symptom is usually mild unilateral weakness, which may evolve slowly over 36 hours. Weakness develops equally in the face, arm, and leg, with sparing of sensation and vision. Pure motor stroke may spare the face or have unequal arm and leg involvement. In some cases, weakness is more proximal than distal. "Large" lacunae usually produce complete hemiplegia, with poor recovery. Most pure motor lacunar syndromes improve within several weeks. As many as 40% of patients have sensory complaints, usually numbness, heaviness, or coldness. Minimal objective sensory abnormalities may be found on examination, however.

Dysarthria–clumsy hand syndrome, marked by arm and hand clumsiness, has been reported with capsular lacunes. Often there is associated dysphagia, facial weakness, and weakness of the hand.

The syndrome of ataxic hemiparesis (initially called homolateral ataxia with crural paresis), is usually caused by a lacunar infarct that affects the corona radiata of the posterior limb of the internal capsule or of the basis pontis. In most cases there is mild-to-moderate weakness of the upper limb and face that is associated with ataxia of the arm and leg on the same side. Truncal ataxia, dysarthria, and nystagmus are present occasionally.

Pure Sensory Stroke

A pure sensory stroke is most commonly caused by a lacuna in the thalamus (usually in the ventral posterior nucleus), although sites in the corona radiata of the posterior limb of the internal capsule have been reported. These lacunae are usually small. The patient complains that the affected body part feels as though it is sunburned or stretched, as if pins are sticking into it, or as if it is heavier, longer, or smaller. These disturbances of sensation can involve the entire side of the body, and symptoms far exceed objective signs. Partial sensory syndromes are most common. Improvement usually occurs within a few weeks.

Basal Ganglia Stroke

Lacunar syndromes have been reported following lacunar infarction of the basal ganglia. Most sites are in the putamen. The infarctions do not result in clinical symptoms, although a few cases of hemichorea–hemiballismus have been reported following lacunar infarction in this region.

Brain Stem Syndromes

Most brain stem lacunar syndromes are caused by atheroma of the basilar artery with stenosis of the lumen of the penetrating vessel. A variety of syndromes may result from brain stem lacunae, including pure motor stroke with or without facial involvement and ataxic hemiparesis.

LABORATORY TESTS

Lacunar strokes greater than 2 mm may be visualized by CT, the diagnostic procedure of choice. Within the first 48 hours, the yield on initial CT is low, but by ten days more than 50% of lacunes that can be visualized by CT are seen. Computed tomography overestimates the size of lacunes by as much as 100%. Lacunes in the pons are difficult to visualize with CT, regardless of their size. Magnetic resonance imaging (MRI) has a much higher sensitivity for demonstrating lacunes, particularly those in the brain stem. The EEG is often normal because the small size of the lacune does not disrupt brain rhythms. Cerebral angiography usually does not permit resolution of smaller penetrating arteries that are occluded. Generalized cerebrovascular disease may be evident, and in some cases, stenosis of the stem of the MCA may be present. Intracerebral tumors, hematomas, and other mass lesions have all been reported to mimic lacunar syndromes, particularly pure motor stroke.

MANAGEMENT

Therapy should be directed at the risk factors for cerebrovascular disease. The role of anticoagulant therapy is controversial. Aspirin is commonly prescribed, but its effect in preventing lacunar strokes is unknown. The most effective way to treat the lacunar syndrome is by controlling risk factors for stroke, particularly diabetes and hypertension. Physical therapy measures are essentially the same as those described above for ischemic stroke. Depression does not seem to complicate lacunar strokes to the degree it does hemispheric stroke, although multiple lacunar strokes may produce a type of dementia. If improvement occurs, it does so more quickly with strokes that are caused by lacunar infarction.

ASYMPTOMATIC CAROTID ARTERY BRUIT

CLINICAL SIGNIFICANCE

The asymptomatic bruit over the carotid artery is often an incidental finding on examination; it provokes much uncertainty regarding what it means and what should be done about it. Localized bruits in the midcervical area are common, present in 4% to 5% of people over age 50. The prevalence is higher in women and patients with hypertension and diabetes. In patients who undergo vascular surgical procedures, the incidence ranges from 8% in coronary artery bypass patients to 20% in those undergoing peripheral vascular reconstruction.

Bruits are a risk factor for stroke, but not for strokes restricted to the arterial territory of the bruit. Approximately 25% of patients with bruits develop a stroke, and 3% develop a TIA per year. There does not appear to be any significant correlation with the bruit and the side of the TIA or stroke, however, because most ischemic events are not in the distribution of the stenotic vessel. Thus, bruits are an indicator of generalized vascular disease.

ETIOLOGY

Not all murmurs auscultated in the neck area are bruits arising from the internal carotid artery. It is estimated that some kind of cervical murmur can be auscultated in as many as one-third of normal adults. Cervical murmurs can be classified by location and acoustic characteristics. Vertebral artery, cardiac, and diffuse murmurs and venous hums may be auscultated as described below.

SYMPTOMS AND SIGNS

Because the bruit discussed here is asymptomatic, the patient does not have any neurological symptoms. However, it is most important to make sure that the bruit is indeed asymptomatic. A detailed, careful neurological history should be obtained, looking for clues of ischemic cerebrovascular disease. A careful neurological examination should be carried out, looking for signs that might suggest that focal ischemia has already occurred (eg, minimal weakness, asymmetrical hyperreflexia). A complete vascular examination should be performed because it may help determine the cause of the cervical murmur.

Venous hums are common in children and occur in as many as 24% of adults. They are heard best at the base of the neck most commonly on the right side. They are low-pitched, roaring, usually continuous, maximal during diastole, and loudest when the patient is upright. Pressure above the point of maximal intensity, Valsalva's maneuver, and a supine position all reduce or abolish the intensity of the murmur.

Murmurs may occur over the course of the *vertebral artery*. They can be heard from the supraclavicular fossa to the mastoid area along the posterior border of the sternocleidomastoid muscle. The murmur is usually systolic, but can extend into diastole. It can be intensified or converted to a continuous sound by compression of the carotid artery.

Diffuse murmurs can be heard over the length of the carotid artery. They are loudest in the supraclavicular area and diminish in intensity as the examiner ascends the neck. They are frequently bilateral, systolic, and not altered by jugular vein compression. Diffuse murmurs are usually caused by transmission of heart sounds, structural changes of the vessels at the base of the neck, or hyperdynamic states (anemia, fever, hyperthyroidism, hemodialysis).

One-third of normal young persons have a short midsystolic bruit of low intensity at the base of the neck. Bruits in this location may also be associated with the thoracic outlet syndrome and giant cell arteritis or Takayasu's arteritis. Aortic stenosis is the most common cause of loud cardiac murmurs transmitted to the carotid artery. Such a murmur is loudest at the base of the heart, radiates into both carotid arteries, and is loudest in their lower portions. The murmur decreases with Valsalva's maneuver.

External carotid artery flow ceases or reverses direction during diastole, whereas flow through the ICA continues. If compression of the superficial temporal, facial, and occipital arteries causes a murmur to become faint or inaudible, stenosis must be in the external carotid artery. If the murmur increases, the ICA is stenosed. Until the cross-sectional area of an artery is reduced by two-thirds, the intensity of the murmur will increase. As stenosis progresses, the intensity decreases. Overall, the higher the pitch, the greater the stenosis. Even if there are no cervical bruits, the carotid artery may be occluded or markedly stenotic.

LABORATORY TESTS

Noninvasive vascular studies should be performed as a screening test in the patient with an asymptomatic bruit. Because not all patients with asymptomatic carotid murmurs have a stenotic carotid artery, noninvasive tests help identify this group of patients. Phonoangiocardiography should be performed because it records characteristics of the bruit. Ophthalmodynanometry allows indirect recording of ICA pressure; Doppler and B-mode studies help determine arterial wall characteristics and flow through the vessel. The EEG may be of value if there is asymmetrical slowing of the brain waves over the hemisphere ipsilateral to the bruit. Computed tomography usually is of no benefit in the asymptomatic patient. It has been suggested that a noncontrast scan might be a reasonable procedure to look for areas of silent infarction, that would suggest that the bruit is not asymptomatic.

Cerebral angiography is the definitive procedure in the evaluation of a carotid artery bruit. It is an invasive procedure, however, and should be reserved for the few patients found to have a tight stenosis by noninvasive studies. Digital subtraction angiography, either intravenous or intra-arterial, also documents the degree of carotid artery stenosis in the cervical area, but it cannot assess more distal areas when used intravenously. If there is a carotid bifurcation lesion, the carotid siphon should also be evaluated because the incidence of distal tandem lesions associated with carotid bifurcation disease is approximately 10%. Indications for angiography are discussed below.

MANAGEMENT

The management of the asymptomatic carotid artery bruit remains controversial. Medical control of risk factors for cerebrovascular disease is important because the increased incidence of stroke occurs in all cerebrovascular territories. Control of hypertension is important; control of cigarette smoking and diabetes mellitus also decreases the progression of the disease. Treatment with aspirin, dipyridamole, or both, has no effect on the natural history of the carotid bruit, but these drugs are widely prescribed. Only 10% to 15% of all ischemic strokes occur ipsilateral to a carotid bruit, and only a small number of patients with asymptomatic bruits develop a subsequent ipsilateral ischemic stroke. In some studies, symptoms were rare when stenosis was less than 80%.

Would any patient benefit from prophylactic carotid endarterectomy for an asymptomatic bruit? Numerous studies have documented that the presence of a carotid bruit in a surgical patient is not a risk factor for perioperative stroke. Most perioperative strokes occur postoperatively and are not associated with carotid occlusion. Avoiding hypotension in this group of patients during and after surgery is necessary. A candidate for coronary artery bypass grafting who has bilateral, high-grade carotid stenosis should probably undergo a prophylactic endarterectomy in a staged procedure before the cardiac bypass graft.

Indications for endarterectomy include large ulcers and progressive stenosis. If noninvasive (B-mode) or invasive studies show an ulcerated plaque that is greater than 0.5 cm in diameter, platelet antiaggregant therapy with aspirin is indicated. The patient should be followed up with periodic noninvasive tests; if symptoms referable to the lesions occur, endarterectomy is necessary. If the vessel lumen is narrowed more than 70% and is associated with an ulcer, endarterectomy is usually indicated. Some experts advocate endarterectomy for stenosed, nonulcerated lesions, but this is controversial. Carotid angiography and surgery should not be performed in asymptomatic patients who do not have evidence of rapid progression of stenosis by noninvasive studies. A conservative approach is best for them.

Bibliography

Ackerman RH: Non-invasive carotid evaluation. *Stroke* 1980; 11:675-680. (Discusses various non-invasive tests for the diagnosis of carotid arterial disease.)

Adams RD, Victor M: Cerebrovascular diseases, in *Principles of Neurology*, ed 3. New York, McGraw-Hill, 1985, pp 569-640. (Good review of cerebrovascular disease, specifically the various stroke syndromes.)

American–Canadian Cooperative Study Group: Persantine aspirin trial in cerebral ischemia. II: Endpoint results. *Stroke* 1985; 16:406-415. (For TIA patients taking aspirin, the addition of dipyridamole gives no additional benefit.)

Barnett HJM; Stein BM, Mohr JP, et al (eds): *Stroke: Pathophysiology, Diagnosis, and Management*. New York, Churchill Livingstone, 1986.(A two-volume book that covers all areas of stroke; the most comprehensive and up-to-date resource for information on stroke. All medical libraries should have this work.)

Canadian Cooperative Study Group: A randomized trial of aspirin and sulfinpyrazone in threatened stroke. *N Engl J Med* 1978; 299:53-59. (Aspirin is effective for reducing stroke in men, but not in women, following TIA.)

Cerebral Embolism Task Force: Cardiogenic brain embolism. *Arch Neurol* 1980; 43:71-84. (State-of-the-art review of cardiogenic embolism; provides guidelines for management.)

Chambers BR, Norris JW: Outcome in patients with asymptomatic neck bruits. *N Engl J Med* 1986; 315:860-865. (Patients with asymptomatic cervical bruits have a higher risk of a cardiac ischemic event than of a stroke. The risk of cerebral ischemic events is highest in patients with severe carotid artery stenosis, but most patients have some warning (TIA) prior to a stroke.)

Easton JD, Hart RG, Sherman DG, et al: Diagnosis and management of ischemic stroke. I: Threatened stroke and its management. *Curr Probl Cardiol* 1983; 7(5):1-76. (A comprehensive, logical, readable review of cerebral ischemia. It should be used in conjunction with Hart et al, below.)

EC/IC Bypass Study Group: Failure of extracranial-intracranial arterial bypass to reduce the risk of ischemic stroke: Results of an international randomized trial. *N Engl J Med* 1985; 1191-1200. (EC/IC bypass offers no benefit in preventing cerebral ischemia in patients with occlusion or severe narrowing of the ICA or MCA.)

Fisher CM: Lacunar strokes and infarcts: A review. *Neurology (NY)* 1982; 32:871-876. (A review of lacunar stroke syndromes by the neurologist who first described most of them.)

Hachinski V, Norris JW. *Stroke*. Philadelphia, F.A. Davis, 1985. (Comprehensive, readable monograph covering all aspects of the stroke syndrome.)

Hart RG, Sherman DG, Miller VT, et al: Diagnosis and management of ischemic stroke. II: Selected controversies. *Curr Probl Cardiol* 1983; 7 (7):1-80. (Comprehensive review of different types of cardiogenic stroke.)

Kistler JP, Ropper AH, Heros RC: Therapy of ischemic cerebral vascular disease due to atherothrombosis. I and II. *N Engl J Med* 1984; 311:27-34, 100-105. (State-of-the-art review of ischemic cerebrovascular disease, including syndromes, laboratory testing, and medical and surgical management; well referenced.)

Ropper AH, Wechsler LR, Wilson LS: Carotid bruit and the risk of stroke in elective surgery. *N Engl J Med* 1982; 307:1388-1390. (In the asymptomatic patient, a carotid bruit is not a significant risk factor for stroke.)

Sandok BA, Whisnant JP, Furlan AJ, et al: Carotid artery bruits: Prevalence survey and differential diagnosis. *Mayo Clin Proc* 1982; 57:227-230. (Prevalence of carotid bruits increase with age; article also has a good discussion of cervical murmurs.)

Shields RW, Laureno R, Lachman T, et al: Anticoagulant-related hemorrhage in acute cerebral embolism. *Stroke* 1984; 15:426-437. (Reviews indications and complications of anticoagulant therapy in acute cerebral embolism.)

Sundt TM Jr, Sandok BA, Whisnant JP: Carotid endarterectomy: Complications and preoperative assessment of risk. *Mayo Clin Proc* 1975; 50:301-306. (Detailed assessment of risk factors for carotid endarterectomy.)

Ueda K, Toole JF, McHenry LC: Carotid and vertebrobasilar transient ischemic attacks: Clinical and angiographic correlation. *Neurology (Minneap)* 1979; 29:1094-1101. (Reviews clinical and angiographic findings in a group of patients with TIA.)

Whisnant JP, Matsumoto N, Elvback LR: The effect of anticoagulant therapy in the prognosis of patients with transient cerebral ischemic attacks in a community: Rochester, Minnesota. 1955 through 1969. *Mayo Clin Proc* 1973; 48:844-848. (Study that showed the high incidence of stroke immediately following TIA, as well as the benefits of anticoagulant therapy.)

Wolf PA, Kannel WB, Verter J: Current status of risk factors for stoke. *Neurol Clin* 1983; 1:317-343. (Comprehensive review of risk factors for ischemic stroke. The entire volume is worth reading because it covers many aspects of clinical relevance.)

21

Brain Tumors

CLINICAL SIGNIFICANCE

Tumors that arise within the cranial cavity may originate from the skull, meninges, cranial nerves, blood vessels, pituitary gland, or the brain parenchyma. The incidence of such tumors can be determined by looking at older neurological studies of patients referred with brain tumor. These series show a predominance of slower-growing tumors, whereas in most general hospitals there is a higher incidence of malignant gliomas and metastatic tumors.

The incidence of intracranial tumors for patients of all ages ranges from approximately 4.2 to 5.4/100,000; approximately 2% of all patients autopsied have a brain neoplasm. In children under the age of 16, the incidence of central nervous system (CNS) tumors is second only to leukemia, accounting for 15% to 20% of all tumors. The incidence in this age group is approximately 2.4/100,000.

In approximately 20% of all patients with tumors, the brain or meninges are involved. In general, intracranial tumors are more common in men; acoustic neuromas and meningiomas, however, are more common in women. As Tables 21-1 and 21-2 show, intracranial tumors that affect adults are commonly supraten-

TABLE 21-1   INCIDENCE OF TYPES OF INTRACRANIAL TUMORS*

TUMOR TYPE	PERCENTAGE
Glioma	43
Meningioma	15
Pituitary adenoma	13
Acoustic neuroma	6.5
Metastatic	6.5
Congenital	4
Blood vessel	3
Miscellaneous	9

*In patients presenting with brain tumors.

Adapted from Rowland LP: Tumors, in *Merritt's Textbook of Neurology*, ed 7. Philadelphia, Lea & Febiger, 1984, p 218.

TABLE 21-2   DISTRIBUTION AND LOCATION OF INTRACRANIAL TUMORS BY AGE

LOCATION	TUMOR TYPE	% OF ALL TUMORS
Birth to 20 years		
Infratentorial		
	Cerebellar:	
	Astrocytoma	15-20
	Medulloblastoma	14-18
	Brain stem glioma	9-12
	Ependymoma	4-8
Supratentorial		
	Hemisphere glioma	10-14
	Craniopharyngioma	5-13
	Ependymoma	3-5
	Choroid plexus papilloma	2-3
	Pinealoma	1.5-3
	Optic glioma	1-3.5
20 to 60 years		
Supratentorial		
	Glioblastoma	25
	Meningioma	14
	Astrocytoma	13
	Metastases	10
	Pituitary	5
Infratentorial		
	Metastases	5
	Acoustic neuroma	3
	Meningioma	1

Adapted from Rowland LP: Tumors, in *Merritt's Textbook of Neurology,* ed 7. Philadelphia, Lea & Febiger, 1984, p 219, and Youmans GP: *Neurology Surgery.* WB Saunders, 1982, p 2685. Used with permission.

torial in location, whereas more than two-thirds of childhood cases are located in the infratentorial space.

This chapter examines general aspects of the brain tumor patient, with short discussions of each common primary tumor type of adults and children. Metastatic disease is not covered in this chapter; it is thoroughly discussed in Chapter 35. Benign intracranial hypertension (pseudotumor cerebri) is also discussed.

SYMPTOMS AND SIGNS

Brain tumors may present in a number of different ways: from minimal non-specific complaints to more profound abnormalities, such as weakness and seizures. Many of the presenting manifestations depend on the location of the tumor. In general, however, no group of symptoms is pathognomonic for brain tumor.

The initial symptoms may be vague. Alterations of mental function include irritability and decreased attention span. Emotional lability or depression are common. This state is called psychomotor asthenia. The patient is slow to respond and may appear apathetic and drowsy. Thought processes are much slower; dullness and somnolence usually increases and may progress to stupor and coma as intracranial pressure increases.

Tumors that usually cause these symptoms are located in frontal, temporal, or callosal areas, but many are related to the increase in intracranial pressure, not to the location of the tumor. The specific triad that suggests an intracranial tumor is headache, vomiting, and papilledema. It is seen predominantly with lesions that obstruct the pathway of cerebrospinal fluid (CSF), and therefore occur more commonly in childhood.

Headache

Approximately one-third of patients who harbor brain tumors develop headaches (Chapter 11). In some patients, the headache is dull and nonspecific. The headache of intracranial tumor is usually intermittent, lasting for as briefly as a few minutes or as long as hours. It may become worse with postural changes or Valsalva's maneuver. Brain tumor headache is most often nonthrobbing, intermittent, and is increased by activity. At times it may be associated with nausea and vomiting. A headache that awakens the patient from sleep suggests increased intracranial pressure and may be a clue to the presence of a possible neoplasm.

As the tumor grows, headache may become more frequent and last longer. It is estimated that more than 90% of patients with brain tumor eventually complain of headache. Generalized headache is believed to result from traction on pain-sensitive fibers. Nausea, vomiting, syncope, and drop attacks may also occur. Rapid head-position change may precipitate a paroxysm, but a change in head position (down or supine) may relieve pain dramatically. This type of headache is often caused by a midline mass that obstructs the ventricular system and causes intermittent or continuous obstruction to CSF outflow. Exertional headache occurs in approximately 10% of patients who have intracranial tumors, usually from those located in the posterior fossa.

Vomiting occurs initially in approximately one-third of brain tumor patients. It is often associated with headaches and is more common in tumors of the posterior fossa. Projectile vomiting (forcible and unexpected) may occur, or the patient may complain of persistent nausea and vomiting. Nonspecific dizziness also occurs, but it is poorly described by the patient and is usually not vertiginous.

Seizures

Focal (partial) or generalized seizures occur in as many as one-third of patients with tumors of the cerebral hemispheres. Seizures may be the first symptom of a brain tumor, so tumor must be considered when any adult has a first seizure. In general the longer the tumor has been present, the more likely it is to produce a seizure; 70% of vascular brain tumors are associated with seizures, whereas 25% of rapidly growing tumors (glioblastoma) are associated with seizures. Focal seizures (jacksonian, uncinate, visual) that occur for the first time in an adult strongly suggest intracranial tumor or other space-occupying lesion.

Some tumors may cause increased intracranial pressure without lateralizing signs, particularly colloid cyst of the third ventricle, medulloblastoma, ependymoma of the fourth ventricle, pinealoma, and craniopharyngioma. False-localizing signs may be present because of increased intracranial pressure. The drowsiness and dullness of affect and cognitive functions fall into this category.

Ataxia of gait and urinary incontinence may also be seen with hydrocephalus of any cause.

Unilateral or bilateral abducens nerve palsies may occur as a result of stretching of cranial nerve VI from increased intracranial pressure. Other false localizing signs include ipsilateral hemiplegia caused by compression of the cerebral peduncle against the tentorium on the side opposite the tumor. Homonymous hemianopia may occur on the same side of the tumor because of an infarct in the distribution of the posterior cerebral artery. A third-nerve palsy contralateral to the tumor may occur with the same mechanism as that of ipsilateral hemiplegia.

Papilledema is present in 50% to 90% of brain tumors, depending on the location and stage of the tumor. Those tumors that obstruct CSF outflow (see above) produce a high incidence of papilledema. Tumors that are confined to the cerebral hemispheres do not produce papilledema unless they grow large enough to produce increased intracranial pressure.

LABORATORY TESTS

Skull x-rays usually add little to the diagnosis and are not cost-effective. Usually, any positive information they yield needs to be further evaluated by other neurodiagnostic tests. Calcification may be seen within a tumor (craniopharyngioma, oligodendroglioma). Bony changes such as hyperostosis of adjacent bone may be seen in 50% of meningiomas. Pituitary tumors may cause erosion of the sella turcica; chronic increased intracranial pressure increases the convolutional markings of the skull, with erosion of the dorsum sellae. Computed tomography (CT) is the most sensitive and readily available test for the diagnosis of brain tumor. In cases of suspected tumor, noncontrast and contrast scans should be performed. Depending on the presumed anatomic localization of the tumor, the CT scan can be angulated through precise areas (eg, pituitary fossa, internal auditory meatus). The scan helps localize the lesion and gives information regarding associated edema, hemorrhage, calcification, or hydrocephalus.

Focal changes may be seen on the electroencephalogram (EEG) (slow waves, spikes) in the presence of a unilateral tumor of the cerebral hemisphere. Tumors that are deeply situated and those in the posterior fossa may be associated with generalized slowing of brain rhythms. Although sensitive for detecting CNS electrical abnormalities, the EEG does not give specific information for diagnosis. In most centers, EEG is not inexpensive; combined with a skull x-ray, its cost approaches that of a CT scan. The CT scan, however, provides more information about brain tumors than do the skull x-ray and EEG together.

Computed tomography has replaced angiography for localizing most brain tumors, but angiography still has a role in the differential diagnosis of mass lesions, as well as in planning a surgical approach to a mass lesion. Lumbar puncture is rarely indicated for the diagnosis of brain tumor; it may be hazardous in the presence of increased intracranial pressure or a posterior fossa mass lesion. The patient with papilledema and a normal CT scan, however, may have pseudotumor cerebri, in which case lumbar puncture (LP) (following a contrast CT) is both diagnostic and therapeutic. If meningeal spread of tumor is suspected, lumbar puncture with cytologic analysis might be a reasonable diagnostic test, but it is best to have a neurological consultant involved before proceeding with an LP.

Radionuclide brain scanning is used rarely nowadays, but it remains a diagnostic test in centers where CT is not available. The CT scan is highly superior to the radionuclide brain scan, especially when contrast is utilized.

Nuclear magnetic resonance imaging (MRI) is a superb diagnostic tool. It is excellent for detecting small extra-axial masses as well as brain stem and posterior fossa lesions. In certain cases, MRI combined with a contrast CT scan has a high yield for the diagnosis of CNS lesions. Occasionally, tumors that were not visualized by CT will be seen on MRI.

DIAGNOSIS

Whenever focal and generalized neurological symptoms—particularly new headaches or seizures—develop over a few weeks or months, a brain tumor should be considered as a cause of the symptoms. Brain tumors usually produce slowly progressive neurological deficits, but abrupt, "stroke-like" syndromes may also occur, usually as a result of infarction or bleeding into an occult tumor.

A careful neurological exam should be performed, looking for evidence of focal disease of the nervous system and increased intracranial pressure. Careful examination of visual fields and optic fundi is necessary. Differential diagnosis includes vascular disorders, infections, demyelination, postictal states, and subdural hematoma.

MANAGEMENT

The treatment of the patient with a brain tumor is directed first by the mode of presentation. If a mass lesion is evident on a CT scan and is associated with edema, then treatment with corticosteroids to reduce the edema should be begun. Dexamethasone, 4 mg bid to qid, or methylprednisolone, 24 mg bid to qid, may be used. Methylprednisolone has an advantage over dexamethasone in this setting; there does not appear to be any interaction between methylprednisolone and the various anticonvulsants, whereas dexamethasone and phenytoin interact in a way that phenytoin increases the metabolism of the dexamethasone and reduces its anti-edema efficacy.

If rapid neurological deterioration occurs, osmotic agents such as 20% mannitol solution and furosemide may need to be infused to acutely reduce cerebral edema and intracranial hypertension. In certain patients who have obstructive hydrocephalus, emergency ventriculostomy may be lifesaving.

Surgical decompression and histologic diagnosis of the tumor are necessary. Extirpation of the tumor in some cases is curative (eg, meningioma); in others it is palliative (eg, glioma). Depending on the diagnosis, chemotherapy (systemic, intrathecal, or intra-arterial) might be indicated. Individual treatment plans will depend on the histological type of tumor.

WHEN TO CONSULT

The patient with a slowly progressive or apoplectiform presentation of neurological dysfunction warrants a neurologic consultation. If a patient has neurological symptoms and the CT scan documents intracranial pathology, referral to a neurosurgeon or neurologist is indicated. Whether referral is to a neurologist or neurosurgeon depends in part on the underlying type of tumor or clinical presentation.

PEDIATRIC BRAIN TUMORS
Infratentorial
Medulloblastoma

Medulloblastoma is one of the most common posterior fossa tumors of childhood. It constitutes 5 to 10% of intracranial gliomas and 25 to 40% of all posterior fossa tumors. In 75% of cases, the child is less than 16 years of age. Medulloblastoma usually presents with signs and symptoms of increased intracranial pressure and cerebellar dysfunction (predominantly ataxia of gait). A CT scan is diagnostic, often showing a hyperdense midline mass in the posterior fossa that is enhanced by contrast and that is associated with hydrocephalus.

Treatment begins with surgical removal of the tumor, followed by postoperative radiation. Medulloblastoma is highly radiosensitive; 4500 to 5500 rads should be delivered to the posterior fossa, and approximately 3500 to 4000 rads to the spinal cord. Neuraxis radiation is necessary because medulloblastoma frequently disseminates throughout the CSF pathways.

Children with recurrent medulloblastoma often have a good response to chemotherapy, eg, methotrexate, bischloroethylnitrosourea (BCNU), vincristine (VCR), procarbazine, or chloroethylcyclohexylnitrosourea (CCNU); prolonged symptom-free intervals have been reported. Less clear at the present time is the role of adjuvant chemotherapy in children with newly diagnosed medulloblastoma. Children with complete surgical resection of the tumor have better rates of survival than those with biopsy or subtotal resection. In cases in which the tumor has not involved the brain stem, survival is longer. Children older than 2 years of age at diagnosis also have prolonged survival. Five-year survival in some studies has reached 50 to 60%. Medulloblastoma can metastasize outside the CNS, primarily to the bone or lymph nodes. These extraneural lesions may respond to local radiation therapy and chemotherapy, thereby improving the quality of life for the child.

Cerebellar Astrocytoma

Cerebellar astrocytoma, the second most common posterior fossa tumor in children represents 13% to 15% of all childhood brain tumors. It occurs most often between the ages of 7 and 15 years. It usually arises from the vermis (midline) or the hemisphere and is often cystic with a mural nodule, but it may be solid. The clinical presentation is similar to that of medulloblastoma: combined cerebellar signs and evidence of increased intracranial pressure (headache, papilledema). A CT scan is usually diagnostic, demonstrating a cystic lesion often associated with a mural nodule and secondary hydrocephalus. The treatment of cerebellar astrocytoma is surgical. If surgical removal is complete, the cure rate approaches 100%; partial resection is associated with recurrence. Postoperative radiation therapy is now utilized only for partially resected or recurrent tumors. Chemotherapy is usually not necessary.

Brain Stem Glioma

Brainstem glioma constitutes 10% of pediatric brain tumors, accounting for 75% of brain stem tumors in patients under 20 years of age. They are most commonly diagnosed between the ages of 6 and 10. Multiple cranial nerve palsies with long-tract signs are commonly seen. Increased intracranial pressure and papilledema do not occur unless there is obstruction of the aqueduct of Sylvius. Unilateral or bilateral cranial nerve VI paresis is the most common sign, followed by facial nerve paresis, deafness, palatal weakness, and contralateral corticospinal signs. The clinical syndrome is often diagnostic. A CT scan with posterior fossa views may show enlargement of the brain stem. Metrizamide cisternography may be required to delineate brain stem involvement. MRI is the most imaging technique for diagnosing brain stem glioma. Lumbar puncture and angiography are not necessary, although ventriculography was needed to demonstrate the brain stem mass in the past.

Surgery is not recommended for these tumors unless there is predominant cyst formation or an exophytic mass. They seed the neuraxis more rarely than other malignant brain tumors of childhood. Radiation (5000 to 5500 rads to the posterior fossa) is the treatment of choice. Children with a tumor in the lower pons and medulla tend to die sooner than those with a tumor in the upper pons and midbrain. Chemotherapy is ineffective.

The rate of survival for children with brain stem glioma is not good. Conservative five-year survival is approximately 17%; in the best study, five-year survival was 30%.

Ependymoma

Ependymoma represents approximately 10% of all intracranial neoplasms of childhood. Most tumors are diagnosed between birth and 4 years of age. These tumors commonly arise from the floor of the fourth ventricle. The clinical presentation is a combination of brain stem and cerebellar signs, at times in association with increased intracranial pressure caused by obstructive hydrocephalus. A CT scan often shows an intraventricular mass, occasionally with an exophytic component or hydrocephalus. Approximately 11% of ependymomas seed the subarachnoid space; in those cases, CSF cytologic analysis will be positive, and myelography may be abnormal. The treatment of choice is surgical excision followed by craniospinal radiotherapy. Chemotherapy is not effective. The five-year survival rate is about 27%; children less than 2 years of age have a five-year survival of only 12%.

Supratentorial Tumor
Astrocytoma, Grades 1 and 2

Approximately 20% of brain tumors in children are supratentorial astrocytomas. They grow slowly and tend to cause focal signs without evidence of increased intracranial pressure, in contrast to the presentation of cerebellar astrocytoma. A CT scan localizes the lesion and guides the biopsy. Surgical excision is usually not possible, but partial resection is associated with a better prognosis than biopsy alone. The use of postoperative radiation therapy remains controversial in the patient with low-grade astrocytoma; recent evidence does favor the use of radiation therapy, which appears to be palliative only. Five-year survival of children with a low-grade astrocytoma of the cerebral hemispheres is approximately 50%. The role of chemotherapy is unclear.

Astrocytoma, Grades 3 and 4

Twelve percent of childhood brain tumors are anaplastic astrocytomas (grade 3) and glioblastoma multiforme (grade 4). The modes of presentation are the same as for those of lower-grade astrocytoma, although grades 3 and 4 carry a poorer prognosis. Gross tumor resection, followed by radiation therapy, improves survival. Chemotherapy is not of benefit. Five-year survival rates for children with grade 3 astrocytoma are 15% to 20%; five-year survival rates for grade 4 astrocytomas are 5% to 10%.

Optic Nerve Glioma

Three to five percent of childhood intracranial tumors involve the visual pathway. Children with neurofibromatosis have a 10% incidence of optic nerve gliomas by the end of the first decade of life (Chapter 26). This tumor usually involves a single nerve, although it can be bilateral and can invade the optic chiasm. These tumors usually cause painless impairment of vision; they may also grow into suprasellar areas and cause neuroendocrine abnormalities or hydrocephalus.

The CT scan with orbital views often demonstrates an increased size of the optic nerve foramen or deformity of the sella turcica. Visual evoked potentials are abnormal on the involved side. The natural history of optic nerve glioma is not known. The child should be followed clinically with neuro-ophthalmologic exams and visual field examinations. If there is involvement posteriorly into the chiasm or superiorly into the hypothalamus, biopsy should be performed, followed by radiation therapy of 5000 to 6000 rads. Five-year survival is the rule. Treatment of recurrence with chemotherapy is unrewarding.

ADULT BRAIN TUMORS

Brain tumors are the fourth leading cause of cancer-related death in middle-aged men. In the adult, the likelihood of developing a brain tumor increases steadily with age until the eighth decade. In the adult, most brain tumors are supratentorial. The more common brain tumors of adults are discussed by histologic type.

Astrocytoma (Glioma)

Approximately 50% of intracranial tumors are gliomas that arise from primitive forms of glial cells. Such tumors are usually classified from grade 1 (least malignant) to grade 4 (most malignant). Astrocytomas constitute approximately 25% of all intracranial gliomas.

Low-grade astrocytomas (grades 1 and 2) grow slowly and cause focal neurological abnormalities and seizures without evidence of increased intracranial pressure. A CT scan usually shows a low-density abnormality that at times may be cystic. The survival for patients with grade 1 astrocytoma is 76%; the five-year survival for grade 2 astrocytoma is only 58%. There is controversy regarding treatment of low-grade gliomas. Radiation therapy improves survival; 67% of tumors that recur become malignant.

Anaplastic astrocytoma (grade 3) and glioblastoma multiforme (grade 4) are the most common primary brain tumors of the cerebral hemispheres in adults. The peak incidence of glioblastoma is 7.5/100,000. It occurs in the 50 to 59 age group. Glioblastoma multiforme represents 50% of all gliomas; and it is usually located in the frontal and temporal lobes, but approximately 4% are multicentric.

On microscopic examination, the tumor is associated with characteristic vascular changes and areas of necrosis. Patients frequently have a combination of increased intracranial pressure and focal neurological changes that depend in part on the location of the tumor. Thus, there is frequently a combination of headache, intellectual change, seizures, and weakness. A CT scan usually demonstrates a low-density lesion that enhances following the administration of contrast and that is associated with marked edema. Angiography usually demonstrates neovascularity with early-draining veins. Histologic diagnosis is made during surgery.

Glioblastoma has a poor prognosis: only 10% of patients are alive 18 to 24 months after conventional therapy. Radiotherapy allows survival into the second year in some cases. Median survival after maximal surgery and radiation is 9.2 months, but is only four months following surgical resection alone. Chemotherapy (BCNU) benefits patients the most who have survived one year (and who have been given chemotherapy). The most significant prognostic factor is the patient's age. Patients older than 50 years of age have a shorter survival regardless of therapy. In one study, median survival of patients younger than 40 years of age was 100 weeks; for patients older than 65 years of age, median survival was only 48 weeks. Patients younger than 50 years of age are also more responsive to BCNU and can tolerate the drug much better than older patients.

Corticosteroids are necessary to control peritumoral edema. As much as 96 mg of dexamethasone daily may be necessary to control symptoms. Biopsy of the lesion should be performed in almost all cases for pathological confirmation. When possible, the tumor should be debulked. Postoperative radiotherapy is indicated, and chemotherapy with BCNU also prolongs survival—particularly in the younger patient. Spread of the tumor to the spinal leptomeninges is probably not rare; irs clinical recognition and incidence are increasing.

There are many novel neurosurgical and chemotherapeutic approaches to malignant astrocytoma. These include (1) localized hyperthermia of the tumor; (2) interstitial radiation implants; (3) immunotherapy with interferon or interleukin; (4) monoclonal antibodies for both diagnosis and treatment; and (5) intra-arterial chemotherapy into the artery supplying the tumor. Intra-arterial chemotherapy allows the use of higher concentrations of the chemotherapeutic agent with less systemic toxicity. Side effects are not infrequent, and functional survival is prolonged. In addition, multiple daily fractions of radiation therapy and neutron- or proton-beam therapy are used to make the tumor more sensitive to therapy. Unfortunately, regardless of the type of treatment, survival beyond three years is exceptional. Therapy should be individualized for each patient in an attempt to prolong functional survival.

Oligodendroglioma

Oligodendroglioma represents approximately 5% of gliomas. It is found primarily in the cerebral hemispheres and predominantly in the frontal lobes. Calcification is seen in 50% of cases. The clinical course is usually prolonged, and seizures commonly occur. A CT scan localizes the tumor, which should be totally excised if possible. The five-year survival rate in oligodendroglioma approximates that of lower-grade astrocytoma (ie, 60% five-year survival). Because most of these tumors are more malignant at the time of first recurrence, especially after age 50, postoperative radiation therapy is recommended. Meningeal seeding may occur, particularly in children.

Meningioma

Fourteen to twenty percent of adult brain tumors arise from the meninges. Symptoms of meningioma are usually caused by compression. Meningiomas rarely invade the brain substance but commonly invade bone and cause localized hyperostosis. The peak incidence is at approximately the age of 45; meningiomas are more common in women. The most common location is the parasagittal or falx area; the second and third most commmon sites are the convexity of the cerebral hemisphere and the sphenoid ridge. Other locations include the olfactory groove, suprasellar area, posterior fossa, middle fossa, and intra-ventricular areas. As a rule, these tumors are solitary; multiple meningiomas occur in fewer than 1% of cases. When tumors are multiple they usually occur in association with other tumors or are secondary to von Recklinghausen's syndrome (Chapter 26).

Symptoms and signs are usually of long duration and are similar to those of other tumors. Tumors located in the parasagittal or falx area (25%) may present with seizures, headache, or progressive gait disturbances. In meningiomas that arise from the convexity (20%), seizures and focal neurological signs are most common. Tumors of the sphenoid ridge (20%) may be associated with seizures, exophthalmos, and ophthalmoplegia—usually with involvement of the outer sphenoidal ridge. Those that involve the inner sphenoid ridge may be associated with unilateral visual loss, secondary optic atrophy, exophthalmos, visual field deficits, ophthalmoplegia, and numbness of the forehead. Meningiomas that arise from the olfactory groove (10%) may grow to a large size before they are detected; unilateral anosmia and visual loss are common signs. When a meningioma arises from the suprasellar area (10%), initial symptoms are usually visual; frequently, bitemporal hemianopia is evident. Rarely, involvement of the pituitary stalk will lead to diabetes insipidus.

Posterior fossa meningiomas (10%) may arise from the tentorium, the surface of the petrous bone, the clivus, or the cerebellar convexity. Tumors that arise from the tentorium often produce hydrocephalus and signs of increased intracranial pressure, often (but not always) associated with cerebellar signs. Because of occipital lobe compression, tentorial meningioma may produce a visual field deficit (homonymous hemianopia) or reading disturbance. Meningiomas that arise from the petrous bone classically produce abnormalities of lower cranial nerves and can mimic tumors of the acoustic nerve if they are located in the cerebellopontine angle.

Intraventricular tumors are rare (2%), and usually produce chronic increased intracranial pressure that is occasionally associated with focal CNS disturbances.

Plain skull x-rays may reveal evidence of localized hyperostosis. A CT scan of the head with and without contrast is 95% accurate for detecting meningiomas. A small tumor may be difficult to visualize. Arteriography helps define the vascular supply of the tumor. Both intracranial and extracranial vascular supply is common.

MANAGEMENT

Although most meningiomas are histologically benign, they frequently are in anatomically malignant locations. They tend to grow slowly and may be quite large when first diagnosed. In general, surgery for gross tumor removal is indicated most often, but because the tumor can be locally invasive and vascular, surgical mortality is approximately 5%. Preoperative embolization or ligation of external carotid vessels benefits some patients and clearly reduces surgical blood loss. Radiotherapy is indicated for histologically malignant meningiomas or those that occur in vital areas that cannot be removed surgically. Tumor recurs in 10% to 30% of patients, depending on the location of the tumor and the type of surgical procedure. The average interval for recurrence is five years.

Acoustic Neuroma

Five to ten percent of intracranial tumors are acoustic neuromas, and 80% to 90% of them occur in the cerebellopontine (CP) angle. They occur most commonly in patients between the ages of 20 and 50 years. When they occur in younger patients or when they are bilateral, they often are associated with neurofibromatosis. These tumors arise from Schwann cells of the vestibular branch of cranial nerve VIII, and grow into the CP angle and the internal auditory meatus. They grow slowly and may not become symptomatic until they are quite large.

Otological symptoms and signs are most common; hearing loss, disequilibrium, and tinnitus occur in more than 70% of patients. Headache, ataxia, vertigo, and facial numbness are less common, and usually are caused by larger tumors. In patients with smaller tumors, impaired hearing is most common and may be associated with nystagmus and diminished trigeminal sensation (with decreased corneal reflex). If the tumor is large it may produce papilledema and pyramidal and cerebellar signs.

A plain skull x-ray may show widening of the internal auditory meatus, but does not demonstrate small lesions. Computed tomography is the most useful technique, demonstrating tumors larger than 2 cm. If a smaller tumor is suspected, MRI or metrizamide cisternography are indicated. Brain stem auditory evoked potentials and audiometric examinations are abnormal in a high percentage of patients, as are caloric testing and electronystagmography. Pure high-frequency tone hearing loss is common, and speech discrimination is usually impaired.

Surgical removal using an operating microscope is indicated. Facial nerve function can usually be preserved with this technique.

Pituitary Tumor

CLINICAL SIGNIFICANCE

Approximately 10% of brain tumors are localized in the pituitary gland. Pituitary tumors are most common in the third and fourth decades of life; both sexes are affected equally. Pituitary tumors are divided into secreting and nonsecreting types. Secreting tumors produce hormones, including growth hormone, gonadotropins, prolactin, and adrenocorticotropin. Most pituitary tumors are secretory. A pituitary tumor confined to the sella turcica is termed intrasellar, but if it extends out of the sella, it is extrasellar (and occasionally suprasellar). Invasive adenomas are tumors that invade the floor and the sella. Tumors smaller than 10 mm in diameter are known as microadenomas.

SYMPTOMS AND SIGNS

The clinical presentation of pituitary tumors is the result of growth of the tumor causing compression of adjacent neural structures, or of endocrine abnormalities that the tumors produce. If the tumor expands superiorly, the optic chiasm is compressed and visual field defects arise. If growth continues, the suprasellar cisterns are filled and secondary hydrocephalus may result because of obstruction of the foramina of Monro. If lateral extension occurs, the cavernous sinuses can be involved, resulting in oculomotor disturbances. If the tumor grows anteriorly, it can invade the frontal lobes.

Frontal or vertex headaches are common. Visual symptoms are common, particularly in cases with suprasellar extension. Vision may be blurred; bitemporal hemianopia is the most common visual field defect. Unilateral visual loss is quite uncommon. Papilledema is rare, but optic atrophy may occur in patients with visual symptoms. In 5% to 15% of cases, there is oculomotor dysfunction that produces diplopia because of lateral extension of the tumor into the cavernous sinus. Partial or complete ophthalmoplegia may be present as may facial hypesthesia secondary to involvement of cranial nerve V in the cavernous sinus.

If the tumor is large and extends into the suprasellar area, diabetes insipidus may result because of hypothalamic dysfunction. Seizures may occur when the tumor extends into the frontal or temporal lobes. Frontally invasive tumors may produce dementia or personality changes. Approximately 5% of patients with pituitary tumors develop pituitary apoplexy, which mimics subarachnoid hemorrhage (sudden onset of headache, nuchal rigidity, nausea, vomiting, diplopia, and progressive visual loss).

Hypersecreting Tumors
Prolactin-Secreting Adenomas

Seventy-five percent of hypersecreting pituitary tumors secrete prolactin. They classically produce amenorrhea and galactorrhea, although almost all men and many women do not develop galactorrhea. Large tumors that secrete prolactin may compress the optic chiasm. Pituitary microadenoma usually occurs in women of childbearing age, causing infertility. Diagnosis is made on the basis of the clinical syndrome, an increased prolactin level, and CT demonstration of a microadenoma.

Growth Hormone-Secreting Adenoma

Overproduction of growth hormone produces acromegaly after the bony epiphyses have closed, and gigantism prior to their closure. The typical acromegalic patient has coarse facial features: prominent supraorbital ridges; a large, protruding mandible with separated teeth; and large, thick lips. Patients may complain of headache, visual disturbances, and hand paresthesias of carpal tunnel syndrome.

ACTH-Secreting Tumor

Of patients with Cushing's syndrome, approximately 70% have bilateral adrenal hyperplasia; 25% have adrenal gland tumors; and 5% have ectopic ACTH production by lung tumor. Only 50% of cases with adrenal hyperplasia have a demonstrable pituitary tumor, even though it is accepted that adrenal hyperplasia is caused by overproduction of ACTH by the pituitary gland.

Hyposecreting Tumors

Destruction of the stalk of the pituitary deprives the anterior pituitary gland of hypothalamic regulatory hormones. All anterior pituitary hormones are then reduced in the blood—except prolactin which is increased. Diabetes insipidus suggests hypothalamic involvement. With nonfunctioning pituitary tumors, impaired secretion of gonadotropins leads to amenorrhea and irregular menstrual periods in women, and to decreased libido and potency in men. Axillary and pubic hair are decreased, and signs of hypothyroidism are commonly present (lethargy, cold intolerance, constipation, weakness). Acute adrenal insufficiency in response to stress may also develop.

LABORATORY TESTS AND DIAGNOSIS

Radiologic examination of the sella and parasellar areas is mandatory. Plain skull x-rays may reveal enlargement of the sella turcica and thinning of the dorsum or floor of the sella. Computed tomography with and without contrast usually demonstrates the presence of a pituitary tumor. With x-ray reconstruction of coronal CT images, microadenomas may also be evident.

Because aneurysms sometimes simulate a pituitary adenoma, cerebral angiography is sometimes necessary. Formal visual field examination is indicated in patients with visual complaints or in those with large suprasellar tumors. Measurement of anterior pituitary hormones should be performed, including growth hormone, prolactin, ACTH, luteinizing hormone (LH), and follicle-stimulating hormone (FSH). A glucose tolerance test with growth hormone determinations may be necessary to prove hypersecretion of growth hormone. In patients with Cushing's disease caused by ACTH hypersecretion, measurement of the serum cortisol level in the morning and after overnight dexamethasone suppression is necessary, in addition to a urinary corticosteroid determination. Thyroid function tests and serum electrolyte determinations should also be performed.

MANAGEMENT

Treatment modalities include hormonal replacement, surgery, radiation therapy, and bromocriptine. Treatment should be directed first at hormone replacement, particularly thyroid and steroid hormones. Patients with secreting tumors should have the tumor removed surgically. In nonsecreting tumors (so called even though many secrete some hormone), tumor excision is indicated to decompress the visual pathways. Smaller tumors can be removed by transphenoidal surgery, but large tumors may require craniotomy. The mortality of a transphenoidal approach is 1% to 2%, compared with 3% to 5% following craniotomy. In patients with secreting microadenomas, the transphenoidal approach allows selective removal of the tumor. Low-dose bromocriptine (a dopamine agonist drug) usually restores fertility.

Radiation therapy with conventional doses (approximately 5000 rads) is usually advised for the patient who is a poor surgical risk, or at times in the patient with a small tumor but without visual impairment. Radiotherapy is also used following subtotal resection of the tumor. Proton beam therapy is highly effective, but it is restricted to centers with particle accelerators.

PSEUDOTUMOR CEREBRI

CLINICAL SIGNIFICANCE

The syndrome of pseudotumor cerebri (PC, or benign intracranial hypertension) is characterized by headache and papilledema from increased intracranial pressure in the absence of intracranial mass lesions and obstructive hydrocephalus.

ETIOLOGY

Psuedotumor cerebri has many causes (Table 21-3) but its pathogenesis is unclear. Increased intracranial pressure is believed the result of reduced absorption of spinal fluid or of cerebral edema. The reduced CSF absorption hypothesis is based on CSF infusion studies. In some animals, hypervitaminosis A results in decreased spinal fluid absorption. There is evidence of primary cytotoxic brain edema from increased cellular swelling, and of interstitial edema from passage of CSF from the ventricular space into the brain. Estrone, a product of estrogen metabolism, can stimulate CSF secretion; this may cause pseudotumor cerebri in the obese woman with menstrual difficulties.

Increased intracranial pressure secondary to occlusion of an intracranial venous sinus usually occurs as the result of otitis media, as the infection extends into the petrous bone and into the lateral sinus (otitic hydrocephalus). It may

TABLE 21-3 PSEUDOTUMOR CEREBRI: ETIOLOGIC FACTORS

Metabolic and Endocrine Disorders

    Obesity with or without menstrual irregularities
    Pregnancy
    Menarche
    Addison's disease
    Hyperparathyroidism
    Hypercorticolism

Drugs and Toxins

    Vitamin A
    Female sex hormones
    Nalidixic acid
    Tetracycline
    Adrenal steroids
    Chlordane (Kepone)

Hematologic and Connective Tissue Disorders

    Iron-deficiency anemia
    Infectious mononucleosis
    Polycythemia
    Systemic lupus erythematosus
    Wiskott–Aldrich syndrome
    Behçet's syndrome

Intracranial Venous Sinus Thrombosis

    Pregnancy and postpartum
    Progestational drugs
    After head trauma
    Mastoiditis and lateral sinus thrombosis
    Idiopathic sinus thrombosis
    Marantic sinus thrombosis
    Cryofibrinogenemia

High Cerebrospinal Fluid Protein Level

    Spinal cord tumors
    Guillain–Barré syndrome

Miscellaneous

    Familial
    Sydenham's chorea
    Empty sella syndrome
    Pulmonary (pickwickian syndrome, hypoventilation)

Idiopathic

occur as a complication of both subacute and chronic infections. Thrombosis of the superior sagittal sinus is also related to oral contraceptives, malignancy, dehydration, hypercoagulable states, and connective tissue diseases, including Behçet's syndrome. It usually presents with stupor, seizures, and lower-extremity weakness.

Pseudotumor cerebri has occurred in some patients who were taking corticosteroids—usually when the steroid dose had been reduced. Excessive vitamin A consumption (as low as 25,000 units per day), use of outdated tetracycline, oral contraceptives, and nalidixic acid have also been reported as causes of pseudotumor cerebri.

Symptoms and Signs

The typical patient is a young, obese woman with menstrual irregularities. Almost all patients with PC have headache. Onset is abrupt, especially in the younger patient; the older patient has a more protracted course. Headache is usually generalized, episodic, often throbbing, worse in the morning, and aggravated by change in position, straining, and coughing. Nausea may occur, but vomiting is uncommon.

Visual symptoms are noted in one-third to one-half of patients. Blurred vision is the most common ocular complaint, but transient obscurations of vision may occur and may progress to permanent visual loss. Visual blurring lasts minutes or hours, and may increase with change of position, most commonly in the morning. Patients with PC look well and only rarely present with transient visual obscurations *without* headache.

Diplopia occurs in as many as one-fourth of patients with PC because of unilateral or bilateral 6th cranial nerve palsies, which are false localizing signs caused by increased intracranial pressure. Peripheral facial nerve palsies have been reported in the course of PC, but their etiology is uncertain.

Virtually all patients with PC exhibit ophthalmoscopic evidence of increased intracranial pressure. Papilledema is usually evident, but loss of spontaneous venous pulsations may be the only sign of increased intracranial pressure. Papilledema is always bilateral but may be asymmetrical. Visual acuity is rarely decreased, but visual field examination usually shows enlargement of both blind spots and constriction of visual fields. Central or paracentral scotomas may be seen, especially when optic nerve hemorrhage occurs. Permanent visual loss has been reported in 4% to 23% of patients with PC.

Laboratory Tests

Computed tomography with and without contrast is usually normal or may show slitlike ventricles. If saggital sinus thrombosis is suspected, a digital subtraction angiogram or MRI can be diagnostic.

Diagnosis of PC requires lumbar puncture. The opening pressure is elevated, frequently in the range of 300 to 400 mm H_2O. The fluid is characteristically acellular, and the glucose concentration is normal. The protein level is often decreased. Abnormalities of CSF are not part of the pseudotumor cerebri syndrome and should lead one to suspect an alternative diagnosis. Cultures and cytologic examination of CSF are normal. The EEG is usually normal but may show mild, generalized slowing.

During lumbar puncture, an opening pressure should be obtained and enough fluid removed so that the closing pressure is normal. Sometimes the pressure fluctuates and may be only mildly elevated when measured during puncture.

Diagnosis

There are four major criteria for the diagnosis of PC: (1) increased intracranial pressure, measured by CSF pressure, greater than 200 mm of H_2O; (2) normal CSF composition; (3) symptoms and signs of increased intracranial pressure only (headache, visual changes); and (4) normal radiographic studies.

MEDICAL MANAGEMENT

Lumbar puncture is both diagnostic and therapeutic: many patients become symptom-free after the first lumbar puncture. Because the spontaneous remission rate is high, it is unclear whether the lumbar puncture itself is the cause of many remissions. Repeated lumbar punctures (every few days) can be the first mode of therapy for PC. The opening pressure should be recorded, and enough CSF fluid withdrawn (usually 20 to 30 mL) to lower the pressure to normal.

Many patients note improvement immediately following a single lumbar puncture. It should be repeated at least once before starting any other treatment. Almost one-quarter of patients have normal pressure by the time of a second lumbar puncture. The patient should have serial visual field examinations during the time the CFS pressure remains elevated.

For the patient who does not respond to serial lumbar punctures, therapy with steroids is indicated. Prednisone, 20 to 60 mg per day is begun. Often a response is noted by the fourth or fifth day, and treatment usually can be stopped within two weeks.

Acetazolamide (Diamox), a carbonic anhydrase inhibitor that reduces CSF secretion, can reduce intracranial pressure. Many neurologists prescribe acetazolamide at 250 mg tid to qid, but this dosage has a very short efficacy: CSF pressure usually falls for about two hours, then reaches the original elevated state thereafter. Sustained release acetazolamide might be a preferable agent. Chlorthalidone is also of some benefit. Weight loss during PC is often associated with remission, but there have been no controlled studies of its efficacy.

SURGICAL MANAGEMENT

Most patients with PC can be controlled with medical therapy. If symptoms are inexorable, however, or if there is documented decrease in visual acuity, surgery may be necessary. In the past, subtemporal decompression was favored, but it was associated with high morbidity. Shunting of CSF is now a widely used surgical therapy. Ventriculojugular or ventriculoperitoneal shunts are used, but lumboperitoneal shunting is preferable. Surgical incision of optic nerve sheaths is recommended to treat impending visual loss; it often reduces intracranial pressure to normal levels, so that shunting procedures are no longer the first line surgical therapy.

Pseudotumor cerebri is usually a self-limited disease. The major concern of therapy should be preservation of vision. If vision is deteriorating, as determined by the history, physical examination, or visual field testing, the patient should be hospitalized. If vision deteriorates in spite of aggressive medical therapy, surgical treatment (optic nerve sheath decompression) is necessary.

WHEN TO CONSULT

The patient who develops papilledema or transient visual obscurations should be referred immediately to a neurologist or neurosurgeon.

PSEUDOTUMOR CEREBRI IN CHILDHOOD

Pseudotumor cerebri is uncommon in childhood; 50% of affected children are younger than 6 years of age. In the past, the most common cause was otitis media with probable lateral sinus occlusion. In one recent review, however, 26% of cases were associated with malnutrition or cystic fibrosis. Five percent of children with PC have peripheral facial nerve weakness. Initial lumbar puncture causes remission in about one-third of children. Because morbidity from steroids is not acceptable in the young patient, it is best to use diuretics first (acetazolamide, or chlorthalidone). Very few children need more aggressive treatment.

Bibliography

Ahlskog JE, O'Neill BP: Pseudotumor cerebri. *Ann Intern Med* 1982; 97:249-256. (Reviews all aspects of this syndrome.)

Cohen ME, Duffner PK: *Brain Tumors in Children: Principles of Diagnosis and Treatment.* New York, Raven Press, 1984. (Comprehensive review of brain tumors in childhood, including diagnosis and management.)

Couch R, Camfield PR, Tibbles JAR: The changing picture of pseudotumor cerebri in children. *Can J Neurol Sci* 1985; 12:48-50. (Reviews childhood pseudotumor cerebri.)

Donaldson JO: Pathogenesis of pseudotumor cerebri syndromes. *Neurology (NY)* 1981; 31:877-880. (Good summary of the possible mechanisms that cause pseudotumor cerebri.)

Rowland LP (ed). Tumors, Chapter 5, in *Merritt's Textbook of Neurology,* ed 7. Philadelphia, Lea and Febiger, 1984, pp 217-253. (Excellent reviews of major groups of intracranial tumors; well referenced and current.)

Tomita T, McClone DG: Brain tumors during the first twenty-four months of life. *Neurosurgery* 1985; 17:913-919. (Reviews tumors that occur in this age group.)

Walker MD (ed): *Oncology of the Nervous System.* Boston, Martinus Nijhoff, 1983. (Multi-authored monograph covering many aspects of CNS tumors, including malignant glioma and pituitary neoplasms.)

Wilson CB: Brain tumors. *N Engl J Med* 1979; 300:1469-1471. (Reviews therapy of several adult and childhood tumors.)

Wilson CB, Gutin PH: New therapeutic approaches for brain tumors. *Cancer* 1984; 54:2702-2705. (Reviews newer therapies for brain tumors.)

22

Central Nervous System Infections

This chapter deals with the major infections of the central nervous system, based on the anatomy involved and the type of infectious process. Infection of the meninges, both septic (bacterial) and aseptic (viral), will be discussed, followed by brain abscess, chronic meningitis, encephalitis, and Reye's syndrome.

BACTERIAL MENINGITIS

CLINICAL SIGNIFICANCE

Acute bacterial meningitis is considered a medical emergency because prompt diagnosis and therapy is lifesaving. Approximately one in three patients with bacterial meningitis dies, many because of error and delay in recognizing and treating the bacterial infection. Meningitis can develop in several ways. The most common route of access to the nervous system is by the hematogenous route. Occasionally, the infection arises secondary to a parameningeal focus that then seeds the meninges, or as a result of direct inoculation of the organisms into the CSF after penetrating trauma or surgery.

ETIOLOGY

The age of the patient determines which bacterial species is likely to be the cause of meningitis (Table 22-1). Neonatal meningitis (Chapter 26) is most commonly caused by group B streptococci and enteric gram-negative rods. Beyond the first few months of life and up to the age of 5 or 6, *Hemophilus influenzae* is the most common cause of bacterial meningitis. *Neisseria meningitidis* and *Streptococcus pneumoniae* must also be considered in this age group. In the adolescent and young adult, *N meningitidis* is a common cause of meningitis; in adults, *S pneumoniae* is a frequent cause.

Meningitis caused by gram-negative rods frequently occurs in the patient with head trauma or following neurosurgical procedures. Asplenic patients or those with certain immune deficiency states are susceptible to systemic meningococcal disease, although most people with meningococcal meningitis do not have altered

TABLE 22-1 BACTERIAL MENINGITIS; COMMON MICROORGANISMS BY HOST AGE

ORGANISM	PRESCHOOLER	CHILD/YOUNG ADULT	ADULT
Hemophilus influenzae	+ + +	+	+
Neisseria meningitidis	+ +	+ + +	+ +
Streptococcus pneumoniae	+ +	+ + +	+ + +
Staphylococcus aureus	+	+	+
Staphylococcus epidermidis	+	+	+
Listeria monocytogenes	+	+	+
Gram-negative bacilli	+	+	+
Group B streptococcus	+	n	n

+ + + = Common cause.
+ + = Intermediate cause.
+ = Occasional cause.
n = Almost never occurs in this age group.

From Durack DT, Perfect JR: Acute bacterial meningitis, in Wilkins RW, Rengachary SS: *Neurosurgery.* New York, McGraw-Hill, 1984, p 1921.

immune systems. In general, 80% to 90% of meningitis is caused by *H influenzae, N meningitidis,* and *S pneumoniae. Listeria monocytogenes* is the fourth most common cause of bacterial meningitis.

SYMPTOMS AND SIGNS

The clinical presentation of septic (bacterial) meningitis in the adolescent or adult is fever with severe headache, vomiting, depressed level of consciousness, nuchal rigidity, and generalized convulsions. In the neonate and in the aged the manifestations may be more subtle: slight fever, lassitude, confusion, hypothermia or seizures. A high index of suspicion is necessary to diagnose meningitis in these age groups.

In the acute presentation of meningitis, symptoms and signs are present for less than 24 hours and are rapidly progressive. The death rate in this group is approximately 50%, but such an *acute* presentation is seen in only 10% of patients with bacterial meningitis. In the *subacute* presentation, symptoms and signs will have been present for one to seven days. The death rate in this group is 25%; almost 75% of patients with bacterial meningitis have this type of presentation.

During the initial stages of infection, the patient may experience chills and fever. There may be symptoms and signs pointing to the original site of infection (eg, otitis media, pneumonia). Certain clinical features may correlate with the underlying bacterial cause of the meningitis.

Pneumococcal meningitis is usually preceded by infection of the ears, lungs, or sinuses. It occurs with increased frequency in the alcoholic or splenectomized patient, in patients with sickle cell anemia, and in those who have a basilar skull fracture.

Neisseria meningitis should be suspected when the evolution of the disease is rapid, when it is associated with epidemics of meningitis, and when there is an associated petechial or purpuric rash. Approximately 50% of patients with meningococcal meningitis have petechiae, purpura, or both. Systemic disease frequently accompanies meningococcemia and may lead to infarction of the adrenal glands (Waterhouse–Friederichsen syndrome) with resultant shock. Global changes in neurological function may be evident, with alterations in the level of consciousness. Photophobia is common. Focal findings are minimal and may represent a transient postictal state, or are the result of cerebritis or vascular occlusion.

The signs of meningeal irritation can be elicited by attempting to flex the neck passively (Brudzinski's sign) or by extending the knees with the hips flexed (Kernig's sign); these maneuvers will be resisted and will cause pain in the neck and lower back in the presence of meningeal irritation. However, these signs of meningeal irritation may be absent in the very young or the stuporous or comatose patient. Seizures may occur (focal or generalized) and are more common with *H influenzae* meningitis. Cranial nerve abnormalities (extraocular muscle weakness, facial palsy) may occur, but do so primarily with pneumococcal disease. Papilledema is unusual, and the presence of papilledema or profound focal findings on presentation should alert the physician to a possible alternative diagnosis, such as a brain abscess or other parameningeal infection.

Laboratory Tests

The diagnosis of bacterial meningitis frequently can be suspected on the basis of the history and physical examination. A lumbar puncture should be performed promptly in patients suspected of having bacterial meningitis. Those with predominant focal signs or with papilledema should have a CT scan prior to the lumbar puncture. However, therapy should NOT be delayed. The first consideration in the patient with the presentation of acute meningitis is therapy, then specific diagnosis.

Lumbar puncture in the patient with bacterial meningitis will usually reveal turbid CSF that is under elevated pressure (Table 22-2). Pleocytosis is present, with the number of leukocytes varying from 1000 to 100,000/mm^3. The usual white blood cell count is 1000 to 10,000/mm^3 with polymorphonuclear (PMN) leukocytes predominating. Some studies have shown that lymphocytosis may occur and account for as much as 50% of the total WBC count. Rarely, the CSF (in early cases) will be without elevated protein content or pleocytosis. Protein levels are elevated in more than 90% of cases, with most in the range of 100 to 500 mg/dL. The glucose content is usually lower than 40 mg/dL or less than half the simultaneous

TABLE 22-2 CSF FINDINGS IN CENTRAL NERVOUS SYSTEM INFECTIONS

	BACTERIAL MENINGITIS	VIRAL MENINGITIS	CHRONIC MENINGITIS	ENCEPHALITIS	PARAMENINGEAL FOCUS (E.G. BRAIN ABSCESS)
WBC	usually > 1000 (10 to 50,000)	usually < 1000 (10 to 2000)	usually < 1000 (10 to 1000)	usually < 1000 (10 to 2000)	usually < 200
RBC	< 100	< 100	< 100	> 100†	< 100
Predominant cell type	PMNs	Mononuclear*	Mononuclear	Mononuclear*	Mononuclear
Glucose	Low	Normal	Low	Normal to low	Normal (rarely low)
Protein	Elevated	Normal or elevated	Elevated	Elevated	Normal or elevated

PMN = polymorphonuclear leucocyte.

*Early on there are mostly PMN's followed by mononuclear pleocytosis.

†Usually only in cases caused by herpes or *Naegleria*.

peripheral blood glucose level. The CSF lactate dehydrogenase (LDH) level is usually increased in cases of bacterial meningitis, predominantly fractions 4 and 5. The CSF lactate level is often elevated.

A Gram's stain of centrifuged CSF should be performed immediately. In 75% of cases the organism will be seen on the smear. Pneumococci and *H influenzae* are identified more readily than meningococci. Bacteriologic cultures for both aerobic and anaerobic bacteria should be performed; a positive culture will occur in 70% to 90% of patients with bacterial meningitis. In patients with prior antibiotic therapy, a positive Gram's stain may be seen only as often as 60% of the time and may be associated with a negative culture. In this setting, or when Gram's stain is negative, countercurrentimmunoelectrophoresis may be quickly performed and will detect the bacterial antigen.

Blood cultures should be obtained because they are positive in many patients with *H influenzae,* meningococcal, or pneumococcal meningitis, and sometimes are the only clue to the causative bacteria. CBC, platelet count, BUN, calcium, electrolytes, and liver function tests should be performed in all patients. X-Ray examinations of the chest and sinuses should be obtained, they may help document the initial source of the infection. If there are focal signs or papilledema, a CT scan should be performed. Hydrocephalus is rarely seen early, but with the use of intravenous contrast material diffuse cortical enhancement may be seen, and an abscess can be excluded.

DIAGNOSIS

The diagnosis of bacterial meningitis is usually not difficult; it is based on the clinical presentation and the CSF examination. Usually the WBC count will be greater than 1200/mm^3, the glucose level less than 40 mg/dL, and the protein level greater than 150 mg/dL. These findings, coupled with the clinical features, suggest bacterial meningitis.

MANAGEMENT

Because bacterial meningitis is a life-threatening infection, prompt recognition and treatment is necessary. If it is suspected on clinical grounds, antimicrobial therapy based on the most likely organism *must* be started within one-half hour of seeing the patient—even prior to the lumbar puncture (Tables 22-3 and 22-4). Drugs must be selected that cross the blood–brain barrier. The organism must be susceptible to the antibiotic.

In the patient aged 2 months to 6 years of age, *H influenzae* is the most common organism, so initial treatment should be with ampicillin, 50 mg/kg IV q 4h, and chloramphenicol, 25 mg/kg IV q 4h. In the patient more than 6 years of age, meningococcus and pneumococcus are the most frequent organisms, so therapy is with penicillin, 50,000 units/kg IV q 4h. In the patient with penicillin allergy, chloramphenicol, 25 mg/kg IV q 4 to 6h should be used. Patients with meningitis who have sustained a head injury or had a recent neurosurgical procedure are at risk for *S aureus, Staphylococcus epidermidis,* and gram-negative rod infection. Empiric therapy should be begun with a penicillinase-resistant penicillin such as nafcillin, 25 mg/kg IV q 6h (or cloxacillin), plus a third-generation cephalosporin (cefotaxine). If *Pseudomonas* meningitis is strongly suspected, an aminoglycoside such as tobramycin 5 to 6 mg/kg/day IV and 5 mg q

TABLE 22-3 ANTIBIOTIC SELECTION FOR ACUTE BACTERIAL MENINGITIS: EMPIRIC TREATMENT

Age	First Choice	Second Choice
2 mo to 10 yr	Ampicillin 50 mg/kg q 4h IV PLUS Chloramphenicol 25/kg q 6h IV	Cefuroxime 50 mg/kg q 6h IV OR Cefotaxime 200 mg/kg/day (in 6 divided doses)*
Over 10 yr	Penicillin G 50,000 U/kg†	Chloramphenicol 1 g q 6h IV
Over 10 yr with risk factors‡	Ampicillin 50 mg/kg q 4h IV (12 g/day in adults) PLUS 3rd generation cephalosporin (cefotaxime 200 mg/kg/day in 6 divided doses)*	

*12g/day in adults. †24 million U/day in adults. ‡Alcoholic, immunosuppressed, elderly.

Adapted from Bolan G, Barza M: Acute bacterial meningitis in children and adults: A perspective. *Med Clin N Am* 1985; 69(2):236. Used with permission.

12h by the intrathecal or intraventricular route, plus ticarcillin, 250 to 250 mg/kg/day should be used.

After the lumbar puncture is performed and the results of Gram's stain, countercurrent immunoelectrophoresis, or (later) culture are available, changes in antibiotics can be made as dictated by the sensitivities of the organism. Peripheral foci of extracerebral infection should be identified so definitive therapy can be undertaken. Most cases should be treated for 10 to 14 days, with all antibiotics given by the intravenous route. Repeat lumbar punctures are usually not necessary in the child or adult, as long as there is satisfactory clinical progress.

Raised intracranial pressure may complicate the course of bacterial meningitis. Dehydrating therapy with mannitol may be necessary. Dexamethasone, 4 mg qid, or methylprednisolone 24 mg qid, may be used in this setting and may have benefit, but they can decrease resistance to the septic process. Seizures may develop and should be treated with intravenous anticonvulsants. Lorazepam can be used initially to stop active seizures and phenytoin thereafter to prevent further seizures. Seizures most commonly occur in the pediatric patients.

Cerebral herniation is a rare complication of bacterial meningitis. It may be temporally related to the lumbar puncture but can occur 12 to 24 hours after the lumbar puncture; thus, the causal relationship is not clear. If signs of herniation develop (Chapter 36), mannitol infusion, intravenous furosemide, and hyperventilation to a pCO_2 level of 25 mmHg is necessary. Subsequent intracranial pressure monitoring may be indicated.

Septic shock, which may complicate bacterial meningitis, should be treated with steroids, fluids, and vasopressors. Disseminated intravascular coagulation may occur with bacterial meningitis; clotting factors must be analyzed and abnormalities replaced by fresh frozen plasma and platelets. The syndrome of inappropriate secretion of antidiuretic hormone (SIADH) occasionally complicates bacterial meningitis. Limiting fluid intake alone may correct hyponatremia. If acute deterioration occurs (increased intracranial pressure, seizures), 0.9% sodium chloride infusion plus furosemide, with measurement of urine sodium levels and subsequent replacement will be necessary. An infusion of 3% sodium chloride solution may also be utilized to correct the hyponatremia.

TABLE 22-4 ANTIBIOTIC TREATMENT FOR ACUTE BACTERIAL
MENINGITIS: BASED ON GRAM STAIN*

Organism	First Choice	Alternative
Gram-positive cocci		
S pneumoniae and other streptococci	Penicillin G 50,000 U/kg q 4h IV (24 million U/day in adults)	Chloramphenicol 25–100 mg/kg/day
S aureus & other coagulase negative staphylococci	Cloxacillin 200 mg/kg/day (maximum)	Nafcillin; Vancomycin 20–40 mg/kg/day
Gram-positive rods		
Listeria monocytogenes (rarely diphteroids, clostridia or Bacillus species)	Ampicillin 50 mg/kg q4 h IV (12 g/day in adults)	Trimethoprim-sulfamethoxazole OR chloramphenicol
Gram-negative cocci		
Neisseria meningitides or cther Neisseria	Penicillin G 50,000 U/kg q4 h IV (24 million U/day in adults)	Chloramphenicol
Gram-negative rods		
Hemophilus influenzae		
Beta-lactamase +	Chloramphenicol 25 mg/kg q 6h IV (4 g/day in adults)	3rd generation cephalosporin*
Beta-lactamase −	Ampicillin 50 mg/kg q 4h IV (12 g/day in adults)	3rd generation cephalosporin*
Pseudomonas	Tobramycin 5–6 mg/kg/day PLUS 5 mg/q12 h intrathecal AND Ticarcillin 250–350 mg/kg/day	Trimethoprim-sulfamethoxazole; 3rd generation cephalosporin*

*Cefotaxime 200 mg/kg/day IV in 6 divided doses; 12 g/day in adults.

Adapted from Bolan G, Barza M: Acute bacterial meningitis in children and adults: A perspective. *Med Clin N Am* 1985; 69(2):236. Used with permission.

The prognosis depends, in part, on the underlying organism. The mortality rate for *H influenzae* and meningococcal meningitis is 5% to 15%. The mortality rate for pneumococcal meningitis is higher—approximately 15% to 30%. The mortality rate for gram-negative rod meningitis is approximately 50%. The presence of coma, seizures, or associated alcoholism, diabetes mellitus, and head trauma all make the prognosis worse.

Residual neurological deficits are noted in 10% of children with *H influenzae* meningitis, and in as many as 30% of those with pneumococcal meningitis. Almost one-third of children with pneumococcal meningitis are left with permanent sensorineural hearing loss. Hemiplegia, hydrocephalus, or blindness may also complicate meningitis, particularly that caused by *H influenzae.*

WHEN TO CONSULT
Consultation with a neurologist and infectious disease specialist (if available) should be obtained for the patient with suspected meningitis. However, time must

not be wasted in waiting for a consultant to arrive. Immediate antibiotic coverage (as discussed above) should be instituted. A neurologist will also help evaluate and treat the various complications that may arise during the course of bacterial meningitis.

PATIENT EDUCATION

A vaccine derived from capsular components of *N meningitidis* type A and C should be considered for adults during epidemics of these types of meningitis and for close contacts of patients with sporadic disease caused by them. Rifampin should be given prophylactically to persons susceptible to meningococcal disease as soon as the index case is documented (10 mg/kg; maximum 600 mg bid for two days). Preschool contacts of patients with *H influenzae* type B meningitis have a 5% to 6% chance of developing an associated disease, and should be considered for prophylaxis with rifampin (20 mg/kg; maximum 600 mg once daily for four days). An *H influenzae* type B vaccine is available and may be widely used in the pediatric population with the goal of reducing the incidence of this form of meningitis.

VIRAL (ASEPTIC) MENINGITIS

CLINICAL SIGNIFICANCE AND ETIOLOGY

Aseptic meningitis is a symptom complex produced by a number of infectious and noninfectious agents. Most cases of aseptic meningitis are caused by viruses. Enteroviral infections are most often caused by echovirus and coxsackie viruses. Mumps, herpes simplex virus (HSV) type 2, lymphocytic choriomeningitis virus, and adenovirus infections are also seen. Viral meningitis usually occurs in the summer, particularly July through September. Bacterial meningitis, particularly when partially treated, and parameningeal infections may also present as aseptic meningitis. Aseptic meningitis is rarely fatal.

SYMPTOMS AND SIGNS

The clinical syndrome of aseptic meningitis consists of fever, headache, and other signs of meningeal irritation. CSF analysis reveals a predominantly lymphocytic pleocytosis with a normal glucose concentration. Frequently there is sudden onset of headache accompanied by vomiting and fever (38° to 40° C). Consciousness is almost always preserved, but drowsiness or confusion may occur. Photophobia and pain on movement of the eyes are common complaints. Neck stiffness is often present, but Kernig's and Brudzinski's signs are usually absent, and headache is worse than neck stiffness. Other signs may be present on examination, depending on the type of viral infection. One-third of patients with enteroviral infections have an associated maculopapular rash, noted peripherally and predominantly in the hands. Coxsackie B virus infection may produce pleurodynia or pericarditis.

LABORATORY TESTS

Aseptic meningitis usually produces a lymphocytic mononuclear cell pleocytosis (Table 22-2). During the first 24 to 48 hours of a viral infection there can be a predominance of polymorphonuclear leukocytes. In general, the total WBC count is less than 1000/mm^3. The protein level is mildly elevated (100 to 150mg/dL) and the glucose level is almost always normal. On rare occasions, mumps virus, lymphocytic choriomeningitis virus, or herpes simplex type 2 virus infections have been associated with depressed CSF glucose levels. If viral meningitis is suspected, attempts should be made to culture the virus from the throat, stool, and CSF. Serum should be sent for acute and convalescent viral titers. CT scan is normal in cases of viral meningitis, and the EEG is often normal, or may have mild nonspecific abnormalities.

DIAGNOSIS

A combination of the clinical syndrome and the findings of CSF analysis are usually sufficient to diagnose viral meningitis. The differential diagnosis includes chronic meningitis, encephalitis, parameningeal infections, and neoplastic disorders, Because a polymorphonuclear pleocytosis may occur in the CSF early in the course of viral meningitis, confusion may arise in distinguishing a viral from a bacterial cause. In the patient with viral meningitis, repeat lumbar puncture in 12 to 24 hours will reveal CSF with predominant lymphocytes.

MANAGEMENT

Aseptic meningitis caused by viral infections is usually a self-limited disease. Analgesic and antipyretic medications may be necessary to make the patient comfortable. In most patients, symptoms clear in two to five days, frequently following the lumbar puncture. In the occasional patient with a predominance of polymorphonuclear leukocytes in CSF, the suspicion of possible bacterial meningitis may require empiric therapy with antibiotics. Such patients should undergo repeat CSF analysis in 8 to 12 hours with cultures and countercurrentimmunoelectrophoresis.

WHEN TO CONSULT

There is usually no need to consult a neurologist for the patient with viral meningitis. Occasionally, consultation will be necessary to help clarify abnormal CSF patterns, especially if there is doubt about the diagnosis.

PARAMENINGEAL INFECTIONS
Brain Abscess

CLINICAL SIGNIFICANCE

A brain abscess is a focal suppurative process within the brain parenchyma. They are not common and occur more often in children and young adults. Males develop abscesses about twice as often as do females. The incidence of brain abscess has not changed in the antibiotic era.

ETIOLOGY

Pyogenic organisms usually reach the brain from a contiguous source of infection. Forty percent of brain abscesses are caused by disease of the middle ear, mastoid cells, and paranasal sinuses. Abscesses arising from the ear or from the paranasal sinuses usually reach the nervous system by direct extension or by extension of associated thrombophlebitis. Middle ear infections may erode into the temporal lobe, or, less often, mastoid air cells erode into the cerebellum. Approximately one-third of abscesses from otic disease lie in the cerebellum; the remainder lie in the middle and inferior parts of the temporal lobe. Sphenoid sinusitis leads to frontal or temporal lobe abscess. Frontal sinusitis may lead to frontal lobe abscess formation.

About one-third of brain abscesses are of hematogenous origin. Abscesses from hematogenous spread may be located anywhere in the brain and are commonly multiple. The middle cerebral artery distribution is the principal site, and most of these are caused by a primary septic process in the lung or pleura (bronchiectasis, abscess). Congenital heart disease or pulmonary arteriovenous fistulas with right-to-left shunting also account for a large percentage of brain abscesses. Bacteremia is frequently complicated by brain abscess formation. In 20% of brain abscesses, the source is not determined.

Anaerobic bacteria are found in as many as 50% of brain abscesses. In cases caused by chronic sinusitis, anaerobes are often found, usually *Bacillus fragilis* and anaerobic streptococci. Abscesses arising from the ear are caused by anaerobes as well as aerobes (*Enterobacter cloacae* and streptococci). Bacterial organisms seen with lung infection include various streptococci and *Fusobacterium* species. *Nocardia* and *Actinomyces* may be causative organisms. In patients with endocarditis, *Staphylococcus aureus* is the most common organism; in those with congenital heart disease *Streptococcus* is most common.

SYMPTOMS AND SIGNS

Most cases of brain abscess occur in the cerebral hemispheres; symptoms and signs depend on the location of the abscess. Clinical manifestations may be caused by increased intracranial pressure or destruction of brain tissue. Focal or generalized headache is the most common symptom. Altered levels of consciousness, confusion, lethargy, focal or generalized seizures, and focal motor and sensory findings are often present. In patients with chronic lung, ear, or sinus infections, recent exacerbation of infection usually precedes the onset of symptoms. Occasionally nuchal rigidity accompanies headache, suggesting a diagnosis of meningitis. Symptoms of increased intracranial pressure may precede focal neurological abnormalities by days or weeks. Papilledema may develop early or late in the disease.

An abscess in the temporal lobe may produce a visual field deficit or (if in the dominant hemisphere) aphasia. An occipital lobe abscess will produce a homonymous hemianopsia or reading difficulty (dyslexia, if the dominant hemisphere is involved). A parietal lobe lesion may present with variable contralateral sensory findings with mild weakness. A frontal lobe abscess may produce mental dullness, hemiparesis, aphasia, and focal motor seizures. A cerebellar abscess may present with periauricular headache, nystagmus, ipsilateral cerebellar ataxia, and increased intracranial pressure. When abscesses are multiple, multifocal abnormalities will be present on examination. Fever may *not* be present, particularly in the late stage. When systemic symptoms are present, they are often the result of underlying infection (eg, sinusitis). The clinical course may evolve slowly or may be rapidly progressive; patients who seem stable may suddenly deteriorate.

LABORATORY TESTS

The erythrocyte sedimentation rate (ESR) may be elevated, and peripheral leucocytosis is often present. Plain x-rays of the chest, skull, paranasal sinuses, and mastoids should be performed to look for a possible source of infection. Blood cultures should be obtained.

A CT scan with contrast enhancement is the diagnostic procedure of choice. An abnormality appears as a central area of decreased density with a surrounding zone of contrast enhancement. The CT is useful for diagnosis of a brain abscess and for follow-up of the lesion. Abscesses of the posterior fossa are more difficult to visualize by CT. Angiography is rarely necessary. Magnetic resonance imaging (MRI), where available is excellent for localizing an abscess, particularly those located in the posterior fossa.

In general, lumbar puncture with CSF analysis should not be performed in the patient with a suspected brain abscess because of the possibility of cerebral herniation resulting from raised intracranial pressure and a shift of intracranial contents. If CSF is examined (Table 22-2), the pressure is often elevated and few cells are present. The protein concentration is usually slightly increased, and the glucose level is normal. If the abscess does not communicate with the CSF, Gram's stain and cultures will be negative.

DIAGNOSIS

In the patient with clinical findings and CT verification of a brain abscess, diagnosis is usually straightforward. However, the infectious source may not be known. An abscess must be differentiated from tumor, infarction, and herpes simplex encephalitis.

MANAGEMENT

If there is evidence of significant mass effect or increased intracranial pressure, dehydrating therapy should be instituted. Mannitol can be given (0.25 to 1.5 g/kg), as well as corticosteroids (dexamethasone or methylprednisolone). Seizures can be treated with phenytoin. The advent of CT has shown that many suppurative nervous system infections can be cured medically, although surgical decompression is still often necessary.

Treatment should be started as soon as the diagnosis is made. Because most brain abscesses are caused by Bacteroides or other anaerobic streptococci, a combination of penicillin G, 20 to 24 million units daily combined with chloramphenicol, 4 to 6 g/day, can be started. The same medications are used if the primary site of infection is known to be the sinuses. If the heart is the likely primary site, therapy will be based on blood culture results. Initial treatment should include a staphylococcus-sensitive, penicillinase-resistant drug (nafcillin, cloxacillin), rather than penicillin G. An abscess that follows penetrating head trauma or neurosurgical procedures can be treated with cloxacillin, 2 g IV q 4h, and chloramphenicol, 1 g IV q 4 to 6h.

If there is evidence of significantly increased intracranial pressure or signs of developing herniation, surgical therapy should be considered to excise the mass lesion. If the abscess does not resolve with antimicrobial therapy, surgery is also indicated, with biopsy and drainage of the abscess cavity. Antibiotics are continued for six to eight weeks, and the lesion is monitored by CT. The mortality of brain abscess is 5% to 10%, with almost one-third of patients having significant residual neurologic abnormalities. Focal seizures are the most common neurological sequela of brain abscess.

WHEN TO CONSULT
Neurological consultation should be obtained whenever a brain abscess is suspected clinically. The neurologist can treat the secondary complications of brain abscess medically, and will help determine if surgery is indicated.

Subdural Empyema

CLINICAL SIGNIFICANCE
Subdural empyema is an extracerebral suppurative collection located between the dura and the arachnoid. It occurs more commonly in males.

ETIOLOGY
Most cases of subdural empyema are from infection involving the paranasal sinuses. The frontal and ethmoid sinuses are most often responsible; mastoid and middle ear infections are responsible less often. Subdural infections are rarely the result of a distant infection or bacteremia. Disease of sinus origin predominates in adolescents and young men. Numerous organisms have been associated with subdural empyema. Aerobic and anaerobic streptococci and *Bacteroides* are the most common organisms. Less often, *S aureus, Escherichia coli,* and *Pseudomonas* are responsible. In approximately 50% of cases, no organism can be isolated.

SYMPTOMS AND SIGNS
There is usually a history of chronic sinusitis or mastoiditis, with recent exacerbation. Fever and headache are often present, with the headache lateralized to the side of the empyema. When the sinus is infected, pain is present over the brow or between the eyes, with percussion tenderness over these areas. General malaise may also result. Increased intracranial pressure can develop, with resultant vomiting and stupor that may progress rapidly to coma. Focal neurological signs develop, including hemiparesis, aphasia, focal seizures, and abnormalities of gaze. By this stage the neck is often stiff.

LABORATORY TESTS
Skull x-ray examination may demonstrate the site of infection. Blood cultures should be obtained, in addition to routine laboratory tests that include CBC, electrolytes, BUN, glucose, and clotting studies. As with brain abscess, lumbar puncture is potentially dangerous and should *not* be performed. CSF findings (Table 22-2) are those of a parameningeal infection, with pleocytosis of 50 to 1000 cells (predominantly PMNs), an increased protein level, and a normal glucose level. Gram's stain and cultures are usually negative. A CT scan should be performed with contrast; it will localize the infection to the subdural space. If CT is not available, angiography is necessary to localize the lesion.

DIAGNOSIS
Any patient with a history of sinusitis or mastoiditis who develops focal neurological abnormalities should be considered to have subdural empyema. A CT scan will document the site of pathology and will help exclude brain abscess. If CT is negative, CSF analysis is necessary to exclude meningitis or encephalitis.

MANAGEMENT
The initial treatment of subdural empyema is surgical drainage through burr holes. Empyema fluid should be sent to the laboratory for microbiological analysis. Antibiotic coverage should be started with penicillin G, 24 million U/day and chloramphenicol, 4 to 6 g/day. If *Staphylococcus* is suspected, a penicillinase-resistant penicillin such as nafcillin or cloxacillin, 12 g/day, can be used. If intracranial pressure is increased, mannitol or corticosteroids can be given to reduce cerebral edema.

Without antimicrobial therapy and surgery, most patients die in 7 to 14 days. Those who are treated promptly usually make a good recovery without significant neurological sequelae.

WHEN TO CONSULT
As with the brain abscess, neurological consultation is advised for the patient with fever and focal neurological findings. If CT demonstrates a subdural empyema, immediate neurosurgical consultation is necessary. An infectious disease consultant may be able to help select the proper antibiotic.

CHRONIC MENINGITIS

CLINICAL SIGNIFICANCE AND ETIOLOGY
Chronic meningitis differs from acute forms of meningitis because it has a subacute-to-chronic onset of symptoms, more prolonged course, and less severe inflammatory response. A number of diseases may cause a chronic meningitis syndrome; most of them are of infectious origin (Table 22-5). CNS involvement by most of these diseases is associated with high morbidity and mortality. If symptoms and signs of meningoencephalitis are persistent for at least four weeks and are associated with an inflammatory CSF, the syndrome of chronic meningitis is present.

By definition, chronic meningitis is persistent, but it must be differentiated from recurrent meningitis. Patients with recurrent meningitis frequently have recurrent episodes of acute meningitis, followed by symptom-free periods during which CSF is normal and the patient is asymptomatic. Causes of recurrent meningitis are listed in Table 22-6. Most cases of chronic meningitis are caused by mycotic organisms or tuberculosis.

SYMPTOMS AND SIGNS
In the patient with suspected chronic meningitis, a careful exposure history should be obtained in an attempt to implicate infectious diseases. The onset is insidious, with chronic symptoms that wax and wane; episodic exacerbations may occur as a result of associated seizures, hydrocephalus, or hyponatremia. The CSF abnormalities, however, are persistent. This discussion focuses on tuberculous

TABLE 22-5 CAUSES OF CHRONIC MENINGITIS

Infectious

Tuberculosis*
Cryptococcosis*
Coccidiodomycosis
Candidiasis
Histoplasmosis
Brucellosis
Nocardiosis
Actinomycosis
Toxoplasmosis
Cysticercosis
Sporotrichosis
Leptospirosis

Noninfectious

Sarcoidosis
Behçet's disease
Neoplasm (meningeal carcinomatosis)*
Granulomatous angiitis
Chronic benign lymphocytic meningitis

*Most common.

TABLE 22-6 CAUSES OF RECURRENT MENINGITIS

Bacterial meningitis
Aseptic meningitis
Mollaret's meningitis
Parameningeal focus of infection
Epidermoid cyst (parameningeal)
Systemic lupus erythematosus
Neoplasm
Subarachnoid hemorrhage

meningitis and cryptococcal meningitis, the most common varieties of chronic meningitis.

Tuberculous Meningitis

CLINICAL SIGNIFICANCE

The incidence of tuberculous meningitis has declined over the past few decades, corresponding to the reduction of the incidence of tuberculosis. Tuberculous meningitis may occur at any age. In the past in the United States, tuberculous meningitis was more common in young children than in adults. Today, it is more common in adults. In under-developed countries, tuberculous meningitis is still common in infants and young children. In the U.S., approximately 20% of cases develop before the age of 5, and more than 80% occur before the age of 40.

ETIOLOGY

The acid-fast organism *Mycobacterium tuberculosis* is the usual cause of tuberculous meningitis, although *Mycobacterium bovis* is the causative agent in a few cases. Tuberculous meningitis is usually a complication of systemic tuberculosis; it results from hematogenous spread of the bacilli to the meninges. The tubercles that develop in these areas eventually rupture into the subarachnoid space, producing meningitis.

Symptoms and Signs

The clinical course of tuberculous (TB) meningitis is divided into three stages. The first, lasting one to two weeks, begins with fever, nausea, and vomiting. Apathy, drowsiness and anorexia may then develop. More than 50% of patients develop headache, and nuchal rigidity is common. In young children and infants, apathy or hyperirritability, unexplained vomiting, and seizures are the usual symptoms; nuchal rigidity is often absent.

The second stage develops with the abrupt onset of cranial nerve symptoms. Approximately half of the patients will have symptoms for longer than two weeks. Extraocular muscle palsies (frequently of cranial nerve VI) are found in 30% to 70% of cases.

In the third stage, signs of meningeal irritability may become prominent, and progressive stupor or coma may develop. Occasional focal neurological deficits may develop, or the patient may present with unexplained hydrocephalus. Generalized or focal seizures may also develop. Stage 3 is characterized by severe clouding of consciousness, stupor, and coma. Seizures may develop in the adult during this stage, but they can occur in all stages.

The physical findings of each stage are those of meningeal irritation, ie, irritability, fever, and nuchal rigidity. Papilledema or other cranial nerve signs (strabismus, facial palsy) are usually present as the disease progresses. If unrecognized or untreated, tuberculous meningitis progresses to stupor and coma associated with increased intracranial pressure and focal neurological signs. Death usually occurs in six to eight weeks. With early diagnosis and treatment, the recovery rate is 90%. Almost 75% of patients have had a history of contact with tuberculosis.

Laboratory Tests

A CT scan of the head, performed prior to the lumbar puncture if there are signs of increased intracranial pressure or focal neurological signs, may demonstrate hydrocephalus. With contrast infusion, there may be diffuse enhancement of the basal cisterns or cortical surfaces. Lumbar puncture usually reveals CSF under increased pressure. The CSF is usually cloudy, with 50 to 500 WBC/mm^3, predominantly lymphocytes. The protein content is always elevated, usually at 100 to 200 mg/dL. The glucose content is often reduced to levels in the range of 20 to 40 mg/dL.

The diagnosis is established by the recovery of organisms from CSF. Cultures are positive in 40% to 90% of cases. Smears of CSF will demonstrate acid-fast bacilli in 10% to 20% of patients after a single examination. The yield of organisms is related to the amount of CSF withdrawn: the more fluid collected, the greater the likelihood of recovering the organism. With repeated examinations the yield is increased to greater than 75%. Sputum and gastric washings are positive in up to 50% of patients. The TB skin test (PPD) is positive in 90% of patients. Chest x-ray evidence of primary TB is also present in over 90% of children with TB meningitis. The ESR is elevated in 80% of cases.

DIAGNOSIS

Because it may take three or four weeks to grow mycobacteria, initial diagnosis is presumptive. Empiric treatment is appropriate, because of the natural history of undiagnosed disease. Tuberculous meningitis needs to be differentiated from other types of meningeal reactions. If acid-fast organisms are seen on the smear, the diagnosis is firm.

Cryptococcal meningitis may produce an identical clinical picture. CSF findings help to differentiate these conditions. Cryptococcal meningitis has a positive india ink smear or a positive test for cryptococcal antigen. In cases of meningeal inflammation of other causes, the CSF glucose is normal (except in leptomeningeal carcinomatosis). If these two diagnoses have been excluded, antituberculous therapy should be started immediately. Meningeal biopsy is rarely necessary.

MANAGEMENT

Treatment should start before bacteriologic culture confirmation. The treatment of TB meningitis consists of triple-drug therapy with isoniazid (INH), rifampin, and ethambutol. These drugs all penetrate the CSF well. INH is given at 5 mg/kg for adults and 10 mg/kg for children. Neuropathy may develop; it is treated with pyridoxine, 50 mg daily. If hepatitis develops, the drug should be discontinued. Rifampin is given at 600 mg daily for adults or 15/mg/kg for children. The dosage of ethambutol for children is 15 mg/kg/day and for adults it is 750 to 1000 mg in divided doses. Corticosteroids are usually given if there is evidence of cerebral edema or hydrocephalus, but they should not be given as the only drug therapy. Therapy is continued for 18 to 24 months. The syndrome of inappropriate secretion of antidiuretic hormone (SIADH) may develop, and if chronic should be treated with lithium carbonate or demeclocycline.

The mortality of tuberculous meningitis is approximately 10%, predominantly in the elderly and in infants. With early diagnosis and treatment, the recovery rate is approximately 90%, but any delay in diagnosis is often associated with progression of neurological deficits and a poorer prognosis. Confusion, lethargy, cranial nerve signs, and an increased CSF protein level are all associated with a poor prognosis, but the presence of tuberculosis in other organs does not affect prognosis. Almost one-third of survivors develop residual CNS damage, including psychomotor and intellectual retardation, psychiatric disturbances, seizures, deafness, visual and oculomotor abnormalities, and hemiparesis.

WHEN TO CONSULT

The patient with CSF evidence or clinical evidence of chronic meningitis should be evaluated by a neurologist.

Fungal Infections

Fungal infections that produce chronic meningitis are seen primarily in chronically ill or immunosuppressed patients, such as those with AIDS, leukemia, or an organ transplant, or those on chronic immunosuppressive therapy with antineoplastic drugs or corticosteroids. Fungal meningitis develops insidiously, with symptoms and signs similar to those produced by tuberculous meningitis. The patient is often afebrile; CSF changes are similar to those produced by tuberculous meningitis. Cryptococcosis, mucormycosis, candidiasis, and coccidioidomycosis all produce chronic meningitis.

_____

Cryptococcal Meningitis

CLINICAL SIGNIFICANCE AND ETIOLOGY
Cryptococcus neoformans is the most common fungal pathogen of the CNS. It is a saprophyte distributed throughout the world. Pigeons are known to harbor the organism and release it in their excrement. Males account for two-thirds of patients; most patients are 30 to 70 years of age. The respiratory tract is often the portal of entry, although the skin and mucous membranes may be the primary sites of infection. One-third to one-half of cases of cryptococcal infection are associated with debilitating illnesses. CNS infection may occur with evidence of systemic disease, or it may occur independently. The cryptococcal organism infiltrates the meninges and may spread throughout the brain.

SYMPTOMS AND SIGNS
The exposure history is of little value because of the widespread distribution of the fungus. Early complaints are headache, nausea, and vomiting. Mental status changes are present in 50% of cases. In some patients, these symptoms are absent (including nuchal rigidity); instead, the patient has dementia, focal CNS signs, or evidence of increased intracranial pressure as a result of hydrocephalus. Cranial nerve palsies may be present, predominantly involving the facial nerve or extraocular muscles. Meningovascular lesions may produce a stroke-like picture; however, the course is usually chronic and progressive.

LABORATORY TESTS
The CSF findings are similar to those of tuberculous meningitis. CSF is usually under increased pressure, with a pleocytosis of 10 to 400 cells/mm^3, lymphocytes predominating. The protein level is increased, and the glucose level is decreased, frequently to values below 40 mg/dL. A positive india ink stain will be present in 30% to 50% of patients. More than 85% of patients will have a positive cryptococcal polysaccharide antigen in CSF. As with tuberculous meningitis or other fungal meningitides, the more CSF that is withdrawn and analyzed, the greater the likelihood of diagnosis. CSF cultures will be positive initially in three-quarters of patients. If cryptococcal meningitis is strongly suspected and the CSF obtained from the lumbar area is not diagnostic, obtaining fluid from the cervical area (by a cisternal puncture) will increase the likelihood of isolating the organism. Urine, sputum, and blood cultures should also be obtained. Cryptococcal antigen should be tested in the serum. The latex agglutination test on CSF for cryptococcal antigen can be positive when cultures and india ink smears are negative and will be present in the serum of more than 50% of patients with cryptococcal meningitis. Urine harbors the organism in approximately one-third of cases. CT may reveal evidence of hydrocephalus with or without basilar meningeal contrast enhancement. Serum electrolyte levels may show evidence of hyponatremia caused by SIADH.

DIAGNOSIS

The subacute course, combined with the results of the CSF analysis, should suggest the possibility of cryptococcal meningitis. The differential diagnosis is the same as that listed for tuberculous meningitis. The lack of other systemic signs, as is often true of tuberculous meningitis, may also strengthen the diagnosis of cryptococcal meningitis. The presence of encapsulated organisms in the CSF sediment is diagnostic.

MANAGEMENT

Amphotericin B, 1 to 1.5 mg/kg/day IV, is the treatment of choice for cryptococcal meningitis. The drug may need to be given intrathecally if there is no response to therapy, which happens usually in the seriously ill patient or in those who have relapsed after the first course of treatment. Treatment usually lasts for at least six weeks, although the optimal duration of therapy is not clear. Clearing of the CSF or a significant fall in the cryptococcal antigen is evidence that therapy is successful. Lumbar puncture should be performed one to two times a week; CSF analysis should include WBC, protein, glucose, culture, and cryptococcal antigen determinations. Approximately 50% of patients will be cured with a single course of therapy; 12% will relapse but will be cured when retreated. Twenty-five percent of patients will die from the cryptococcal meningitis and 10% will die from associated illnesses. Nephrotoxicity is a common side effect; thrombocytopenia, fever, and anemia may also occur. 5-Fluorocytosine is often combined with amphotericin B to treat cryptococcal meningitis. Used alone it is inadequate. There is, however, no conclusive evidence that therapy with amphotericin B and 5-fluorocytosine is more effective than only amphotericin B in standard doses. However, prevailing evidence suggests that both drugs should be utilized because the relapse rate appears to be lower with combination therapy.

Untreated cryptococcal meningitis is usually fatal within a few months, although some patients may have a course with intermittent exacerbations and remissions. Most relapses occur during the first 12 months but have been reported as long as 29 months after treatment.

WHEN TO CONSULT

Recommendations for neurological consultation are the same as those given for tuberculous meningitis.

ENCEPHALITIS

CLINICAL SIGNIFICANCE

Encephalitis differs from primary meningitis in that there is primary infection of the brain parenchyma with resultant neurological symptoms and signs. Often there is evidence of both meningitis and encephalitis, hence the term meningoencephalitis. Most cases of encephalitis are caused by viral diseases. This section will deal with primary viral encephalitides and will focus on herpes simplex encephalitis. The syndrome of acute viral encephalitis is manifested by an acute febrile illness, often with signs of meningeal involvement and with evidence of dysfunction of the brain parenchyma manifested by convulsions, delirium, stupor or coma, aphasia, hemiparesis, involuntary movements, ataxia, or cranial nerve palsies.

ETIOLOGY

Some of the viruses responsible for the encephalitis syndrome are listed in Table 22-7. Death occurs in 5% to 20% of all patients with acute encephalitis, and neurological sequelae occur in a similar percentage. However, certain encephalitides have been associated with high mortality: 50% of patients with herpes simplex (HSV) encephalitis die, and 80% to 90% of those who survive are left with severe residual neurological sequelae (although with current effective antiviral medications, the morbidity and mortality rates are lower than these percentages).

WHEN TO CONSULT

A neurological consultation is appropriate for all patients with suspected encephalitis. This is particularly true in the case of suspected HSV encephalitis, for which there is effective antiviral therapy. The neurologist can help identify HSV encephalitis.

Togaviruses

CLINICAL SIGNIFICANCE AND ETIOLOGY

Togaviruses are also known as arboviruses because they are arthropod-borne. The most frequent mosquito-borne diseases are the arthropod-borne encephalitides

TABLE 22-7   COMMON CAUSES OF ENCEPHALITIS

Viral

Togaviruses (Arboviruses)
    Eastern equine
    Western equine
    St. Louis
Bunyaviruses
    California
Herpesviruses
    Herpes simplex
    Varicella-zoster
    Epstein–Barr
    Cytomegalovirus
Picornaviruses
    Echovirus
    Coxsackie virus
    Poliovirus
Paramyxoviruses
    Mumps
    Measles

Nonviral

Collagen vascular diseases
Mycobacterium tuberculosis
Mycoplasma pneumoniae
Rickettsia rickettsii
Leptospirosis
Legionella species
Lyme disease (spirochetal)
Toxoplasmosis

(eastern equine, western equine, St. Louis, and California types). They occur in temperate zones and their incidence corresponds with the period of mosquito activity. Such activity begins in early June, peaks by late summer and early fall, and ceases by November.

SYMPTOMS, SIGNS, AND LABORATORY TESTS

The illness runs from a mild meningoencephalitis to a fulminant encephalitis leading to coma and death. Typically, patients have a clinical syndrome that suggests moderate encephalitis. Fever and headache followed by disorientation, a depressed level of consciousness, altered memory, frequent seizures, and focal signs are common. The illness may last from one to four weeks. A mild lymphocytic pleocytosis (up to 1,000 cells mm^3), increased protein, and normal glucose are typical CSF findings. The peripheral white blood count may also be elevated. CT is frequently normal, but may demonstrate focal areas of hypodensity with associated edema. The EEG is often abnormal, with slowing and focal epileptiform discharges.

DIAGNOSIS

Togavirus encephalitis tends to be more severe than encephalitis caused by enteroviruses. Western and eastern equine encephalitis outbreaks may be preceded by deaths of horses in the endemic areas. Viral isolation is difficult. Diagnosis is based primarily on serological testing. Hemagglutination-inhibiting and -neutralizing antibodies appear first.

MANAGEMENT

There is no specific antiviral therapy for togavirus encephalitis. Fluid and electrolyte balance should be maintained. Excessive fluid intake should always be avoided because of the danger of cerebral edema. Seizures should be treated with an anticonvulsant.

St. Louis Encephalitis

St. Louis encephalitis is the most common and widely distributed arbovirus encephalitis in the United States. Large epidemics, particularly in the elderly, occur in urban areas throughout the United States and Canada. The virus is carried by the *Culex* species of mosquito. Frequent associated medical symptoms include urinary problems (dysuria, pyuria) and muscle aching. The disease is usually not fatal (8% of patients die), but the majority who die are elderly. Most patients recover completely, although many complain of subjective nervous system problems (irritability, memory loss).

Western Equine Encephalitis

Western equine encephalitis is the third most common cause of arbovirus encephalitis, but it is the most common arbovirus encephalitis in horses. Most cases occur in rural localities in the western two-thirds of the United States; it rarely occurs in the East. Disease in horses precedes human cases. Most infections are subclinical, and the disease appears to be more common in males. Seizures are common during the acute illness in young children. Overall mortality rate is

3%, but western equine encephalitis can be a devastating illness of infants. Most adults recover completely; approximately 20% have residual sequelae (tremor, headache, tremulousness). Brain damage occurs in 37% to 64% of children with disease prior to 1 year of age. Childhood sequelae include mental retardation, motor damage, extrapyramidal dysfunction, and seizures.

Eastern Equine Encephalitis

Eastern equine encephalitis is the most severe arbovirus encephalitis. Hot, wet weather resulting in a large population of mosquitoes is necessary for an outbreak. Infection in horses may warn of the development of the disease in humans. The onset is abrupt and fulminant, with progression to a coma-like state in one to two days. Fifty percent of patients die, although the mortality rate is slightly lower in children.

California Encephalitis

More than 90% of the cases of California encephalitis occur in children under the age of 15. Cases have been reported in the eastern half of the United States and Canada; the highest concentration occurs in the north central states. California encephalitis is the most benign form of arboviral encephalitis. Seizures are common in affected children. Approximately 25% have focal neurological findings. Death is rare, occurring in fewer than 1% of cases. Behavioral problems may be the only sequela, although persistent seizures sometimes result. As with other togavirus infections, the differential diagnosis is that of summertime meningoencephalitis. Mild cases resemble enteroviral infections, but often there is no rash.

HERPES SIMPLEX ENCEPHALITIS

CLINICAL SIGNIFICANCE

Herpes simplex virus encephalitis is the most common sporadic encephalitis. There is no seasonal trend to HSV encephalitis, which is in contrast to the other encephalitides. Mortality is quite high, varying from 30 to 70%, with a morbidity equally as high. Rapid diagnosis and treatment of HSV encephalitis decreases mortality and morbidity. Because of its frequency and presentation, it is important to recognize HSV encephalitis, for therapeutic intervention may be lifesaving.

ETIOLOGY

In contrast to the neonate, most adult cases of HSV encephalitis result from infection with HSV type 1. How the encephalitis develops is unknown. It has been postulated that HSV encephalitis might result from olfactory spread through the cribiform plate, with spread to the base of the brain. It is likely that HSV encephalitis occurs in individuals with a prior history of HSV infection and results from a reactivation of latent brain infection. In the patient without a previous HSV infection, encephalitis probably results from a direct spread to the brain.

SYMPTOMS AND SIGNS

Patients with HSV encephalitis often have fever, malaise, and headache. Behavioral and focal neurological symptoms develop subsequently. Focal symptoms include seizures, which may be focal or generalized. An olfactory aura may herald the onset of the seizure disorder. Aphasia and hemiparesis also develop, depending on the location of the encephalitic process. Damage usually occurs to the limbic system, including the frontal and temporal lobes. At times the disease may have a subacute course, with initial behavioral disturbances and memory impairment. Coma or stupor usually results within six days after onset of the infection. A variety of symptoms and signs may occur, although the encephalitic process, once developed, is usually inexorably progressive and results in brain swelling and destruction.

LABORATORY TESTS AND DIAGNOSIS

The EEG is the most sensitive test. It may suggest a focal infectious brain disturbance or may help to establish the diagnosis. Periodic lateralized epileptiform discharges (PLEDs) are highly suggestive of the disease, but their absence does not exclude it.

CT is the primary neuroradiologic procedure for the diagnosis of HSV encephalitis. Low-density abnormalities associated with mass effect may be present in the temporal lobes. The technetium-99m brain scan may also be abnormal early in the disease, but such a scan is now rarely necessary with the presence of high-resolution CT scanners.

The CSF in most cases is usually under elevated pressure and contains 500 to 1000 WBC/mm³, with lymphocytes predominating. Early in the course of the disease polymorphonuclear leukocytes may be present in high numbers. Red blood cells or xanthochromia may be present because of the hemorrhagic nature of the lesions. Protein levels are usually elevated and may be as high as 1000 mg/dL, although they often average 80 to 100 mg/dL. CSF glucose levels are usually normal, but hypoglycorrhachia has been reported. There have been rare biopsy-proven cases of HSV encephalitis in which CSF was entirely normal. Early in the course of the disease, CSF antibody titers to HSV may be elevated, as are the CSF-to-serum ratios. These tests are not widely available, however, and they may take a long time to perform. Such time cannot be wasted waiting for a laboratory test result.

Brain biopsy of the involved area (usually the medial temporal or frontal lobe) provides tissue for immunofluorescent studies, with results usually available in two to four hours, and for virus isolation, with results provided in 24 to 72 hours. Light microscopy and electron microscopy should be performed; intranuclear inclusion bodies may be present.

There has been much debate as to whether or not a brain biopsy should be performed in the critically ill patient with suspected HSV encephalitis. If the clinical course and other laboratory tests strongly suggest the diagnosis, biopsy is probably not necessary. If the diagnosis is less strongly considered, a biopsy might be needed. With the introduction of less neurotoxic antiviral drugs, however, risks of biopsy may outweigh the benefits. The differential diagnosis of HSV encepha-litis includes other encephalitides, brain abscess, stroke, neoplasm, and other CNS infections.

MANAGEMENT

The sooner the diagnosis is made and therapy started, the greater the likelihood for survival with decreased mortality and morbidity. Supportive treatment includes control of respirations and fever and proper fluid balance. Overhydration should be avoided because it may exacerbate cerebral edema. Increased intra-cranial pressure may develop; it can be controlled with hyperventilation, furosemide, or mannitol. The use of corticosteroids is unclear, but they probably have benefit in reducing cerebral edema and intracranial pressure. Seizures should be controlled with lorazepam initially and with phenytoin over the long term. Close attention should be paid to electrolyte balance, as SIADH may complicate HSV encephalitis and may exacerbate cerebral edema.

Specific antiviral therapy with adenine arabinoside (Ara-A) or acyclovir de-creases morbidity and mortality, particularly if the patient is not already comatose. Ara-A reduces the mortality of acute HSV encephalitis from 70% to 30%. Administration of Ara-A requires large volumes of fluid, which may exacerbate cerebral edema. Toxicity of the drug is not minor at the suggested effective doses (15 mg/kg/day), and treatment needs to be continued for 10 days.

Acyclovir (10 mg/kg/q 8h) has recently been shown to be superior to Ara-A for the treatment of HSV encephalitis. Toxicity is not a problem, and acyclovir does not have to be given in large volumes of fluid. Mortality in acyclovir-treated patients was 19% in one study, compared to 50% mortality in the group treated with Ara-A. Fifty-six percent of the acyclovir-treated patients returned to normal life, compared to only 13% of the Ara-A patients. Because acyclovir is an effective and relatively safe drug for HSV encephalitis, the need for brain biopsy is not as great with it as it is with Ara-A.

WHEN TO CONSULT

Any patient with suspected HSV encephalitis should be evaluated by a neurologist. An emergency evaluation is necessary, for the sooner treatment is started, the better the prognosis. The seizures and increased intracranial pressure that can complicate HSV encephalitis can be handled by the neurologist.

REYE'S SYNDROME

CLINICAL SIGNIFICANCE

First described in 1963, Reye's syndrome is an uncommon neurological disorder with an incidence of 0.3 to 0.6/100,000 children. It represents one of the primary causes of death for young children in the United States. It is principally a disease of childhood, but adult cases have been reported.

ETIOLOGY

There is a relationship between the varicella and influenza viruses and Reye's syndrome. Epidemic forms of Reye's syndrome follow influenza infections, and those cases that are sporadic tend to follow infections from varicella. One-quarter of patients with Reye's syndrome have had varicella as an antecedent illness. Most other patients had influenza as the antecedent infection, although other viruses have been implicated. Numerous investigators have looked at the possibility of environmental factors such as toxins, but none has been discovered. Injury to mitochondria is apparent, but the relationship between viral infection and mitochondrial injury is unclear. Injury to mitochondria can explain metabolic abnormalities seen in Reye's syndrome. Encephalopathy may result from hepatic dysfunction and the subsequent accumulation of ammonia. Excessive amounts of free fatty acids may also account for encephalopathy.

The evidence for an association between salicylates and Reye's syndrome includes the following: (1) Salicylate intoxication and Reye's syndrome are similar, with hepatic dysfunction and encephalopathy occurring in both. (2) Acid-base disturbances and coagulopathy also occur in both disorders. (3) There is a statistical association between salicylate intake and Reye's syndrome. (4) Salicylates can damage mitochondrial function.

SYMPTOMS AND SIGNS

Reye's syndrome can occur in children of all ages, with rare cases reported in infants and adults. The severity of the preceding viral infection does not correlate with the intensity of the encephalopathy. Usually, there is an antecedent upper respiratory infection with cough, sore throat, and rhinorrhea. Recovery usually occurs, lasting a few days to a few weeks, followed by the abrupt onset of neurological symptoms. Vomiting followed by stupor, coma, and seizures is common. A delirious stage often precedes the development of coma, and tends to follow the onset of vomiting. This delirious–hyperexcitable state is associated with nervous system hyperactivity with fever, tachycardia, sweating, tachypnea, and pupillary dilation. In general, the disease that affects the nervous system can be divided into five stages (Table 22-8).

TABLE 22-8 CLINICAL STAGES OF REYE'S SYNDROME

STAGE	LEVEL OF CONSCIOUSNESS	PAIN RESPONSE	RESPIRATORY PATTERN	PUPILLARY REACTION
1	Lethargy and drowsiness; responsive to commands; vomiting	Normal	Normal or hyperventilation	Normal
2	Delirium with disorientation and combative behavior; unresponsive to command; verbalizes inappropriately	Purposeful	Hyperventilation	Dilated, responsive
3	Obtundation or coma	Decorticate	Hyperventilatory or Cheyne–Stokes	Dilated, briskly responsive
4	Comatose	Decerebrate	Hyperventilation, irregular or absent	Dilated; responds slowly or nonresponsive
5	Comatose	Absent	Absent	Absent

From Bohan TP, Roe CR: Reye's syndrome, in Conn RB: *Current Diagnosis*. Philadelphia, WB Saunders, ed 7, 1985, p 943. Used with permission.

The encephalopathy tends to last 24 to 96 hours. The stage of the illness on admission to the hospital tends to correlate with the likelihood of recovery. The outcome correlates with the clinical stage. If the disease does not progress beyond stage 3, complete recovery can be expected. Progression to stage 4 or 5 usually results in death or significant neurological disability.

Physical findings on admission include changes in mental status, irritability, lethargy, coma, hyperpnea, and hepatomegaly. Muscle tone may be increased, and diffuse hyperreflexia results. Focal neurological signs and jaundice are absent.

LABORATORY TESTS

Abnormal tests of liver function are universally present. Serum transaminase enzymes are elevated, and hypoprothrombinemia and hyperammonemia are present. Creatine phosphokinase (CPK), lactate dehydrogenase (LDH), glutamate dehydrogenase (GDH), amylase, and lipase levels may also be elevated. Serum glucose and phosphorus levels are decreased and arterial pH tends to be normal. The serum cholesterol level is decreased and the very-low-density lipoprotein (VLDL) concentration is often reduced. The CSF is normal but may be under increased pressure, and the CSF glucose level may be reduced. The EEG demonstrates diffuse slowing. CT scan is normal or demonstrates "slit-like" ventricles resulting from generalized increased intracranial pressure.

DIAGNOSIS

The initial differential diagnosis of Reye's syndrome includes bacterial or viral meningoencephalitis, drug intoxications (salicylates, amphetamines, valproic acid), and metabolic disorders (systemic carnitine deficiency, inherited defects of amino acid metabolism). An increased WBC count and protein content in the CSF should raise doubt about the diagnosis of Reye's syndrome. In general, the abnormalities on neurological examination associated with systemic hypoglycemia, elevated liver function tests, and clotting abnormalities are quite diagnostic for Reye's syndrome.

MANAGEMENT

Early recognition is important if therapy is to be effective. Management depends on the neurological stage of the patient. All patients with Reye's syndrome should be hospitalized because early vigorous treatment can limit progression of the disease. All patients who progress beyond stage 1 should be hospitalized in a center where neurosurgical services are available. Children in stage 1 should be observed and treated with oral or intravenous fluids. Children in stage 2 must be observed in an intensive care unit (ICU), and should be treated with intravenous hydration with a 10% hypertonic glucose solution combined with multivitamins sufficient to maintain the serum glucose between 150 and 200 mg/dL. Serum glucose determinations should be obtained every two to four hours, and serum electrolytes and osmolarity should be measured every four hours. Intravenous fluids are administered at a rate of 1600 to 1800 mL/M^2/day. (M^2 represents square meters of surface area.) Vitamin K is given every 24 hours (1 mg IV or 5 mg IM). Approximately 90% of patients admitted in stage 2 remain stable and do not progress.

In the ICU, frequent monitoring of vital signs and neurological functions is mandatory. Agitation or combativeness in early stages can be controlled by IV administration of a short-acting barbiturate (eg, sodium pentobarbital, 1 to 2 mg/kg every one to two hours). Urine output should be maintained at 0.75 to 1.0 mL/kg/h. Children in stages 3 through 5 require more intensive management. The child should be placed on a cooling blanket and paralyzed with pancuronium bromide (Pavulon), 0.1 to 0.2 mg/kg), intubated, placed on assisted ventilation, and hyperventilated, maintaining a pCO$_2$ of 25 mm Hg. A nasogastric tube, arterial line, central venous pressure (CVP) line and Foley catheter are necessary. In stages 3 through 5 the IV solution should include 200 g glucose, 40 mEq Na Cl, 15 mEq potassium acetate, 15 mEq potassium phosphate, and one ampule of multivitamins added to each liter. This solution (Reye's solution) is infused at the rate given above (1600 to 1800 mL/M^2/day). The constant infusion of glucose should not be interrupted.

Increased intracranial pressure is the most serious and life-threatening complication during acute stages of Reye's syndrome. Initial management is by the administration of 20% hypertonic mannitol solution. An epidural pressure monitor should be placed in all grade 3 patients to allow prompt recognition (and subsequent therapy) of intracranial hypertension. Usually, the epidural catheter is placed through a burr hole overlying the right frontal (nondominant) lobe. The intracranial pressure monitor can be placed in the ICU by the neurosurgeon using local anesthesia. Boluses of IV 20% mannitol solution (0.25 to 0.5 g/kg) are enough to control the intracranial hypertension. The dose is administered every 3 to 20 minutes and repeated as often as necessary. Larger doses (1.0 to 2.0 g/kg) can be administered, usually over 10 to 30 minutes.

The child should be placed on a cooling blanket to keep the core body temperature down. Acetaminophen can also be used to control fever. Suctioning of secretions should be performed carefully, and should be preceded by a dose of IV thiopental to prevent elevations of intracranial pressure. The CVP should be maintained between 4 and 8 mm Hg. In the child with elevated intracranial pressure who does not respond to medical management, IV pentobarbital will be necessary in a dose of 1 to 5 mg/kg IV every four to eight hours to achieve a plasma concentration of 30 to 50 μg/L. Complete blood count, coagulation profile, osmolarities, ammonia, and liver function tests should be performed every 24 hours. Blood glucose, lactate, pH, and phosphorus levels, and arterial blood gases should be tested every four hours.

Most children so managed improve clinically (and as measured by laboratory tests) in 24 to 72 hours. When consciousness is regained, the IV solution should be decreased by 25% decrements every eight hours. The patient is then extubated. Overall, the outcome is satisfactory in 85% to 90% of patients.

WHEN TO CONSULT
A child or adult who has the clinical picture of Reye's syndrome should undergo an immediate neurological consultation. If neurological and neurosurgical consultants are not readily available, the patient should be treated as described above and transferred to a center where such services are available.

Bibliography

Devivo D: How common is Reye's syndrome? *N Engl J Med* 1983; 309:179-181. (Summarizes epidemiologic data.)

Devivo D: Reye syndrome. *Neurol Clin* 1985; 3:95-115. (Most up-to-date review of this syndrome available.)

Ellner J, Bennett J: Chronic meningitis. *Medicine* 1976; 55:341-369. (Brief overview of the major infectious causes of chronic meningitis; illustrative case vignettes.)

Garvey G: Current concepts of bacterial infection of the central nervous system. Bacterial meningitis and bacterial brain abscess. *J Neurosurg* 1983; 59:735-744. (Good review of brain abscesses.)

Heubi JE, Daugherty CG, Partin JS, et al: Grade 1 Reye's syndrome: Outcome and predictors of progression to deeper coma grades. *N Engl J Med* 1984; 311:1539-1542. (Reviews course of a large series of grade 1 patients; with prompt diagnosis and therapy few progressed to other stages.)

Mandell LA, Ralph ED (eds): *Essentials of Infectious Diseases.* Boston, Blackwell, 1985. (Concise, well-written textbook of infectious diseases, with excellent chapters on septic and aseptic meningitis.)

Meythaler JM, Varma RR: Reye's syndrome in adults: Diagnostic considerations. *Arch Intern Med* 1987; 147:61-64. (A reminder that Reye's syndrome may occur in adults.)

Molavi A, LeFrock JL (eds): Infections of the central nervous system. *Med Clin N Am* 1985; 69. (A comprehensive monograph covering all aspects of CNS infection; easily accessible.)

Reye RDK, Morgan G, Baral J: Encephalopathy and fatty degeneration of the viscera: A disease entity in childhood. *Lancet* 1963; 2:749-752. (First description of the clinical and pathological features of Reye's syndrome.)

Skoldenberg B, Alestig K, Burman L, et al: Acyclovir for the treatment of herpes simplex encephalitis: A Swedish multicenter study. *Lancet* 1984; 2:707-711. (Study that showed that acyclovir was more effective with essentially no toxicity when compared to Ara-A for treatment of HSV encephalitis.)

Stillman A, Gitter H, Shillington D, et al: Reye's syndrome in the adult: Case report and review of the literature. *Am J Gastroenterol* 1983; 78:365-368. (A reminder that Reye's syndrome can occur in the adult.)

Whitley RJ, Alford CA, Hirsch MS, et al: Vidarabine versus acyclovir therapy in herpes simplex encephalitis. *N Engl J Med* 1986; 314:144-149. (Confirms the Swedish study (Skoldenberg et al, above) that acyclovir is the best drug for treating herpes simplex encephalitis.)

Whitley RJ, Soong SJ, Dolin R: Adenine arabinoside therapy of biopsy proved herpes simplex encephalitis. *N Engl J Med* 1977; 287:289-294. (Cooperative study that demonstrated the effectiveness of Ara-A in reducing mortality from 70% to 30% in HSV encephalitis.)

23

Demyelinating Diseases

The most common central nervous system (CNS) demyelinating diseases are multiple sclerosis (MS) and optic neuritis. These disorders share the pathologic feature of primary loss of the myelin sheath that surrounds central nervous system axons. The myelin sheath requires three principal anatomic systems for its formation and continued health: (1) oligodendrocytes, the central nervous system glial cells responsible for producing and maintaining myelin; (2) an adequate blood supply; and (3) an intact axon within the myelin sheath. Myelin breakdown can occur when any system is disrupted. It is believed that oligodendrocytes are damaged in demyelinating diseases. Dysmyelinating disorders, an unrelated group of childhood diseases in which myelin formation is congenitally abnormal, are discussed in Chapter 27.

MULTIPLE SCLEROSIS

CLINICAL SIGNIFICANCE

Multiple sclerosis can be defined clinically and pathologically. Clinically, it is a chronic disease of young and middle adulthood that is characterized by remitting and relapsing symptoms and signs indicative of multifocal central white matter dysfunction. Pathologically, MS is characterized by the presence of scattered, widespread, discrete plaques of demyelination in the white matter of the brain, spinal cord, and optic nerves. These demyelinating plaques later develop gliosis in their margins, giving the disease its name. Multiple sclerosis is a major cause of acquired neurological disability in young adults, ranking second after brain and spinal cord trauma.

ETIOLOGY

The precise etiology and pathogenesis of MS are unknown, but two major theories—slow viral infection and autoimmunity—are widely accepted. According to the slow viral theory, a neurotropic virus infects oligodendrocytes during childhood. This virus remains dormant until activated during adulthood by unknown factors. Then oligodendrocytes are episodically damaged by direct viral action or by an induced inflammatory response against the persistent virus. During each phase of damage, demyelination results from the inability of damaged oligodendrocytes to synthesize and maintain myelin.

According to the autoimmune theory, a childhood viral infection induces an autoimmune state in which lymphocytes previously sensitized to viral antigens cross react with oligodendroglial surface receptor proteins. Clones of sensitized lymphocytes are episodically released during adulthood, accounting for the phasic nature of the illness.

Multiple sclerosis is marked by genetic and environmental predispositions. Observations that persons with certain HLA subtypes (eg, DW-2) have a propensity for the disease and that MS is very rare in certain ethnic groups (Eskimos, Japanese, African blacks) suggests host factor determinants. Environmental determinants are suggested by the variable incidence of MS in different geographic latitudes, the reported epidemics, and the fact that the risk of developing the disease corresponds to the average risk in the geographic area in which the person lived the first 15 years of his life.

SYMPTOMS AND SIGNS

Multiple sclerosis usually begins in young adulthood. The mean age at onset is 33 years, and women are affected slightly more often than men. The symptoms at onset are variable in distribution, type, and duration. The initial course is one of spontaneous, unpredictable relapses and remission at irregular intervals. As the disease progresses, complete remission becomes less likely and new neurological deficits tend to be added to the older ones, producing a cumulative deficit. The various courses of MS are listed in Table 23-1.

Weakness, usually involving the arm and leg on the same side or involving both legs, is the most common presenting complaint. Examination confirms a pyramidal pattern of weakness that is worse in the extensors of the arm and the flexors of the leg. Tone is increased in the weak limb, and deep tendon reflexes are hyperactive. Pyramidal lesions in MS often produce spasticity that is out of proportion to weakness. Babinski's sign is usually present; abdominal cutaneous reflexes are lost. The responsible lesion is in the spinal cord, brain stem, or cerebral hemispheres. Patients frequently also complain of generalized fatigue and markedly reduced exercise endurance.

Numbness and paresthesias are the next most common presenting symptoms. These sensory complaints usually take the form of vague, nagging, prickly feelings in one or more limbs, but they may also produce burning pain and, rarely, trigeminal neuralgia. Examination often confirms loss of vibration sensation and impairment in graphesthesia and two-point discrimination. The sensory examination may be normal, however, despite sensory complaints. The plaque that

TABLE 23-1 CLINICAL COURSE OF MULTIPLE SCLEROSIS

Benign	Mild relapses with complete recovery
Mild	Moderate relapses with gradually accumulating neurological deficit
Progressive	Steady progression without remission
Severe	Frequent severe relapses with only partial recovery

produces sensory symptoms may be in the spinal cord, hemisphere, or brain stem. L'Hermitte's sign, a painful electric-shocklike sensation radiating into all extremities when the head is suddenly flexed, suggests demyelination in the posterior columns of the cervical cord.

Visual symptoms include monocular visual loss, blurred vision, and diplopia. Monocular visual loss, caused by optic neuritis, will be discussed later. Blurred vision and diplopia are the result of plaques in the brain stem's vestibular–ocular connections. A characteristic syndrome is internuclear ophthalmoplegia caused by a plaque in one or both median longitudinal fasciculi. On attempted lateral gaze, the patient loses the ability to adduct. Attempts to abduct produce coarse horizontal nystagmus of the abducting eye. In a young person, the presence of internuclear ophthalmoplegia alone highly suggests the diagnosis of MS.

Incoordination of limbs and clumsiness when walking are common complaints of MS. Examination discloses cerebellar ataxia of affected limbs and cerebellar tremor on attempted fine movements. Tandem gait is made impossible by truncal ataxia.

Urinary urgency or incontinence is a common symptom in established cases but is rarely a presenting complaint. Similarly, dysarthria, dysphagia, and vertigo may be seen later in the illness.

Symptoms and signs of MS are exacerbated by elevated temperature and emotional stress. Elevation of body temperature impairs central nerve conduction in already demyelinated neurons. Decompensation from fever or summertime overheating may induce a relapse. Whether emotional stress exacerbates MS by an immunologic mechanism or by other means, these stresses often precede exacerbation of the disease.

LABORATORY TESTS

While there is no specific laboratory test to prove or disprove the diagnosis of MS, there are several helpful confirmatory tests. The laboratory workup for suspected MS should include cerebrospinal fluid (CSF) immunoelectrophoresis, computed tomography (CT) brain scanning, and multimodality sensory evoked potentials. Where available, magnetic resonance imaging (MRI) should be performed in place of CT scanning.

Cerebrospinal fluid immunoelectrophoresis shows an oligoclonal pattern of IgG banding in about 90% of patients. If immunoelectrophoresis is unavailable, CSF protein electrophoresis reveals an elevation of the gamma globulin fraction in about two-thirds of patients. The CSF concentration of myelin basic protein may be elevated in acute MS, but generally has poor correlation with disease activity.

Computed tomography brain scans may reveal plaques as transient zones of increased uptake after a double contrast dose and a one-hour delay. Magnetic resonance imaging (MRI) is at least a magnitude more sensitive than CT; it reveals a multitude of plaques, most of which are asymptomatic.

Multimodality sensory evoked potentials help identify central white matter demyelination. Visual evoked responses can identify a former optic neuritis, which was forgotten by the patient or never realized. Similarly, brain stem auditory evoked responses can disclose past or present demyelinating plaques in the brain stem white matter. Somatosensory evoked responses test for plaques from the posterior columns of the spinal cord to the thalamus.

DIAGNOSIS

Multiple sclerosis remains a clinical diagnosis with the diagnostic criterion of "dissemination of central white matter lesions in space and time." Thus, MS cannot be diagnosed in a purely monophasic illness, or in an illness in which all signs and symptoms can be accounted for by a single lesion. The diagnosis is suggested when a young adult has a history of evanescent, fluctuating, multifocal neurological symptoms. Examination corroborates the multifocal nature of the lesions and often discloses more signs than the patient described. Laboratory investigation can confirm the multifocal nature of central white matter lesions. The laboratory is most useful when it discloses a completely new lesion unanticipated by history or examination.

MANAGEMENT

The three categories of management of the MS patient are (1) general principles, (2) specific therapies, and (3) symptomatic therapies. A general principle is that a clinician should tell the MS patient his diagnosis when it is made. The patient also should be told the level of confidence with which the diagnosis is made. He should be reassured that many cases are mild and that what he probably knows about the disease is slanted by news media toward the most severe cases. Withholding diagnostic information and using euphemisms to describe the disease are discouraged, except in exceptional circumstances.

A multiple sclerosis patient should be followed at regular intervals, and should be reassured that the physician will not abandon him despite his "untreatable" illness. Each follow-up examination should consist of a history of new and old symptoms and a neurological exam. Both proven and experimental therapies should be discussed. The patient should be permitted to "fine-tune" medication dosages and participate in planning his therapy.

The patient with MS should be urged even more strongly than the usual patient to take proper care of his general health. He must receive proper nutrition, regular exercise, and adequate sleep. Blood pressure and weight should be normal. The patient should refrain from using cigarettes and alcohol. He should avoid becoming overheated in hot weather and, if necessary, purchase air conditioners for the home and automobile.

Specific therapies designed to alter the course of MS have been mostly unsuccessful. Adrenocorticotropic hormone (ACTH) and synthetic glucocorticoids are the only specific agents to be of widely accepted benefit. Even these agents are not believed to alter the prognosis; rather, they are used to shorten the duration of a sudden relapse. They are usually used in conjunction with bed rest in one of three regimens:

1. ACTH, 40 units intramuscularly twice daily for seven days; 20 units twice daily for four days; 20 units once daily for three days.

2. Prednisone, 60 mg orally daily for seven days; 40 mg daily for two days; 20 mg daily for two days.

3. Methylprednisolone, 500 mg intravenously (by Soluset) once daily for three to five days.

Steroids should not be continued for more than two weeks and should never be injected intrathecally because this frequently produces seizures and arachnoiditis. At least one month should separate successive courses.

Cytotoxic immunosuppressive therapy is under investigation in an attempt to improve the long-term course of MS. Of the various agents tried, intravenous cyclophosphamide (Cytoxan) has produced the most impressive results. A multicenter trial of Cytoxan is underway to determine what dosages may help improve the prognosis of MS in which patients.

COMPLICATIONS

There are effective therapies for specific complications of MS. For spasticity, the drug of choice is baclofen (Lioresal), which works at the spinal cord level to reduce spasticity from corticospinal tract lesions. It should be started orally as follows: baclofen 10 mg, ½ tablet three times daily for three days; 1 tablet three times daily for three days; 1½ tablets three times daily for three days; then two tablets three times daily. Daily dosage should not ordinarily exceed 90 mg. Side effects of drowsiness and dizziness are more common in older, debilitated patients.

Dantrolene sodium (Dantrium) reduces spasticity by a dose-related paralysis of the muscle membrane. It is a less useful agent than baclofen because it induces weakness as the dosage is increased and is often associated with fatal hepatotoxicity. If this agent is prescribed, pretreatment baseline liver function tests and frequent liver function testing should be performed during the course of treatment. The drug should be stopped at the first signs of elevated levels of hepatocellular enzymes.

Diazepam (Valium) helps reduce spasticity when used with baclofen. Diazepam 2 to 5 mg should be added to the baclofen dosage at the point in the day when the patient has the most severe spasticity. Diazepam alone is not an adequate antispasmodic in MS because it produces drowsiness in the same dosage range as it reduces spasticity.

Patients often have paroxysmal symptoms of transient paresthesias, ataxia, dysarthria, pain, and tonic muscle contractions. Carbamazepine (Tegretol) helps reduce them in the same dosage range as its anticonvulsant action. Cerebellar tremors may respond to propranolol (Inderal) or occasionally to isoniazid (INH). Management of bowel, bladder, and sexual dysfunction is discussed in Chapter 17.

Psychiatric complications of MS are common. Euphoria is seen late in the course, reflecting periventricular plaques deep in the hemispheric white matter that "core out" the frontal lobes. This state is a saving grace for patients with advanced MS: they are happy and carefree despite their debilitation. Depression is more common early in MS and should be diagnosed and treated promptly. The physician should question the patient about his appetite, interests, sleep patterns, morbid thoughts, and mood. Depression should be treated by psychotherapy and with tricyclic antidepressants in the form of nighttime doses of amitriptyline (Elavil), imipramine (Tofranil), or doxepin (Sinequan).

Patients who use unproven therapies complicate their medical management. Faced with a progressively deteriorating and essentially untreatable disease, many patients turn to alleged cures about which they have heard from family, friends, or the news media. These "cures" range from special diets and vitamins to toxic injections and removal of dental fillings. They waste money at best and are harmful at worst. The physician must tactfully and compassionately counsel the patient about what has been scientifically proven about these regimens and about their risks. A valuable reference to consult in this regard is *Therapeutic Claims in Multiple Sclerosis* (see Bibliography).

Securing the services of rehabilitation professionals is essential in the management of MS. The advice and programs of a physical therapist and an occupational therapist should be followed. Exercise regimens, walking aids, orthoses, and devices to aid activities of daily living enhance the quality of life for the MS patient.

When the patient's health can be improved no more, his environment should be altered. Rehabilitation professionals can advise on changes in home construction to permit wheelchair use and to build specially equipped bathrooms.

When an invalid patient is living at home, his caregiver should get attention. Were it not for this person, the patient would certainly be consigned to a nursing home. The caregiver needs tremendous support, reassurance, and encouragement. If the physician perceives that the caregiver needs a vacation, he should arrange to have the patient admitted to an extended-care facility for a few weeks to allow the caregiver a respite.

WHEN TO CONSULT

A neurologist should be consulted initially to make the diagnosis of MS. Whether the patient is followed at regular intervals by a neurologist is optional: it depends on the neurologist's availability and on the preferences of the generalist and the patient. Most symptomatic treatment of MS, as well as periodic courses of ACTH or glucocorticoids, can be administered by a generalist. The neurologist should be reconsulted if (1) the patient responds poorly to symptomatic therapy or if (2) the patient wants to try an experimental therapy such as cyclophosphamide.

PATIENT EDUCATION

The patient should be taught about MS to the extent that he is interested and is able to comprehend. Investing a few extra minutes to explain the rationale of a particular therapy is likely to yield a return of better compliance.

Patients should be encouraged to buy one of the two good patient education books (see Bibliography). They provide detailed but understandable explanations of the illness and its treatment.

Patients should be told about the National Multiple Sclerosis Society and given the address and telephone number of the local chapter. For information about local chapters, write to: National Multiple Sclerosis Society, 205 East 42nd Street, New York, NY 10017. Local chapters provide numerous services for the patient— from education and counseling to furnishing wheelchairs. They can also enroll patients and their families in MS community support groups. Here patients can share experiences, ideas, and other information.

OPTIC NEURITIS

CLINICAL SIGNIFICANCE

About 40% of MS cases begin with unilateral or bilateral optic neuritis (ON). Of those patients with acute ON, 20% to 40% were once believed to later develop multiple sclerosis (depending on the length of follow-up). Recent studies show, however, that as many as 75% of patients with acute ON develop MS when followed for 15 years.

ETIOLOGY

Acute ON is a demyelinating plaque of the optic nerve, optic chiasm, or both. Its etiology is unknown but experts believe it to be the same as that of MS.

SYMPTOMS AND SIGNS

Optic neuritis presents with a subacute (over 4 to 48 hours) loss of visual acuity in the affected eye(s). Both optic nerves may be involved, but often days to weeks elapse between the time one eye and the other is affected. Pain in the eye and eyeball tenderness are common. Loss of vision may be profound and usually is worst for central and color vision. Eye movements may produce the hallucination of bright flashing lights (visual phosphenes).

Examination discloses a central or centrocecal (fovea and blind spot) scotoma in the involved eye(s). Color vision is absent, but peripheral visual fields may be normal. If the plaque in the optic nerve is near the retina, the optic disc may appear inflamed with indistinct margins (optic papillitis). If the plaque is closer to the optic chiasm (retrobulbar neuritis), the disc appears normal. Satisfactory recovery of vision in 4 to 12 weeks occurs in most cases. Residual central scotoma and persistent impairment of color vision, impaired acuity, and increased visual evoked response latency are usual sequelae. Optic disc pallor or atrophy may be present after optic neuritis resolves—most often in the temporal portion of the optic disc.

LABORATORY TESTS

The visual evoked response shows a characteristic latency delay that is permanent. Formal visual field testing with a perimeter or tangent screen reveals a central or centrocecal scotoma, which can be seen particularly well with a small, red target object.

DIAGNOSIS

The sudden or subacute loss of monocular vision is the syndrome of acute optic neuropathy. In addition to ON, the differential diagnosis includes vascular insults to the optic nerve complicating atherosclerosis or temporal arteritis (acute ischemic optic neuropathy); compressive lesions of the optic nerve or chiasm (tumors); toxic optic neuropathies from ingested drugs or poisons; and Leber's hereditary optic atrophy. In the young, otherwise healthy person, subacute monocular visual loss is likely to be caused by ON.

The patient should be examined for signs of other demyelinating central white matter lesions. If none are found, laboratory tests to diagnose MS are probably not valuable. Such tests should be performed, however, if the history or exam provides evidence of other plaques.

MANAGEMENT

Untreated, the prognosis for spontaneous recovery from optic neuritis is very good. The patient should be reassured that most vision will return. Treatment with ACTH or glucocorticoids is unnecessary. Based on the history and neurologic examination, the patient should be given the diagnosis of idiopathic ON or of ON resulting from MS.

WHEN TO CONSULT

A neurologist or ophthalmologist can confirm the diagnosis. If the screening neurologic history and exam are positive for other CNS lesions in space or time, a neurologist should be consulted.

PATIENT EDUCATION

The patient should be told the nature of optic nerve demyelination and that permanent, but usually mild, impairment of visual acuity and color vision may result. He should be told about the relationship of ON to MS but reassured that many cases never proceed to MS.

Bibliography

Ellison GW: Multiple Sclerosis. *Ann Intern Med* 1984; 101:514-526. (Current discussion of immunology of MS.)

Hallpike JF, Adams CWM, Tourtellote WW, (eds): *Multiple Sclerosis: Pathology, Diagnosis and Management.* Baltimore, Williams & Wilkins, 1983. (A competitor for the McAlpine book, this book is current and very thorough.)

Hauser SL, Dawson DM, Lehrich JR, et al: Intensive immunosuppression in progressive multiple sclerosis. *N Engl J Med* 1983; 308: 173-180. (The paper that showed the benefit of cyclophosphamide in MS.)

Hutchinson WM: Acute optic neuritis and the prognosis for multiple sclerosis. *J. Neurol Neurosurg Psychiatry* 1976; 39:283-289. (The paper reporting that the incidence of MS following acute optic neuritis increases with time.)

Kurtzke JF: Optic neuritis or multiple sclerosis. *Arch Neurol* 1985; 42:704-710. (Scholarly review of studies of the frequency with which MS progresses to ON. Has many helpful tables.)

Mattews WB, Acheson ED, Batchelor Jr et al: *McAlpines's Multiple Sclerosis.* London, Churchill Livingstone, 1985. (The most recent update of the complete and classic MS textbook.)

McFarlin DE, McFarland HF: Multiple sclerosis. *N Engl J Med* 1982; 307: 1183-1188, 1246-1251. (A good current review of MS etiologies.)

Scheinberg LC (ed): *Multiple Sclerosis: A Guide for Patients and Their Families.* New York, Raven Press, 1983. (A well-written and very popular patient education book.)

Therapeutic Claims in Multiple Sclerosis. The International Federation of Multiple Sclerosis Societies, 1983. (An excellent source book containing scientific critiques on all alleged MS cures and treatments. Available from the National Multiple Sclerosis Society, 205 East 42nd Street, New York, NY 10017.)

Wolf JK (ed): *Mastering Multiple Sclerosis: A Handbook for MSers and Families.* Rutland, VT, Academy Books, 1984. (Another readable patient education book comparable to the Scheinberg book.)

24

Movement Disorders

Disorders of movement are classified as hyperkinetic, in which there are excessive involuntary movement, or hypokinetic, in which there is a paucity and slowness of movement. Tremor is the most common hyperkinetic disorder, and Parkinson's disease is the most common hypokinetic disorder.

Neurotransmitters such as dopamine, acetylcholine, and gamma-aminobutyric acid (GABA) in the basal ganglia and substantia nigra are the neurochemical modulators of movement. Lowering the dopamine level results in a hypokinetic movement disorder such as Parkinson's disease, whereas excessive dopamine concentrations result in a hyperkinetic movement disorder such as Huntington's disease. Deficiencies in the levels of acetylcholine and/or GABA also lead to a hyperkinetic movement disorder; an excess of those neurotransmitters produces hypokinesia. Thus, a balance exists between the cholinergic and dopaminergic systems that facilitate muscle control and movement. Diseases or chemicals that affect these neurotransmitters produce clinical states of abnormal movements, but, by replacing the defective neurotransmitter, control of the abnormal movement is possible. Only in the past 20 years have effective modulation and control of the various movement disorders been possible, thanks to a better understanding of the neurochemical anatomy of the brain.

PARKINSON'S DISEASE

Parkinson's disease, first described by James Parkinson in 1817, is one of the most common disorders of the basal ganglia and one of the leading causes of neurologic disability in patients over 60 years of age. It has an incidence of 20 cases per 100,000 population, with a prevalence rate of 100 to 150 per 100,000.

Parkinson's disease is a disorder of middle and late life. It usually begins between the ages of 50 and 65 years, although there is a rare juvenile form of the disease. Parkinson's disease usually begins insidiously with gradual progression and a slow clinical course. The disease manifests four major clinical features: tremor, bradykinesia, rigidity, and disturbances of posture.

The tremor of Parkinson's disease results from the alternating contraction of a muscle group and its antagonist. A rest tremor of 4 to 7 Hz results, occurring more distally than proximally. It may be referred to as "pill-rolling" by the thumb and forefinger. It often disappears with intention (purposeful movements) and during sleep, and increases with anxiety and stress. An action tremor may also be present, noted only with postural movements.

Tremor and other manifestations of Parkinson's disease may occur unilaterally and may remain confined to one side, even when other manifestations are bilateral. Tremor may not be a prominent part of the disease, and its absence often causes diagnostic confusion. Tremor may also lead to the incorrect diagnosis. Essential (senile) tremor is the disease most frequently mislabeled Parkinson's disease; 5% of patients with essential tremor are incorrectly diagnosed initially as having Parkinson's disease. Senile tremor is not present at rest, usually is bilateral, and may involve the head, voice, and legs. The ingestion of alcohol may reduce senile tremor, but it has no effect on parkinsonian tremor. The differential diagnosis of tremor is considered further in Chapter 12.

Rigidity of muscles is present in nearly all patients with Parkinson's disease. It may initially involve only a few muscles, but it gradually progresses to other areas. Stiffness in Parkinson's disease is usually caused by rigidity, which also causes the feeling of weakness noted by many patients. Although rigidity frequently occurs bilaterally, the presence of unilateral rigidity often results in a delayed diagnosis. In one study, 60% of patients with unilateral rigidity (caused by Parkinson's disease) received an incorrect initial diagnosis. Cogwheel rigidity is the resistance to passive motion of an extremity caused by increased tone with superimposed resting tremor.

The stooped posture of the patient with Parkinson's disease is the result of rigidity. This posture is characterized by flexion of the trunk, drooping of the shoulders, flexion of the arms at the elbows, and flexion of the knees; thus, the center of gravity is displaced forward. The small-stepped "festinating" accelerating gait results from a combination of this forward displacement of the center of gravity, akinesia, and other postural changes. The typical parkinsonian gait consists of stooped posture, difficulty in starting the first step, and shuffling associated with small steps. A tendency of the patient to run (propulsion) thereby results.

Bradykinesia is one of the most disabling features of Parkinson's disease, but it is infrequently an initial complaint. Bradykinesia consists of three components: (1) the marked poverty of spontaneous movements, (2) the slow initiation of all voluntary movements, and (3) the loss of normal associated movements. Routine activities of daily living take much longer to perform. The infrequent blinking and paucity of facial expression of the patient are in part the result of bradykinesia. Low-volume monotonous speech may result and may be associated with stuttering. Micrographic handwriting often results from bradykinesia. Bradykinesia may progress to periodic akinesia, in which the patient is seemingly frozen and unable to move.

Autonomic signs may also be seen in Parkinson's disease. Hyperhidrosis, orthostatic hypotension, and bowel and bladder dysfunction may develop. Intellectual deterioration (dementia) also occurs. In some patients dementia is caused by co-existent Alzheimer's disease. Not all patients with Parkinson's disease have signs of significant intellectual deterioration, and two forms of Parkinson's disease apparently exist: one associated with progressive dementia, the other without loss of higher brain functions.

Following the epidemic of von Economo's encephalitis lethargica from 1919 to 1926, postencephalitic Parkinson's disease was a prominent sequela. It was often associated with oculogyric crises. Parkinsonism usually immediately followed the acute infection, but some cases did not develop for ten years.

Arteriosclerotic disease is a rare cause of a syndrome resembling Parkinson's disease. The etiology is usually multiple small lacunar infarcts caused by hypertensive disease. The onset may be insidious, however, and the classical description of multifocal episodes (infarcts) with stepwise deterioration is rarely seen. Dementia, dysarthria, and pseudobulbar palsy are also often present, and gait disturbance may be predominant. Tremor is rare, and this disease is usually more rapidly progressive than typical idiopathic Parkinson's disease.

Drug-induced parkinsonism is becoming more prevalent because of the widespread use of potent dopamine receptor-blocking neuroleptic drugs to control psychiatric disorders and to control the nausea and vomiting from cancer chemotherapy. Antihypertensive medications that contain reserpine may lead to a parkinsonian state (caused by dopamine depletion) and may be confused with a vascular cause. Symptoms include tremor, akinesia, and rigidity. With the neuroleptic agents, however, dystonic movements and akathisia (state of constant movement) also may result, and with metoclopramide, dystonic movements of the face may be seen. With neuroleptic-induced parkinsonism, rigidity tends to be more evident than tremor, the opposite of which is true for idiopathic Parkinson's disease. Parkinsonian symptoms usually disappear within a few days of the drugs being stopped, but they may persist for as long as six months to two years.

TREATMENT

Pharmacologic therapy (Table 24-1) is designed to (1) restore central dopamine to the basal ganglia and substantia nigra; (2) stimulate intact dopamine receptors; or (3) block central acetylcholine to produce a more favorable balance between the dopaminergic and cholinergic systems. When the signs and symptoms of the

TABLE 24-1 PHARMACOLOGIC TREATMENT OF PARKINSON'S DISEASE

Anticholinergic Drugs
  Benztropine (Cogentin): 0.5 to 4.0 mg bid
  Trihexyphenidyl HCl (Artane): 1 to 5 mg tid
  Biperiden (Akineton): 1 to 2 mg tid
  Ethopropazine (Parsidol): 10 to 20 mg tid
Amantadine (Symmetryl): 100 mg bid to tid
Dopaminergic drugs (presynaptic)
  L-dopa: 500 to 1000 mg tid to qid
  Sinemet: 10/100, 25/100, 25/250 mg sizes; initial dosage
    of 10/100 tid, gradually increasing to maximum
    of 25/250 four to five times daily
Dopaminergic drugs (post-synaptic)
  Bromocriptine (Parlodel): 2.5 mg daily, gradually increasing by 2.5 mg
    weekly to a dose of 15 to 30 mg daily in divided doses (tid).
  Pergolide (not approved by FDA)

disease are minimal and the disability is slight, it is usually best to withhold drugs. Anticholinergic drugs that block central and peripheral acetylcholine receptors may produce moderate improvement in the patient with Parkinson's disease. They are indicated in patients with mild but bothersome parkinsonism, particularly when tremor is present. Rigidity tends to respond less well. The most common peripheral side effects include visual impairment (blurred vision due to mydriasis and cycloplegia), dryness of the mouth, constipation, and urinary retention. These drugs may precipitate glaucoma in the susceptible patient. Central nervous system side effects include confusion, hallucinations, delusions, and psychosis. No one drug has any major advantage over another, although tremor seems to respond better to benztropine and rigidity responds more to trihexyphenidyl. It is best to use the drug with which the physician is most familiar and to start slowly titrating the dosage to the patient's clinical response or to the appearance of significant side effects. The production of confusion has limited the effectiveness of the anticholinergics in patients over 70 years of age; they should be used very cautiously in this age group. Anticholinergic drugs are best used for temporary control because they eventually fail to modify the patient's symptoms.

Amantadine, an antiviral drug used for influenza prophylaxis, exhibits both central and peripheral anticholinergic activity, yet it is often combined with an anticholinergic for more effective action. The usual dosage is 100 mg bid; 30% to 40% of patients fail to maintain any benefit from the drug beyond two months. Side effects are similar to those produced by the anticholinergics, including confusion and alteration of mood, nausea, and edema. Livedo reticularis may occur with Amantadine therapy.

Usually within two to three years after diagnosis, bradykinesia or postural difficulties cause increasing difficulties that do not respond to anticholinergics and amantadine. At this time dopamine replacement therapy is necessary.

L-dopa is the greatest single advance in therapy for Parkinson's disease. It replaces striatal dopamine that is depleted in parkinsonism. L-Dopa can be given alone or with carbidopa. Carbidopa is a dopa-decarboxylase inhibitor that reduces the peripheral side effects of L-dopa, such as nausea, vomiting, cardiac arrhythmias, and postural hypotension. It allows more of the ingested L-dopa to reach the brain.

Sinemet, the combination of L-dopa and carbidopa, is available in 10:1 and 4:1 ratios, a daily dosage of 100 mg is needed to saturate the peripheral enzyme. Sinemet improves all of the symptoms of Parkinson's disease, although bradykinesia and rigidity respond more than tremor. Treatment is usually started with low doses, 10/100 mg bid to tid, with the dosage gradually increased by 10/100 mg every three to four days. Because many patients develop nausea or vomiting, it is best to give the medication after meals, or after the patient has eaten a light snack. Absorption of the Sinemet will be less than if given on an empty stomach, but compliance will be greater if side effects do not occur or are minimal. Most patients begin to improve when they have reached a total daily dose of 50/500 mg. Most patients end up taking 25/250 mg tablets tid or qid. If gastrointestinal upset persists during the initial therapy, a switch to the 25/100 mg tablet may be of greater benefit, reducing the nausea by providing more peripheral decarboxylation of the L-dopa. The confusion and psychosis that may result from Sinemet therapy responds to a dosage reduction, or to discontinuance of the medication. Sinemet is best avoided in patients with dementia, melanoma, hypotension, or gastric ulcer. Approximately 20% of patients respond poorly regardless of the dose or plasma concentration; 20% have a dramatic response; 60% improve somewhat. The lack of any response should arouse the suspicion that the patient is not taking the medication, that the diagnosis is incorrect, or that he has a parkinsonian variant.

Abnormal involuntary movements are the most frequent limiting side effects of L-dopa. Unilateral or bilateral choreic movements or severe generalized dyskinesias and dystonic movements may result. These movements are usually dose-related and occur more frequently in the patient who has been taking high doses for a long time. In general, they occur after the first year of treatment if they have not developed during the initial phase of L-dopa therapy. Slowly reducing the dosage until the movements cease and the parkinsonian symptoms are controlled is necessary, but not always possible. Many patients prefer minor dyskinesias to the akinesia and rigidity. End-of-dose akinesia (wearing-off effect) is best treated by smaller and more frequent doses of Sinemet or by the addition of a dopamine agonist (bromocriptine). Akinesia that is present upon awakening in the morning is best treated with a dose of Sinemet at this time or by the addition of bromocriptine.

The "on–off" response is characterized by sudden fluctuations in parkinsonian symptoms; the patient has no symptoms ("on") then suddenly becomes markedly parkinsonian ("off"). The on–off reaction usually has no relation to the timing of the medication, and it may seem to occur as an end of dose akinesia. On–off effects usually occur after at least one year of therapy and in more than 50% of patients who have been receiving therapy for more than ten years. Smaller and more frequent Sinemet doses are necessary; they may provide temporary control. The addition of amantadine, 100-mg bid, may provide some benefit, but again the response is only temporary. The addition of bromocriptine is somewhat helpful in reducing the frequency and severity of these on–off reactions.

Depression occurs in 50% of patients treated with Sinemet; it is best controlled with tricyclic antidepressants. Nightmares and hallucinations may respond at first to a reduction in or altered timing of Sinemet therapy. After six years of L-dopa, 50% of patients fail to maintain benefit or cannot tolerate its side effects.

Physical therapy, with an emphasis on gait training and balance, is often useful, especially when combined with pharmacologic replacement therapy. The patient should be advised to exercise, particularly walking or bicycling. Psychotherapy may be necessary for the patient who feels incapacitated by the disease and may be useful for treating the associated depression. Amitriptyline has a dual effect of improving the depression and (because of its anticholinergic activity) the symptoms of the parkinsonism.

Neurosurgical procedures, common in the pre-L-dopa era, are now rarely performed. Stereotaxic thalamotomy is the most common procedure. The patient with unilateral tremor and rigidity seems to benefit the most and may not need antiparkinsonian medications postoperatively. Transplantation of dopaminergic-rich fetal implants to the brain is an exciting area for future research. If this technique is shown to be effective, then control of the disease could be easier and some complications of chronic therapy (on–off reaction) might be obviated.

The patient should be given the address of the Parkinson's Disease Foundation and support groups (see Appendix).

PROGRESSIVE SUPRANUCLEAR PALSY

Approximately 4% of patients with parkinsonian findings on examination manifest clinical features of progressive supranuclear palsy (PSP). PSP usually occurs in the sixth decade of life and more often in men than in women. Bradykinesia, postural instability, and rigidity are commonly associated manifestations, as in parkinsonism. However, in PSP the rigidity predominantly affects the axial muscles, often resulting in hypertonic neck extension (axial dystonia). Tremor, common in Parkinson's disease, is uncommon in PSP. The gait of PSP patients is more wide-based and stiff, in contrast to the small-stepped, shuffling gait of patients with typical Parkinson's disease. Patients with PSP usually look worried or surprised, in contrast to the paucity of facial expression in parkinsonism.

The clinical hallmark of PSP is the supranuclear paralysis of vertical gaze. Downgaze is commonly affected first, which may contribute to the severe, constant extension of the neck. Voluntary vertical gaze may be absent, but reflex movements such as the oculocephalic response and Bell's phenomenon are intact. Reflex eye movements persist because nuclear and infranuclear pathways are intact, thereby localizing the defect to the supranuclear control of vertical eye movements. Within three years of the onset of symptoms, almost all patients exhibit supranuclear ophthalmoparesis. Because not all patients have a vertical gaze disorder when first seen, their condition is often diagnosed as idiopathic Parkinson's disease.

Almost all patients with PSP develop pseudobulbar palsy with dysarthria, dysphagia, hyperactive gag reflex, and emotional hyperreactivity. Horizontal ocular movements may also be diminished, blinking may be decreased, and blepharospasm and apraxia of lid opening may develop. Dementia may develop, but akinesia and atypical facial appearance may give a false appearance of dementia in an intellectually intact patient. Tremor is conspicuously absent in the patient with PSP.

LABORATORY TESTS
Laboratory tests are often normal in the patient with PSP, although computed tomography (CT) and nuclear magnetic resonance imaging (MRI) may reveal brain stem atrophy, particularly of the midbrain. An electroencephalogram (EEG) reveals generalized, nonspecific slowing in most patients.

TREATMENT
The pharmacologic management of PSP includes those drugs that benefit the patient with Parkinson's disease. Initial therapy with anticholinergics, amantadine, or Sinemet may benefit some patients with PSP, although these medications do not provide as much relief for the patient with PSP as they do for the parkinsonian

patient. Bromocriptine provides the patient with PSP the greatest benefit. Doses are in the 1 to 30 mg range (daily total) and patients respond who are not also taking L-dopa. Methysergide (Sansert) and pergolide may also be effective in some patients with PSP. Amitriptyline and other tricyclic antidepressants are useful, particularly in the patient who is depressed. Physical and speech therapies are also useful, and may help the patient cope with the gait and speech disability present in almost all patients with PSP.

Unfortunately, any response to therapy is often limited. The course of the disease is that of gradual progression with death usually occurring by the eighth year of symptoms.

HUNTINGTON'S DISEASE

Huntington's disease, a progressive hereditary neurological disorder, is characterized by a movement disorder (choreoathetosis) and dementia and is associated with an autosomal dominant pattern of inheritance. Its prevalence is 4 to 8 per 100,000. New, spontaneous mutations are rare or possibly do not occur. The characteristic features of the movement disorder and mental deterioration may occur together at the onset, or one may precede the other. The usual age of onset is in the fourth or fifth decade, but 10% of patients are affected before the age of 20. When onset occurs in childhood an akinetic-rigid state may develop with associated mental abnormalities and convulsions. The childhood form is rapidly progressive, with a fatal outcome usually in less than 10 years. Ninety percent of childhood cases are inherited from the father.

In the adult, disturbances of mood and behavior are common and depression frequently develops. Intellectual deterioration develops, with progressive memory failure and inattention. Emotional outbursts are common and may reach the proportion of psychosis. Abnormal motor movements may develop insidiously. Choreic movements are rapid and may involve proximal, distal, and axial muscles. Dyskinesias are seemingly purposeless, may be increased by emotional stimuli, and may cease during sleep. Clumsiness develops and walking may be associated with abnormal movements. There is a high suicide rate among patients with neuropsychiatric manifestations.

Pathologically, there is atrophy of the caudate and putamen, with a moderate amount of frontal-temporal atrophy. Neurochemically, striatal GABA and acetylcholine levels are reduced.

The main difficulty diagnosing Huntington's disease occurs in patients who lack a definite family history. Sometimes the family history is not complete, or the illness of a family member was misdiagnosed. Neuroleptic-induced tardive dyskinesia, systemic lupus erythermatosus, or Sydenham's chorea must be considered in patients who seemingly lack a family history or those who are without intellectual deterioration.

Diagnostic tests are usually of no help, especially in the patient with minimal disease. A CT scan may show increased bicaudate diameter or generalized atrophy. There are no currently available predictive tests that are acceptable from an ethical or pharmacological standpoint.

TREATMENT

Although there is a central deficiency of the neurotransmitter GABA in patients with Huntington's disease, drugs that facilitate GABA or acetylcholine have not been successful in modifying the disease. Choreic movements can be treated with drugs that deplete dopamine (reserpine, tetrabenazine) or those that block dopamine receptors (phenothiazines, butyrophenones). In this regard, haloperidol (Haldol) and perphenazine (Trilafon) are the most useful. In addition to helping the dyskinesias the neuroleptic agents may also control some of the behavioral changes and emotional outbursts. Usually, as the disease advances, confinement to a psychiatric facility will be necessary. Death usually ensues 15 to 20 years after onset.

SENILE CHOREA

Choreic movements may begin in the person older than 60 years, usually not associated with other symptoms. These movements are usually mild, slowly progressive, and involve the limbs. There are no associated mental disturbances nor is there a family history of dementia or a movement disorder. Some cases appear acutely and then resolve, often associated with hyperglycemia. Although at some times considered a variant of Huntington's disease, senile chorea is probably a separate entity. Usually the symptoms are mild and treatment is not necessary. Neuroleptic drugs (perphenazine, haloperidol) may be used to reduce the chorea if it is troublesome. Serum calcium, phosphorus, and glucose levels and liver function tests should be tested. A CT scan of the head should be performed to exclude a space-occupying lesion (tumor, subdural hematoma, AVM) or lacunar infarction.

HEMICHOREA AND HEMIBALLISMUS

Ballistic movements are more violent than chorea; they are characterized by almost continuous flailing movements of the proximal extremity and axial musculature. Movements are quite violent and forceful, and biballism (bilateral ballismus) occasionally occurs. Hemichorea, in which choreic movements are confined to the arm or leg on one side of the body, usually develops suddenly in middle-aged or older persons. Both hemichorea and hemiballism have an abrupt onset, and are often associated with vascular disease. Infarction of the sub-thalamic nucleus is the most common cause of hemiballismus. Hemichorea often results from infarcts in the caudate-basal ganglia area. Both types of movements can be associated with tumors, subdural hematomas, and transient hyperglycemia.

Hemiballismus, because of its violent nature, may tax the elderly patient's cardiovascular system. Immediate therapy is mandatory, usually with haloperidol or phenothiazines, although reserpine may be of benefit. Most patients are controlled pharmacologically, but chronic hemiballismus that is unresponsive to medication can be treated neurosurgically by ventrolateral thalamotomy. A metabolic profile test should be performed on all patients with hemichorea or hemiballismus; in cases associated with hyperglycemia, return of the blood glucose level to normal may be associated with a resolution of the movement disorder. A CT scan should be performed in an attempt to identify a structural cause for the abnormal movements.

SYDENHAM'S CHOREA

Also known as St. Vitus dance and rheumatic chorea, Sydenham's chorea is a disease of childhood that begins between the ages of 3 and 13, occurring more often in girls. A first attack after the age of 15 is uncommon, except when a patient uses oral contraceptives or is pregnant. An old maxim states that a child with Sydenham's chorea is punished three times before the diagnosis is made: once for general fidgetiness, once for breaking crockery, and once for making faces at his grandmother. Involuntary movements affect mainly the face, hands, and arms. Onset is abrupt and of short duration, gradually becoming more frequent and extensive and disappearing during sleep. Weakness may be present and is often profound. Speech is often jerky; diffuse hypotonia is often present. The wrist is often flexed and the metacarpophalangeal joints overextended (choreic hand); the child is unable to maintain a continuous muscular contraction, manifested by waxing and waning of the grip (milkmaid sign). Eighteen percent of patients exhibit hemichorea. The child is often fearful and apathetic. The duration of the chorea usually ranges from one month to two years. One-third of patients have an isolated attack, the remainder having as many as five or more recurrences. Complications of Sydenham's chorea are rare. They include occlusion of the central retinal artery and pseudotumor cerebri. Complete recovery is usual, but minor neurological signs may persist.

Approximately 75% of patients exhibit other manifestations of rheumatic disease; patients with rheumatic chorea have antibodies that react with subthalamic and caudate nuclei neurons. The erythrocyte sedimentation rate and C-reactive protein level are usually normal, and the CSF also is often normal, except for rare pleocytosis.

Manifestations of rheumatic infection may occur at any time in relation to the chorea. Cardiac involvement, usually endocarditis, occurs in 20% of cases; myocarditis and pericarditis are less common. Rheumatoid nodules, erythema nodosum, and purpura may also develop. Acute chorea is usually benign; and complete recovery is usual, although mortality is approximately 2% (as a consequence of cardiac complications).

TREATMENT

There is no specific treatment for Sydenham chorea. As soon as the diagnosis is made, a course of penicillin is indicated with a single IM dose of 1.2 million units penicillin G benzathine (Bicillin) or with an oral penicillin 250 mg qid for 10 days. Phenothiazines or butyrophenones may be utilized to reduce the dyskinesias. In addition, bed rest and sedation may be necessary to control the chorea.

WILSON'S DISEASE

Hepatolenticular degeneration (Wilson's disease) is an inborn error of copper metabolism which is associated with degenerative changes in the basal ganglia and cirrhosis of the liver. It is transmitted as an autosomal recessive trait. The prevalence is 5 to 30 per million, and the gene frequency of heterozygotes varies from 1 in 200 to 1 in 400. The disease appears to be caused by decreased copper excretion into the bile. Copper accumulates in the liver in the first five years of life. When that organ is saturated, copper is released into the serum and accumulates in other organs, principally the brain, kidney, bone, and blood. The majority of patients show a markedly diminished serum ceruloplasmin concentration, with low serum copper levels and increased urinary copper excretion. Aminoaciduria may be present, more so during the later stages. Hemolytic anemia often complicates the course of Wilson's disease. Liver disease results in the form of acute hepatitis, fulminant hepatitis, chronic active hepatitis, or cirrhosis associated with portal hypertension.

In the brain, the basal ganglia show the most striking abnormalities. Degenerative (often cystic) changes occur in the putamen, and the globus pallidus and caudate become atrophic. Copper may be seen deposited within astrocytes. Copper is also deposited in the cornea, and in the periphery of the cornea the copper appears as golden-brown or greenish discolorations in the zone of Descemet's membrane in the limbic region of the cornea (Kayser–Fleischer rings).

The neurological manifestations commonly appear between 12 and 30 years of age. Onset in the fifth and sixth decades have been reported. Adults tend to have a more benign course than do children. One of the most frequent early symptoms is difficulty in speaking or writing, often leading to poor performance in school. Tremors and rigidity are common early signs, and cerebellar symptoms may predominate. Tremor may be resting (parkinsonian-like) or of intention-type. Usually the tremor is localized to the arms and described as "wing-beating"; this form of tremor is absent at rest and begins after the arms are extended. Changing the posture of the arms may reduce the tremor. Although the tremor may affect both arms, it is usually more severe in one. Muscle rigidity is common and may affect all muscles. Dystonic movements such as torticollis are common.

Dysphagia, dysarthria, and excessive salivation are common. Psychiatric manifestations may be prominent. Patients with Wilson's disease may present in adolescence with an adjustment reaction, or they may develop an affective disorder or psychosis. The Kayser–Fleischer ring may be evident to the naked eye or may require slit-lamp examination to be seen. It is present in 75% of patients with hepatic symptoms, and in virtually all patients with cerebral symptoms.

Laboratory Tests

The biochemical diagnosis of Wilson's disease is usually based on a low serum level of ceruloplasmin; however, approximately 15% of patients have normal levels. Serum copper levels in patients with Wilson's disease may be high, normal, or low, depending on the disease stage so are not diagnostic. Urinary excretion of copper is increased, and the hepatic copper level (obtained from a liver biopsy) is usually elevated to greater than 250 μg/dry weight. The finding of a normal hepatic concentration excludes the diagnosis of Wilson's disease. A CT scan of the head in advanced cases may show cystic changes in the lenticular nuclei; and magnetic resonance scanning shows changes in the basal ganglia much earlier in the course of the disease than CT.

TREATMENT

The basic therapy for Wilson's disease is directed toward decreasing the tissue accumulation of copper. A low copper diet (less than 1.5 mg/day) is helpful, and may allow a lowering of the dose of chelating agents. D-Penicillamine (Cuprimine), 1 to 3 g/day in divided doses, promotes the urinary excretion of copper. Neurological and hepatic symptoms may improve and survival may be prolonged with treatment.

Bibliography

Ballard PA, Tetrud JW, Langston JW: Permanent human parkinsonism due to 1-methyl-4-phenyl-1,2,3,6-tetrahydropyridine (MPTP). *Neurology* (Cleve) 1985; 35:949-956. (MPTP is a meperidine analog and one of the most potent neurotoxins; future research with this drug may help determine the cause of parkinsonism.)

Calne DB: Progress in Parkinson's disease. *N Engl J Med* 1984; 310:523-524. (Editorial that reviews the direction in treatment of Parkinson's disease.)

Calne DB, Langston JW: Aetiology of Parkinson's disease. *Lancet* 1983; 2:1457-1459. (A recent review of possible etiologies of Parkinson's disease.)

Cotzias GC, Papavasiliou PS, Gellene R: Modification of parkinsonism—chronic treatment with L-DOPA. *N Engl J Med* 1969; 280:337-345. (Study that showed the effectiveness of chronic treatment with L-DOPA; a "classic.")

Jackson JA, Jankovic J, Ford J: Progressive supranuclear palsy: Clinical features and responses to treatment in sixteen patients. *Ann Neurol* 1983; 13:273-278. (Synopsis of a study of a group of patients with PSP; bromocriptine is of benefit.)

Jankovic J (ed): Movement disorders. *Neurol Clin* 1984; 2:415-634. (Covers many aspects of frequently encountered movement disorders.)

Kolata G: Grafts correct brain damage. *Science* 1982; 217:342-344. (Briefly discusses the experimental and clinical studies on intracerebral implantation of dopamine-rich tissue.)

Martin JB: Huntington's disease: New approaches to an old problem. *Neurology* (Cleve) 1984; 34:1059-1072. (Reviews clinical and experimental aspects of Huntington's disease.)

Nausieda PA, Grossman BJ, Koller WC, et al: Sydenham's chorea: An update. Neurology (NY) 1980; 30:331-334. (A review of the records of 240 patients between 1951 and 1976; documents the decline of the disease, and that one-third of patients had coexisting heart disease.)

Nutt JG, Woodward WR, Hammerstad JP, et al: The "on–off" phenomenon in Parkinson's disease: Relation to levodopa absorption and transport. *N Engl J Med* 1984; 310:484-488. (Food reduces absorption of levodopa, and neutral amino acids compete with levodopa transport across the blood–brain barrier—likely causes for most (but not all) cases with "on–off" reactions.)

Osborne JP, Munson P, Burman D: Huntington's chorea. *Arch Dis Child* 1982; 57:99-103. (Huntington's disease presents a different clinical picture in childhood.)

Ross ME, Jacobson IM, Dienstag JC, et al: Late-onset Wilson's disease with neurological involvement in the absence of Kayser-Fleischer rings. *Ann Neurol* 1985; 17:411-413. (Stresses that Wilson's disease should be considered in the patient of any age with chronic degenerative extrapyramidal or cerebellar symptoms, especially if there is evidence of hepatic dysfunction.)

Stephen PJ, Williamson J: Drug-induced parkinsonism in the elderly. *Lancet* 1984; 2:1082-1083. (Fifty-one percent of new cases of parkinsonism were associated with medication; the paper points out the frequency of drug-induced (iatrogenic) parkinsonism.)

Teychenne PF, Bergsend D, Racy A, et al: Bromocriptine: Low-dose therapy in Parkinson's disease. *Neurology* (NY) 1982; 32:577-583. (Low-dose bromocriptine (7.5 to 15 mg) is of therapeutic benefit.)

Todes C: Inside parkinsonism...A psychiatrist's personal experience. *Lancet* 1983; 1:977-978. (A psychiatrist recounts his struggle with Parkinson's disease, diagnosed when he was 39 years old.)

25

Hereditary and Degenerative Diseases

The degenerative diseases of the nervous system usually begin slowly, after a long period of normal nervous system function. They tend to follow a progressive course over few to many years. Because many degenerative disorders depend on genetic factors, they are sometimes referred to as heredodegenerative diseases.

The onset of a degenerative disease is usually insidious and is not associated with a particular precipitating event. Often the disease has been present for some time when minor stress or trauma seemingly brings it to light clinically. Because many degenerative diseases are familial, an attempt should be made to ascertain whether other family members have the disease. Occasionally, families may not realize that a disease is hereditary, or they may attempt to cover up the fact that it has been passed from generation to generation.

Most degenerative diseases of the nervous system run an inexorably progressive course, although some may be associated with long periods of stability. Many degenerative diseases are bilaterally symmetric. Occasionally (especially at the onset), the disease may appear asymmetric, only to eventually become symmetric. The more common neurodegenerative syndromes are discussed in this chapter. Dementia and movement disorders are discussed in Chapters 13 and 24, respectively.

MOTOR NEURON DISEASE

Diseases that affect the motor neuron tend to be characterized by selective damage to the systems that mediate voluntary movement. Because of the restricted motor system involvement, there tends to be a lack of involvement of other neural systems; sensation, autonomic function, and cognition tend to be unaffected.

Amyotrophic Lateral Sclerosis

CLINICAL SIGNIFICANCE

Although uncommon, amyotrophic lateral sclerosis (ALS), popularly known as Lou Gehrig's disease, is not rare. Its incidence is 0.8 to 1.2/100,000 and its prevalence is 4 to 6/100,000. The death rate is approximately 50/100,000 population. Thus, primary care practitioners occasionally encounter patients with ALS.

ETIOLOGY

The etiology of ALS is not known. In 5% to 10% of cases, it is a definite genetic tendency with an autosomal dominant pattern. No definite environmental factor has been identified for sporadic cases. A viral cause has been postulated, but no virus has ever been recovered from postmortem tissue. One current theory proposes that ALS results from a deficiency of DNA enzymes and subsequent accumulation of abnormal DNA in motor neurons. Recently, an antibody was found in the serum of patients with ALS that inhibits the sprouting of neurons and the subsequent reinnervation of skeletal muscle. Clinical correlation of this sprouting inhibition is not known, nor is it known yet if these antibodies are of primary pathogenic importance.

SYMPTOMS AND SIGNS

Amyotrophic lateral sclerosis is a disease of middle and late life, although it does occur rarely in patients less than 30 years of age. The initial manifestations depend upon whether the upper motor neuron system or the lower motor neuron system is involved. Limb weakness, predominantly of the hand, often is the first manifestation. This is associated with fasciculation and atrophy of the hand muscles. Cramping may also occur, and muscle bulk often diminishes. Although the deficit may be asymmetric at the outset, it frequently becomes symmetric within a few months. Gait disturbances, dysarthria and dysphagia may also develop, the latter signifying bulbar involvement.

The abductors, adductors, and extensors of the fingers and thumb become weak before the long flexors, and the dorsal interosseous spaces become hollow. The arms may be involved prior to the onset of lower-extremity abnormalities. Tongue atrophy and fasciculations are common, and the atrophic process frequently spreads to the neck, laryngeal, and pharyngeal muscles and eventually to the lower extremities. Sphincteric function, extraocular movements, sensation, and gait are usually maintained. In general, the usual triad of atrophic weakness of the hands and arms associated with generalized hyperreflexia and normal sensation is most suggestive of ALS. Respiratory insufficiency, although usually a late manifestation may be an early symptom with rapid onset.

The disease is progressive; half of the patients die within three years; 90%, within six years. Death usually occurs within five years of onset, particularly when there are both upper and lower motor neuron signs. Patients with bulbar involvement tend to die sooner, in part due because of the complications of aspiration; these patients also tend to be older.

Progressive Muscular Atrophy

Progressive muscular atrophy is a variant of ALS in which weakness and atrophy occur in the absence of corticospinal tract dysfunction. Wasting of the intrinsic hand muscles is often the first sign; eventually, there is involvement of proximal upper-extremity structures. It is uncommon for the proximal parts of the limbs to be affected before the distal parts are. Deep-tendon reflexes are diminished or absent. Patients with lower motor neuron disease have a much longer survival than patients with classical ALS; they may live 15 years or longer after onset. If upper motor neuron signs do not develop within two years, it is unlikely that ALS will develop. At this stage it is best to refer to this condition as spinal muscular atrophy.

Progressive Bulbar Palsy

Some patients with ALS have symptoms and signs that arise from weakness of the bulbar innervated muscles; dysarthria and dysphagia are presenting symptoms. There is an early deficit in articulation, especially in the pronunciation of lingual (*l,n,r*), and labial (*f,b,m,p*), dental (*d,t*) and palatal (*k,g*) consonants. A raspy, nasal quality to the voice may develop. Atrophy and fasciculation of the tongue are early manifestations. Eventually, deglutition and mastication are involved. Reflux of food and liquids into the nose or trachea occurs. The jaw jerk is often exaggerated when the muscles of mastication are weak, and clonus of the jaw may result.

The outcome for patients with bulbar palsy is less favorable than in the usual case of ALS; most patients die within two or three years of respiratory insufficiency. Approximately one-fourth of cases of motor neuron disease (ALS) begin with bulbar symptoms, and almost always other manifestations of ALS become evident within a few months.

LABORATORY TESTS

Routine blood and radiologic studies are normal; so are the electroencephalogram (EEG) and evoked potentials. Creatine kinase levels may be elevated as high as 1000 to 1500 IU, especially in cases in which denervation is rapid or in cases of progressive muscular atrophy. The CSF usually remains normal, as does the CT scan of the head. Electromyographic (EMG) alterations are usually evident from the outset, they vary with the extent and degree of disease. Diffuse (or at times localized) sharp waves and fibrillations or fasciculations are seen; they are present almost universally in patients with advanced disease. In cases with purely corticospinal involvement, denervation is not seen.

Motor and sensory nerve conduction velocities are normal or slightly slowed. Muscle biopsy demonstrates evidence of a neurogenic process. Because of a possible association of ALS with paraproteinemia or heavy metal intoxication, patients should be screened for lead toxicity and paraproteinemia. Myelography is often performed in patients with primary corticospinal signs but without clinical involvement above the foramen magnum, although magnetic resonance scanning (MRI) may be of greater value as a noninvasive test to exclude a compressive lesion.

DIAGNOSIS

Few diseases cause a combination of lower motor neuron and upper motor neuron signs with intact sensation. Because patients with ALS have a progressive and essentially untreatable illness, an investigation of treatable causes is indicated.

Cervical spondylosis or a cervical cord tumor can simulate ALS; in these cases there is usually pain, often some limitation of neck movement, and sensory symptoms and signs. Peroneal muscle atrophy is familial and is associated with distal sensory loss and significant slowing of motor nerve conduction velocities. Occasionally, patients with multiple sclerosis present with a distal amyotrophy and corticospinal signs, which may be difficult to distinguish from ALS at first.

Progressive diabetic amyotrophy or polymyositis may also be initially confused with ALS. Patients with a history of poliomyelitis may present with deterioration in motor function and any increase in pain, cramps, and atrophy. The exact cause of this "post polio" syndrome is not known, but it bears a resemblance to the progressive muscle atrophy form of ALS. Bulbar palsy may occur with myasthenia gravis, but the presence of atrophy and a negative Tensilon test make that diagnosis untenable.

The clinical findings, coupled with the EMG examination are usually sufficient to make the diagnosis of ALS, although early in its course the signs and symptoms can be confusing.

MANAGEMENT

There is no specific treatment for ALS. Many therapies have been tried (without success) including snake venom, plasmapheresis, immunosuppression, and guanadine. Recently, thyroid releasing hormone (TRH), injected parenterally or intrathecally, has been reported to improve motor function—albeit transiently— in patients with ALS. Multicenter studies are underway in an attempt to learn whether TRH therapy is effective and feasible. Baclofen, an antispasticity medication, can be of benefit in patients with prominent upper motor neuron signs; it also benefits patients with muscle cramps. Because sialorrhea may develop and is a prominent symptom, anticholinergic agents (atropine, amitriptyline, trihexyphenidyl) may be effective and of some benefit for this problem. Cricopharyngeal myotomy may benefit some patients with prominent dysphagia caused by upper motor neuron disease. Vocal cord injections with polytef (Teflon) can reduce the risk of aspiration.

The patient and his family should have a basic understanding of the disease. Because respiratory insufficiency is invariable and dysphagia may be predominant, the patient should be informed about tracheostomy, with or without ventilator support, or a feeding gastrostomy. Some patients prefer to have a tracheostomy and gastrostomy but do not want to be placed on a ventilator. When the disease is progressing the patient must decide whether his life should be prolonged by mechanical means.

WHEN TO CONSULT

It is best to have the neurologist involved from the onset of the illness. Because patients with ALS present in a variety of ways, it may be difficult for the primary care physician (and the neurologist) to diagnose the disease initially. Sometimes the patient is referred after an EMG has documented findings compatible with ALS. A careful neurological examination and a review of diagnostic tests by the neurologist can help clarify the diagnosis. Most ALS patients and their families want a second opinion; this is reasonable because ALS is always a fatal disease. Intermittent consultation to help quantify the degree of progression of the disease is advisable.

PATIENT EDUCATION

There is a national ALS society (see Appendix) and in many communities, local ALS societies provide support to patients and their families.

Primary Lateral Sclerosis

Primary lateral sclerosis features spastic paresis without evidence of lower motor neuron dysfunction (atrophy, fasciculations). If evidence of lower motor neuron dysfunction is not present within two years after the onset of symptoms, ALS is unlikely and the patient should be assigned a diagnosis of primary lateral sclerosis.

This disease is very slowly progressive and uncommon. Symptoms most frequently begin in the lower extremities with a spastic gait. Eventually, the disease spreads to the arms, and suprabulbar paresis results in dysphagia and dysarthria. Bladder dysfunction is common; vibration and position sensation loss may be evident.

Because this is such an uncommon disease, primary lateral sclerosis tends to be a diagnosis of exclusion. Other diseases should be ruled out, including cervical cord tumors or herniated discs and syringomyelia. Furthermore, it is not uncommon for multiple sclerosis to begin with a midlife gait disturbance. Cervical myelography and CSF analysis are often necessary for diagnosis, and a CT scan of the head should be performed to rule out a parasagittal lesion. Evoked potential and MRI studies may also be of benefit. There is no specific treatment, but physical therapy and antispasticity medication such as baclofen are often of benefit.

SPINOCEREBELLAR DEGENERATIONS

The spinocerebellar degenerations are a group of usually hereditary disorders in which ataxia is the predominant sign. The cerebellum and its connections are the major site of the disease, although there also may be involvement of the pyramidal tracts, posterior columns, basal ganglia, and other regions of the brain. The classification of the spinocerebellar degenerations has long been a matter of dispute. Because none of these disorders is very common, it is hard to gather large numbers of patients for analysis and classification.

In general, the spinocerebellar degenerations can be classified as those associated with a known metabolic or other cause and as those of unknown etiology. The disorders of unknown etiology are more common; they can be subdivided further on the basis of whether the onset is before or after 20 years of age. Virtually all the disorders with an early onset have an autosomal-recessive mode of inheritance, and those with a late onset are autosomal-dominant. Although the spinocerebellar degenerations are uncommon, the differential diagnosis in any patient who presents with ataxia includes these disorders. A discussion of only the more commonly encountered spinocerebellar degenerations follows.

Friedreich's Ataxia

CLINICAL SIGNIFICANCE

Friedreich's ataxia is the most common spinocerebellar degeneration. It is one of the more common hereditary diseases of the nervous system.

ETIOLOGY

The etiology of Friedreich's ataxia is unknown. It is usually inherited as an autosomal-recessive disorder, but some patients do not have a family history. It is more common in males, and all races are affected. Reduced levels of pyruvate dehydrogenase and lipoamide dehydrogenase have been documented in the platelets and cultured skin fibroblasts of most patients with Friedreich's ataxia, but the significance of this chemical abnormality is not known. Pathologically, there is degeneration of the spinal cord, primarily involving the posterior columns, the dorsal and ventral spinocerebellar tracts, and the lateral corticospinal tract. The cerebellum and basal ganglia are usually normal, although at times areas of cerebellar degeneration are found.

SYMPTOMS AND SIGNS

The onset of symptoms is usually between the ages of 6 and 16 years. Symptoms may begin in infancy or may be delayed until the third decade. Ataxia of gait is usually the initial symptom; both legs are commonly affected. Difficulties in standing or running are noticed early; within a few years ataxia of the arms and trunk develops, and dysarthric speech appears after the arm involvement. Movements are jerky and poorly controlled. Intention tremor is common in the arms, and may also involve the trunk. Speech is slow, often slurred, at times explosive, and it eventually becomes unintelligible. Athetoid and choreic movements of the limbs may be noted. Weakness of muscles is common, more so distally. Dementia or psychosis occur infrequently.

On examination, ataxia of gait is evident, often associated with limb ataxia and tremor. Deep-tendon reflexes in the legs are almost always absent, but the plantar response is usually extensor. About 75% of patients have loss of vibration and joint-position sense. Optic atrophy occurs in one-third of patients; horizontal nystagmus is usually seen at some stage of the disease in almost all patients. Kyphoscoliosis is seen in 80% of patients; pes cavus deformity occurs in over 50%. A cardiomyopathy occurs in over half of patients.

In general, the mean age at which the patient loses the ability to walk is 25 years. Most patients die in the fourth or fifth decades of life. Cardiac involvement is of major clinical importance. Symptoms are those of progressive congestive heart failure or of cardiac arrhythmias. Such cardiac symptoms usually develop some years after neurological deterioration has occurred. It has been suggested that most patients with Friedreich's ataxia die from cardiac complications; in one series, more than 50% died of heart failure. Death from cardiac causes is uncommon in childhood and usually occurs in the third or fourth decade of life. Diabetes mellitus also is associated with Friedreich's ataxia and is present in about 10% of patients.

LABORATORY TESTS

Laboratory tests are usually normal and do not help with diagnosis. As mentioned above, deficiencies of platelet pyruvate dehydrogenase and lipoamide dehydrogenase have been reported. The ECG shows generalized T-wave inversion or signs of left ventricular hypertrophy. Cardiac arrhythmias occur, including atrial tachycardia, fibrillation, or extrasystoles. Variable degrees of cardiomegaly, left ventricular hypertrophy, or pulmonary congestion can be seen on x-rays; scoliosis is evident on thoracic x-ray. The fasting blood sugar may be elevated. A CT scan of the head is of limited value, but helps exclude hydrocephalus or neoplasm as a cause of the gait disturbance. Nerve conduction studies may reveal slowing of motor nerve conduction velocities, with predominant abnormalities of sensory nerve conduction.

DIAGNOSIS

In most cases, the diagnosis of Friedreich's ataxia is not difficult. The combination of pes cavus deformity, kyphoscoliosis, areflexia, ataxia, and Babinski's sign is almost pathognomonic. Atypical forms of the disease tend to be difficult to distinguish from some other types of spinocerebellar degeneration unless there is a similar condition in other family members.

MANAGEMENT

There is no basic treatment for Friedreich's ataxia, although a diet high in fat and carbohydrate has been reported to cause improvement in some patients. Physical therapy is of some benefit; treatment of cardiac abnormalities is often necessary. Surgical procedures on deformed feet are often indicated to prolong the ability to walk for as long as possible. Because a group of spinocerebellar degenerations is associated with Vitamin E deficiency, many neurologists treat all such patients with vitamin E, 400 IU daily.

WHEN TO CONSULT

Neurological consultation is usually indicated when the patient has ataxia of unknown origin. Because not all cases are associated with a family history, the diagnosis of Friedreich's ataxia may be unclear. When other family members are affected, neurological consultation may be of less benefit.

Early Onset Cerebellar Ataxia with Retained Deep-Tendon Reflexes

Progressive cerebellar ataxia associated with mild-to-moderate dysarthria, pyramidal signs in the limbs, normal or increased knee jerks, ankle areflexia, and occasional sensory loss is an uncommon disease that resembles Friedreich's ataxia. The lack of predominant sensory loss or generalized areflexia and of optic atrophy, severe skeletal deformities, diabetes, and cardiac abnormalities distinguishes this disease from Friedreich's ataxia. Patients with this condition remain ambulatory for at least ten years longer than those with Friedreich's ataxia. The inheritance pattern probably is not autosomal recessive.

OLIVOPONTOCEREBELLAR DEGENERATION

CLINICAL SIGNIFICANCE

The olivopontocerebellar degenerations (OPCD) are a form of late-onset cerebellar ataxia in which there is striking atrophy of the cerebellum, pons, and inferior olives. There are familial and sporadic forms of OPCD. Most of the cases encountered in clinical practice are sporadic and present to the practitioner as unexplained ataxia.

ETIOLOGY

As with most other spinocerebellar degenerations, the etiology of OPCD is not known. The hereditary type is usually an autosomal dominant trait, but occasionally it is inherited in a recessive fashion. A reduction of levels of the enzyme glutamate dehydrogenase has been found in a number of patients with the recessive form.

SYMPTOMS AND SIGNS

Onset typically occurs after the fifth decade of life. Progressive cerebellar ataxia of the limbs and trunk develops, with gait ataxia, dysarthria (often with scanning speech), nystagmus, and tremor of the head and trunk. Extrapyramidal symptoms and signs are often evident, including rigidity and resting tremor. Deep-tendon reflexes may be normal, but frequently there is distal areflexia with Babinski's sign. Dementia is common; sphincteric disturbances may occur. Orthostatic hypotension and other signs of autonomic failure may be evident.

LABORATORY TESTS

There are no specific laboratory tests. Platelet pyruvate dehydrogenase levels may be decreased. A CT scan reveals evidence of brain stem and cerebellar degeneration, but these changes do not occur early in the disease. The scan does help exclude a space-occupying lesion as a cause of the symptom complex, however. Nuclear magnetic resonance imaging is also of diagnostic value early in cases of OPCD.

DIAGNOSIS

The diagnosis of OPCD may be difficult at the onset because often a family history of the condition is lacking. Some patients are first given the diagnosis of Parkinson's disease because of dominant extrapyramidal symptoms. OPCD has a much later onset and fewer spinal cord signs than Friedreich's ataxia. A posterior fossa neoplasm or cerebellar degeneration of unknown cause may be considered at first because of primary cerebellar features.

MANAGEMENT

There is no effective therapy. Physical therapy and gait training may be of limited benefit. Treatment with antiparkinson medications may reduce rigidity and tremor temporarily; a combination of carbidopa and levodopa is most effective. A discussion of the management of postural hypotension can be found in the section on multiple-system degeneration at the end of this chapter.

WHEN TO CONSULT

Because patients usually present later in life with progressive ataxia or an atypical extrapyramidal syndrome, neurological consultation is usually warranted to help determine the exact nature of the disease process.

Hereditary Cerebellar Ataxia

Hereditary cerebellar ataxia is a cerebellar degeneration that differs from Friedreich's ataxia in that onset of symptoms occurs later, and characteristic spinal and skeletal signs are lacking. Autopsy reveals primary cerebellar degeneration and atrophy without brain stem or spinal cord lesions.

CLINICAL SIGNIFICANCE

The hereditary cerebellar ataxias are considered rare diseases that have a late-life onset. Ataxia has clinical significance because the presentation of cerebellar disease in the elderly patient may be associated with a potentially treatable condition (e.g., neoplasm).

ETIOLOGY

The etiology is not known. The condition is sometimes hereditary—commonly autosomal dominant—but sporadic cases have occurred.

SYMPTOMS AND SIGNS

Onset is usually between the fourth and sixth decades of life. It can be abrupt in onset but is usually insidious with slow progression. Gait ataxia is most common. Tremors of the head and hands, and slow, dysarthric speech are often present. Nystagmus is uncommon; optic atrophy occurs in some patients. Deep-tendon reflexes may be reduced or increased; extensor plantar responses are sometimes found. Mentation is usually preserved.

LABORATORY TESTS

There are no specific laboratory tests. A CT scan may reveal generalized cerebellar atrophy, and helps exclude other causes of cerebellar dysfunction (eg, neoplasm, stroke).

DIAGNOSIS

If there is a family history, the diagnosis is easier than if the case is sporadic. There tends to be a paucity of spinal cord signs; this observation, with the late onset, makes Friedreich's ataxia unlikely. Other OPCDs must be excluded, however, as must cerebellar neoplasms and paraneoplastic conditions.

MANAGEMENT

There is no known therapy, but physical therapy with gait training may be of benefit; nevertheless, the disease tends to be slowly progressive.

WHEN TO CONSULT

When the patient presents with unexplained cerebellar ataxia, a neurological consultation is usually in order to help determine the exact nature of the neurological disturbance.

PHAKOMATOSES

The phakomatoses are a group of neurocutaneous diseases of genetic origin that involve the skin and the nervous system. Common to these diseases are anomalies in structures of ectodermal origin, which includes the central and peripheral nervous systems and the skin. Cutaneous stigmata are often present at an early age, frequently allowing the diagnosis to be made prior to the onset of neurological symptoms. Genetically determined phakomatoses are autosomal dominant traits, but there is a high mutation rate. The clinical spectrum ranges from the characteristic disorders to frequent abortive forms (formes frustes).

Neurofibromatosis (von Recklinghausen's Disease)

CLINICAL SIGNIFICANCE

Neurofibromatosis is one of the most common genetic disturbances that affect the central nervous system. The main features of this syndrome are multiple tumors that arise from elements of the peripheral nervous system and/or the central nervous system, and multiple cutaneous hyperpigmented skin lesions (*café au lait* patches). The prevalence of neurofibromatosis is approximately 30 to 40 per 100,000, with an incidence of one case in every 3,000 births. Neurofibromatosis is therefore one of the common degenerative diseases encountered by the primary care physician. Because its symptoms may result from lesions in the skin, bone, or nervous system, it is important for the physician to have a basic knowledge of this disease and its neurological complications.

ETIOLOGY

Neurofibromatosis is a genetic disorder with an autosomal dominant inheritance pattern. Approximately 50% of patients have affected relatives; the remaining 50% are likely spontaneous mutations. Males and females are affected equally. The pathogenesis is obscure, but in part may involve the abnormal production and distribution of nerve growth factor.

SYMPTOMS AND SIGNS

There are both cutaneous and neurological features of neurofibromatosis.

Cutaneous

The café au lait spot is the pathognomonic lesion and the hallmark of the disease. It is a light brown, macular patch that may occur anywhere but is most common over the trunk. Spots tend to spare the face; they are usually present at birth and become more numerous with increasing years. Six or more café au lait spots larger than 1.5 cm in diameter are said to be diagnostic of neurofibromatosis. Brown axillary freckles or freckles in the intertriginous areas are frequently observed. Multiple subcutaneous tumors (neurofibromas) tend to appear first in late childhood.

Cutaneous lesions in the dermis are often soft, firm, and flesh-colored, ranging in size from a few millimeters to a few centimeters. They can be flat, pedunculated, or sessile or can have other shapes. Patients may have a few of these lesions or thousands of them. Subcutaneous nodules are often multiple and may be attached to a nerve (plexiform neuroma) or may result in overgrowth of subcutaneous tissue.

Neurofibromas usually become evident when the patient is between the ages of 10 and 15. They may increase in size and number during the second and third decades of life. Congenital neurofibromas tend to be vascular and invasive, and often are located in the orbital, periorbital or cervical areas. A hyperpigmented plexiform neuroma that extends to the midline often is an indication of an intraspinal tumor at that level. Pigmented iris hamartomas (Lisch nodules), present in most patients older than 16 years of age, tend to increase in number with age. The Lisch nodule is present in 94% of patients older than 6 years of age and in 28% younger than 6.

Neurological

Neurological manifestations of this disease are related to the effects of various tumors that can involve peripheral nerves and intraspinal or intracranial structures. Mental retardation, precocious puberty, and seizures (the incidence of which is 20 times as great as that of the general population) are also related to neurofibromatosis. Occlusive cerebral vascular disease may occur, often presenting as acute hemiplegia associated with occlusion of the supraclinoid carotid artery.

Acoustic neuromas, optic nerve gliomas, neurilemmomas, meningiomas, and astrocytomas occur with a frequency of approximately 10% in all patients with neurofibromatosis. Optic nerve glioma tends to occur in children under 10 years of age and usually presents with failing vision or unilateral nystagmus. This optic nerve glioma is usually multicentric, tends to be slowly progressive, and has a better prognosis than similar tumors not associated with neurofibromatosis.

Central neurofibromatosis with bilateral acoustic neuromas, usually associated with mild cutaneous changes, is a distinct syndrome. Symptoms usually begin by the age of 20 and include tinnitus, hearing loss, headache, and ataxia. Spinal tumors occur with higher frequency in neurofibromatosis, and are usually meningiomas. If a neurofibroma involves the spinal cord, it usually arises from nerve ganglia or roots/trunks and spreads centripetally. Macrocephaly may occur, usually with a postnatal onset and tends to be an incidental finding.

Approximately 20% of patients with neurofibromatosis have kyphoscoliosis, which becomes manifest between 5 and 15 years of age and is progressive. Other skeletal defects include anomalies of the posterior superior wall of the orbit, with pulsating exophthalmos, dural ectasia with enlargement of the spinal canal, and pseudoarthrosis, with the tibia involved most often, followed by the radius. (Fifty percent of all congenital pseudoarthrosis is caused by neurofibromatosis.) At least 40% of patients are handicapped, with frank mental retardation occuring in 2% to

5% of patients with the disease. Speech impediments occur in 30% to 40% of patients, clinically manifested as hoarseness, hypernasality, or vocal tremor.

LABORATORY TESTS

The laboratory diagnosis of neurofibromatosis is not yet possible. Any laboratory investigation should be directed individually. All persons with neurofibromatosis or those at risk for it should probably undergo evaluation to confirm the diagnosis and identify complications. Evaluation should be individualized and should include neuropsychological testing; EEG; audiometry; slit-lamp ocular examination; cranial CT scan with and without contrast and with orbital, optic chiasmal, and internal auditory meatus views; radiologic skeletal survey; and measurement of 24-hour urinary excretion of epinephrine and norepinephrine. Each of these procedures yields information that helps substantiate the diagnosis or influence the management of at least 10% of patients. Serum levels of nerve growth factor have not been useful in distinguishing patients with classical neurofibromatosis from normal subjects, although nerve growth factor levels do help differentiate classical neurofibromatosis from the acoustic form of the disease.

DIAGNOSIS

The diagnosis of neurofibromatosis is based on clinical criteria. A history of similar illness in a family member makes recognition of the disease more certain. Difficulties arise when there is no family history in the patient who has acoustic or other CNS neurofibromas but few or no skin lesions. The tendency for central neurofibromatosis to be accompanied by few cutaneous neurofibromas, however, is well recognized. Eighty percent of patients with neurofibromatosis can be diagnosed by the presence of six or more café au lait spots measuring more than 1.5 cm. The remaining 20% of patients over 21 years of age have multiple axillary freckles or cutaneous tumor and few pigmented spots. In patients under the age of 21 with only a few café au lait spots and dermal tumors, a positive family history and the radiographic demonstration of bone lesions help make the diagnosis.

MANAGEMENT

There is no specific treatment for neurofibromatosis. Close follow-up of the patient is necessary for the recognition of surgically treatable conditions. Surgical removal of cutaneous neurofibromas usually is reserved for those that are functionally compromising or disfiguring. Speech defects may require speech therapy. Neoplasms of the CNS should be dealt with on a case-by-case basis, usually by surgery or radiation therapy. All patients probably should be reevaluated at least every twelve months. Surgical intervention may be necessary for progressive kyphoscoliosis.

WHEN TO CONSULT

When neurological signs or symptoms begin to develop or if neurodiagnostic tests are abnormal, it is generally best to obtain a neurological consultation.

PATIENT EDUCATION

Genetic counseling is indicated for the younger patient with neurofibromatosis. Psychotherapy is often necessary. Patients can be referred to local support groups or to the national neurofibromatosis society (see Appendix). The patient must realize the importance of close follow-up by the physician.

Tuberous Sclerosis

CLINICAL SIGNIFICANCE

Tuberous sclerosis is a hereditary, progressive disease characterized by the triad of adenoma sebaceum, epilepsy, and mental retardation. It has an incidence of 5 to 7 per 100,000 and occurs with the same frequency in both sexes and in all races.

ETIOLOGY

Tuberous sclerosis is a genetic disease with an unknown pathogenesis. One-third of cases are inherited as an autosomal dominant trait; the remaining cases probably are caused by gene mutation. The frequency of the gene ranges from 1 in 20,000 to 1 in 50,000. Characteristic lesions evolve from both ectodermal and mesodermal subtypes, but why they arise is not known. Neuropathologically, there are numerous tubers or sclerotic patches on the surface of the brain cortex that vary in size but are seldom greater than 20 mm in diameter. They often show greatly increased numbers of astrocytic nuclei. Bizarre giant cells can be found in these lesions, and calcification is often seen in the tubers. The lining of the lateral ventricles is frequently the site of numerous small nodules that project into the ventricular cavity (candle gutterings).

SYMPTOMS AND SIGNS

Neurological

The neurological presentation is usually mental retardation or seizures. A common presentation is the development of infantile spasms between four and seven months of age: the child may have been normal to the time of the seizures, or there may have been obvious developmental delay. The older child or adult usually has generalized tonic–clonic or temporal lobe seizures. Retardation rarely occurs without seizures, and acquisition of developmental milestones is delayed. Mental functions continue to deteriorate slowly. Behavioral and affective abnormalities may also occur. Retinal phakomas, which arise near the optic disc, are present in 20% of children with tuberous sclerosis, and in 50% of all patients who are studied closely.

Cutaneous

Hypomelanotic (ash-leaf) macules are the earliest skin lesions and are often present at birth. They may be visible only with the aid of a Wood's lamp. Most macules are leaf-shaped, and they sometimes follow a dermatomal pattern. Three or more macules that measure more than 1 cm in length makes the diagnosis of tuberous sclerosis likely.

Adenoma sebaceum is the best known skin manifestation of the disease. Characteristically, it is a papular, acneform rash over the "butterfly area" of the face. It is usually red and symmetrically distributed and does not involve the upper lip. These lesions gradually increase in size and become yellowish. Adenoma sebaceum is rarely detectable under the age of 2. It is present in 53% to 90% of children by the age of 5, and is present in almost all patients by the age of 35.

A rarer cutaneous sign of the disease is the shagreen patch, which is rarely present in infancy and becomes evident after the first decade of life. Shagreen patches are raised, irregular, yellow-brown areas of "rough" skin. Café au lait spots and vascular nevi are more common in tuberous sclerosis than in the general population, occurring in about 5% of cases.

Visceral

Kidneys are affected more than other viscera (a frequency of about 80%). Angiomyolipomas and renal cysts are common, usually multiple, bilateral, and occult. Cardiac rhabdomyomas occur more commonly in patients with tuberous sclerosis than in the general population: in one series the incidence was as high as 50%. Pulmonary involvement with small numerous cysts is seen more often in females than males and may cause spontaneous pneumothorax.

LABORATORY TESTS
Skull x-rays usually reveal small intracranial calcifications. A CT scan is often diagnostic when there are numerous calcified cortical nodules or calcified subependymal nodules in the lateral ventricle. The EEG often has multiple abnormalities, ranging from multifocal spike waves and sharp waves to generalized spike- and sharp-wave complexes. Renal angiomyolipoma is usually asymptomatic, but it may be detected by CT or ultrasound of the kidneys. Likewise, renal cysts, which are often multiple, may be associated with azotemia or increased blood pressure, and an intravenous pyelogram (IVP) may be diagnostic.

DIAGNOSIS
When the full triad is present (usually in the child or adult), there is little difficulty in diagnosing tuberous sclerosis. In infancy, the diagnosis may be more difficult to make. It is suggested by infantile spasms and by the presence of three or more of the characteristic skin lesions. Calcified subependymal nodules seen on a head CT scan also help establish the diagnosis. Epilepsy alone is not diagnostic because it is nonspecific. When the finding of epilepsy is coupled with abnormal skin lesions or a suggestive CT scan, the diagnosis can be established.

MANAGEMENT
Anticonvulsant therapy for seizures is necessary. Corticosteroids, adrenocorticotropic hormone (ACTH) or valproic acid may be given for infantile spasms. Focal and generalized seizures can be treated with phenobarbital or carbamazepine. There is usually no reason to excise cutaneous lesions. Renal cystic disease or angiomyolipoma eventually may cause renal compromise, so that excision may be necessary. Myocardial symptoms can be controlled with medication; if congestive heart failure develops, diuretics, digitalis, and a low-salt diet may be indicated. If the cardiac rhabdomyosarcomas are obstructive, surgery is necessary.

The disease tends to advance slowly. Of patients who are severely affected, approximately 30% die before the fifth year of life; 50% to 75% die before reaching adulthood. Mental disturbances are common. Malignant transformation of the cerebral subependymal tumor, renal or pulmonary compromise, or cardiac disease may all lead to the demise of the patient. Status epilepticus was once a cause of many deaths, but the advent of anticonvulsants has reduced the death rate from continuous seizures.

WHEN TO CONSULT
Depending on the expertise of the primary care physician, the infant may need to be referred to a neurologist for evaluation of infantile spasms or abnormal neurological development. Referral also may be necessary when seizures develop in the older patient or if malignant transformation of the subependymal brain tubers occurs.

PATIENT EDUCATION
Genetic counseling should be provided for parents of afflicted children, although many cases occur from spontaneous mutation.

Sturge–Weber Syndrome

CLINICAL SIGNIFICANCE
Sturge–Weber syndrome is a rare, often sporadic disorder in which there is a large cutaneous vascular nevus of the face that is associated with contralateral hemiparesis and hemiatrophy, seizures, glaucoma, and mental retardation.

ETIOLOGY
The etiology is not known, but the nevus is clearly congenital and related to the cutaneous distribution of the trigeminal nerve. It tends to be genetically transmitted in an autosomal recessive pattern.

SYMPTOMS AND SIGNS
Convulsions are the earliest symptoms, commonly beginning in the first year of life—often in the neonatal period. The seizures may be of any type, including focal motor, generalized, or partial complex. They frequently occur contralateral to the nevus and are often intractable, with frequent episodes of status epilepticus and progressive mental deterioration. Hemiparesis and hemiatrophy also develop contralateral to the nevus. The facial nevus (port-wine in appearance) commonly involves the forehead; it is rarely bilateral. Raised intraocular pressure is found in one-third of patients with Sturge–Weber syndrome. Buphthalmos results from an antenatal rise in intraocular tension. Homonymous hemianopia is a common visual sign, invariably caused by occipital lobe involvement.

LABORATORY TESTS
The pathognomonic x-ray finding is intracranial calcification with a double contour (trolley-track) that has a gyriform distribution. This is not evident on plain skull x-ray examination in patients under 2 years of age, but becomes detectable and denser later. It can be demonstrated earlier by a CT scan, which

usually also demonstrates atrophy of the involved hemisphere. The EEG usually reveals diffuse epileptiform activity with voltage reduction and paucity of epileptiform discharges over the calcific area.

DIAGNOSIS

The diagnosis is based on the presence of the facial port-wine nevus, seizures, contralateral hemiparesis, hemiatrophy, mental retardation, and glaucoma. The plain x-ray appearance or the CT scan confirms the diagnosis. On rare occasions, otherwise typical Sturge–Weber features occur without the facial nevus but with typical intracranial calcifications.

MANAGEMENT

Treatment is directed mainly toward the seizures, which may be difficult to control even with anticonvulsant medications. Lobectomy or hemispherectomy are necessary occasionally to control seizures. Glaucoma may need to be medically or surgically treated. Special schooling is often necessary because these children have both physical and learning disabilities. Physical therapy is necessary because of hemiplegia; vocational training can be attempted. Often behavioral abnormalities are present and require treatment with psychotropic medications.

WHEN TO CONSULT

The manifestations of Sturge–Weber syndrome are readily apparent and usually do not require confirmation by a neurologist. Because the seizures are often difficult to treat, however, neurological consultation may be necessary to optimally treat the seizure disorder.

MULTIPLE SYSTEM ATROPHY

CLINICAL SIGNIFICANCE

The term multiple system atrophy (MSA) is applied to a group of diseases in which progressive autonomic failure is associated with symptoms and signs of nervous system disease. In general, the neurological diseases that occur with MSA have features of OPCD or striatonigral degenerations. Neuropathologically, MSA differs from Parkinson's disease in its widespread neuronal loss that includes the anterior and lateral horns of the spinal cord. The association of autonomic failure and neurological manifestations is also known as Shy–Drager syndrome, first described by Shy and Drager in 1960.

ETIOLOGY

The pathogenesis of MSA is not known. Biochemical studies reveal marked depression of dopamine beta-hydoxylase concentrations in sympathetic ganglia.

SYMPTOMS AND SIGNS

Patients with MSA tend to develop signs of autonomic failure as the first manifestation of disease. Impotence may be the initial symptom in men. Bladder involvement is manifested clinically as urinary frequency or increased residual urine in the bladder; such involvement tends to occur early in the course of the disease. Constipation can develop. Symptoms of orthostatic hypotension invariably develop. Nonspecific complaints such as weakness, dizziness, and blurred vision may be early symptoms. Postural syncope frequently develops; loss of the ability to sweat often develops in many patients.

Patients with MSA tend to manifest neurological signs within a few years following the onset of autonomic dysfunction, although the neurological symptoms may precede the onset of autonomic dysfunction. Men are affected twice as often as are women, and the disease rarely starts before the fifth decade of life. A parkinsonian-like disorder primarily comprising bradykinesia, rigidity, and tremor is common; it has features of either a disease known as striatonigral degeneration (bradykinesia, rigidity, and loss of postural associated functions with minimal tremor) or of OPCD (predominant limb ataxia, dysarthria, and intention tremor). There is a definite overlap with the symptoms of Parkinson's disease; some patients have features common to both striatonigral degeneration and OPCD.

Dysphagia is common. Intellectual functions are usually retained until the later stages of the disease. Corticospinal tract signs and Babinski's sign also may be evident. Signs of autonomic dysfunction are evident on examination. Orthostatic hypotension, with a fall of blood pressure of greater than 30/20 mm Hg, is an almost universal finding. Horner's syndrome, fixed and dilated pupils, and anhidrosis may be evident. Death usually occurs within seven to ten years after onset of the neurological dysfunction.

LABORATORY TESTS

The majority of laboratory tests utilized document autonomic dysfunction. In patients with MSA that overlaps with OPCD, brain stem and cerebellar atrophy may be evident on a CT scan or MRI. The CSF is usually normal, as are motor nerve conduction velocities. Plasma catecholamines are usually normal when the patient is supine, but they fail to increase with postural changes. Levels of urinary norepinephrine metabolites are reduced, particularly normetanephrine; vanillyl-mandelic acid (VMA) levels are normal.

Bedside diagnostic physiologic tests also help document the level of autonomic dysfunction. These include Valsalva's maneuver and the cold pressor test. An abnormally attenuated response to the intravenous infusion of norepinephrine occurs because of denervation hypersensitivity.

DIAGNOSIS

The degree of autonomic insufficiency can usually be determined easily. Its coexistence with symptoms and signs of parkinsonian-like diseases makes the diagnosis of MSA likely. True Parkinson's disease may be associated with a degree of orthostatic hypotension, but other signs of autonomic dysfunction are usually absent, and there is a lack of pyramidal tract or brain stem signs. Furthermore, when orthostatic hypotension accompanies Parkinson's disease it usually manifests a few years after the neurologic symptoms, not prior to the neurological disturbance—as is common in MSA.

A variety of peripheral neuropathies are accompanied by dysautonomia, including those caused by diabetes mellitus, alcohol, amyloidosis, porphyria, and Guillain-Barré syndrome. The alcoholic or diabetic parkinsonian patient may develop autonomic dysfunction as part of his neuropathic disease and not because of Parkinson's disease. Time determines if a degenerative process such as MSA is present.

365

MANAGEMENT

Treatment is directed toward both the neurologic and autonomic symptoms and signs. Dopaminergic drugs such as L-dopa, bromocriptine, and pergolide usually do not produce neurological improvement; they may exacerbate the orthostatic hypotension. Anticholinergic medications such as benztropine and triphenhexidyl produce some short-lived benefit, as does amantadine. The treatment of orthostatic hypotension (which can be quite disabling) is usually the principal therapy in the patient with MSA. Treatment does not alter the underlying degenerative process, but it may greatly improve the quality of life of the patient.

Treatment modalities for orthostatic hypotension are listed in Table 25-1. Nonpharmacological means of controlling blood pressure are usually of benefit when the magnitude of the blood pressure fall and the resulting symptoms are not severe. Rapid postural shifts, excessive straining, and extreme heat should be avoided. Sleeping in the reverse Trendelenberg position will increase renin secretion and blood pressure. Increased sodium and fluid intake may also help reduce the orthostatic fall in blood pressure. Antigravity stockings can be used to help prevent pooling of blood in the lower extremities when the patient is standing. Atrial tachypacing by means of a transvenous pacemaker also helps reduce the magnitude of the postural blood pressure drop.

A number of medications can be utilized to treat orthostatic hypotension. Flurohydrocortisone has been used for the longest time. It acts by increasing sodium and fluid retention (thereby expanding plasma volume), and it may

TABLE 25-1 TREATMENT OF ORTHOSTATIC HYPOTENSION

Nonpharmacological

Mechanical measures
  Reverse Trendelenberg position of bed
  Elasticized body garment
  Atrial tachypacing via transvenous pacemaker
Plasma and extracellular fluid volume expansion
  High-salt diet
Patient education
  Avoidance of rapid shifts of body position
  Avoidance of excessive heat

Pharmacological

Plasma and extracellular fluid volume expanders
  9α-Flurohydrocortisone
  Prednisone
Vasoconstrictor drugs
  Ephedrine
  Amphetamine
  Methylphenidate
  Vasopressin
  Monoamine oxidase inhibitors
  Propranolol
  Indomethacin
  Dihydroergotamine
  Midodrine
Other drugs
  Clonidine
  Metoclopramide
  Caffeine

sensitize vascular α-adrenergic receptors. The usual dosage is 0.1 to 1.0 mg per day. However, as the autonomic insufficiency increases, flurohydrocortisone often does not control the blood pressure.

Indomethacin, 25 to 50 mg three times daily, has been used successfully to treat orthostatic hypotension; it also benefits the patient with Parkinson's disease (without MSA) who has developed postural hypotension. Indomethacin apparently inhibits the action of certain vasodilatory prostaglandins.

Vasoconstrictor agents, such as amphetamines, ephedrine, and methylphenidate, may control blood pressure transiently, but supine hypertension may develop. Midodrine, an investigational α-adrenergic agonist, and dihydroergotamine are effective for controlling orthostatic hypotension. They do not cause supine hypertension.

WHEN TO CONSULT

It is often advisable to have the neurologist involved with the care of the patient with a movement disorder. Because not all patients with MSA have parkinsonian symptoms, however, referral is *necessary* for those who present with symptoms and signs of an occult neurological disease. In the patient with isolated orthostatic hypotension, a neurological referral may be of value because a careful neurological examination may reveal evidence of nervous system dysfunction. The neurologist can also help evaluate the hypotension and may be able to aid in its treatment.

Bibliography

Engel WK, Siddique T, Nicoloff JT: Effect on weakness and spasticity in amyotrophic lateral sclerosis of thyrotropin-releasing hormone. *Lancet* 1983; 1:73-75. (Original article concerning the beneficial effect of TRH.)

Gomez MR (ed): *Tuberous Sclerosis.* New York, Raven Press, 1979. (Comprehensive review of tuberous sclerosis.)

Harding AE: Classification of the hereditary ataxias and paraplegias. *Lancet* 1983; 1:1151-1155. (A recent attempt to classify the spinocerebellar degenerations; with excellent, succinct discussions.)

Harding AE: Friedreich's ataxia: a clinical and genetic study of 90 families with analysis of early diagnostic criteria and intrafamilial clustering of clinical features. *Brain* 1981; 104:589-620. (An accessible report that defines well the clinical spectrum of Friedreich's ataxia.)

Harding AE, Matthews S, Jones S, et al: Spinocerebellar degeneration associated with a selective defect of vitamin E absorption. *N Engl J Med* 1985; 313:32-35. (Reviews patients with vitamin E-deficient spinocerebellar degeneration.)

Polinsky RJ: Multiple system atrophy: clinical aspects, pathophysiology, and treatment. *Neurol Clin.* 1984; 2:487-489. (Current review that details all aspects of MSA; well referenced.)

Riccardi VM: von Recklinghausen neurofibromatosis. *N Engl J Med* 1981; 305:1617-1627. (State-of-the-art discussion of all aspects of neurofibromatosis.)

Ropper AH: Case records of the Massachusetts General Hospital (#23). *N Engl J Med* 1983; 308:1407-1414. (CPC in a patient with MSA syndrome; superb discussion of this syndrome and its associated conditions.)

Rowland LP (ed): *Human Motor Neuron Diseases.* New York, Raven Press, 1982. (A good overview of human motor neuron diseases.)

Rowland LP: Looking for the cause of amyotrophic lateral sclerosis. *N Engl J Med* 1984; 311:979-981. (An up-to-date discussion of the etiology and treatment of motor neuron disease.)

Shy GM, Drager GA: A neurological syndrome associated with orthostatic hypotension. *Arch Neurol* 1960; 2:511-527. (The classical article that defines a syndrome of autonomic dysfunction with neurological signs that is frequently called Shy–Drager syndrome as a result of this publication.)

Thomas JE, Schirger A, Fealey RD, et al: Orthostatic hypotension. *Mayo Clin Proc* 1981; 56:117-125. (Excellent article dealing with the evaluation and treatment of patients with orthostatic hypotension. Fairly easy to read, and it makes sense.)

26

Congenital and Neonatal Disorders

INTRACRANIAL HEMORRHAGE

The premature neonate has an increasingly favorable chance for survival because of increased technologies available in the neonatal intensive care unit. Consequently, more infants of low gestational age are seen with hemorrhagic intracranial disorders. Intracranial hemorrhage is now at least as common as neonatal asphyxia. This section examines the types of neonatal intracranial hemorrhage seen in the premature and the term infant.

Periventricular–Intraventricular Hemorrhage

CLINICAL SIGNIFICANCE

Intracranical hemorrhage in the premature infant is becoming more apparent with the aid of the CT scan and cranial ultrasound. These intracranial hemorrhages can now be diagnosed readily, ranging from those that are relatively silent to ones that are life-threatening. Periventricular–intraventricular hemorrhage (PVH–IVH) in the preterm baby occurs in approximately 40% to 70% of births in which the infant weighs less than 1500 grams or is under 35 weeks' gestational age. The mortality of PVH–IVH has ranged from 27% to 55%. In general, infants with hemorrhage have higher mortality than those without hemorrhage. These hemorrhages may also occur in the term neonate, but they are quite uncommon (1/1000 births).

ETIOLOGY

In most cases, hemorrhage arises in the vascular germinal plate over the head of the caudate nucleus at the level of the foramen of Monro. Periventricular hemorrhage may be confined to this matrix area or can extend into the lateral ventricles or brain parenchyma. The germinal matrix is highly vascularized and tends to resorb at 35 weeks' gestation. Bleeding may be of arterial or venous origin, and many factors may be responsible for hemorrhage. Hyaline membrane disease in an infant who requires assisted ventilation is commonly seen in premature infants with PVH–IVH. These infants are usually quite sick because of their prematurity and pulmonary disease. In contrast, the site of hemorrhage in the term infant with PVH–IVH is the choroid plexus of the ventricle.

SYMPTOMS AND SIGNS

In the premature infant bleeding usually occurs within 24 to 48 hours after birth, although rarely it is delayed or occurs in utero. With the advent of the CT scan for diagnosis, it is apparent that many hemorrhages are asymptomatic. In one study, 70% of surviving neonates with CT-documented PVH–IVH had no clinical evidence of hemorrhage, whereas 20% of infants without hemorrhage had signs that suggested hemorrhage.

Symptoms may be mild, with irritability or lethargy occurring in the infant with a minimal hemorrhage. In infants with larger hemorrhages (with enlargement of the ventricles or extension into the brain) signs include apnea and bradycardia, extensor posturing, convergent or divergent ocular deviation, nystagmus, lack of oculocephalic or pupillary response, a full and bulging anterior fontanelle, and decreased muscle tone. Clonic limb movements may also be present.

The onset of symptoms in the term neonate with PVH–IVH usually occurs acutely within the first four days of life; 90% of infants, however, have the onset within 24 hours. A delayed onset (10 to 21 days) also has been reported. Seizures are the prominent symptom in almost all term infants with this type of hemorrhage.

LABORATORY TESTS

In infants with larger hemorrhages, inappropriate fall of the hematocrit (by 10% or more) or failure of the hematocrit to rise after transfusion may be evident. Hypocalcemia, acidosis, hypo or hyperglycemia also may be present. Lumbar puncture usually reveals xanthochromic cerebrospinal fluid with increased numbers of red blood cells; however, lumbar puncture is not always diagnostic. A CT scan is the most reliable test for detecting hemorrhage in the high-risk preterm infant. Ultrasonography, using a portable B-mode, real-time scanner is also a reliable noninvasive method for detecting these hemorrhages, especially in the critically ill infant who would be difficult to transport to the CT scan.

DIAGNOSIS

The diagnosis is suspected in the preterm infant who develops signs of central nervous system dysfunction. Many of these hemorrhages are clinically silent and can only be diagnosed by CT or ultrasound.

MANAGEMENT

The asymptomatic infant or one with limited hemorrhages has a good prognosis and an 80% to 90% survival rate; treatment is usually unnecessary. Brain tissue can be damaged by hemorrhage, by increased intracranial pressure with resultant decreased cerebral arterial perfusion, or by resultant posthemorrhagic hydrocephalus. Posthemorrhagic hydrocephalus occurs in 20% to 36% of surviving infants with PVH–IVH. Ventricular enlargement is usually far advanced before clinical signs of hydrocephalus are present (head enlargement, split cranial sutures, full fontanelles). CT or ultrasound can detect such hydrocephalus at least two to four weeks before it is clinically evident.

Repeated lumbar punctures have been utilized to control hydrocephalus. Acetazolamide, which decreases the formation of CSF, has produced improvement in some infants. A high morbidity is associated with using traditional shunt placement in the premature infant, so attempts should be made to avoid a shunt until the infant has grown and matured. Furthermore, spontaneous resolution of hydrocephalus has been noted to occur in six to eight weeks in one-third to one-half of infants with posthemorrhagic hydrocephalus.

WHEN TO CONSULT
It is usually not necessary to consult a neurologist for evaluation and treatment of the infant with PVH–IVH because the neonatologist and pediatrician are usually well-versed in dealing with this problem.

Primary Subarachnoid Hemorrhage

CLINICAL SIGNIFICANCE
Primary subarachnoid hemorrhage is hemorrhage within the subarachnoid space that is not related to a primary source of bleeding in the subdural or epidural space and is not an extension of an intracerebral or intracerebellar hemorrhage. Primary subarachnoid hemorrhage is a common variety of neonatal intracranial hemorrhage. This category includes many newborns who have several hundred red blood cells in their cerebrospinal fluid.

ETIOLOGY
Primary subarachnoid hemorrhage can occur with hypoxia, particularly in the preterm infant. It may result from trauma (precipitous birth, forceps delivery), too.

SYMPTOMS AND SIGNS

The clinical presentation of primary subarachnoid hemorrhage in the neonate is variable. Three major syndromes have been described:

1. Few or no signs of hemorrhage. Minor degrees of hemorrhage occur, predominantly in preterm infants, who account for 75% of infants with primary subarachnoid hemorrhage.

2. Seizures. These occur especially in the full-term infant. They usually appear on the second or third day of life. Interictally these infants appear well. In premature infants, recurrent apneic spells may develop.

3. Massive subarachnoid hemorrhage with marked neurological deterioration and (usually) a rapidly fatal course. These infants often have sustained severe perinatal asphyxia.

LABORATORY TESTS AND DIAGNOSIS
Subarachnoid hemorrhage is often detected by an increase in the number of red blood cells in the spinal fluid, which is usually obtained for some other reason

(eg, to rule out meningitis). Subarachnoid hemorrhage from other sources can be excluded only with the aid of a CT scan. Thus, the diagnosis of primary subarachnoid hemorrhage tends to be a diagnosis of exclusion.

MANAGEMENT

Most infants require no specific treatment. An anticonvulsant can be given to the unusual infant in whom seizures recur. Repeated lumbar puncture is reportedly useful to prevent posthemorrhagic hydrocephalus. In general, the prognosis for infants with the noncatastrophic type of primary subarachnoid hemorrhage is good; more than 90% of full-term infants, in whom seizures are the only manifestation of hemorrhage, are normal on follow-up examination.

WHEN TO CONSULT

Usually it is not necessary to consult a neurologist because the neonatologist or pediatrician are trained to deal adequately with this problem. It is usually not necessary to consult a neurosurgeon, although if persistent hydrocephalus develops shunting may be necessary at a later date.

Cerebellar Hemorrhage

CLINICAL SIGNIFICANCE

The incidence of intracerebellar hemorrhage is increasing as more premature infants survive as a result of technologies available in the neonatal intensive care unit. Of infants less than 32 weeks of gestation or 1500 grams body weight, 15% to 25% develop this form of nervous system hemorrhage. It becomes rare after 32 weeks gestation.

ETIOLOGY

A large percentage of cerebellar hemorrhages seem to be related directly to intraventricular or subarachnoid bleeding. Traumatic laceration of the cerebellum or rupture of major veins, hemorrhagic (venous) infarction, and primary intra-cerebellar hemorrhage occur less commonly.

SYMPTOMS AND SIGNS

Asphyxia and respiratory distress syndrome are common symptoms. Most of these infants have had a catastrophic course, with progressive apnea, bradycardia, falling hematocrit, and bloody spinal fluid. Signs of brain stem dysfunction may also be present, including nystagmus, ocular bobbing, and abnormalities of the oculovestibular reflex. The onset is usually within 48 hours of birth, and death usually results in 12 to 36 hours following the onset of symptoms. The diagnosis is difficult to make on clinical grounds alone. Brain stem signs and bloody CSF should lead to the clinical suspicion of cerebellar hemorrhage.

LABORATORY TESTS AND DIAGNOSIS

If the diagnosis is suspected, a lumbar puncture should *not* be performed because it carries a risk of cerebellar herniation. A CT scan of the head should be performed on an urgent basis; it localizes the hematoma and provides information on the status of the ventricular system (hydrocephalus is common).

MANAGEMENT

As is the case in the adult, the sooner the diagnosis is made and definitive treatment started the better the prognosis for the child. Most cerebellar hemorrhages cannot be managed medically; surgical decompression and evacuation of the clot are necessary. Mannitol or furosemide may help decrease the mass effect and brain stem compression as the infant is being readied for surgery. Because of the concomitant hydrocephalus that may be persistent, a shunt is often necessary.

WHEN TO CONSULT

IF the diagnosis of a cerebellar hemorrhage is considered clinically or confirmed by CT, a neurosurgeon should be consulted immediately.

HYDROCEPHALUS

CLINICAL SIGNIFICANCE

The term hydrocephalus, as the lay expression "water on the brain" indicates, refers to an increase in CSF volume associated with dilatation of the ventricular system. The CSF is produced largely by the choroid plexus of the ventricles. It circulates through the foramina of Monro, third ventricle, aqueduct of Sylvius, and foramina of the fourth ventricle (Luschka's and Magendie's) to enter the subarachnoid space. Most CSF passes over the basal and ambient cisterns to reach the subarachnoid space over the surface of the cerebral hemispheres, where it is absorbed through the arachnoid villi into the cerebral venous sinuses. Hydrocephalus is classified in Table 26-1.

Hydrocephalus is *active* when there is a progressive course and evidence of increased intracranial pressure; it is *occult* when there are no symptoms or signs of increased intracranial pressure; it is *arrested* when ventricular enlargement ceases. Obstructive hydrocephalus refers to obstruction of either the ventricular or extraventricular pathways of CSF flow. In communicating hydrocephalus, obstruction to CSF flow is at the level of absorption through the arachnoid villi.

ETIOLOGY

Although hydrocephalus can result from excessive formation of CSF, most cases are produced by lesions that cause abnormalities of the circulation or absorption of CSF. Obstructive hydrocephalus is the most common form of hydrocephalus.

TABLE 26-1 HYDROCEPHALUS

Obstructive
> Mass lesions (eg, posterior fossa tumors)
> Congenital malformations (eg, Arnold–Chiari malformation)
> Postinflammation (eg, meningitis)
> Posthemorrhage (eg, subarachnoid hemorrhage)

Communicating
> Increased CSF production (eg, choroid plexus palpilloma)
> Defective absorption (eg, normal pressure hydrocephalus)
> Defective venous drainage (eg, lateral sinus thrombosis)

Hydrocephalus *ex vacuo*

Obstruction may occur at any of the sites of CSF flow. In obstruction of the extraventricular CSF pathways, reduction of CSF flow may occur at the subarachnoid spaces of the brain or over the convexities.

Congenital malformations associated with obstructive hydrocephalus include Arnold–Chiari malformation, Dandy-Walker deformity, and aqueductal stenosis. Arnold–Chiari malformation is often associated with hydrocephalus and myelomeningocoele; there is downward displacement of the medulla and cerebellar tonsils into the foramen magnum, which obstructs free flow of CSF. Dandy–Walker deformity results from occlusion of the foramina of the fourth ventricle; the cerebellum is often hypoplastic with a distended fourth ventricle.

Aqueductal stenosis may occur as a sex-linked recessive trait or more commonly as a developmental defect. A gliotic membrane may occlude the aqueduct, or it may be kinked. Postmeningitic ependymitis and tumors of the aqueductal-midbrain area may also lead to an acquired form of aqueductal stenosis.

Midline tumors may cause obstructive hydrocephalus. In children, posterior fossa neoplasms (medulloblastoma, cystic astrocytoma) cause fourth-ventricular obstructon. Suprasellar neoplasms (craniopharyngioma), posterior third ventricular tumors (pinealoma), and colloid cysts of the third ventricle all obstruct CSF flow. Chronic meningeal reactions from bacterial infections or subarachnoid bleeding produce defective absorption of CSF and obliteration or blockage of CSF pathways. A choroid plexus papilloma may produce large volumes of CSF, resulting in communicating hydrocephalus. Chronic otitis media in children may produce thrombosis of the lateral sinus, with hydrocephalus resulting from defective venous drainage.

SYMPTOMS AND SIGNS

The infant with hydrocephalus usually has a large head. Whereas it is usually not difficult to recognize gross enlargement of the head, lesser degrees may be overlooked unless the head circumference is measured and checked against figures for normal children. The hydrocephalic head is abnormal in shape and size. The face, although of normal size, seems small compared to the head. The eyes appear to be displaced downwards. The sclera can be seen between the upper lid and the iris (the "setting-sun" sign). The scalp appears stretched and thin, and scalp veins are prominent.

Abducens nerve palsies may be present, with decreased ocular abduction. Papilledema is uncommon in infants and young children, but retinal hemorrhages and optic atrophy are sometimes seen. The anterior fontanelle is large and may feel tense on palpation. Separation of the cranial sutures often can be palpated. Percussion of the skull may result in a cracked-pot sound (Macewen's sign).

If the progression of hydrocephalus is slow, the child may do well and have few symptoms. If rapid, the child does poorly, with irritability, vomiting, lethargy and seizures. Lower-extremity spasticity or hypertonus is frequently present, and Babinski's sign may be present bilaterally. Visual failure secondary to optic atrophy is a late finding. Chronic hydrocephalus produces motor and intellectual retardation.

LABORATORY TESTS AND DIAGNOSIS

Hydrocephalus is not usually difficult to diagnose in the infant. X-ray of the skull may show evidence of increased intracranial pressure but is not diagnostic. A CT scan is the procedure of choice; it demonstrates the type of hydrocephalus (communicating or obstructive) and associated intracranial abnormalities. Isotope or metrizamide cisternography is usually not necessary in children. The diagnosis of hydrocephalus in the neonate can usually be made from the history and examination, with confirmation by CT.

MANAGEMENT

Pharmacological therapy is usually of limited value in the patient with hydrocephalus. Acetazolamide is of some value for reducing CSF production, but its effect is often short-lived. The treatment is usually surgical.

In most patients, shunting of CSF is necessary. A ventriculoperitoneal shunt is usually the safest and most effective shunt for children. If a tumor or other mass lesion is producing obstructive hydrocephalus, surgical removal of the lesion may be curative, although frequently hydrocephalus persists. Shunts may occasionally occlude as a result of infection or foreign matter; if obstruction occurs, symptoms and signs are usually those of increased intracranial pressure. On occasion, the shunt must be replaced as the child grows. In general, the outcome of hydrocephalus in the child depends on how promptly the diagnosis is made and how severe the underlying disease process is.

WHEN TO CONSULT

The neurologist may be of value to help evaluate the child with possible hydrocephalus. Most pediatricians, however, are well versed in the diagnosis and management of the condition so that neurological consultation is often unnecessary. A neurosurgeon should be consulted, however, when hydrocephalus is diagnosed to help outline a surgical plan.

PERINATAL INFECTIONS

Clinical manifestations of neurological disease are often inconspicuous in the neonate. Prompt recognition of CNS infection of the newborn infant depends on the physician's index of suspicion and predisposing clinical factors. Nervous system infections in the neonate can be acquired during the perinatal period (usually bacterial diseases) or in utero (viral and protozoal diseases). This section examines more common perinatal infections. They are classified by bacterial and nonbacterial origin in Table 26-2.

Bacterial Infections
Bacterial Meningitis

CLINICAL SIGNIFICANCE

Neonatal meningitis is the most common bacterial infection of the nervous system in the neonate. Meningitis is more common in the premature infant than in the full-term infant. There is a close association between neonatal sepsis and neonatal meningitis; approximately 30% of cases of neonatal sepsis spread to the meninges.

TABLE 26-2 PERINATAL NERVOUS SYSTEM INFECTIONS

Bacterial Infections
 Bacterial meningitis
  early onset (within 48 hr of birth)
  late onset (after first week of life)
 Brain abscess
 Infantile botulism

Viral or Protozoal Infections
 Toxoplasmosis
 Rubella
 Cytomegalovirus
 Herpes simplex

ETIOLOGY

There are many risk factors for the development of neonatal meningitis. In addition to prematurity, risk factors related to pregnancy and delivery include maternal sepsis, urinary tract infection, and prolonged rupture of the membranes. Neonatal sepsis and meningitis can also be acquired by the infant from contaminated equipment used for resuscitation or mechanical ventilation. Infected indwelling catheters and exposure of the infant to hospital personnel, family members, or other infected infants are other risk factors related to the neonatal environment.

Neonatal meningitis can arise from a variety of gram-positive and gram-negative bacteria. *Escherichia coli* and group B *Streptococcus* are the cause of the majority of cases. Group B *Streptococcus* is responsible for approximately 40% of cases; and *E coli* and other gram-negative organisms *(Proteus, Pseudomonas)* account for another 30% to 40%. Staphylococci have become less common causative agents, but *Listeria monocytogenes* and other rare organisms account for the remainder of cases. Causes of meningitis that are common after 3 months of age *(Streptococcus pneumoniae, Neisseria meningitidis,* and *Hemophilus influenzae)* rarely give rise to neonatal infection.

SYMPTOMS AND SIGNS

Clinical features of neonatal bacterial meningitis can be separated into two syndromes by age of onset; those with an *early* onset (within 48 hours of birth), and those with a *late* onset (after the first week of life).

  Early Onset. Symptoms and signs develop in 24 to 48 hours after birth, usually in the preterm infant born to a mother who has had obstetrical complications. Non-neurological signs are usually the first manifestation of the disease; they are usually related to sepsis and respiratory disease, and include crying, apnea, hypotension, hyperthermia, feeding disturbances, jaundice, and hepatosplenomegaly. The infant may appear lethargic and irritable. Seizures may occur, but bulging of the anterior fontanelle and nuchal rigidity are infrequent.

  Late Onset. Late-onset meningitis is more likely to have neurological, rather than systemic, manifestations. Fever and feeding disturbances are common. Most infants are stuporous; seizures develop in approximately 75% of cases, with focal seizures occurring in 50%. Focal cerebral signs, including hemiparesis and ocular deviation, are common but variable. Extensor rigidity, which may lead to opisthotonus, occurs in as many as 50% of the infants. Cranial nerve signs, predominantly involving cranial nerves III, VI, and VII, are common. A bulging anterior fontanelle is present in one-third to one-half of the infants.

Various events may complicate the course of neonatal meningitis. Intracranial pressure may be increased, usually as a result of cerebral edema or hydrocephalus. Although cerebral or cerebellar herniation rarely occurs as a result of increased intracranial pressure, cerebral perfusion may be decreased. Ventriculitis secondary to inflammation of the ependymal lining frequently occurs and may lead to obstruction of CSF flow. Acute hydrocephalus is common in the survivors of neonatal bacterial meningitis. Obstruction may be caused by associated ventriculitis or arachnoiditis. Clinical signs are those of increased intracranial pressure and rapid acceleration of head growth.

Extracerebral collections of fluid or intracerebral masses occasionally complicate neonatal meningitis. Hemorrhagic infarction can occur; the onset is usually abrupt, with focal findings on examination. Likewise, brain abscess is uncommon and also is associated with focal abnormalities. Increasing head growth and increased intracranial pressure may also be caused by subdural empyema, another uncommon complication of neonatal meningitis.

LABORATORY TESTS AND DIAGNOSIS

When sepsis is suspected in the newborn, meningitis should also be considered. Blood cultures are ordered for the evaluation of sepsis. They should be ordered even for the infant without signs of overt sepsis because positive blood cultures have been found in 70% to 80% of cases of neonatal meningitis. Liver function tests, complete blood count and clotting profile, electrolyte test, and a blood chemistry profile should also be obtained. Diagnosis is made by lumbar puncture and CSF analysis. The CSF pressure may be elevated, and the CSF picture for neonatal bacterial meningitis is an elevated white blood cell count with PMNs predominating, elevated protein concentration, and a low glucose level. Infants with early onset disease or those with a gram-negative enteric infection tend to have more severe CSF abnormalities. Rarely, CSF is completely normal; and if clinical suspicion remains high, lumbar puncture should be repeated.

The CSF should be cultured to determine the causative bacterium. Gram's and methylene blue stains should be performed on CSF; they will demonstrate organisms in more than 75% of cases. Counterimmunoelectrophoresis allows for rapid determination (usually within two hours) of the bacterial antigen, particularly in the infant who has been receiving antibiotics. A CT scan should be obtained initially to determine the degree of cerebral edema, hydrocephalus, or brain infarction. During the course of treatment, CT can be utilized to determine the degree of ventricular dilation and encephalomalacia and the presence of extracerebral or intracerebral abnormalities.

MANAGEMENT

When the newborn infant is found to have CSF abnormalities compatible with bacterial meningitis, antibiotic treatment should be initiated, even before the positive isolation of the bacterium. In general, CSF in meningitis caused by gram-positive organisms (group B *Streptococcus* or *Listeria)* is more easily sterilized than CSF infected with gram-negative bacteria.

The customary approach is to begin treatment immediately with systemic ampicillin and gentamicin; appropriate changes can be made after the organism is isolated. If group B *Streptococcus* is isolated, penicillin G is the drug of choice. It is also the drug of choice for meningitis caused by *S pneumoniae* and infrequent cases caused by group A *Streptococcus* and nonenterococcal group D *Streptococcus.* Ampicillin is the optimal therapy for meningitis caused by *Listeria.* Ampicillin and gentamicin should be administered for infections caused by *E coli* or other gram-negative organisms. Gentamicin may need to be given by intraventricular injection in the infant with gram-negative bacillary infection who has not responded to systemic therapy.

The CSF should be examined every other day for the first week or until it is sterile. Gram-negative infections should be treated for at least two weeks *after* the CSF is sterilized. Gram-positive meningitis should also be treated for two weeks after the CSF has been sterilized, although exceptions can be made in the infant with rapid clinical and bacteriological response. In all cases, a repeat lumbar puncture is indicated 48 hours after antibiotics are discontinued.

Seizures (Chapter 15) should be treated, although they may be difficult to control. Cerebral edema usually can be controlled by maintaining careful fluid balance; dehydrating agents such as mannitol may cause intracranial fluid shifts and are best avoided. Corticosteriods may be dangerous in the face of severe infection. Inappropriate antidiuretic hormone secretion can develop, and can present initially as a gradual deterioration in the level of consciousness, as a result of cerebral edema and increased intracranial pressure secondary to hypo-osmolality and hyponatremia. Fluid restriction is the initial treatment for this syndrome.

Acute hydrocephalus and subdural effusions may also occur, but both are uncommon. Hydrocephalus often needs to be treated by decompression, usually by a ventriculostomy; antibiotics often need to be injected into the ventricles in these cases because hydrocephalus probably arises from ventriculitis. Subdural effusions usually resolve spontaneously. Brain abscess is uncommon, but if one is apparent on the CT scan and is believed to cause clinical problems, drainage is the best therapy, although cases of neonatal brain abscess treated successfully with antibiotics and without surgery have been reported.

WHEN TO CONSULT

Neurological consultation is usually not necessary during the acute phases of neonatal meningitis. If neurological problems develop (intractable seizures, focal deficits), however, consultation with a neurologist may be indicated. Most pediatricians and neonatologists are well trained to handle neonatal neurological infections and their complications. Neurosurgical consultation is necessary if acute hydrocephalus develops because ventriculostomy and intraventricular injections of antibiotics may be necessary.

Brain Abscess

CLINICAL SIGNIFICANCE

Brain abscess formation rarely occurs during the neonatal period. Most occur as a rare complication of neonatal meningitis. A number of cases of brain abscess in the neonatal period have been reported, however, that are not related to meningitis.

ETIOLOGY

Gram-negative organisms (predominantly *Citrobacter, Proteus,* and *Pseudomonas)* cause most neonatal brain abscesses. *Candida* and *Aspergillus* may also cause a necrotizing brain abscess. *Staphylococcus aureus* has not been reported to cause a neonatal brain abscess.

SYMPTOMS AND SIGNS

Two clinical syndromes have been defined: (1) symptoms and signs of increased intracranial pressure or, uncommonly, focal cerebral signs usually are noted in the first few weeks of life; (2) the acute onset of apparent meningitis occurs, differing little from late-onset neonatal meningitis.

LABORATORY TESTS AND DIAGNOSIS

Diagnosis is made by a CT scan, which demonstrates a mass lesion(s) surrounded by edema, and associated with rim enhancement after the administration of intravenous contrast. When CSF analysis is performed, it often reveals a mononuclear pleocytosis of several hundred cells and an elevated protein concentration (75 to 150 mg/100 mL). The glucose level is usually normal, and the offending bacterium will not be present in the CSF unless there is concomitant bacterial meningitis. Peripheral leukocytosis is often common. Aspiration of the brain lesion is often necessary to make a definite diagnosis.

MANAGEMENT

The treatment of brain abscess is usually surgical, with drainage of the abscess cavity. Craniotomy is not always necessary because CT-guided needle aspiration can be performed through a burr hole. In selected cases, brain abscess can be treated medically with antibiotics alone.

WHEN TO CONSULT

Brain abscess is usually diagnosed without the help of a neurologist. Unexplained or focal neurological signs in a neonate may be a reason for neurological consultation, but this depends on the ability of the attending physician to deal with neonatal bacterial infections. When an abscess is diagnosed, a neurosurgeon should be consulted because surgery is probably necessary.

Infant Botulism

CLINICAL SIGNIFICANCE

Infantile botulism was first recognized in the mid-1970's as a cause of neurological deterioration and death in otherwise healthy infants, mimicking, at times, sudden infant death syndrome.

ETIOLOGY

Infantile botulism occurs when spores of *Clostridium botulinum* are ingested by infants (possibly in honey) and multiply in the intestinal tract, producing botulinum toxin. Bacterial flora in the intestinal tracts of infants less than 1 year of age do not inhibit the growth of *botulinum* as well as the flora of older children or adults. Botulinum toxin impairs the release of acetylcholine, thereby causing motor weakness. Ninety-five percent of cases occur between the ages of 1 and 6 months; the mean age of onset is 10 weeks.

SYMPTOMS AND SIGNS

The presenting problem is usually constipation, which frequently lasts three or more days. Within a few days the infant becomes listless and lethargic and does not eat well. The cry becomes weak, and spontaneous movements decrease. Dysphagia, ptosis, drooling, and extraocular muscle weakness may occur. The pupils may be midposition, with a sluggish reaction to light. The infant develops generalized flaccid weakness and poor head control. The baby is floppy, and deep-tendon reflexes, which may be present during the acute phases of the illness, disappear as it progresses. Respiratory insufficiency may develop.

The course of the disease is variable; some children are affected only mildly with constipation and slight weakness; others have a fulminating course leading to a total paralysis within a few hours of onset. The fulminating course may lead to death and mimics sudden infant death syndrome. In general, progression of weakness usually reaches its maximum during the first or second week of symptoms. The infant stabilizes for a few weeks before recovery begins. If infants are hospitalized, fewer than 5% die. Improvement is usually slow but steady.

LABORATORY TESTS

Routine laboratory tests (BUN, CBC, calcium, electrolytes) are usually normal. Muscle enzymes (creatine phosphokinase), CSF protein, and nerve conduction studies are also normal. Augmentation (facilitation) of compound muscle action potential occurs with repetitive stimulation higher than 10 Hz. Electromyography (EMG) frequently shows brief, small-amplitude, abundant motor-action potentials. *C botulinum* spores may be found in the feces; the toxin may be isolated, too.

DIAGNOSIS

Diagnosis is made in the infant with characteristic signs whose feces contain *C botulinum*. Pupillary abnormalities and the incremental response to repetitive nerve stimulation help differentiate infant botulism from myasthenia gravis.

MANAGEMENT

The infant with suspected botulism should be placed in the intensive care unit and monitored carefully. Management is primarily symptomatic, with special attention to pulmonary status. If weakness is progressive and respiratory failure develops, the infant must be intubated and placed on assisted ventilation. He should not be fed by mouth until it is clear that aspiration will not occur; tube feeding may be necessary. Botulinum antitoxin is not of proven benefit, and systemic antibiotics do not eliminate the organism from the gut. Guanidine hydrochloride, which promotes presynaptic acetylcholine release, is also not of benefit.

WHEN TO CONSULT

A neurologist should be consulted when a previously healthy infant develops unexplained neurological signs that include weakness, hypotonia, and cranial nerve abnormalities. The neurologist can also perform necessary electrodiagnostic studies.

Nonbacterial Infections

Most nonbacterial infections in the neonate are caused by the *TORCH* complex: **TO**xoplasmosis, **R**ubella, **C**ytomegalovirus, and **H**erpes simplex. Unlike manifestations of neonatal bacterial meningitis, these diseases can be protean in their presentation. Many are acquired in utero any time between the first trimester and delivery. Collectively, these diseases are a common cause of learning disability and mental retardation.

Toxoplasmosis

CLINICAL SIGNIFICANCE

Congenital toxoplasmosis, caused by the protozoan *Toxoplasma gondii,* results in a high incidence of neurological damage to the infant.

ETIOLOGY

Congenital toxoplasmosis is acquired in utero by transplacental passage of the parasite. A few infants are infected during the first or second trimester (20 to 25%); 65% are infected during the third trimester. The severity of the disease, however, is greater in the infant infected during one of the first two trimesters. Meningoencephalitis and hydrocephalus frequently result. Toxoplasmosis has a predilection for periventricular areas, but diffuse disease can often be found elsewhere. If the disease is severe, cerebral destruction may occur. Microcephaly that occurs in 15% of affected infants is the result of the necrotizing brain process.

SYMPTOMS AND SIGNS

Clinically asymptomatic cases of congenital toxoplasmosis occur more often than symptomatic cases. Approximately two-thirds of symptomatic infants with *Toxoplasma* infection have primarily a neurological syndrome of seizures, signs of meningoencephalitis, hydrocephalus, and diffuse intracranial calcifications or microcephaly. Ninety percent of infected infants have chorioretinitis, which is typically bilateral and prominent in the macular regions. Chorioretinitis is usually present in the newborn infant, but it may be delayed in appearance by several months. The systemic syndrome consists of signs of anemia, hepatosplenomegaly, and hyperbilirubinemia; in these infants CNS involvement is often not evident clinically. Chorioretinitis occurs in two-thirds of patients with systemic involvement.

LABORATORY TESTS

Most cases of congenital toxoplasmosis are identified by serological techniques, including the Sabin–Feldman dye test and the IgM fluorescent antibody test. The latter test is more specific and is the preferred test to document toxoplasmosis. At times, the organism can be identified in concentrated CSF by Wright's stain. An elevated protein level and mononuclear pleocytosis are often present in CSF; the latter indicates meningoencephalitis, which can occur in symptomatic and asymptomatic patients. Diffuse cerebral calcifications are evident on skull x-rays; a CT scan often demonstrates intracranial calcifications, hydrocephalus, and cortical lesions. Serum IgM levels are often increased, and thrombocytopenia and hyperbilirubinemia are evident in patients with systemic disease.

Diagnosis

The diagnosis is usually considered in the newborn with bilateral chorioretinitis, seizures, and intracranial calcifications who may have the other manifestations discussed above. Serological tests help confirm the diagnosis.

Management

In general, the infected infant with signs of the disease is a poor candidate for antimicrobial therapy. However, some damage is reversible and further neurological damage is preventible by therapy directed against the organism. Pyrimethamine and sulfadiazine have been utilized; treatment is usually for 21 days. Folinic acid should also be administered because pyrimethamine is a folic acid antagonist. Patients wtih asymptomatic congenital toxoplasmosis should also be treated with this triple drug regimen. Data from one series suggest that infants so treated have higher IQs than those who are not treated.

Only 9% of infants with congenital toxoplasmosis with prominent neurological manifestations are normal on follow-up examination. The remaining 91% have serious disturbances of higher brain functions, including retardation, spasticity, and seizures; 70% also have significant visual impairment. Congenital toxoplasmosis with prominent systemic signs also has a poor neurological outcome: only 16% of patients remain normal. Of infants with asymptomatic subclinical infection, approximately 25% have chorioretinitis, which may not appear until after the neonatal period. Many of these children develop intellectual deficits that may have been prevented by treatment.

Rubella

Clinical Significance and Etiology

Rubella (German measles) virus is a togavirus that induces chronic, persistent infection in the fetus. Congenital rubella syndrome causes a number of congenital abnormalities (cataracts, cardiovascular lesions) and mental retardation. Infection with rubella virus occurs during intrauterine life by the transplacental passage of the virus. The earlier in pregnancy the infection occurs, the greater the severity of the clinical disease. Neurological deficits are most common with infection that occurs during the first two months; they do not occur with infection that occurs after the fourth month. Meningoencephalitis, vasculopathy, microcephaly, and impaired myelination may occur with congenital rubella infection.

Symptoms and Signs

Approximately two-thirds of infants are asymptomatic in the neonatal period, but most develop evidence of disease in the first few years of life. Intrauterine growth retardation, hepatosplenomegaly, thrombocytopenia, and bony abnormalities are common clinical manifestations. Pulmonic stenosis and patent ductus arteriosus are characteristic cardiac defects.

Neurological features are present in 50% to 75% of cases. Meningoencephalitis, verified by CSF analysis, is present in most infants. Lethargy, hypotonia, and irritability are common features. Opisthotonus and retrocollis may also occur, probably because of meningeal irritation. Seizures appear in approximately 15% of infants. Microcephaly, which develops subsequently, is uncommon at birth. White or pearly cataracts (centrally located) and chorioretinitis (salt-and-pepper appearance) are commonly seen. Hearing loss is present in 20% of infants.

LABORATORY TESTS

The rubella virus can be isolated from the CSF or the nasopharynx. The IgM content of the cord blood is elevated, and can be used as evidence of specific intrauterine infection. The persistence of hemagglutination inhibitor titers after 4 to 6 months of age is diagnostic of congenital rubella infection. Thrombocytopenia, leukopenia, and elevated liver function tests may also be seen. Analysis of CSF reveals a mononuclear cell pleocytosis and an elevated protein level.

DIAGNOSIS

Congenital rubella infection is suspected when there is a history of maternal exposure to or infection by the virus during pregnancy or when physical signs in the newborn suggest the diagnosis. Cataracts, cardiac defects, "salt-and-pepper" chorioretinitis, and CSF pleocytosis suggest the diagnosis and tend to distinguish rubella from other TORCH-complex diseases.

MANAGEMENT

There is no specific treatment for congenital rubella. Attention should be paid to systemic manifestations of the disease. Auditory function should be assessed to see if there is hearing loss, which may be treatable with a hearing aid. Cataract surgery is often necessary to preserve vision. At 18 months of age, only 10% of infants are normal. Delayed neurological deficits and spasticity are present in 50% of infants; 80% have microcephaly and 70% have hearing loss. Behavioral disturbances (hyperactivity, learning disturbances) are present in 50% of infants, necessitating specially structured educational programs for many of them.

Cytomegalovirus

CLINICAL SIGNIFICANCE

Congenital cytomegalovirus (CMV) infection is transplacentally transmitted to the fetus; it is the most common congenital infection. Most infants are asymptomatic, but they may suffer neurological sequelae.

ETIOLOGY

Cytomegalovirus is a DNA-containing virus. During pregnancy, the organism is transmitted to the fetus during maternal infection. Maternal infection is common, occuring from 3% to 6% of pregnancies; the infection is usually asymptomatic, but may be manifested as a mononucleosis-like illness. Significant fetal CMV infection occurs during the first or second trimester. Fifty percent of infants born to mothers infected during pregnancy develop congenital infection. Ten to thirty percent of infants acquire CMV in the first four to eight weeks of life; there is no evidence that CNS disease occurs in these cases. Meningoencephalitis, periventricular necrotizing inflammation (resulting in periventricular calcifications), microcephaly, and disturbances of neuronal migration are seen on pathologic examination.

Symptoms and Signs

Ninety-five percent of cases of CMV infection are asymptomatic in the neonatal period. The most common neurological findings are meningoencephalitis (documented by CSF examination), microcephaly, and periventricular calcifications; seizures may also occur. Hepatosplenomegaly, petechiae, and ecchymoses are common non-neurological manifestations.

Laboratory Tests

Biochemical abnormalities of liver dysfunction and hemolytic anemia are commonly present. The virus is readily isolated from the nares and throat. Complement fixation and fluorescent antibody tests are useful serological tests for diagnosis. A persistently elevated titer of IgG immunoglobulin suggests infection. The CSF is often marked by mononuclear pleocytosis and an elevated protein level. Skull x-rays demonstrate periventricular calcifications, which are readily apparent on CT.

Diagnosis

Periventricular calcifications or microcephaly, CSF pleocytosis, and intrauterine growth retardation suggest congenital CMV infection. Serological studies or virus isolation also help make the diagnosis.

Management

There are no effective chemotherapeutic agents for treating congenital CMV. Treatment is convervative, with attention paid to hematological and hepatic dysfunction. Because the infected infant sheds CMV in his saliva or urine, he is a threat to other infants in the nursery; isolation precautions should be instituted. Of infants with the symptomatic neurological syndrome, approximately 95% have major neurological sequelae (mental retardation, seizures) or die. Of infants with systemic signs but without neonatal neurological deficits, approximately 50% are normal and 16% exhibit major neurological sequelae or die. In the asymptomatic group, approximately 13% of children develop sensorineural hearing loss, which often is not discovered until language development is impaired; a lower IQ has been reported in asymptomatic patients.

When to Consult

A neurologist is frequently not consulted for the child with CMV, toxoplasmosis, or rubella. If seizure control is difficult to achieve, however, or if the child has a learning disability, a neurologist may be of help.

Herpes Simplex

CLINICAL SIGNIFICANCE

Neonatal herpes simplex virus (HSV) infection occurs in approximately 1 of every 7500 deliveries; 40% of those will occur in the premature infant. In contrast to other TORCH diseases, HSV infection uniformly produces clinical disease.

ETIOLOGY

Neonatal herpes infection is usually acquired by direct contact of the infant's eyes, skin, or mouth with herpetic lesions in the mother's infected birth canal. Less commonly, transplacental passage of the virus causes intrauterine infection. Seventy-five percent of neonatal infections are caused by herpes simplex virus type 2. The virus usually causes significant CNS involvement. Meningoencephalitis and associated Cowdry type A intranuclear inclusions, areas of multifocal brain necrosis, and subsequent multicystic encephalomalacia are common neuropathological findings.

SYMPTOMS AND SIGNS

Neonatal herpes simplex infection may be disseminated or local; disseminated disease accounts for 50% to 70% of all cases and usually occurs at the end of the first week of life. Fever, vomiting, and feeding difficulties may be the first symptoms, followed (in 50% of infants) by a neurological syndrome characterized by irritability, stupor, and seizures that often progresses to opisthotonus and coma. In 50% of cases neurological involvment is not evident. In either syndrome, hepatomegaly, jaundice and bleeding are common; skin vesicles are present in 50% of cases of disseminated disease.

Localized herpes infection occurs in the absence of systemic involvement. Nervous system involvement in localized disease occurs later than it does with disseminated involvement—on the average of 11 days later. Irritability and stupor, seizures, and eventually coma commonly occur. Almost all localized cases have visible herpetic lesions, usually of the skin, but abnormalities of the eye or oral cavity may develop.

LABORATORY TESTS

The virus often can be isolated from scrapings of vesicular lesions and when stained, multinucleated giant cells and intranuclear inclusion bodies are evident. Serological studies are less useful for diagnosis. Analysis of CSF reveals meningoencephalitis with pleocytosis (commonly mononuclear) and increased protein levels; in severely affected infants, the glucose level is low and red blood cells may be present. A CT scan may demonstrate multifocal areas of hypodensity, often in the temporal lobes. The EEG may be slowed diffusely or focally, with evidence of epileptiform discharges that at times occur in a periodic fashion.

DIAGNOSIS

The clinical pattern of neonatal HSV infection is usually distinctive: vesicular rash, keratoconjunctivitis, seizures, and CSF evidence of meningoencephalitis. The lack of microcephaly, intracranial calcifications and hydrocephalus differentiates it from other TORCH-related diseases.

MANAGEMENT

Prevention of the disease should be attempted because virtually all cases of neonatal HSV infection are acquired at the time of delivery. Cesarean section should be performed on all pregnant women with genital herpes; if the membranes have ruptured, however, cesarean section within four hours of rupture is associated with a low risk of neonatal infection, but it is greater than 80% if delayed for more than six hours. Fluid overload should be avoided in the infected infant because infection causes cerebral edema. The benefits of mannitol and steroids are unclear. The antiviral drugs adenine arabinoside (Ara-A) and acyclovir are somewhat effective for decreasing morbidity and mortality, especially if disease is localized to the CNS. Mortality is 60% to 80% in patients with disseminated disease; 50% of survivors suffer significant neurological deficits. Sixty percent of patients with localized nervous system disease survive, but two-thirds of them suffer serious neurological sequelae. Thirty to fifty percent of infants with HSV infection that is clinically localized to the skin or eye have neurological sequelae on follow-up examination.

WHEN TO CONSULT

When faced with an infant with or without vesicular lesions but with neurological symptoms, neurological consultation may be indicated, especially if neonatal HSV infection is suspected. In general, the neonatologist or pediatrician can diagnose and treat any neonatal infection, although some neurological complications may need to be evaluated by a neurologist.

CEREBRAL PALSY

Cerebral palsy refers to motor manifestations of nonprogressive brain damage sustained during prenatal or postnatal life. Classification is based on the neurological signs listed in Table 26–3. In general, there are four major types of cerebral palsy; at times, two or three types occur in the same patient.

CLINICAL SIGNIFICANCE

Cerebral palsy is not rare. Although the incidence is variable in study to study because of recognition and reporting, it is estimated to occur in one to three of every 1,000 live births. Incidence probably has decreased over the last 20 years,

---

TABLE 26-3 CLINICAL CLASSIFICATION OF CEREBRAL PALSY

Spastic

    Monoplegia (1 limb involved)
    Paraplegia (legs only)
    Diplegia (same limbs bilaterally)
    Hemiplegia (1 side of body)
    Triplegia (3 extremities)
    Quadriplegia (all 4 extremities)

Dyskinetic

    Athetotic
    Mixed

Ataxic

Mixed

---

especially with dyskinetic and diplegic forms. The hemiplegic type now accounts for a higher percentage of the total cases than it once did.

ETIOLOGY

There is usually no single underlying cause of cerebral palsy. Anoxia and ischemia commonly are implicated. A birth weight of less than 2,500 grams is the single most frequent factor associated with cerebral palsy. Any complication of childbirth may predispose the infant to the development of cerebral palsy. Approximately 70% to 90% of cases of spastic hemiplegic cerebral palsy are congenital and are the result of brain damage in the perinatal period. Definite perinatal abnormalities are seen in 40% of these infants; unknown factors account for the remaining 30% to 50% of cases. Ten to thirty percent of hemiplegic cerebral palsy is acquired as a result of inflammation, trauma, or vascular causes.

The quadriplegic type is often associated with perinatal factors, including hypoxia and asphyxia; a prolonged or precipitous delivery is common. Diplegic forms are almost always congenital, with 50% of infants having been born prematurely or having a low birth weight. A common causative factor in the mature neonate is preeclampsia; in the premature infant, antepartum hemorrhage is implicated. The dyskinetic type is usually caused by ataxia or hyperbilirubinemia. The ataxic form is commonly associated with hydrocephalus, although in almost 40% of cases the cause is unknown.

SYMPTOMS AND SIGNS

Spastic forms of cerebral palsy are most common; they occur in two-thirds of all patients. Thirteen percent of patients with cerebral palsy have the mixed type.

Spastic Cerebral Palsy
Quadriplegia (Tetraplegia)

This form of cerebral palsy accounts for 5% of cases. It usually includes some of the most severely handicapped children. Spasticity is the prominent symptom; usually, the legs are impaired more than the arms. The infant usually exhibits a paucity of movement of all the extremities. Dysarthria and feeding difficulties are common, and drooling is often a significant problem. Recurrent aspiration pneumonia often occurs, particularly during the first two years of life. Convulsions occur in at least 50%. Most children remain at a neonatal stage of development; their IQ is often less than 50.

The posture of the infant with spastic quadriplegia is flexion of the upper extremities with the hands held tightly fisted and the legs hyperextended. In addition to spasticity, ankle clonus is often present with bilateral Babinski's sign. Contraction of the lower extremity in the equinovarus position, and of the wrists and elbows in the flexed posture, are common.

Hemiplegia

Seventy to ninety percent of cases of hemiplegic cerebral palsy are congenital; the rest are acquired postnatally. Infants with spastic hemiplegia have involvement of the limbs on one side of the body. The right side is involved in more than two-thirds of cases. The arm is affected more often than the leg is; the face is rarely affected.

The characteristic posture of these children is flexion of the arm with the hand held in a fisted position and the leg extended. One-third of children with this form of cerebral palsy will have a seizure disorder, and almost one-third have some degree of mental retardation. Motor milestones are delayed. Hand preference is demonstrated early on, almost always before 12 months of age. Sitting balance develops late; walking is delayed. When the child does walk, it is with a hemiplegic gait: dragging of the affected leg with the foot held in an equinovarus position and with reduced or absent arm swing. Spastic limbs may be smaller and thinner than the other extremities. Hyperreflexia, ankle clonus, and Babinski's sign are common.

Diplegia

Spastic diplegia usually consists of bilateral spasticity of the arms or legs. In most cases the legs are involved more often than the arms. Spastic diplegia is found more frequently in premature infants. The child may have normal early developmental milestones, but walking is commonly delayed.

Examination reveals increased tone in the legs: thighs held in an adducted posture, extension of the lower extremities, and equinovarus posturing of the feet. When the child is suspended upright the legs tend to cross ("scissoring") because of increased tone and spasticity of the adductors. Hyperreflexia, ankle clonus, and Babinski's sign are common. The gait is clumsy and dyscoordinated, with a tendency to toe-walking. The arms may have a variable degree of involvement; associated movements may be reduced when walking, and occasionally the arms are weak.

Atonic diplegia is a variant of this type in which hypotonicity and weakness of the legs are present and are associated with normal or increased deep-tendon reflexes. In general, children with spastic diplegia do not have significant intellectual impairment; and most develop speech at a normal rate.

Dyskinetic

The dyskinetic type is dominated by involuntary movements. Athetosis is the form of dyskinesia most often seen, in which movements affect mainly the distal limbs. They are slow, writhing, and purposeless, involving agonist and antagonist muscle groups and increased by attempted voluntary movement. Choreiform movements may also be present, often with athetosis. Choreiform movements are quicker, more jerky, and most marked proximally. The combination of choreic and athetoid movements usually results in rapid movements of the distal extremity, with persistent hypertonicity and writhing movements of the limb; dyskinesias cease with sleep. These movements typically are not seen in the neonatal period; they usually appear as soon as a few months or as long as a few years after birth.

Coordination of body movements is difficult. Difficulty with swallowing and articulation are common. There is difficulty controlling the head; facial grimacing and drooling are frequently observed. Many patients also have spasticity, but seizures and intellectual deterioration are not common.

Ataxic

As many as 10% of cases of cerebral palsy are the ataxic type. Most are congenital and are not diagnosed during early life. Most of these children have normal intelligence, but they may be delayed in reaching motor milestones. Ataxia may occur alone, or may be associated with spasticity of the legs. Patients with ataxic cerebral palsy are usually floppy as infants. Because hydrocephalus can be a cause, head enlargement may be evident. Hypotonia tends to decrease by 12 weeks of age; soon after, the legs become spastic. Sitting ability is delayed and is often associated with head titubation. Ataxia may be asymmetrical, but usually involves arms, legs, and the trunk. In some children, spasticity is absent in the arms. Cerebellar speech may also develop.

Mixed

Some patients with cerebral palsy have a combination of forms of cerebral palsy. Dyskinetic and spastic features may coexist in quadriplegic and hemiplegic patients. Because multiple areas of nervous system damage often account for the cerebral palsy, multifocal features are not unexpected or uncommon.

LABORATORY TESTS

Laboratory tests are of limited value for the diagnosis of cerebral palsy. The EEG may be abnormal, with diffuse or focal slowing; epileptiform discharges may be evident. A wide range of abnormalities can be demonstrated by CT, depending on the type of cerebral palsy. Porencephalic cysts, infarcts, or other developmental abnormalities may be seen. Hydrocephalus may be evident, primarily in the patient with the ataxic or diplegic type.

DIAGNOSIS

The diagnosis of cerebral palsy is based primarily on neurological examination and the child's development history. Crucial to the diagnosis is that the course of cerebral palsy is not progressive even though clinical manifestations can change. Distinction between progressive and nonprogressive disorders is made on clinical grounds, particularly by the history. Because cerebral palsy encompasses many conditions, no test or CT finding is specific for it. Hereditary and metabolic disorders also must be considered.

MANAGEMENT

Management of the child with cerebral palsy is multidisciplinary. The goals of therapy should be to improve function, provide education and vocational support, and help the patient adjust emotionally to his disability. In infancy, range-of-motion exercises can be the first form of therapy. An attempt should be made to help the child develop head and balance control and truncal stability. The infant with poor motor function should not be allowed to lie in a crib all day. A specially designed infant seat (with padding on the sides and head guards) allows the child to sit up and be exposed more to the surroundings. For older children, a similar type of wheelchair may be useful.

Some children with spastic hemiplegia have one leg that is shorter than the other, usually resulting in a noticeable limp. An orthopedic shoe with a raised sole

389

will equalize the length of the legs and permit easier ambulation. Severe spasticity can result in fixed posturing of the limbs; surgical procedures are of some benefit in reducing spasticity and contraction deformities. Baclofen can be used to reduce spasticity. Diazepam or L-dopa may reduce the dyskinetic movements. Cerebellar stimulation by implanted electrodes reduces spasticity in some children and adults with cerebral palsy, but this procedure is not widely accepted or performed. Attention to the child's education is important; often, he needs a special school or classroom.

WHEN TO CONSULT

At some point—early or as part of the multidisciplinary evaluation—a neurologist should be involved with the care of the infant or child with cerebral palsy. Management of seizures or spasticity can be directed by the neurologist. Once the diagnosis is made and complications controlled as much as possible, however, the role of the neurologist is limited.

PATIENT EDUCATION

Parents should be counseled about their child's problem. An early initiation of physical therapy is important. Some communities have local support groups, and the National Cerebral Palsy Foundation offers services to patients and their families (see Appendix).

Bibliography

Bell WE, McCormick WF: *Neurologic Infections in Children,* ed 2. Philadelphia, W.B. Saunders, 1981. (Comprehensive review of pediatric nervous system infections.)

Pickett J, Berg B, Chaplin E, et al: Syndrome of botulism in infancy: Clinical and electrophysiological study. *N Engl J Med* 1976; 295:770-772. (Article that called attention to infant botulism.)

Russell HM. *Observations on the Pathology of Hydrocephalus.* London, Her Majesty's Printing Office, 1949. (A classical monograph on the subject of hydrocephalus.)

Schwartz JF, Ahmann PA, Dykes FD, et al: Neonatal intracranial hemorrhage and hypoxia, in *Neurologic Emergencies in Infancy and Childhood.* Philadelphia, Harper & Row, 1984, pp 37-46. (Up-to-date reference on pediatric emergencies; well referenced, comprehensive, and easy to read.)

Swaiman KF: Cerebral palsy-perinatal motor impairment, in Swaiman KF, Wright FS (eds): *The Practice of Pediatric Neurology,* ed 2. St Louis, C.V. Mosby, 1982, vol 1, pp 444-471. (Comprehensive review of cerebral palsy in the Bible of pediatric neurology.)

Volpe JJ: in *Neurology of the Newborn.* Philadelphia, W.B. Saunders, 1981, pp 141-298. (In-depth review of neonatal hemorrhage.)

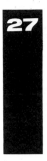

Diseases of the Spinal Cord

Spinal cord diseases (myelopathies) have a wide variety of causes (Table 27-1). The most common are cord compressions caused by cervical spondylosis (Chapter 9), spinal cord injuries (Chapter 38), and epidural metastatic carcinoma (Chapter 40). Less common, but occasionally encountered in outpatient practice are the disorders considered in this chapter: subacute combined degeneration, acute transverse myelopathy, spinal cord tumors, spinal cord infarction, and syringomyelia.

SPINAL CORD SYNDROMES

A careful history and physical examination can often localize a patient's disorder to a spinal cord syndrome. Three particular symptoms and signs immediately suggest a spinal cord lesion: severe motor and/or sensory disturbance in both legs that spares the arms, acute new urinary retention or incontinence, and a bilateral thoracic sensory level.

The presence of Brown–Séquard syndrome immediately localizes the lesions to the spinal cord. In this functional hemisection of the cord, the patient develops (below the level of the lesion) ipsilateral upper motor neuron motor signs: ipsilateral loss of vibration and position sensation and contralateral loss of pain and temperature sensation. Some patients have segmental sensory loss or segmental lower motor neuron dysfunction at the level of the lesion.

In the cervical cord syndrome, there is lower motor neuron dysfunction (eg, atrophy, fasciculations) in the arm, hand or shoulder muscles at the level of the lesion and dermatomal sensory loss of the affected cervical segments. Below the level of the lesion, there is upper motor neuron dysfunction (eg, spastic, hyperreflexic legs, upgoing toes), and there may be a "sensory level" (reduced sensation to all modalities below the level of the lesion). There may be radicular pain in the upper extremities.

TABLE 27 ETIOLOGY OF MYELOPATHY

Infection	**Mechanical compression**
Bacterial	Cervical spondylosis
Pyogenic abscess	Rheumatoid arthritis
Tuberculoma	Ankylosing spondylitis
Syphilitic myelitis	Acute intervertebral disc protrusion
Fungal	
Aspergillosis	**Neoplasms**
Blastomycosis	Primary
Candidiasis	Metastatic
Coccidioidomycosis	Remote effects
Cryptococcosis	
Parisitic	**Physical agents**
Echinococcosis	Decompression sickness
Cysticercosis	Electrical injury
Paragonimiasis	Radiation
Schistosomiasis	
Viral	**Toxins and drugs**
Poliomyelitis	Nitrous oxide
Other enteroviruses	Intra-arterial contrast agents
Herpes zoster	Myelographic contrast agents
Rabies	Spinal anesthetics
Parameningeal	Cresyl phosphates
Acute epidural abscess	Iodochlorhydroxyquinolone
Chronic epidural abscess	
	Metabolic and nutritional
Immunological	Diabetes mellitus
Postinfectious	Pernicious anemia
Postviral	Pellagra
Postexanthematous	Chronic liver disease
Post vaccination	
Acute transverse myelitis	**Vascular**
Multiple sclerosis	Infarction
	Epidural hematoma
Trauma	Arteriovenous malformations
Cord compression or contusion	Hematomyelia
Cord transection	
Hematomyelia	**Inflammatory**
	Systemic lupus erythematosus
Developmental	Mixed connective tissue disease
Spina bifida	Arachnoiditis
Syringomyelia	Acute necrotizing myelitis

Adapted from Kincaid JC, Dyken ML: Myelitis and myelopathy, in Baker AB, Joynt RJ (eds): *Clinical Neurology*, vol 3. Philadelphia, Harper & Row, 1986, chapter 48. Used with permission.

In the thoracic cord syndrome, the arms are spared. The legs exhibit upper motor neuron signs as in the cervical cord syndrome, but the sensory level is on the trunk. There may be thoracic radicular pain in the chest, back, or abdomen.

In the lumbosacral cord syndrome, because of frequent concomitant involvement of the cauda equina, there is a mix of upper motor neuron and lower motor neuron signs in the legs and segmental sensory loss. Bowel and bladder dysfunction is an early sign. Pain often radiates into the legs. Table 27-2 lists the signs that differentiate a syndrome of the cauda equina and a syndrome of the lumbosacral spinal cord (conus medullaris).

In the central cord syndrome—as seen in syringomyelia, intramedullary spinal cord tumors, and in spinal cord trauma—the most important sign is dissociation

TABLE 27-2 CLINICAL FEATURES OF CAUDA EQUINA AND CONUS MEDULLARIS LESIONS

	CONUS MEDULLARIS	CAUDA EQUINA
Spontaneous pain	Not common or severe; bilateral and symmetric; in perineum or thighs	May be most prominent symptom; severe; radiating; may be unilateral or asymmetric; in perineum, thighs and legs, back or bladder; distribution of sacral nerves
Sensory changes	Saddle distribution; bilateral, usually symmetric; dissociation of sensation	Saddle distribution; may be unilateral and asymmetric; all forms affected; no dissociation of sensation
Motor changes	Symmetric; not marked; fasciculations may be present	Asymmetric; more marked; may be atrophy; usually no fasciculations
Reflex changes	Only Achilles reflex absent	Patellar and Achilles reflexes may be absent
Bladder and rectal symptoms	Involvement early and marked	Involvement occurs late and is less marked
Trophic changes	Decubiti common	Decubiti less marked
Sexual functions	Erection and ejaculation impaired	Involvement less marked
Onset	Sudden and bilateral	Gradual and unilateral

Adapted from DeMyer W: Anatomy and clinical neurology of the spinal cord, in Baker AB, Joynt RJ (eds): *Clinical Neurology*, vol 3. Philadelphia, Harper & Row, 1986, p 20. Used with permission.

of sensory loss. Because of the central cord location of the segmentally decussating spinothalamic fibers, there is loss of pain and temperature sensation at the level of the lesion. Position and vibration sensations are spared because these sensory modalities ascend uncrossed in the posterior columns and decussate in the brain stem.

ACUTE TRANSVERSE MYELOPATHY

Acute transverse myelopathy (ATM) is a rare disorder with an approximate annual incidence of 1 to 2 per million. Because it is untreatable, its principal significance lies in its differentiation from acute myelopathies that can be treated.

The etiology of ATM is unknown, but about one-third of cases develop after a viral illness. Pathologically, the spinal cord undergoes an inflammatory demyelination that in the most severe cases progresses to frank necrosis.

The initial symptoms of ATM are usually leg paresthesias, leg weakness, and/or back pain. The disorder progresses for over seven to ten days before it produces its maximal deficit, which usually includes bowel and bladder sphincter disturbances and varying degrees of paralysis and sensory loss below the level of the lesion. The midthoracic region is affected most often. After 10 to 14 days, most patients begin to improve. About half of patients have a good outcome, regaining sphincter control and the ability to walk. Half of the remaining group recover incompletely, and the other half do not recover at all.

Laboratory test findings are nonspecific. Occasionally a peripheral leukocytosis is present. Cerebrospinal fluid is often normal, but one-third of cases are marked by CSF mononuclear pleocytosis and/or an elevated CSF protein. CSF IgG and gamma globulin levels are rarely elevated.

The diagnosis is made using myelography or magnetic resonance imaging (MRI) to exclude other types of acute myelopathy. All patients should undergo an emergency total myelogram to exclude spinal cord compression. The patient who develops acute myelopathy but has a normal myelogram fits the diagnostic criteria for acute transverse myelopathy.

Management is supportive and expectant. Evidence does not suggest that ACTH or oral glucocorticoid therapy is beneficial—although both are used widely. "Minidose" heparin (5,000 U subcutaneously every 12 hours) should be used to counter calf thrombophlebitis, a common complication. Contrary to what is often written, there is a low incidence (around 7%) of patients who develop multiple sclerosis after having an attack of ATM.

SPINAL CORD TUMORS

Neoplasms originating in or compressing the spinal cord are always part of the differential diagnosis in the patient presenting with a progressive myelopathy. The classification of spinal cord tumors is listed in Table 27-3. Primary spinal cord tumors (except for epidural metastatic carcinoma) are rarer (about one-sixth as common) than primary brain tumor. Metastatic carcinoma that produces epidural cord compresson is more common (Chapter 40). Spinal cord tumors are particularly rare in patients under the age of 20.

TABLE 27-3 CLASSIFICATION OF SPINAL CORD TUMORS

Intramedullary
  Astrocytoma*
  Oligodendroglioma
  Ependymoma*
  Metastatic carcinoma

Extramedullary but intradural
  Meningioma*
  Neurolemmona*
  Ependymona

Extradural
  Metastatic carcinoma, sarcoma, lymphoma*
  Lipoma
  Hemangioma
  Neurolemmona
  Epidermoids
  Cysts
  Primary bone tumors
  Chordoma

*Most common

The symptoms and signs of spinal cord tumors depend on the tumor's origin: within the cord or outside the cord and compressing it. The signs and symptoms of both presentations are compared in Table 27-4.

Myelography is essential to make the diagnosis of spinal cord tumors. A myelogram shows a spindle-shaped enlargement of the cord in cases of intramedullary cord tumor. It shows characteristic abnormalities in cases of extradural compression and extramedullary intradural compression. The CSF protein level is usually elevated in cases of cord tumors, rising as high as 300 to 2,000 mg/dL when the tumor completely blocks the spinal cord. Magnetic resonance imaging (MRI) in the sagittal plane is a sensitive and noninvasive test to disclose spinal cord tumors.

Spinal cord tumors should be treated by neurologists and neurosurgeons who have experience doing so. In general, surgical removal is attempted in all extramedullary tumors. Patients with intramedullary tumors usually receive radiation therapy, too. Glucocorticoid therapy is given initially to reduce edema.

The outcome is contingent on the location, extent, and type of the tumor. Patients should be followed at regular intervals by their neurologist or neurosurgeon.

SUBACUTE COMBINED DEGENERATION

The spinal cord is affected out of proportion to other parts of the nervous system in vitamin B_{12} deficiency. The term subacute combined degeneration (SCD) refers to the concomitant degeneration of both the posterior columns and corticospinal tracts of the spinal cord. The spinal cord tract degeneration features both dissolution of the axon and myelin sheath.

Pernicious anemia induces a state of vitamin B_{12} deficiency because there is a lack of intrinsic factor to transfer dietary vitamin B_{12} across the intestinal mucosa.

TABLE 27-4 CLINICAL DIFFERENTIATION OF INTRAMEDULLARY AND EXTRAMEDULLARY SPINAL CORD TUMORS

Symptom	Intramedullary Tumor	Extramedullary Tumor
Sensory loss	Begins just below, and predominates near, level of lesion; loss may be dissociated at tumor level; perianal sparing may be seen	Begins well below, and extends upward to, lesion level; upper border of sensory loss or complaints tends to be sharper
Pyramidal signs	Usually present late	Usually present early
Lower motor neuron signs	Often prominent and widespread	Often absent, but segmental when present
Root pains	Often absent	Often the first symptom
Spinal block	Develops late in clinical course	May develop early in clinical course
Fasciculations	Rare	Common
Incontinence	Early	Late
Spasticity	Later and less severe	Earlier and more severe
Trophic changes in skin	Common	Rare
Local vertebral pain or sensitivity	Rare	Common
CSF protein increase	Infrequent or slight in early stages	Commonly increased in early stages

Adapted from DeMyer W: Anatomy and clinical neurology of the spinal cord, in Baker AB, Joynt RJ (eds): *Clinical Neurology*, vol 3. Philadelphia, Harper & Row, 1986, p. 15. Used with permission.

In pernicious anemia, the neurological syndrome may precede the hematologic syndrome or may dominate it, particularly if the diet is supplemented with folate. In almost all cases of SCD, however, a Wright-stained peripheral blood smear discloses hypersegmentation of polymorphonuclear leukocytes.

The typical patient with SCD develops numbness and paresthesias in the distal limbs followed by impaired gait. Examination discloses marked loss of vibration and position sensation, pyramidal signs in the legs (eg, upgoing toes, increased reflexes), and sensory gait ataxia with Romberg's sign. There may be some mental slowness and visual impairment from brain and optic nerve involvement, respectively, but these are not typical presenting signs.

The diagnosis is confirmed in the laboratory. Serum levels of vitamin B_{12} should be tested. Low-normal or depressed levels should be followed by a Schilling test. The patient with the classic clinical presentation should probably undergo a Schilling test regardless of the results of the serum B_{12} determination. The CSF is usually normal, but the EEG often shows nonspecific slowing of background rhythms.

Patients are treated with parenteral vitamin B_{12}, 1000 μg per month for life. The patient treated early in the course will make a satisfactory recovery. Even when treatment is delayed, parenteral vitamin B_{12} prevents further progression. Many neurologists treat all undiagnosed progressive myelopathies with vitamin B_{12} because SCD is the most treatable degenerative myelopathy.

SYRINGOMYELIA

Syringomyelia is a rare degenerative myelopathy in which there is progressive enlargement of a cavity (syrinx) within the gray matter of the cord, extending rostrally or caudally for many segments. In about one-sixth of cases, the syrinx is related to a contiguous intramedullary spinal cord tumor. In rare cases, the syrinx develops rostral to a previous cord injury by trauma or arachnoiditis. There is an increased incidence of craniocervical junction abnormalities (eg, Arnold–Chiari Type 1 malformation).

Syringomyelia produces the central cord syndrome of dissociation of sensory loss. Because the syrinx usually involves the cervical and upper thoracic cord segments, the patient has dense loss of pain and temperature sensation on the hands, arms, and over a "cape" distribution on the shoulders and upper trunk. Areas of anesthesia are subject to accidental burns and other trauma. Sensation may be normal above and below involved dermatomes giving rise to the "suspended sensory level." Neuropathic pain in the involved limbs is common, despite the anesthesia. There is a lower motor neuron syndrome with weakness, atrophy, areflexia, and fasciculations of hand and arm muscles caused by anterior horn cell damage by the expanding syrinx. Segmental thoracic lower motor neuron weakness predisposes patients to kyphoscoliosis. Brain stem signs can develop if the syrinx extends to the medulla (syringobulbia).

Laboratory tests of value include intrathecal metrizamide CT scanning and MRI. In CT, metrizamide is injected into the lumbar intrathecal space; a scan is performed an hour later. The syrinx may be visualized as an enlargement of the cord and because of the delayed entry of the metrizamide into the syrinx itself.

MRI scanning is less invasive and is exquisitely sensitive to produce an image of a syrinx.

Management of these cases should be restricted to experienced neurologists and neurosurgeons. Shunting the syrinx cavity into the subarachnoid space is commonly performed; in the best hands, this technique arrests the progression. Radiation therapy of the syrinx cavity is of no value.

SPINAL CORD INFARCTION

Spinal cord infarction usually occurs in the area of the single anterior spinal artery and only rarely in the areas of the paired posterior spinal arteries. Because the anterior spinal artery perfuses the entire cord except for the posterior columns and a portion of the posterior horns, anterior spinal artery infarction produces a nearly transverse myelopathy. The most common etiologies are atherosclerosis, abdominal aortic aneurysm, and emboli from the heart and aorta. Some cases have occurred during contrast angiography. Occasionally, a spinal cord arteriovenous malformation produces hematomyelia, mimicking the suddenness of a spinal cord infarction.

The patient suddenly develops back pain, paralysis of the legs, dissociated sensory loss below the lesion, and bowel and bladder dysfunction. The syndrome commonly evolves over minutes, but may grow worse over a few hours. There is incomplete, spontaneous recovery over the next few months.

Myelography or MRI should be performed to exclude treatable forms of acute myelopathy. Management is directed toward rehabilitation.

Bibliography

Barnett HJM, Foster JB, Hudgson P: *Syringomyelia*. Philadelphia, Saunders, 1973. (Authoritative and thorough reference work. Contains original descriptions of post-traumatic syrinxes.)

DeMyer W: Anatomy and clinical neurology of the spinal cord, in Baker AB, Joynt RJ (eds): *Clinical Neurology*. Philadelphia, Harper & Row, 1986, chapter 43. (An excellent review of spinal cord anatomy with clinical correlations; many clinical pearls.)

Herrick M, Mills PE Jr: Infarction of the spinal cord. *Arch Neurol* 1971; 24:228-234. (Discusses clinical features.)

Kincaid JC, Dyken ML: Myelitis and myelopathy, in Baker AB, Joynt RJ (eds): *Clinical Neurology*. Philadelphia, Harper & Row, 1986, chapter 48. (Reviews obscure myelopathies. Source of Table 1.)

Mulder DW, Dale AJD: Spinal cord tumors and disks, in Baker AB, Joynt RJ (eds): *Clinical Neurology*. Philadelphia, Harper & Row, 1986, chapter 44. (Excellent descriptions of spinal cord tumors; well illustrated.)

Ropper AH, Poskanzer DC: The prognosis of acute and subacute transverse myelopathy based on early signs and symptoms. *Ann Neurol* 1978; 4:51-59. (Reviews clinical features and prognosis of ATM.)

Scott JM, Wilson P, Dinn JJ, et al: Pathogenesis of subacute combined degeneration. A result of methyl group deficiency. *Lancet* 1981; 2:334-337. (Discusses pathophysiology of SCD, with companion paper on methyl folate trap on pp 337-340 of same issue.)

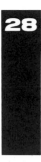

Diseases of Peripheral Nerves

Diseases of the peripheral nerves are referred to generically as peripheral neuropathies. An older term suggesting inflammation, "peripheral neuritis," is misleading and should be abandoned. The most useful classification of peripheral neuropathies is into the major presenting syndromes of polyneuropathy and mononeuropathy. Polyneuropathy is the generalized, symmetric, usually distal dysfunction of all the peripheral nerves. Mononeuropathy is the localized dysfunction of a particular nerve or of several individual nerves (multiple mononeuropathies or "mononeuropathy multiplex").

Each syndrome may have predominant signs and symptoms of motor, sensory, or autonomic dysfunction, or any combination thereof. In general, the polyneuropathies are produced by systemic disorders of metabolic, toxic, or hereditary causes. The mononeuropathies, on the other hand, are caused by localized nerve dysfunction that results from trauma, infarction, or compression.

This chapter examines the polyneuropathies, the mononeuropathies, and Guillain-Barré syndrome. Emphasis is on the common office disorders of the peripheral nervous system, including Bell's palsy, postherpetic neuralgia, causalgia, and the reflex sympathetic dystrophy syndrome. Trigeminal neuralgia is discussed in Chapter 8. Carpal tunnel syndrome and other upper-limb entrapment neuropathies are discussed in Chapter 11.

POLYNEUROPATHIES

Clinical Significance

Polyneuropathies share the features of widespread, generalized involvement of all the nerves in the body. They can be further classified into three groups on the basis of the site of dysfunction within the peripheral nerve.

1. *Axonopathies:* Axonal degeneration occurs because of failure of axonal transport. There may be secondary segmental demyelination.

TABLE 28-1 CLASSIFICATION OF POLYNEUROPATHIES

Axonopathies
Metabolic
    Diabetes mellitus
    Chronic renal failure
    Hypothyroidism
    Porphyria
Toxic
    Drugs
        Vincristine
        Nitrofurantoin
        Phenytoin
        Sulfonamides
        Isoniazid
        Cis-platinum
    Heavy metals
        Arsenic
        Lead
        Mercury
        Thallium
    Poisons
        Industrial solvents
        Pesticides
Deficiency
    Thiamine
    Pyridoxine
    Vitamin B_{12}
Genetic
    Hereditary motor–sensory neuropathies, types 1 to 3
Paraneoplastic
    Small-cell carcinoma of the lung
    Multiple myeloma and other dysproteinemias
    Amyloid

Myelinopathies
Immunological
    Guillain-Barré syndrome
    Chronic relapsing inflammatory polyneuropathy
    Chronic inflammatory polyneuropathy
Toxic
    Diphtheria
    Buckthorn
Genetic
    Refsum disease
    Metachromatic leukodystrophy

Neuronopathies
Motor
    Infectious (poliomyelitis)
    Genetic (hereditary motor neuronopathies)
    Unknown (amyotrophic lateral sclerosis)
Sensory
    Infectious (herpes zoster)
    Paraneoplastic (sensory neuronopathy syndrome)
    Toxic (pyridoxine)
    Unknown (subacute sensory neuronopathy syndrome)
Autonomic
    Genetic (hereditary dysautonomia)

Adapted from Schaumburg HH, Spencer PS, Thomas PK: *Disorders of Peripheral Nerves.* Philadelphia, F.A. Davis, 1983, p 8. Used with permission.

2. *Myelinopathies:* Myelin breakdown occurs as a result of a defect in the functioning of the Schwann cell.

3. *Neuronopathies:* The nerve cell body is damaged primarily, producing a pure motor, sensory, or autonomic neuropathy.

ETIOLOGY

The anatomic and etiologic classification of polyneuropathies is given in Table 28-1. Diabetic polyneuropathy is discussed in Chapter 31.

SYMPTOMS AND SIGNS

Polyneuropathies usually have a gradual onset and slow progression. In general, the longest and largest axons are affected first, and there is a "dying-back" of their endings that progresses proximally toward the cell body. The characteristic "stocking-glove" pattern of polyneuropathic sensory loss is produced as the distal axonal segments are most severely involved. Patients note numbness, tingling, prickling (paresthesias), or burning pain (dysesthesias) in the hands and feet. There may be distal weakness when the sensory loss is profound.

Examination discloses a reduction to sensation over the hands and feet and absent or reduced ankle jerks. In primarily "small-fiber" polyneuropathies, pain is prominent because of the selective damage to small, unmyelinated C fibers. There is more loss of pain and temperature sensation than loss of position or vibration. Autonomic disturbances are prominent, and reflexes are preserved. In primarily "large-fiber" polyneuropathies, selective dropout of large myelinated A fibers results in a greater loss of vibration and position sensation. Distal reflexes are diminished, and spontaneous pain is less common.

Overall, there is a gradual change from impaired to normal sensation as the examiner marches the sensory stimulus proximally up the extremity. Occasionally, there is a hypesthetic zone in a shield distribution around the sternum, representing the most distal segments of the intercostal nerves.

LABORATORY TESTS

Electroneurography and electromyography can confirm the presence of a polyneuropathy and can differentiate the axonopathies from the myelinopathies. The cerebrospinal fluid protein level is often elevated in polyneuropathies. Muscle and nerve biopsy may be of diagnostic value in selected cases. None of these tests is usually necessary, however, because the syndrome is readily diagnosed clinically.

The patient with a newly diagnosed polyneuropathy needs a laboratory diagnostic workup. If the history does not disclose the cause (alcohol/nutritional, hereditary, toxin, or drug exposure) the patient should undergo the following screening tests:

1. Two-hour postprandial glucose test or fasting blood glucose test to screen for diabetes; if elevated, check hemoglobin A1C to assess chronicity and severity.
2. BUN and creatinine tests for uremia.
3. Erythrocyte sedimentation rate for malignancy.
4. Serum protein electrophoresis for dysproteinemia.

5. Thyroid function tests for hypothyroidism.
6. Chest x-ray for small-cell carcinoma.
7. Urine heavy-metals to screen for arsenic, lead, etc.
8. Serum vitamin B_{12} level.

DIAGNOSIS

The onset of sensory symptoms of greater severity than motor symptoms in the hands and feet, with evidence of multimodality distal limb sensory and reflex impairment, is diagnostic of the syndrome of polyneuropathy. Laboratory workup reveals the etiology in only about 50% of cases.

MANAGEMENT

Specific causes of polyneuropathy (eg, diabetes mellitus) should be specifically treated. If the cause cannot be determined, members of the patient's family should be interviewed and, if possible, examined because a high percentage of otherwise undiagnosed polyneuropathy syndromes are hereditary.

If the cause cannot be determined, most neurologists treat patients empirically with therapeutic B vitamins on the presumption that there may be a partial deficiency. Dysesthetic pain in polyneuropathies can be treated with anticonvulsant doses of phenytoin (Dilantin) or carbamazepine (Tegretol) or with a small nighttime dose of a tricyclic antidepressant. Physical and occupational therapy improves function and prevents contractures.

WHEN TO CONSULT

A neurologist should be consulted for the patient with a progressive polyneuropathy whose laboratory workup does not reveal a primary cause or if control of neuropathic pain becomes difficult. Orthopedic surgical referral may be useful to determine if paralysis or deformities would benefit from orthotics or tendon transplants.

MONONEUROPATHIES

CLINICAL SIGNIFICANCE

Mononeuropathies are produced by ischemic, infiltrative, compressive, or immunologic local effects on nerve trunks or nerve twigs. Entrapment mononeuropathies are encountered very often in office practice. Carpal tunnel and cubital tunnel syndromes (Chapter 11) are responsible for much suffering and many lost employment hours.

ETIOLOGY

The causes of mononeuropathies are listed in Table 28-2. Entrapment mononeuropathies of the upper limb are considered in Chapter 11; diabetic mononeuropathies, in Chapter 31.

Ischemia is the major mechanism of nerve dysfunction in mononeuropathies of diabetes and vasculitis. Because of a plentiful collateral circulation, nerve trunks are usually spared in large-vessel occlusive disease. An occlusion of the arterioles ("vasa nervorum") that produces a nerve trunk infarction is the mechanism in vascular mononeuropathies.

TABLE 28-2 CLASSIFICATION OF MONONEUROPATHIES

Ischemia	Physical Injuries
Diabetes mellitus	Severance
Polyarteritis	Focal crush
Other vasculitis	Compression
Rheumatoid arthritis	Stretch and traction
	Entrapment
Infiltration	
Leukemia	**Immunological**
Lymphoma	Brachial plexus neuropathy
Granuloma	Lumbosacral plexus neuropathy
Schwannoma	
Amyloidosis	

Adapted from Schaumburg HH, Spencer PS, Thomas PK: *Disorders of Peripheral Nerves*. Philadelphia, F.A. Davis, 1983, p 8. Used with permission.

Infiltration is the mechanism of single nerve dysfunction in amyloidosis, leprosy, sarcoidosis, leukemia, and lymphoma. In the infiltrative disorders, there is a physical compression as well as an inflammatory injury.

Physical injury to nerves is the mechanism in acute and chronic nerve trauma. In Class 1 injuries (neurapraxia) conduction block occurs; recovery is the rule, however, because the axon and nerve sheath are maintained. In Class 2 injuries (axonotmesis), the axon is interrupted but the Schwann-cell basal lamina and connective tissue endoneurium remain intact. Recovery is common, but incomplete. In Class 3 nerve injuries (neurotmesis), there is the total severance of the nerve fiber, Schwann-cell basal lamina, and endoneurium connective tissue sheath. Spontaneous recovery is uncommon, and neuroma growth is common.

Symptoms and Signs

The typical case of a vascular mononeuropathy is marked by local pain at onset, probably from ischemia of the nervi nervorum. The neurological deficit is greatest at onset, and is usually total, with motor and reflex loss more conspicuous than sensory loss. Over several weeks or months there is a slow, gradual recovery of nerve function as the damaged axon regenerates at a rate of about 1 mm/day. The pain usually resolves within days or weeks. There is incomplete, but generally acceptable, return of muscle bulk and power.

In entrapment neuropathies, sensory symptoms tend to predominate over motor symptoms because most of the fibers in the distally entrapped nerves are sensory. The symptoms of numbness, tingling, and pain are frequently positional and are exacerbated by exercises that further stretch the entrapped nerves. In late cases, there is dense anesthesia in the sensory distributions of such nerves and severe atrophy in the motor distribution.

Laboratory Tests

Electroneurography and electromyography are valuable to localize the level of nerve dysfunction. Screening laboratory tests of value include (1) a two-hour postprandial blood glucose or fasting blood glucose test to screen for diabetes mellitus; and (2) an erythrocyte sedimentation rate to screen for rheumatoid arthritis, occult neoplasm, and vasculitis.

Nerve and muscle biopsy may be of value in selected cases, but the decision to order them should probably be made by a neurologist.

Diagnosis

It is important to distinguish syndromes of the multiple mononeuropathies from the polyneuropathies. If more than a single nerve territory is involved in the former, the nerves are usually affected asymmetrically and with more motor than sensory dysfunction. There is not the symmetric, generalized, widespread, distal sensory loss characteristic of a polyneuropathy. The clinician is advised to consult textbooks of neurological examination (see books by the Mayo Clinic, DeJong, Medical Research Council, and Wolf in the Bibliography of Chapter 1) to see if the assessed areas of the patient's neurological dysfunction correspond to the motor, reflex, and sensory distribution of a particular nerve.

Management

The underlying disease must be identified and treated. In most cases of vascular mononeuropathy, there is adequate spontaneous recovery over several months. Physical therapy may be helpful to prevent contractures in the interim.

In compression mononeuropathies, the patient is first treated with medical means to reduce inflammation and relieve chronic compression. These include wearing splints or protection pads, local injections of depot-steroid preparations, and prevention of subsequent trauma by instructing the patient how to avoid causing further injury (Chapter 11). If these measures fail, surgical release of entrapped nerves is usually curative.

When to Consult

A neurologist may be consulted to perform electroneurography or detailed neurological examination on patients with newly diagnosed mononeuropathies. Most entrapment neuropathies can be managed by the primary physician. An occupational therapist knowledgeable about limb entrapment mononeuropathies can be very helpful in counseling the patient.

GUILLAIN-BARRÉ SYNDROME

Clinical Significance

The Guillain–Barré Syndrome (GBS) is a subacute progressive demyelinating polyneuropathy; it produces a paralytic state that worsens over days or weeks and then gradually resolves. A progressive decrease and loss of deep-tendon reflexes, but only mild polyneuropathic sensory loss, accompanies the paralysis.

Guillain–Barré syndrome strikes with an annual incidence of about 1/100,000 in the United States. Young adults are affected primarily, but middle-aged persons are also susceptible. In the era before mechanical ventilation, the disease was frequently fatal. Today, mortality is about 5%.

Etiology

The main pathologic feature of GBS is an endoneurial infiltration by mononuclear inflammatory cells and a subsequent widespread segmental demyelination. After several weeks, Schwann cells begin to proliferate and new myelin is made to repair the demyelination. A pathologically and clinically similar disease, experimental allergic neuritis, can be produced by injecting a laboratory animal with peripheral nerve extract.

Because of these findings, and the observation that in humans the disease tends to occur a few weeks after viral illness or vaccination, it is widely believed that GBS is an autoimmune disorder of delayed hypersensitivity. There is probably a cross-reactivity between a viral antigen and an antigenic site on peripheral nerve myelin. Thus, lymphocytes previously sensitized to the viral antigen unwittingly attack the patient's own peripheral myelin. Nearly identical acute polyneuropathy syndromes can follow infectious mononucleosis, viral hepatitis, and porphyria.

Symptoms and Signs

Patients with GBS note the onset of weakness or numbness in the legs, which progresses inexorably over hours to days to involve all limbs and usually the face. Motor signs and symptoms predominate over sensory and facial movements. Swallowing, speaking, and breathing are frequently impaired. At the syndrome's worst, there may be a total flaccid quadriplegia and bulbar paralysis; at the least, only mild distal weakness. Even in the presence of severe paralysis, however, sensory symptoms and signs are only those of a mild, large-fiber polyneuropathy.

Deep-tendon reflex loss is a constant feature and of great diagnostic value. Often, reflexes disappear as the weakness progresses; in other cases, they are absent at the first examination.

Autonomic dysfunction is common and accounts for many of the associated fatalities. Labile hypertension alternating with hypotension and a variety of bradyarrhythmias and tachyarrhythmias may be seen. Raised intracranial pressure and papilledema may also be present.

Guillain–Barré syndrome reaches its functional nadir at one to three weeks after onset and then begins to improve. It has been estimated that 85% of patients are again ambulatory at six months. Most patients make a good recovery; only 16% are permanently disabled. Careful examination discloses some permanent damage to the peripheral nervous system in more than half of patients. The presence of distal atrophy is correlated with incomplete recovery.

Several variants of GBS occur. Fisher's syndrome features deep-tendon areflexia with ophthalmoplegia and severe cerebellar ataxia. Chronic relapsing inflammatory polyneuropathy is like GBS, except that it is marked by repeated relapses and responds to steroid therapy. Chronic inflammatory polyneuropathy is like a slow, protracted GBS; it also responds to steroid therapy.

Laboratory Tests

The diagnosis of GBS is a clinical one; laboratory tests are unnecessary. Cerebrospinal fluid findings are confirmatory; they reveal a steady climb of the CSF protein level from day four of the illness over several weeks to levels in the 150 to 400 mg/dL range. Despite the protein level elevation, only a few mononuclear cells are present in the CSF (albuminocytologic dissociation).

Electroneurography of proximal nerve segments can demonstrate slowing of motor nerve conduction velocities, which is consistent with a proximal demyelinating polyneuropathy.

DIAGNOSIS

The progressive onset of widespread flaccid paralysis and areflexia is diagnostic of GBS. Acute transverse myelopathy is distinguished by early bowel and bladder dysfunction, upper motor neuron signs in the legs, and a spinal sensory level. Myasthenia gravis is distinguished by variability in weakness, early ptosis and ophthalmoplegia, and retained deep-tendon reflexes. Acute poliomyelitis is distinguished by fever, headache, muscle pain, asymmetric involvement, and CSF pleocytosis. Acute botulism is distinguished by early bulbar palsy and pupillary dysfunction, absence of sensory involvement, and a normal CSF protein level. Acute hypokalemia can be excluded by measuring serum electrolyte levels.

MANAGEMENT AND WHEN TO CONSULT

The patient should be admitted and a neurologist should be consulted. Frequent pulmonary function tests, especially of inspiratory force, should be performed, and the patient should be placed on a ventilator at the first evidence of deterioration. The usual measures for the treatment of paralyzed patients should be instituted, including nasogastric feeding tubes, urinary catheter, "minidose" subcutaneous heparin, and skin care. All possible attempts should be made to communicate with the patient. Glucocorticoid therapy is not generally helpful, although some neurologists still prescribe it. In some reported cases, plasma exchange has been beneficial, but it must begin within the first week of symptoms to be helpful.

BELL'S PALSY

CLINICAL SIGNIFICANCE

Spontaneous unilateral dysfunction of the facial nerve (Bell's palsy) is the second most common cranial neuropathy after superior laryngeal nerve palsy. Bell's palsy generally has a favorable prognosis, but the clinician must be able to differentiate it from similar conditions and to institute appropriate therapy in a timely fashion.

ETIOLOGY

Spontaneous unilateral lower motor neuron facial paralysis occurs as idiopathic Bell's palsy in 73% of cases, from herpes zoster oticus (Ramsay Hunt syndrome) in 13%, from trauma in 5%, from otitis media in 2%, at birth in 2%, and from other causes in 7% (Adour, 1982). In idiopathic (Bell's palsy) cases, the bulk of evidence suggests that facial nerve dysfunction is from a virally induced inflammatory demyelination, perhaps caused by herpes simplex virus. In most cases, there is evidence of mild dysfunction of other cranial nerves, particularly the trigeminal and vagus. There is no evidence that Bell's palsy results from swelling and subsequent infarction of the facial nerve as it passes through the bony fallopian canal, despite the plausibility of such a theory.

Ramsay Hunt syndrome is herpes zoster of the geniculate ganglion. The facial nerve is damaged incidentally by the virus as it passes through the infected geniculate ganglion.

SYMPTOMS AND SIGNS

Bell's palsy usually presents with a mild aching auricular or retroauricular pain, followed by sudden dysfunction of the muscles on one side of the face. The suddenness and deformity of a unilateral lower motor neuron facial paralysis lead many patients to incorrectly conclude that they have suffered a stroke. The patient drools from the corner of his mouth and cannot close his eye on the paralyzed side. When chewing food, the patient must manually dislodge food from between his lower lip and gums on the affected side. In about 20% of cases, there is a numb sensation over the affected face or ear.

Examination discloses a marked facial deformity with total loss of facial expression, forehead creases, and eye closure on the affected side. The magnitude of the deformity is exaggerated when the patient closes his eyes or smiles. With attempted eye closure, the globe rotates superiorly, presenting the sclera inferior to the cornea (Bell's phenomenon).

Examination of the exposed cornea may disclose small ulcerations by particulate foreign bodies unable to be washed away because of dry eyes (sicca) and an absence of blinking. Some patients have dry mouth and loss of taste on the anterior two-thirds of the tongue because of involvement of the chorda tympani nerve. Hyperacusis in the ipsilateral ear may be present as a result of denervation of the stapedius muscle in the middle ear. Eye dryness may be caused by denervation of the lacrimal gland by involvement of the greater superficial petrosal nerve. Objectively determined sensory loss over the face, head, or neck may be present.

Premonitory auricular discomfort also occurs before the onset of facial palsy in Ramsay Hunt syndrome. Careful examination discloses zoster vesicles in the external auditory canal. Sometimes they do not become apparent, however, until several days after facial paralysis begins.

LABORATORY TESTS AND DIAGNOSIS

Laboratory evaluation is usually not necessary. By taking a history and performing a physical examination, the clinician should be able to classify the facial paralysis as central or peripheral. Upper motor neuron facial weakness is much more pronounced in the lower half of the face because of bilateral supranuclear innervation of the upper face; these patients can always close their eyes. If paralysis is of the lower motor neuron, the presence of vesicles in the ear canal distinguishes Ramsay Hunt syndrome. It is important to assess hearing, taste, salivation, and lacrimation to determine the extent of the seventh nerve lesion.

MANAGEMENT

Adour (1982) distinguishes two groups of patients with Bell's palsy: incomplete (group I) and complete (group II) facial paralysis. The two forms are treated somewhat differently.

Prednisone should be given to patients with either form because it lessens pain and leads to a more satisfying recovery if begun within the first 48 hours. The patient is started on a dose of 1 mg/kg/day in two divided doses and is reexamined on the fifth or sixth day after the onset of the paralysis. If the paralysis remains incomplete (Group I), the prednisone is tapered to zero over the next five days. If the paralysis is complete (Group II), the prednisone is continued at full dosage for another ten days and then is tapered to zero over five more days (Adour, 1982). Prednisone is also recommended for the patient with Ramsay Hunt syndrome unless the patient is immunosuppressed or has disseminated herpes zoster.

Eye care is designed to prevent corneal abrasions that are likely to occur because of sicca and inability to blink. Adour (1982) recommends wearing dark glasses during the day, using artificial tears if sicca is present, and using a bland eye ointment at night. The eye can be taped shut if there is a high probability of airborne particles striking the cornea.

There is no evidence that electrical stimulation of the facial muscles is helpful. Surgical decompression of the facial nerve in its bony canal is not advisable because the procedure is risky and does not improve the prognosis.

COMPLICATIONS

Findings that correlate with a poor prognosis for recovery include sicca, hyperacusis, diabetes, hypertension, ear or face pain, and age over 60 years. All patients in Group I and about 75% in Group II make a good recovery. Prednisone therapy is believed to speed recovery in Group I patients and increase the percentage of recovery in Group II patients.

Facial synkinesias caused by aberrant regeneration of the facial nerve complicate some healed cases. Eye closure on the affected side may occur with smiling. The syndrome of "crocodile tears" is unintentional lacrimation that is provoked by a gustatory stimulus. Permanent facial deformity may be improved by plastic surgery. Hypoglossal nerve–facial nerve anastamosis can restore some facial muscle function. Affected men often choose to wear beards to hide the facial asymmetry.

WHEN TO CONSULT

A neurologist should be consulted only if findings on exam raise the question of neoplasm, Guillain-Barré syndrome, or neurological disorders other than Bell's palsy. A neurosurgeon experienced in hypoglossal nerve–facial nerve anastamosis should be consulted if there is a poor cosmetic result.

PATIENT EDUCATION

Patients need reassurance that their disfigurement is temporary and that they will likely recover spontaneously. They must be taught the importance of protecting their eye until voluntary eye closure returns.

POSTHERPETIC NEURALGIA

CLINICAL SIGNIFICANCE

Herpes zoster may be followed by a syndrome of severe, spontaneous neuropathic pain in the territory of the healed vesicular eruption. This syndrome, known as postherpetic neuralgia (PHN), is one of the most difficult and severe pain syndromes physicians are called upon to treat. The incidence of PHN increases with age: it is rarely a sequela of herpes zoster in patients under the age of 50.

Thereafter, it increases from a rate of about 10% of zoster cases in the sixth decade to nearly one-half of cases in the ninth decade. It has a much higher incidence following ophthalmic zoster, regardless of age.

ETIOLOGY
The hemorrhage and inflammation produced in the dorsal root ganglia during the active vesiculation phase is later replaced by fibrosis. It is believed that spontaneous impulse generators in the dorsal root ganglia are thus created, which produce the PHN.

SYMPTOMS AND SIGNS
Postherpetic neuralgia pain is classically neuralgic: it is a steady, constant, tearing, burning, searing background discomfort upon which is superimposed a paroxysmal, sudden, lancinating, jabbing, excruciating pain. Some patients also complain of an itching or crawling sensation. Patients carefully guard the involved skin area and do not allow anything, including clothing, to touch the area.

Examination usually discloses silvery-white scars with lightly pigmented borders that result from the healed reddish skin of the vesicular eruption. The scars and pain occur in the involved dermatomes—usually a thoracic dermatome arching from back to chest. Although the scars are hypesthetic to touch, the entire dermatome is exquisitely sensitive to pain and can experience severe pain with the slightest stimulus.

About two-thirds of patients have spontaneous resolution of PHN within a year. Treatment is necessary during the short term for this group and over the long term for the unlucky one-third of patients with persistent pain.

LABORATORY TESTS AND DIAGNOSIS
PHN is a purely clinical diagnosis made in the elderly patient with healed zoster who continues to experience severe spontaneous neuropathic pain in the involved dermatomes.

MANAGEMENT AND WHEN TO CONSULT
A variety of drug regimens and neurosurgical ablative treatments have been used with some success to treat PHN. The regimen of Watson et al (1986) described below seems to have the greatest efficacy.

1. Amitriptyline is begun as soon as the diagnosis of PHN is made. If the patient is under 65 years of age, the starting dosage is 25 mg at bedtime; if over 65 years, start with 10 mg at bedtime. The dosages are then slowly increased, as tolerated, using drowsiness and confusion as evidence of toxicity.

2. If this treatment does not provide adequate relief, fluphenazine (Prolixin), 1 mg daily, is added to the amitriptyline.

3. If this regimen fails, a transcutaneous electrical nerve stimulation (TENS) unit is applied.

4. If these measures fail, contact a neurosurgeon who has experience in creating dorsal root entry zone (DREZ) lesions in the spinal cord. The DREZ lesions are made at each spinal segment that receives input from the affected dermatomes.

There is evidence that a ten-day course of prednisone (20 mg tid for six days, 20 mg bid for two days, and 20 mg qd for two days) during the onset of herpes zoster prevents PHN in some cases. Physicians should only consider preventive PHN treatment measures in patients at high risk—namely those over the age of 60 and those of any age who have ophthalmic zoster.

REFLEX SYMPATHETIC DYSTROPHY SYNDROME AND CAUSALGIA

CLINICAL SIGNIFICANCE
Dysfunction of the autonomic nervous system plays an important role in the production of many pain syndromes. In reflex sympathetic dystrophy syndrome (RSDS, shoulder–hand syndrome, or Sudeck's atrophy) there are autonomic dysfunction, pain, atrophy, and trophic changes in a distal limb following a seemingly trivial injury. Causalgia is a special type of RSDS, in which a partial nerve injury was the inciting factor. Treatment of these syndromes must take into account the important role played by autonomic nervous system dysfunction.

ETIOLOGY
The establishment of automatic pain following a limb injury or a partial nerve injury has been explained in two ways. Spontaneous impulse generators may be created in injured nerves, which continue to send pain impulses to the brain in the absence of peripheral pain-provoking stimuli. Alternatively, there may be a formation of "ephapses" or artificial synapses in injured nerves, which allow impulses in sympathetic efferent fibers to be shunted to somatic afferent fibers. Experimental data support both theories.

SYMPTOMS AND SIGNS
Reflex sympathetic dystrophy syndrome follows minor injuries to the limbs, including trauma, burns, infections or any source of inflammation, or it occurs following myocardial infarction or cervical degenerative joint disease. In the acute stage, lasting several weeks after the inciting event, there is spontaneous pain; warm, dry, red skin that later becomes cold, sweaty, and blue; dependent rubor; and decreased range of motion in the joints.

The dystrophic stage lasts until about six months after the injury and features persistent pain; edema; cracked, grooved, or ridged nails; osteoporosis; muscle atrophy; and continued decreased range of motion in joints. In the atrophic stage, which occurs after six months, the pain is less prominent, but the trophic changes are worse: skin, nail, subcutaneous tissue, and muscle atrophy; frozen joints; pale-blue, cool skin; periarticular bone demineralization; and sweating abnormalities.

Causalgia is a kind of RSDS that occurs after partial nerve injury. It has the essential features of RSDS as described above, but the pain is more prominent and the vasomotor, sudomotor, bone, and joint sequelae are less prominent. The pain has the neuralgic quality of burning, tearing, and searing, with superimposed paroxysms of lancinating pain. The pain occurs after a partial nerve injury to a proximal nerve trunk, such as to the median or the sciatic. The nerve can be injured by laceration, by crush, or iatrogenically during surgery as a result of traction, compression, or laceration.

LABORATORY TESTS AND DIAGNOSIS

Reflex sympathetic dystrophy syndrome and causalgia are clninical diagnoses, but the diagnosis can be confirmed by several tests. Plain X-rays of affected limbs should be studied for periarticular bone resorption. Skin temperature can be measured and regional limb blood flow can be assessed by thermography or bone scan to disclose vasomotor changes. Diagnostic sympathetic blockade is useful when effective, but is not always effective. If pain and other symptoms improve temporarily during sympathetic blockade, the diagnosis is secured.

MANAGEMENT AND WHEN TO CONSULT

The patient should be referred to an anesthesiologist who has experience in sympathetic blockade for a series of sympathetic nerve blocks. If there is temporary, but not sustained, improvement, surgical sympathectomy may be helpful.

Physical therapy should be instituted with range of motion exercises to prevent contractures and frozen joints. Medication, including alpha- and beta-blocking sympatholytic agents, nonsteroidal anti-inflammatory drugs, and tricyclic anti-depressant drugs, have been used with varying success. Transcutaneous electrical nerve stimulation (TENS) units help some patients but are most effective when the electrodes are placed on the skin overlying the nerve trunk proximal to the site of injury. Biofeedback conditioning strategies are helpful in some cases. Neurosurgery to create DREZ lesions is the most successful surgical treatment.

Bibliography

Adour KK: Diagnosis and management of facial paralysis. *N Engl J Med* 1982; 307:348-351. (Authoritative review of Bell's palsy, based on the author's personal experience with more than 3000 cases.)

Criteria for the diagnosis of Guillain–Barré syndrome. *Ann Neurol* 1978; 3:565-566. (Useful outline of GBS diagnostic criteria.)

Dawson DM, Hallett M, Millender LH: *Entrapment Neuropathies.* Boston, Little, Brown, 1983. (Authoritative and practical guide to common nerve entrapments and their management; recommended.)

Dyck PJ: The causes, classification, and treatment of peripheral neuropathy. *N Engl J Med* 1982; 307:283-286. (Current but disappointingly incomplete descriptions and references.)

Dyck PJ, Thomas PK, Lambert EH, et al: *Peripheral Neuropathy,* (ed2). Philadelphia, Saunders, 1984. (The ultimate reference work for the most detailed descriptions and reference lists.)

Rizzi R, Visentin M, Mazzetti G: Reflex sympathetic dystrophy. *Adv Pain Res Ther* 1984; 7:451-464. (Contains useful tables comparing RSDS and causalgia.)

Schaumburg HH, Spencer PS, Thomas PK: *Disorders of Peripheral Nerves.* Philadelphia, F.A. Davis, 1983. (A short, fact-filled current reference work with excellent organization, practical information, and a good current bibliography.)

Sunderland S: *Nerves and Nerve Injuries* (ed 2). New York, Churchill Livingstone, 1978. (The encyclopedia of nerve injury diagrams and treatment by the master.)

Watson PN, Evans RJ: Postherpetic neuralgia: A review. *Arch Neurol* 1986;43:836-840. (Reviews the clinical features, pathology, pathogenesis, and treatment of postherpetic neuralgia.)

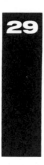

Diseases of Muscle

The skeletal muscle fiber is the primary site of pathology in a large number o diseases that are generically referred to as myopathies. The advent of moderr muscle pathological techniques—particularly enzyme histochemistry and elec tron microscopy—has permitted an improved classification and better under standing of the miscellany of primary muscle disorders. A simplified classification of the myopathies appears in Table 29-1.

The patient with a myopathy must have his condition diagnosed by a neurologist with special expertise in muscle diseases. On the other hand, most patients can be managed satisfactorily on a day-to-day basis by the generalist. Of all the myopathies, only polymyositis, the muscular dystrophies, and myasthenia gravis occur with sufficient frequency to be of concern to the generalist.

EVALUATION

The diagnosis of a myopathy in the patient with suspected muscle disease challenges the clinical skills of the physician. Unlike most neurological disorders, the symptoms and signs of myopathies are purely motor. Weakness is the major symptom of primary muscle disease. The clinician should take care to communicate effectively with the patient regarding his symptoms. Many patients use the term "weakness" to refer to fatigue or lassitude, (Chapter 10) rather than loss of muscle power on attempted contraction. Other patients use the term "numbness" to refer to true weakness rather than to sensory loss.

The patient with facial weakness complains of droopy eyelids, an expressionless face, or a snarling expression when he attempts to smile. Whistling and sucking liquids through a straw are impossible. Extraocular muscle weakness produces diplopia. Weakness in the muscles of mastication produces chewing difficulties. The patient with marked jaw weakness sits with one palm supporting the sagging jaw. Lingual and palatal weakness produce dysarthria and dysphagia, respectively. Myopathic (and all other types of lower motor neuron) dysphagia typically is worse when the patient drinks liquids than when he eats solid food, and the patient complains of nasal liquid regurgitation.

The patient should be questioned about limb weakness. Proximal arm and shoulder weakness impair the ability to comb the hair and reach for high objects. Distal arm and hand weakness reduce grip strength and dexterity and impair such simple activities as turning a doorknob and unscrewing a jar. Proximal leg and hip weakness impairs the ability to rise from a chair, climb steps, and get off the toilet. Distal leg and foot weakness produce difficulty in descending stairs and in walking as a result of foot drop.

Muscle fatigability is an important sign of disorders of the neuromuscular junction, particularly myasthenia gravis. Patients note tremendous fluctuations in weakness during the day and improvement with rest. Complaints of muscle pain and tenderness should be solicited because they occur in about one-third of patients with polymyositis. If the patient's syndrome has a marked sensory component, the diagnosis is not a myopathy or there are two coexisting syndromes.

Examination of the muscles begins with inspection for atrophy, hypertrophy, and fasciculations. In myopathies, atrophy is late and is commensurate with the degree of weakness. Fasciculations suggest a denervating process and are uncommon in myopathies. Muscle hypertrophy may be seen in Duchenne-type dystrophy.

Muscle tone and strength are assessed (Chapter 1) with attention to documenting true weakness and assessing the distribution of weakness. In most myopathic disorders (except for myotonic dystrophy, distal myopathy, and occasional cases of polymyositis), weakness is proximal and diffuse. Thus, weakness in myopathies is usually most profound in the neck flexors, shoulder girdle, and pelvic girdle muscle group. Careful testing usually also discloses weakness of the orbicularis oculi and other facial muscles.

The patient should be observed walking, arising from a low chair, and arising from the floor. The patient should be observed climbing three nine-inch steps. If no weakness is obvious, the patient steps up on a chair whose seat is 18 inches from the floor. Normal strength is required for this maneuver.

Gowers' sign should be watched for as the patient arises from the floor. In this sign of trunk weakness, the patient lifts his buttocks first, then uses his palms to climb progressively up his thighs (as if they were a ladder) until his back is erect.

Muscle tendon reflexes in myopathic disorders are unaffected or are reduced commensurately with the reduced muscle mass. Only in thyrotoxic myopathy are the tendon reflexes exaggerated.

The syndrome of myopathy can be diagnosed clinically in the patient who complains of diffuse muscle weakness in whom the clinician confirms a pattern of diffuse proximal weakness without sensory impairment and with no more than modest reduction in deep-tendon reflexes.

Laboratory assessment for myopathy should include tests of serum creatine kinase (CK) and aldolase to assess the degree of active muscle fiber degeneration. The erythrocyte sedimentation rate (ESR) is often elevated in inflammatory myopathies. Complete electromyography, electroneurography, and muscle biopsy should be performed by a neurologist trained in these techniques (Chapter 4). The extent of endocrine evaluation depends on associated signs suggestive of the endocrinopathies listed in Table 29-1.

TABLE 29-1 CLASSIFICATION OF MUSCLE DISEASES

Genetic

Muscular dystrophies
  X-linked recessive
      Duchenne-type
      Becker's
  Facioscapulohumeral
  Scapuloperoneal
  Limb-girdle
  Distal
  Chronic progressive external ophthalmoplegia
  Oculopharyngeal

Congenital myopathies
  Mitochondrial
  Nemaline
  Central core
  Many others

Myotonic disorders
  Myotonic dystrophy
  Myotonia congenita
  Paramyotonia congenita

Glycogen storage diseases
  McArdle's
  Others

Familial periodic paralysis
  Hyperkalemic
  Hypokalemic
  Normokalemic

Myositis ossificans

Traumatic

Physical
Toxic
Drugs

Inflammatory

Infections
    Viral
    Bacterial
    Parasitic

Immunologic
    Polymyositis–dermatomyositis, groups I to V
    Polymyalgia rheumatica
    Sarcoidosis

Endocrine/Metabolic

Thyrotoxicosis
Myxedema
Hypopituitarism
Acromegaly
Cushing's disease
Addison's disease
Hyperaldodsteronism
Hyperparathyrodism
Metabolic bone disease
Calcitonin-secreting medullary carcinoma of the thyroid
Alcoholic
Nutritional
Renal failure

TABLE 29-1 *continued*

Paraneoplastic
  "Carcinomatous"
  Eaton-Lambert
  Embolic
  Carcinoid

Neoplastic
  Rhabdomyoma
  Rhabdomyosarcoma

Myasthenia Gravis

Other
  Acute rhabdomyolysis
  Paroxysmal myoglobinuria
  Amyloid
  Muscle hypertrophy states
  Disuse atrophy
  Muscle cachexia
  Muscle wasting in contralateral parietal lobe lesions

Adapted from Walton JN (ed): *Disorders of Voluntary Muscle*, ed 4. Edinburgh, Churchill Livingstone, 1981, pp 467-479. Used with permission.

The sequence of evaluation, in summary, is: The generalist classifies the patient's syndrome as a myopathy and orders tests of CK, adolase, and ESR. Then the patient should be referred promptly to a neuromuscular center for a complete diagnostic work-up.

POLYMYOSITIS

CLINICAL SIGNIFICANCE

Polymyositis is a related group of immune-system-mediated inflammatory myopathies. When the characteristic skin rash is present, the disorder is referred to as dermatomyositis. Because it is treatable, the polymyositis group of inflammatory myopathies is important to recognize and to distinguish from other myopathies.

Classification of polymyositis into the following five groups is from the work of Bohan, Peter, and Pearson (1975, 1977): group I, polymyositis (34%); group II, dermatomyositis (29%); group III, polymyositis or dermatomyositis associated with malignancy; group IV, childhood polymyositis or dermatomyositis associated with vasculitis; group V, polymyositis or dermatomyositis with associated connective tissue disorder (21% "overlap group").

Polymyositis is a rare disease with an annual incidence of seven cases per million. Males and females are affected equally; familial clustering is not seen. There are two age peaks: between the ages of 10 and 14, and near the age of 50. Patients with associated malignancy have an age peak near the age of 62.

ETIOLOGY

In polymyositis, there is an inflammatory, cell-mediated destruction of muscle fibers, primarily by lymphocytes and macrophages. Muscle biopsy usually reveals a lymphocytic infiltration of muscle fibers with fiber degeneration, necrosis, and regeneration, and with macrophage phagocytosis of cellular debris. The cause of inflammatory infiltration is unknown, but it is likely that a clone of T lymphocytes has been previously sensitized to a surface antigen on skeletal muscle fibers. There is little evidence that humoral immunity is important in the pathogenesis of polymyositis.

SYMPTOMS AND SIGNS

Symmetric proximal weakness, the *sine qua non* of polymyositis, is seen in over 95% of patients. Weakness evolves over weeks to months, as opposed to evolving over years, as is the case in muscular dystrophies and in many other myopathies. The weakness may not be obvious on initial presentation, but almost always occurs by the time the disease is fully developed. Spontaneous remissions and exacerbations of weakness are common. In severe cases, respiratory embarassment and dysphagia occur. Neck flexors are severely involved, but facial muscles are generally only mildly weak. The weakness of all affected muscles is profoundly out of proportion to the degree of atrophy.

The skin rash of dermatomyositis has the following features: a lilac-colored hue of the upper eyelids, periorbital edema, and the constellation of linear streaks or dusky-red patches on the knuckles and other joints, dermal erythema, atrophy, and scaling (Gottron's sign).

In patients with the overlap syndrome, arthralgias, myalgias, and Raynaud's phenomenon are commonly present. Muscle tenderness is often present but is more common in states of massive rhabdomyolysis. Heart block and cardiomyopathy are occasionally present.

Malignancy is associated with polymyositis far less often than is usually stated. The actual frequency of underlying malignancy is probably in the range of 5% to 10%.

LABORATORY TESTS

There is a uniform elevation of muscle enzyme levels, reflecting muscle fiber necrosis. Aldolase and CK are the most sensitive indicators in this regard; one or both are elevated in 98% of patients with polymyositis. Elevations in serum transaminases and lactate dehydrogenase (LDH) are less constant. The ESR is often elevated but is inconstant and does not correlate with the activity of the disease.

Electromyography discloses "myopathic" motor unit potentials (small amplitude, short duration, polyphasic) in 90% of cases. Fibrillations, positive sharp waves, and increased insertional activity are present in about 75%. Muscle biopsy discloses either focal or widespread changes of degeneration, regeneration, necrosis, and/or inflammation in 88% of cases.

DIAGNOSIS

Bohan, Peter, and Pearson (1975, 1977) identify five diagnostic criteria for polymyositis: (1) progressive symmetrical proximal muscle weakness; (2) elevation of skeletal muscle enzymes, particularly CK and aldolase; (3) the electromyographic triad of small, brief duration, polyphasic motor units, fibrillations with positive sharp waves, and increased insertional activity; (4) muscle biopsy evidence of fiber necrosis, degeneration, regeneration, and inflammation; and (5) the classic skin rash of dermatomyositis. Response to prednisone is *not* a diagnostic criterion.

The following exclusions, when present, should raise a question of the diagnosis of polymyositis. These include: evidence of frank denervation on clinical, electrophysiologic, or histopathologic grounds; muscle weakness with a slowly progressive, nonremitting course; positive family history; clinical or biopsy evidence of infection or granuloma; recent exposure to myotoxins or myotoxic drugs; flagrant rhabdomyolysis with myoglobinuria; and endocrinopathies.

MANAGEMENT

Despite the absence of rigorous proof of its efficacy, glucocorticoid therapy remains the cornerstone of the treatment of polymyositis. The patient is started on prednisone, 60 to 100 mg per day in two or three divided doses. During the induction phase of therapy, the patient is followed with examinations of muscle power and testing of CK. Although it is common for the CK (and sometimes the ESR) to fall during induction glucocorticoid therapy, the only definitive response to therapy is a documented improvement in muscle strength.

During the consolidation phase, an attempt is made to convert the patient to alternate-day prednisone therapy to minimize the suppression of the pituitary–hypothalamic axis. During the maintenance phase, as soon as the disease is under control, the alternate-day doses are lowered, and an attempt can be made to discontinue the drug.

In patients who fail trials of high-dose prednisone, several other cytotoxic and immunosuppressant agents have been shown to be of benefit in selected cases. These include courses of methotrexate, cyclophosphamide, azathioprine, chlorambucil, and plasma exchange.

COMPLICATIONS

The prognosis varies with the type of polymyositis; it is best in children and worst in patients who have malignancies. Overall, the five-year survival rate is about 80%. Complications that produce morbidity and mortality include dysphagia with aspiration pneumonia, congestive heart failure, and steroid myopathy. Successful treatment alone of the malignancies in group III often induce an improvement in the accompanying polymyositis.

WHEN TO CONSULT

A neurolgist and/or rheumatologist should be consulted to confirm the clinical diagnosis. An electromyogram and muscle biopsy should be performed at a neuromuscular center to secure the diagnosis. Treatment should be initiated by the neurologist or rheumatologist, but the patient can be followed by a generalist during the consolidation and maintenance phases.

MUSCULAR DYSTROPHIES

CLINICAL SIGNIFICANCE

The muscular dystrophies are a group of related genetic disorders characterized by progressive noninflammatory muscle fiber degeneration and their replacement by connective tissue and fat. The syndromes differ in age of onset, rate of progression, involved muscle groups, and mode of inheritance. For the most severe of the disorders, Duchenne-type dystrophy, identification of the female carrier state and genetic counseling are crucial.

ETIOLOGY

The etiology of the dystrophies remains unknown. In Duchenne-type, the dystophy that has been most thoroughly studied, most current evidence points to a muscle fiber membrane disorder. Abnormalities peculiar to Duchenne-type dystrophy, however, have also been reported in circulating blood platelets, the microcirculation, and catecholamine metabolism. Some experts still embrace a neuropathic etiology suggesting that motor neuron pathology is somehow transferred to the muscle fiber. But the consensus remains that the dystrophies are true myopathies and the pathology is intrinsic to the muscle fiber.

SYMPTOMS AND SIGNS

1. Duchenne-type Dystrophy is inherited as an X-linked recessive trait, so only males are affected. The disorder is transmitted by their essentially asymptomatic mothers. The incidence is 1 case per 3000 to 5000 male births. Because of frequent spontaneous mutations, as many as one-third of mothers of affected sons are not carriers.

The disease first becomes noticeable at about 2 years of age when the child is seen walking clumsily and falling frequently. By the age of 5, it is clear to the parents that the child cannot run well or keep up with other children, and that he is slow to arise from the floor after falling. The child may walk on his toes with his feet rotated externally. Exaggeration of lumbar lordosis is common.

Enlargement of calf muscles then becomes obvious, secondary to infiltration of fat and connective tissue between the muscle fibers (pseudohypertrophy) and is not caused by true fiber hypertrophy. The enlarged muscles have a rubbery consistency when palpated. Despite their impressive appearance, enlarged muscles are weak.

Weakness progresses through childhood and teenage years. After the child is wheelchair-bound, which usually occurs between the ages of 10 and 15, severe contractures develop along with kyphoscoliosis. Death usually occurs early in the third decade from hypostatic pneumonia or congestive heart failure.

Examination in the early disease phase discloses diffuse proximal muscle weakness, calf enlargement, and a positive Gowers' sign. In the later stages, atrophy becomes more marked, with disappearance of deep-tendon reflexes. In the terminal stage, there is widespread, profound, flaccid paralysis.

An almost identical disorder that has a later onset and a more protracted course is Becker's variant of X-linked muscular dystrophy. Such patients usually become symptomatic in the second decade of life and become wheelchair-bound by the fourth decade; they usually die in middle age.

2. Facioscapulohumeral (FSH) Dystrophy is an autosomal-dominant disorder about one-thirtieth as common as Duchenne-type dystrophy. Symptoms begin during early teenage years with facial and shoulder girdle weakness. There is then a slow progression over several decades to other muscle groups.

Examination discloses a "transverse smile," wasting of neck muscles, winging of the scapulae, and "mounding" of the trapezius muscles. There is weakness of face and shoulder muscles. Proximal leg weakness is often present.

3. Scapuloperoneal Dystrophy may be a variant of FSH dystrophy. It is usually inherited as an autosomal-dominant trait and rarely as an X-linked recessive trait. Weakness is confined to the shoulder girdle and peroneal muscles, producing FSH-type arm weakness and bilateral foot drops.

4. Limb-girdle Dystrophy refers to a group of similar disorders with onset usually in the second or third decade, autosomal-recessive or sporadic inheritance, involvement that produces weakness of the hip and the shoulder girdle, and progression to disability within 20 years of onset. Some patients with a very mild form of this disease have onset in middle or late life.

5. Distal Myopathy is a rare, autosomal-dominant dystrophy with onset in midlife. Predominant symptoms include wrist drops, foot drops, and weakness of intrinsic hand muscles.

6. Ocular Myopathies include a spectrum of unusual disorders. Oculopharyngeal dystrophy is an autosomal-dominant disorder seen most commonly in French-Canadians and Mexican-Americans who in midlife develop severe progressive ptosis and dysphagia. Chronic progressive external ophthalmoplegia itself comprises a group of myopathies caused by muscle fiber mitochondrial dysfunction, in which diplopia from progressive bilateral lateral rectus paralysis occurs in midlife.

7. Myotonic Dystrophy is a relatively common neuromuscular and systemic disorder producing characteristic facies and symptoms. It is inherited as an autosomal-dominant trait and has a prevalence of 3 to 5 cases per 100,000. Symptoms usually begin early in the third decade of life and include hand stiffness, the inability to release a grip, and thick speech. Myotonia is demonstrable by contraction or percussion (Chapter 1). Affected patients have "swan neck" and "hatchet face" abnormalities caused by masseter and sternocleidomastoid atrophy. Ptosis is present, cataracts are common, the voice is weak, and males have frontal baldness and testicular atrophy. The weakness is primarily distal in location, unlike most dystrophies. Electrocardiographic abnormalities commonly include bradycardia and an increased PR interval. Endocrinopathy and immunoglobulinopathies are common. Electromyography discloses copious myotonic discharges, which are diagnostic. The disorder progresses slowly; death from pulmonary or cardiac failure usually occurs in the sixth or seventh decade of life.

LABORATORY TESTS

Elevations of serum CK and aldolase are the rule in Duchenne-type dystrophy. Levels of CK above 2,000 are common between the ages of 4 and 8, during the peak of muscle fiber degeneration. Even presymptomatic newborns with Duchenne-type dystrophy almost always have elevated CK levels. Elevations of CK in FSH, limb-girdle, and scapuloperoneal dystrophies are common but are not as high as those in Duchenne-type. In distal myopathy and chronic progressive external ophthalmoplegia, CK levels are normal or only slightly elevated.

Electrocardiographic abnormalities are seen in about 70% of Duchenne-type dystrophy cases and much less commonly in the other dystrophies. The abnormalities include widespread Q waves and tall R waves in V_1 and V_2, and a number of arrhythmias.

Electromyographic abnormalities ("myopathic" potentials), including short-duration, small-amplitude, and polyphasic action potentials, are common in all dystrophies if sampling of a moderately involved muscle is performed. Muscle biopsy specimens analyzed with enzyme histochemistry staining techniques can reveal findings that have some diagnostic specificity for different dystrophies.

DIAGNOSIS AND WHEN TO REFER

The presence of one of the above clinical syndromes with corroborating enzyme, EMG, and muscle biopsy data is diagnostic of one of the muscular dystrophy syndromes. Patients with suspected dystrophy should be referred to a neuromuscular disease center for complete diagnostic evaluation. The Muscular Dystrophy Association will pay all expenses necessary for diagnosis and most of the expenses of treatment for patients who make application.

MANAGEMENT, COMPLICATIONS

There is no cure or specific treatment that will halt the dystrophies, but complications can be avoided by preventive care. The following regimen for the Duchenne-type dystrophy patient is recommended by Brooke (1986).

The patient can be cared for jointly by a neurologist, an orthopedic surgeon, a physical therapist, an occupational therapist, and a social worker. Physical therapy is devoted first to twice-daily passive stretching of the Achilles tendon to prevent equinovarus deformity. Light bivalve casts or splints can be applied at night to further prevent contracture. The iliotibial band is also passively stretched. Children should be encouraged to exercise as much as they wish, but not to the point of producing muscle pain.

Orthopedic surgery may be recommended when the patient is at the threshold of being wheelchair-bound. Palliative procedures to be considered include lengthening of the Achilles tendon and transposition of the posterior tibial muscle. Long leg braces can be supplied with a spring-loaded lock at the knee joint to prevent buckling of the knee.

When the patient is wheelchair-bound, consideration can be given to a full Milwaukee body brace or to a plastic body jacket, designed to prevent kyphoscoliosis. The plastic jacket is usually tolerated better by the Duchenne-type dystrophy patient.

In advanced disease, the patient should use alternating air mattresses to prevent decubiti. Pulmonary care should include postural drainage, cupping and coughing, nighttime oxygen, and a Cuirass respirator, if necessary.

Genetic counseling should be offered to the patient's mother. Carrier detection should be performed on at-risk females, such as the patient's sisters and maternal aunts. Of the many parameters assessed in studies of carrier detection, the serum CK value remains the most useful. Between 70% and 80% of female carriers show a persistent elevation in serum CK levels. Amniocentesis has not been successful in prenatal diagnosis of muscular dystrophy. It has been used successfully only to determine fetal sex to allow elective abortion if the fetus is male.

PATIENT EDUCATION

All muscular dystrophy patients, indeed all patients with neuromuscular diseases—should contact the Muscular Dystrophy Association, 810 Seventh Avenue, New York, NY 10019. The telephone number is 212-586-0808. The MDA can provide a variety of services to the patient, and often will underwrite the expenses of medical care. Most large muscle-disease clinics in the United States are conducted under the auspices and financial support of the MDA.

MYASTHENIA GRAVIS

CLINICAL SIGNIFICANCE

Myasthenia gravis (MG) is a disease of the neuromuscular junction characterized by fluctuating weakness and fatigability of skeletal muscles. Although its prevalence is estimated at only 1 case per 20,000, it is important to recognize because it is an eminently treatable disease that often remains undiagnosed and may be fatal if untreated. Careful neuro-immunologic work on MG during the last 20 years has brought us close to the understanding of its pathophysiology.

Myasthenia gravis occurs in both sexes and at all ages, but it is particularly common in young adult women and in older men. There is occasional familial clustering of cases, but no consistent inheritance pattern has emerged.

ETIOLOGY

Myasthenia gravis is an autoimmune disease in which clones of antibodies, which are specific to the acetylcholine receptor protein of skeletal muscle, are raised in affected patients. Although the antibody may interfere dynamically with receptor functioning, the disease is more likely the result of antibody-induced acceleration of receptor degradation. Longstanding cases of MG reveal a much-reduced acetylcholine receptor surface area.

The stimulus for antibody production is unknown. Possible culprits of abnormal immune response to the stimulus include excessive helper T cell activity, deficient suppressor T cell activity, or B cell hyperactivity. The macrophage also may be implicated to the extent of an improper presentation of the receptor antigen to the helper T cell.

SYMPTOMS AND SIGNS

The hallmark of myasthenic weakness is fatigability. There is marked fluctuation in weakness throughout the day. Weakness becomes worse with repetitive muscle contractions, and strength is improved temporarily by rest.

Certain muscle groups are commonly weak in MG. Ptosis and diplopia are the most common initial symptoms; so frequently are they present that their absence itself casts doubt on the diagnosis of MG. Bulbar muscles are frequently affected, producing dysphagia and dysarthria. Trunk and extremity weakness tend to occur somewhat later. In severe cases, pulmonary failure is produced by respiratory paralysis.

The disease of some patients is restricted to the eyelids and extraocular muscles (ocular myasthenia), although most cases eventually generalize. The course of the disease is unpredictable, and spontaneous remissions are not infrequent, particularly in young women. Most patients have a fluctuating course, with exacerbation related to physical and emotional stimuli.

The thymus gland is abnormal in most patients with MG. Thymic hyperplasia is present in about half of patients; thymoma, in about 10%. Thyroid abnormalities, usually of the thyrotoxic variety, are also present in about 10% of MG patients. There is an increased incidence of other autoimmune disorders, including rheumatoid arthritis, systemic lupus erythematosus, and pernicious anemia.

LABORATORY TESTS

Serologic tests have been developed to assay the level of acetylcholine receptor antibody in the serum. Most myasthenics have an increase in the concentration of this antibody, but the rise is not well correlated to the severity of the disease. An antistriated muscle antibody has been detected in the serum that has a high correlation to the presence of a thymoma.

Electrophysiologic testing of value includes repetitive nerve stimulation and single-fiber electromyography. In the repetitive stimulation test, a nerve is stimulated at 5 Hz, and the amplitude of the resulting compound muscle action potential (CMAP) is measured. Because of fatigability, CMAP amplitudes in myasthenia decrease with repetitive stimulation. In single-fiber EMG, there is an increased variability in the firing of individual muscle fibers of a motor unit ("jitter") when the nerve is stimulated.

The suspected MG patient should undergo plain chest radiographs and a chest CT scan to look for thymoma or thymic hyperplasia. Serum thyroid function tests also should be performed.

DIAGNOSIS

The suspected myasthenic patient should be tested for muscle fatigability and with a Tensilon (edrophonium chloride) test. Fatigability can be assessed by having the patient perform repetitive contractions of symptomatic muscles. To assess development of ptosis or dysconjugate gaze, the patient should stare with an upward gaze at the examiner's finger for 30 to 60 seconds without blinking. The patient can be asked to repeat: "one hundred, one hundred and one, one hundred and two," all the way to two hundred. The examiner assesses for increasing dysarthria. Repetitive squeezing of a hand dynamometer can assess extremity fatigability.

Intravenous edrophonium chloride should produce brief but dramatic improvement in weakness. The muscle response to be measured is first identified and examined to establish a baseline. Then a test dose of Tensilon, 2 mg, is injected, and the patient is reexamined. If there is no obvious change, an additional 8 mg is infused. A positive test produces a noticeable improvement (eg, disappearance of ptosis) 30 to 60 seconds after injection. The test is occasionally negative in definite myasthenia, particularly of the ocular type.

MANAGEMENT

Current therapies for myasthenia include anticholinesterase agents, glucocorticoids, other immunosuppressive agents, thymectomy, and plasma exchange. A neurologist with experience in managing myasthenia gravis should direct the therapy. Medications that make neuromuscular blockade worse should be avoided. (Table 29-2).

Anticholinesterase drugs may be used initially in patients with limited disease. Pyridostigmine (Mestinon) tablets are 60 mg. From ½ to 2 tablets are given every three hours while the patient is awake. The dosage is titrated to the patient's symptoms. Signs of overdose include abdominal cramps, diarrhea, fasciculations, and increasing weakness.

Glucocorticoid therapy with prednisone should be started in the patient with more than mild symptoms. Prednisone, 60 mg in three divided doses, may be initiated, although some experts advocate that the dosage be increased gradually to this level from a lower starting dosage. Occasionally, glucocorticoid induction therapy will induce a temporary exacerbation, so most patients should be admitted to the hospital for induction therapy and observed for seven to ten days. Once myasthenic symptoms are under control, the consolidation phase attempts to convert to alternate-day prednisone therapy. In the maintenance phase, alternate-day dosages are reduced to the minimum acceptable level.

Immunosuppressive therapy with cyclophosphamide, azathioprine, or methotrexate has been used in refractory cases. Plasma exchange has been used with uneven success.

Thymectomy is recommended for all patients with thymoma and for patients (under the age of 40) with thymic hyperplasia. The entire thymus must be excised for the procedure to be of benefit. The transsternal approach is most satisfactory.

TABLE 29-2 DRUGS THAT EXACERBATE MYASTHENIA GRAVIS OR PRODUCE MYASTHENIC-LIKE SYNDROMES

Antibiotics	**Psychotropic Drugs**
Colistin	Chlorpromazine
Gentamicin	Lithium
Kanamycin	
Neomycin	**Anticonvulsants**
Polymyxin B	Phenytoin
Streptomycin	Trimethadione
Tetracyclines	
	Hormones
Cardiovascular Drugs	ACTH
Procainamide	Corticosteroids
Propranolol	Thyroid hormones
Timolol	Oral contraceptives (?)
Practolol	
Oxprenolol	**Other Drugs**
Quinidine	Anticholinesterases
Trimethaphan	Methoxyflurane
	Tetanus antitoxin
Antirheumatic Drugs	
Chloroquine (?)	
D-penicillamine	

Adapted from Argov A, Mastaglia FL: Disorders of neuromuscular transmission caused by drugs. *N Engl J Med* 1979; 301:410. Used with permission.

Patients should first be induced and controlled with prednisone to avoid neuromuscular complications of thymectomy.

PATIENT EDUCATION

Patients should be encouraged to contact the Myasthenia Gravis Foundation for information and services. The address is: Myasthenia Gravis Foundation, 15 East 26th Street, New York, NY 10010. The telephone number is 212-889-8157.

Bibliography

Argov A, Mastaglia FL: Disorders of neuromuscular transmission caused by drugs. *N Engl J Med* 1979; 301:409-415. (Discusses drug-induced myasthenia gravis and myasthenia-like syndromes.)

Bohan A, Peter JB: Polymyositis and dermatomyositis. *N Engl J Med* 1975; 292:344-347, 403-407. (This account provides the basis for current classification of polymyositis.)

Bohan A, Peter JB, Bowman RL, et al: A computer-assisted analysis of 153 patients with polymositis and dermatomyositis. *Medicine* 1977; 56:255-286. (Refines the authors' earlier account.)

Brooke MH: *A Clinician's View of Neuromuscular Diseases, ed 2.* Baltimore, Williams & Wilkins, 1986. (A beautifully written, very readable, and highly personal account from an experienced clinician. Recommended.)

Drachman DB: Myasthenia gravis. *N Engl J Med* 1978; 298:136-142,186-193. (Thorough summary of scientific and clinical data on myasthenia gravis.)

Dubowitz V: The female carrier of Duchenne muscular dystrophy. *Brit Med J* 1982; 284:1423-1424. (Authoritative review of Duchenne-type carrier screening.)

Engel AG, Banker BQ: *Myology.* New ;York, McGraw-Hill, vol 1 and 2, 1986. (The most current and comprehensive reference work covering all aspects of muscle diseases.)

Furukawa T, Peter JB: The muscular dystrophies and related disorders. *JAMA* 1978; 239:1537-1542, 1654-1659. (A brief but accessible review of the dystrophies.)

Mastaglia FL, Ojeda VJ: Inflammatory myopathies. *Ann Neurol* 1985; 17:215-227, 317-323. (Current review of all inflammatory myopathies with comparisons of polymyositis and infectious myopathies.)

Seybold ME: Myasthenia gravis. A clinical and basic science review. *JAMA* 1983; 250:2516-2521. (Less thorough than the Drachman (1978) paper, but reviews literature to 1983.)

Walton JN (ed): *Disorders of Voluntary Muscle, ed 4.* Edinburgh, Churchill Livingstone, 1981. (A comprehensive reference work for detailed explanations and obscure points.)

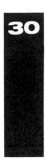

30

Sleep Disorders

The frequency of sleep disorders is usually underestimated by physicians. Surveys have shown that 10% to 15% of adults in the western world complain of a serious or frequent disturbance of the quality or quantity of sleep. As many as 35% complain of at least occasional sleep problems.

THE SLEEP LABORATORY

The classification of sleep disorders has evolved largely from polysomnographic data gathered from studies in sleep laboratories of normal people and those with sleep disturbances. Polysomnography refers to the series of physiologic functions during sleep that can be recorded simultaneously on a polygraph. Most sleep laboratories are equipped to simultaneously measure cardiac rate and rhythm, respiratory rate and rhythm, electroencephalography (EEG), surface electromyography, electro-oculography, and blood oxygen saturation by earlobe oximetry. Specialized studies, including measurements of penile tumescence and esophageal pH, may also be performed. A lengthy paper recording of all functions versus time is then studied by the polysomnographer. Specific patterns of diagnostic value (eg, REM-onset sleep in narcolepsy, sleep apnea) can then be identified.

The operational standards and certification of sleep disorder clinics in the United States and Canada are established under the auspices of the Association of Sleep Disorders Centers. Polysomnography is expensive, usually between $500 and $1200, depending upon the duration of the study. Furthermore, there are relatively few fully equipped sleep laboratories. They are usually located in large medical centers. A complete list of centers can be obtained by writing: The Association of Sleep Disorders Centers, P.O. Box 2604, Delmar, CA 92014.

Sleep disorders can be divided into two major groups: transient situational disorders lasting a few days to one month, and persistent disorders lasting longer than one month. Transient problems can be treated by reassurance and expectant or symptomatic therapy. Only if the sleep disorder has persisted for longer than one month should evaluation by a sleep laboratory be considered.

Sleep Physiology

Normal sleep consists of repetitive cycles in which periods of lighter sleep alternate with periods of deeper sleep. The normal person falls asleep 8 to 10 minutes after retiring and descends to stage 1, then stage 2 sleep. In stage 1, the background alpha activity on the EEG (8 to 13 Hz) becomes replaced by low-voltage theta (4 to 7 Hz) mixed with low voltage beta (14 to 24 Hz). In stage 2 sleep, this activity is joined by high voltage bursts of slower waves followed by 14 Hz rhythmic "sleep spindles" (the "K-complex").

After 30 to 45 minutes, the subject descends to sleep stages 3, then 4 ("slow-wave sleep") in which the background EEG becomes composed of high-voltage 1 to 3 Hz delta activity and 4 to 5 Hz theta activity. After 30 to 45 minutes in slow-wave sleep, the normal subject ascends to stage 2, then stage 1 sleep. When he reaches stage 1, he has rapid eye movements (REM) for 5 to 10 minutes, associated with dreaming and with penile erection in men. Then the cycle repeats—stage 2, slow-wave sleep, stage 2, REM, etc. The first cycle lasts 90 to 100 minutes; subsequent cycles last 85 to 90 minutes. The duration of each REM period increases throughout the night from 5 to about 30 minutes. The duration of slow-wave sleep decreases from 40 to about 10 minutes and then disappears in the final few sleep cycles. The cycle may proceed briefly to full wakefulness once or twice before the subject fully awakens in the morning.

Classification

In 1979, the Association of Sleep Disorders Centers published the Diagnostic Classification of Sleep and Arousal Disorders; it both classifies and provides diagnostic criteria for the disorders. A shortened classification appears in Table 30-1.

In this chapter, we will concentrate on (1) the disorders of initiating and maintaining sleep (insomnias); (2) two major disorders of excessive sleepiness, narcolepsy and sleep apnea; and (3) several of the parasomnias: sleepwalking, sleep terrors, and enuresis.

DISORDERS OF INITIATING AND MAINTAINING SLEEP (INSOMNIAS)

Although complaints of excessive daytime sleepiness are the most frequent reason for referral to a sleep center, the most common sleep disorder is insomnia. Most insomnias are short-lived episodes lasting a few days to a few weeks; they are associated with transient emotional disturbances. When they are persistent, the most common cause is depression, either a bipolar or monopolar affective illness. Personality disorders and psychosis account for smaller numbers of patients with persistent insomnia.

TABLE 30-1 CLASSIFICATION OF SLEEP DISORDERS

Disorder	%
Disorders of Initiating and Maintaining Sleep (Insomnias)	**31.2**
Psychiatric disorders	10.9
Psychophysiologic disorders	4.8
Drug and alcohol dependencies	3.9
Sleep related myoclonus and restless legs syndrome	3.8
Sleep apnea syndromes	1.9
Medical, toxic, or environmental causes	1.2
Childhood-onset insomnia	0.1
Other or no abnormality	4.6
Disorders of Excessive Sleepiness	**50.8**
Sleep apnea syndromes	22.0
Narcolepsy	12.7
Idiopathic CNS hypersomnia	4.5
Psychiatric disorders	1.9
Sleep related myoclonus and restless legs syndrome	1.8
Medical, toxic, or environmental causes	1.4
Drug and alcohol dependencies	0.8
Psychophysiological disorders	0.6
Other or no abnormality	5.1
Disorders of the Sleep–Wake Cycle	**2.9**
Delayed sleep phase syndrome	1.2
Irregular sleep–wake pattern	0.8
Other	0.9
Dysfunctions Associated with Sleep, Sleep Stages, or Partial Arousal (Parasomnias)	**15.1**
Sleep-related convulsive seizures	1.7
Sleep-related gastroesophageal reflux	1.3
Sleepwalking (somnambulism)	0.9
Sleep terror (pavor nocturnus)	0.9
Sleep-related enuresis	0.4
Dream anxiety attack (nightmares)	0.4
Sleep-related cardiovascular symptoms	0.2
Familial sleep paralysis	0.2
Sleep-related head banging	0.2
Sleep-related bruxism, cluster headaches, painful erections, abnormal swallowing, asthma, or hemolysis	0.4
Other, symptomatic polysomnographic findings, or no findings	8.7

Classification is based on Association of Sleep Disorders: *Sleep* 1979; 2:1-137.

Data reproduced, with permission, from Coleman RM, Roffwarg HP, Kennedy SJ, et al: Sleep-wake disorders based on a polysomnographic diagnosis. A national cooperative study. *JAMA* 1982; 247:999-1001. Copyright 1982, American Medical Association. Data on rates of occurrence are based on 4,698 patient referrals to 11 cooperating sleep centers over a two-year period.

Sleep disturbance is a classic feature of depression. Patients complain of intrusive thoughts and the inability to fall asleep at night. They awake early in the morning and cannot fall asleep again. Sleep studies reveal a reduction in the amount of slow-wave sleep and a shortened interval from falling asleep to the first REM episode. When sleep does occur, it is accompanied by restlessness and is not refreshing.

Drug or alcohol dependence can cause sleep disturbances, either during sustained drug use or during withdrawal. There is a reduction of time spent in both slow-wave sleep and in REM sleep. Multiple awakenings at night and restlessness are common symptoms. Almost all prescription sedatives decrease or eliminate REM sleep; consequently, with long-term use they will produce these sleep abnormalities. The rapid-acting benzodiazopines flurazepam (Dalmane), triazolam (Halcion), and temazepam (Restoril) do not decrease REM sleep at their usual dosages and do not induce sleep disorders, even with long-term use. They are, therefore, the preferred agents for use as hypnotics in the patient with insomnia.

Restless Legs Syndrome and Nocturnal Myoclonus

Restless legs syndrome and nocturnal myoclonus are two sleep disorders that are usually seen together and account for difficulty in maintaining sleep and subsequent excessive daytime sleepiness. The patient with restless legs syndrome feels a constant urge to move his legs, stretch his leg muscles, and change leg position because of a profound restless but not exactly painful feeling deep in the lower leg muscles. The new position is achieved, then moments later, the same urge to move begins the cycle anew. Restless legs syndrome is usually idiopathic but is seen with increased frequency in patients with uremia. Sleep studies of patients with restless legs syndrome disclose periodic movements of the legs during non-REM sleep. Sudden, involuntary contractions of the lower leg muscles occur every 20 to 30 seconds and last a few seconds. The movements are termed nocturnal myoclonus incorrectly because contractions last longer than with true myoclonus. The patient is usually not aware of the leg contractions, but the force of the movements and the imparted somesthesia are sufficient to disturb the transition to slow-wave sleep. The patient awakens in the morning unrefreshed. Nocturnal myoclonus is seen in numerous other sleep disorders in addition to restless legs syndrome. Treatment with diazepam (Valium), clonazepam (Clonopin), or baclofen (Lioresal) has had limited success.

DISORDERS OF EXCESSIVE SLEEPINESS (HYPERSOMNIAS)

The most well-known sleep disorders, narcolepsy and sleep apnea syndromes, produce excessive daytime sleepiness. The urge to sleep may be irresistible and may greatly impair daytime functioning. All sleep disorders that reduce the quality and quantity of nighttime sleep induce some degree of excess daytime sleepiness.

Sleep Apnea Syndromes

Sleep apnea syndromes are classified as central (nonobstructive), obstructive, or mixed (with both central and obstructive features). They all share the phenomenon of frequent apneic episodes during sleep, which disturb the quality and quantity of sleep and induce irresistible sleep urges during the day. Sleep recordings in cases of sleep apnea reveal multiple awakenings, essentially no slow-wave sleep, and reduced REM sleep. Patients may lie in bed for eight hours or more but awaken groggy and unrefreshed.

In central sleep apnea, all respiratory effort ceases suddenly. Unlike obstructive sleep apnea, this disorder does not result from mechanical obstruction of the airway, which remains open. After apnea lasting 10 to 60 seconds or longer, the patient usually awakens with a loud snore or gasp then returns to sleep and repeats the cycle in 2 to 30 minutes. The patient is not aware of the multiple awakenings, but the cumulative effect is to greatly reduce slow-wave and REM sleep, those components that seem to be responsible for the refreshing power of sleep.

In obstructive sleep apnea, the usually obese, male, middle-aged patient is known to be a heavy snorer. When he falls asleep, the snoring begins and occurs regularly during normal breathing. Then, because of the collapse of the upper airway, there is a 20 to 50 second pause during which the patient is apneic. The apneic phase ends with several rapid, loud snores as breathing is reinstated. Sleep is disturbed because of the awakenings and the interruption of slow-wave and REM sleep.

Obstructive sleep apnea is produced by airway obstruction. There may be a congenital predisposition in some patients with micrognathia or cleft palate. Numerous acquired ENT disorders, including deviated nasal septum, adenoidal–tonsilar hypertrophy, or palatal abnormalities, may also aggravate the condition. Occlusion of the oropharyngeal airway during sleep occurs as the tongue moves posteriorly and the lateral oropharyngeal walls collapse during sleep. Upon awakening, the oropharyngeal airway is reestablished and loud gasping and snoring accompanies the first breaths.

Sleep apneas are serious because they have many complications. There is an increased incidence of sudden death from ventricular tachyarrhythmias and asystole. Hypertension is common and increases with the hypercapnia induced during apnea. Pulmonary hypertension eventually occurs, producing right-sided congestive heart failure and cor pulmonale. The frequent hypoxic episodes during sleep induce an elevation in hematocrit and hemoglobin concentrations. Aspiration pneumonias may occur during snoring.

Treatment of sleep apnea syndromes first requires elucidation of the type. In all sleep apneas, the patient is urged to lose weight, to discontinue alcohol and any sedating medications, and to cease smoking.

If these measures fail, the patient with obstructive or mixed sleep apnea should undergo a permanent tracheostomy. The tracheostomy stoma can be occluded during the day and opened at night. When the oropharynx collapses during sleep, the stoma provides a sufficient alternative airway to prevent obstruction and promote normal sleep. After normal sleep is reestablished, daytime sleepiness usually resolves, pulmonary hypertension is arrested, and systemic hypertension is usually lowered. Experimental treatments of sleep apneas with tricyclic antidepressant agents, such as clomipramine and progesterone hormones, have had inconsistent benefits. Laryngeal surgical procedures other than tracheostomy have had mixed results.

Sleep apnea in the neonate (Ondine's curse) is prevented with apnea alarms to awaken the sleeping baby and alert the guardian to stimulate the neonate to breathe. Phrenic nerve pacemakers, rocker beds, and other temporary ventilators also can be used during sleep.

Narcolepsy

Narcolepsy is the most dramatic and colorful of the disorders of excessive sleepiness. Its notable features are sleep attacks and cataplexy. In its fully developed form, narcolepsy also causes hypnogogic hallucinations, sleep attacks, disturbed nighttime sleep, and a variety of unusual automatic behaviors.

Its onset is during teenage years or early adulthood. It is not a rare disease: prevalence is 0.4/1000, and it affects men and women equally. There is a strong hereditary basis as an autosomal recessive trait. First-degree relatives of probands have a 60-fold increased incidence of the disease over age-matched nonrelated controls. Almost all patients with classical narcolepsy have the DR2 histocompatibility site in the HL-A group. The disorder remains throughout life.

The *sleep attack* is the most conspicuous symptom. The narcoleptic patient suffers multiple daily attacks of an irresistible urge to sleep. The attacks can occur at any time and often in inappropriate situations for sleep, such as while driving a car, eating, or bathing. The narcoleptic patient soon learns that he or she cannot successfully fight the urge to sleep and must capitulate. Ordinarily he sleeps for only 10 to 15 minutes unless he is lying in bed or on a couch; then he may sleep for a few hours. Although he awakens refreshed temporarily, the patient complains of chronic fatigue and drowsiness.

Cataplexy is the sudden loss of muscular tone induced by a strong emotional state. Attacks of cataplexy occur in 80% to 90% of patients with narcolepsy. A typical attack is induced by laughter at a humorous situation. The patient's head suddenly drops with his chin on his chest, and he may fall to the floor. Unlike syncope or seizure, there is no alteration in consciousness. The loss of muscle tone is transient, lasting only a few seconds, and the patient picks himself up and resumes his activities. Incontinence is rare. Various emotions—anger, fear, surprise, sadness—can trigger an attack and produce loss of tone. Attacks differ in individual patients as to whether the loss of tone is focal or generalized, but the pattern of loss of tone is usually consistent in each patient.

Hypnogogic hallucinations are vivid, colorful dreams that the narcoleptic patient experiences while awake just before falling asleep at night or during a daytime sleep attack. Similar hallucinations occurring just at awakening from sleep are called hypnopompic hallucinations. The patient is awake and knows the hallucinations are dreamlike. They occur in fewer than half of narcoleptic patients.

Sleep paralysis also occurs upon awakening and just before falling asleep in fewer than half of narcoleptics. Although the patient is awake, his limb muscles are totally paralyzed for several seconds to minutes during the attack. Extraocular muscles and breathing are maintained. He becomes frightened and can later recount the fear and frustration. Examination during an attack of sleep paralysis reveals that the patient is mute and his eyes are closed. The limbs are flaccid and the patient appears to be asleep.

Various *automatic behaviors* are encountered in narcoleptics for which they have no memory. These resemble fugue states or symptoms of complex partial seizures but have no epileptiform EEG activity and do not respond to anticonvulsant medication. The patient may stare into space, make stereotyped fumbling finger movements, walk or drive unknowingly, or speak incoherently. Episodes usually last several seconds.

Sleep studies of narcoleptics have disclosed specific findings. In more than 70% of cases, REM occurs at the onset of sleep, unlike the 90 minutes of sleep before the first REM period that usually occurs in the normal person. The brief daytime sleep attacks are almost all REM sleep. In addition to REM-onset sleep, the latency between the time of lying down and that of falling asleep in narcoleptics is 1 to 5 minutes, which is shorter than in normal persons. Anyone who is sleep-deprived or has a chronic sleep disorder has a shortened sleep latency, but only the narcoleptic begins his sleep in REM.

Hypnogogic hallucinations and sleep paralysis are thought to be caused by the intrusion of REM even before the patient is fully unconscious. Muscles are flaccid during REM and much active dreaming occurs during that stage. Cataplexy is believed to be a fragment of REM with concomitant muscle flaccidity that is somehow induced emotionally. Similarly, automatic behaviors may be the intrusion of a sudden REM fragment that temporarily impairs full consciousness.

Sleep attacks of narcolepsy are treated with stimulant medications. The most success has been achieved with methylphenidate (Ritalin), but many neurologists prefer pemoline (Cylert). Dextroamphetamine prevents sleep attacks but has a higher potential for abuse. Patients on these drugs should undergo periodic blood pressure and pulse determinations.

Cataplexy is best treated with tricyclic antidepressants in divided doses. The most experience has been accumulated with imipramine (Tofranil) and protriptyline (Vivactil). One of these medications should be added to the stimulants if cataplexy is symptomatic. The most effective tricyclic agent, clomipramine, is not yet available in the U.S.A. but can be obtained in Canada.

General treatment measures include scheduling naps into the daily regimen to decrease the need for REM sleep. Drug holidays are of value to assess medication needs and to restore medication potency.

DISORDERS OF THE SLEEP–WAKE SCHEDULE

In this group of disorders, there is a disturbance of the circadian rhythms that regulate the timing of sleep–wake cycles and neuroendocrine outputs. Most disorders are transient (jet-lag, change in work-shifts). Occasionally, a persistent problem occurs, such as the delayed sleep-phase syndrome. Here, despite a regular daily schedule, the patient cannot fall asleep until 3 to 6 AM, thereby awakening tired every morning. It may be that such a patient has an "internal biologic clock" that is not on the 24 to 25 hour schedule of most people; he may have a 27 to 28 hour circadian rhythm.

PARASOMNIAS

Dysfunctions associated with sleep, sleep stages, or partial arousals are also known as parasomnias. This is a group of miscellaneous disorders which do not produce insomnia or excessive daytime sleepiness but in which sleep triggers a peculiar symptom.

Parasomnias occur in slow-wave sleep and are more common in children than in adults. They tend to occur early in the night (when more slow-wave sleep occurs) and usually within 60 minutes of going to sleep during the first slow-wave sleep cycle. Multiple parasomnias may occur in the same patient. Patients are difficult to awaken during parasomnias because they are in the deepest plane of sleep (slow-wave sleep). Consequently, they have no memory of the event the next day.

Somnambulism

Somnambulism (sleepwalking) is common in children—15% of children have at least a single episode and 1% to 6%of children have regular episodes. Almost any child can be made to sleepwalk if he is lifted out of bed and placed on his feet during slow-wave sleep.

Ordinarily, the subject will sit up, get out of bed, and wander aimlessly for several minutes. The eyes are open, but there is no communication because the patient is asleep. Sleepwalking is serious only if an injury occurs accidentally, such as falling down the stairs. The episode is terminated by the patient returning to bed or lying down where he is and resuming ordinary recumbent sleep. There is no subsequent memory of the event. Sleep laboratory evaluation is not usually necessary to make the diagnosis, but can help if a nocturnal seizure disorder must be excluded.

Sleep Terror

Sleep terror (pavor nocturnus) is another paroxysmal disorder of slow-wave sleep that occurs mainly in children. In affected children, there is a sudden loud cry or moaning, sometimes compared to a wild animal cry. The child sits bolt upright, continues to moan, and moves his arms. As in sleepwalking, the patient does not talk and does not respond to reassurance. This episode ends after a few minutes with a deep yawn, after which there will be normal sleep. As in sleepwalking, the event usually occurs in the first slow-wave sleep cycle within an hour after going to bed. It is more likely to occur if the child is overtired or has had unusual emotional stresses that day. There is no memory for it the next day, and there is no clear dream content.

Sleep terrors should be distinguished from nightmares that occur in the latter part of the night during REM sleep. Nightmares are merely dreams with a frightening content for which the subject has excellent recall. The person responds to awakening and reassurance.

Medication can suppress those parasomnias that are severe or continuous. Sleep terrors and sleepwalking can be prevented by nighttime doses of diazepam 2 to 5 mg for children, 5 to 20 mg for adults. Imipramine may be tried if diazepam fails.

Enuresis

Bedwetting (enuresis) is a common parasomnia. Surveys of its prevalence showed that 10% of children at age 7, 3% of children at age 12, and 1 to 3% of American and British Navy recruits in World War II had regular enuresis.

As in other parasomnias, enuresis occurs most often in slow-wave sleep; therefore, bedwetting usually happens during the first one-third of a night's sleep. There appear to be spontaneous bladder wall contractions with urethral sphincter relaxations during slow–wave sleep. Some transient arousal to a confused state is common.

The child with primary enuresis (nighttime bladder training never learned) should have congenital urologic conditions excluded by physical examination (urethral obstruction in boys, ectopic urethra in girls). Most children without an organic predisposition can be treated with bladder-training exercises, small nighttime doses of imipramine, and urination alarm systems.

Bibliography

Association of Sleep Disorders Centers: Diagnostic classification of sleep and arousal disorders. *Sleep* 1979; 2:1-137. (The basis for the current classification of sleep disorders. Contains criteria for the diagnosis for each disorder, differential diagnosis, and references.)

Coleman RM, Roffwarg HP, Kennedy SJ, et al: Sleep–wake disorders based on a polysomnographic diagnosis. A national cooperative study. *JAMA* 1982; 247:997-1003. (A survey of the frequency of referral to sleep centers for each type of sleep disorder.)

Guilleminault C, Dement WC (eds): *Sleep Apnea Syndromes*. New York, Alan R. Liss, 1978. (Thorough series of papers on sleep apnea physiology, diagnosis, and treatment.)

Guilleminault C, Lugaresi E (eds): *Sleep–Wake Disorders. Natural History, Epidemiology, and Long-Term Evolution*. New York, Raven Press, 1983. (A series of current papers on various aspects of sleep disorders.)

Hauri P: *The Sleep Disorders*. Kalamazoo, MI, Scope Publications, Upjohn Co, 1977. (An excellent illustrated introduction to the biology and disorders of sleep. Available from the Upjohn Company.)

Kales A, Vela-Bueno A, Kales JD: Sleep disorders: Sleep apnea and narcolepsy. *Ann Intern Med* 1987; 106:434-443. (Contains current tips on the management of the common major sleep disorders.)

Spiegel R: *Sleep and Sleeplessness in Advanced Age*. New York, SP Medical and Scientific Books, 1981. (Discusses special sleep problems of the geriatric patient.)

Weitzman ED: Sleep disorders, in: Rowland LP (ed): *Merritt's Textbook of Neurology*, ed 7. Philadelphia, Lea & Febiger, 1984, pp 652-666. (Concise and current summary of the essentials of sleep physiology and disorders.)

Williams RL, Karacan I (eds): *Sleep Disorders. Diagnosis and Treatment*. New York, John Wiley, 1978. (Standard textbook; thorough descriptions of all sleep disorders).

Neurological Complications of Diabetes

Central and peripheral nervous system complications of diabetes mellitus occur about as frequently as do renal, retinal, and peripheral vascular complications. They are seen in both types I and II diabetes and increase in frequency with the duration of the disease. Table 31-1 lists several presenting neurological syndromes and the specific disorders causing each that must be considered in the diabetic patient. Because diabetic complications striking the central nervous system are discussed in detail elsewhere, this chapter focuses on the complications of diabetes on the peripheral nervous system.

The classification of diabetic neuropathies is listed in Table 31-2. Polyneuropathy syndromes affect the peripheral nerves in a gradually progressive, diffuse, symmetric, and distal more than proximal distribution, consistent with their metabolic basis. Mononeuropathy syndromes affect discrete nerve trunks, singly

TABLE 31-1 NEUROLOGICAL SYNDROMES IN DIABETES

Syndrome	Examples
Stupor, Coma	Hypoglycemia
	Nonketotic hyperglycemia
	Ketoacidosis
	Uremic encephalopathy
Stroke	Thromboembolic brain infarction
	Lacunar infarction
Meningitis	Mucormycosis
	Cryptococcosis
Visual loss	Retinopathy
	Cataract
	Lens changes
Diplopia	Oculomotor nerve palsy
	Abducens nerve palsy
Dysautonomia	Autonomic neuropathy
Lumbar and cervical radicular pain	Diabetic radiculopathy

TABLE 31-2 CLASSIFICATION OF DIABETIC NEUROPATHIES

Polyneuropathy Syndromes

    Mixed sensory–motor–autonomic polyneuropathy
    Predominantly sensory polyneuropathy
        Large-fiber
        Large- and small-fiber
        Small-fiber
    Predominantly motor polyneuropathy
    Predominantly autonomic polyneuropathy
    Rapidly reversible polyneuropathy

Mononeuropathy and Multiple Mononeuropathy Syndromes

    Focal mononeuropathy
    Cranial mononeuropathy
    Proximal motor mononeuropathy (amyotrophy)
    Polyradiculopathy
    Entrapment mononeuropathy

or multiply, with sudden focal dysfunction followed by recovery, consistent with a vascular occlusion etiology. The two neuropathic disorders often coexist in the same patient.

DIABETIC POLYNEUROPATHIES

CLINICAL SIGNIFICANCE

The distal, symmetric, polyneuropathy is the most common diabetic neuropathy. Clinical examination reveals that it is already present in about 10% of newly diagnosed diabetics and is seen in 50% after 25 years. Prevalence figures vary depending upon the means of ascertainment. In asymptomatic diabetics, a careful neurologic examination often discloses reduced fingertip and toe sensation and ankle reflexes. In diabetics with normal neurologic examinations, performance of electromyography and measurements of sensory nerve conduction velocities often reveal abnormalities of early polyneuropathy.

ETIOLOGY

Axonal degeneration is the pathology of the distal, symmetric diabetic poly-neuropathy. Some studies have also shown the presence of independent segmental demyelination. Axonal degeneration is more severe in distal than in proximal nerve segments. It is thought that the axon is poisoned by the accumulation of sorbitol, the sugar that accumulates in the lens of diabetics and leads to cataracts. There is a concomitant reduction in the concentration of myoinositol in the peripheral nerves. These and other metabolic derangements in the diabetic affect the entire peripheral nervous system in a diffuse, symmetric, slowly progressive fashion. The diabetic with poor glucose control generally has a somewhat more severe polyneuropathy than one with tight glucose control, but the correlation is imperfect.

SYMPTOMS AND SIGNS

Polyneuropathies may be predominantly sensory, motor, or autonomic but usually are a combination of these three features. In addition, a mild, rapidly reversible syndrome of painful feet and slowed nerve conduction velocities may be present in newly diagnosed diabetics who have uncontrolled hyperglycemia. With initial regulation of glucose, these symptoms and signs may clear temporarily.

Sensory symptoms and signs often predominate in the patient with a diabetic polyneuropathy. When the large, myelinated A-nerve fibers are principally involved, the signs are more pronounced than the symptoms. The patient experiences reduced sensation in the feet and fingers and may complain of paresthesias of the toes and soles. Examination discloses reduced sensation to light touch and vibration out of proportion to pain and temperature loss in the hands and feet (stocking-and-glove distribution), and absent ankle jerks. When the small, unmyelinated C-nerve fibers are more affected, the symptoms are more pronounced than the signs. Here, foot pain is prominent, often described as boring and burning, and is felt deep in the bones. Examination discloses loss of pain and temperature sensation in the feet and fingers, with relative preservation of vibration and light touch. Ankle reflexes are retained. When both large- and small-fiber involvement is severe, the pseudotabetic form of diabetic polyneuropathy may occur with spontaneous pain, loss of ankle jerks, sensory ataxia from impaired proprioception, positive Romberg's sign, Charcot's joints, and foot ulcers.

Brown and Asbury (1984) have distinguished five different types of pain that may be present in diabetic polyneuropathies. Paresthesias (uncomfortable sensations), the most common, are often described as a "burning" or a "raw sensation like an abrasion." Dysesthesias (contact sensory discomfort) are common in the feet. When walking, the patient feels as if he is walking across broken glass. Causalgia is the most severe form of dysesthesia in which even the slightest touch of the affected area (such as by a bedsheet brushing against the toes) induces excruciating pain similar to that in reflex sympathetic dystrophy syndrome. Deep aching pain, which is boring, burning, or stabbing, may occur in paroxysms, much as it does in a neuralgia. Finally, cramps of the calves or intrinsic foot muscles may be present, resulting from muscle fiber denervation by the neuropathy.

Motor symptoms and signs are unusual except in well-advanced cases when distal hand and foot weakness and atrophy may be present. Occasionally, a syndrome resembling acute post-infectious polyneuropathy occurs during diabetic ketoacidosis. Similar cases, however, are seen in patients critically ill from other causes.

Autonomic disturbances are relatively common, but they predominate only in a small number of young patients with type 1 diabetes. The autonomic dysfunction may strike the gastrointestinal system, the cardiovascular system, and/or the genitourinary system. Gastrointestinal symptoms include slowed esophageal motility, gastroparesis, and episodic nocturnal diarrhea. Cardiovascular symptoms include loss of postural vasomotor reflexes, producing orthostatic hypotension, elevation of resting heart rate, loss of sinus arrhythmia, and sudden death from cardiac arrhythmia. Genitourinary symptoms include difficulty initiating micturition, and in men, retrograde ejaculation and impotence. Abnormalities of pupillary light reflexes and sweating may be seen in autonomic neuropathy.

LABORATORY TESTS

Electromyography and electroneurography may help in surveying the extent and severity of the polyneuropathy, but are not necessary to make the diagnosis. Electromyography reveals evidence of widespread denervation, which is usually symmetric and worse distally. Electroneurography in advanced cases discloses slowing of motor nerve conduction velocities. In milder cases, motor nerve conduction velocities are normal, but sensory action potentials are small and sensory velocities are slowed.

Spinal somatosensory conduction measurements by evoked responses are also slow in the early cases. Cerebrospinal fluid protein level is elevated in most cases, usually in the 45 to 120 mg/dL range. Peripheral nerve biopsy findings are not specific for diabetic polyneuropathy.

DIAGNOSIS

The distal symmetric polyneuropathy of diabetes is diagnosed when the patient notes paresthesias of his hands and/or feet, and the examination discloses reduced ankle jerks and multimodality sensory loss in a stocking-and-glove distribution. Autonomic neuropathy is suspected when the diabetic develops gastrointestinal, cardiovascular, and genitourinary symptoms of autonomic dysfunction. Laboratory evaluation is not necessary for diagnosis.

MANAGEMENT

Although it remains a point of controversy, there is some evidence that optimal glucose control reduces the severity and progression of polyneuropathy. Conversely, with poor control, the polyneuropathy is worse and progresses more quickly. In addition to using insulin or oral hypoglycemic agents, the obese patient with type II diabetes should be strongly encouraged to achieve his or her ideal weight. Specific measures to induce a normal state of peripheral nerve metabolism by treatment with myo-inositol, aldose reductase inhibitors, and gangliosides have been unrewarding. There is no evidence that the B vitamins benefit the diabetic neuropathies, but they are widely prescribed.

Management of pain is the most important therapeutic issue. Because neuropathic pain results from "spontaneous impulse generators" in damaged nerves, anticonvulsant medications have been used with some success. Carbamazepine (Tegretol) and phenytoin (Dilantin) in their usual dosages are the most useful anticonvulsants. If these drugs fail, the patient should be begun on the combination of a low-dose phenothiazine and a low-dose tricyclic antidepressant. Fluphenazine (Prolixin), 1 mg one to three times daily, and amitriptyline (Elavil), 25 to 75 mg nightly, are adequate for most patients. If this regimen fails, amitriptyline should be slowly increased to 150 mg nightly, if tolerated, and fluphenazine continued.

Skin care and foot care are particularly important to prevent trophic ulceration. Patients should be taught to examine their feet and hands frequently for evidence of trauma because they may have wounds that are painless because of the polyneuropathy. Shoes should be ideally fitting and non-chafing. Local debridement and early antibiotic treatment of foot ulcers are desirable. Any unusual joint swelling should be x-rayed to assess formation of Charcot's joints.

Autonomic dysfunction should be recognized and treated. Orthostatic hypotension responds favorably to elastic stockings (if the patient does not have severe peripheral vascular disease), changing positions slowly, and avoidance of alcohol. Sleeping with the head of the bed on six-inch blocks has been shown to improve orthostatic hypotension. When hypotension is severe, fluorinated steroids can be given to increase plasma volume. Gastrointestinal motility problems may respond to codeine, diphenoxylate (Lomotil), or to metoclopramide (Reglan). Bladder and sexual dysfunction therapies are discussed in Chapter 17.

When to Consult
Diabetic polyneuropathies usually do not need to be referred to a neurologist for diagnosis or treatment. Severe cases with pain that is intractable to the usual therapies may be referred to a neurologist or diabetologist who has expertise in this area. Electromyography and electroneurography are not usually necessary for patients with diabetic polyneuropathies. Referral to a podiatrist may be useful for diabetic foot care. Referral to a physical therapist for cane and brace evaluation may be useful if weakness impairs walking. Referral to an occupational therapist for hand aids may be beneficial if the patient has lost fine finger movements.

Patient Education
The patient should be taught the importance of close glucose control and achievement of ideal weight, as well as good foot care as previously described.

DIABETIC MONONEUROPATHIES

Clinical Significance
Sudden impairment of motor, sensory, and reflex functions of a single peripheral nerve trunk is common in diabetics and is known as diabetic mononeuropathy. There is usually a history of longstanding distal symmetric polyneuropathy. The nerves may be affected singly or multiply (multiple mononeuropathy, mononeuritis multiplex). Multiple involvement is usually asymmetric and follows no particular pattern. Nerves may be involved at the level of root, plexus, or distal trunks. Cranial nerves and spinal nerves are also affected.

Etiology.
The pathology of diabetic mononeuropathy is vascular occlusion of the vasa nervorum and consequent nerve infarction. The clinical course, featuring sudden onset of peripheral nerve dysfunction with gradual recovery, is identical to the course of vascular mononeuropathy in polyarteritis nodosa. Experimental models and the pattern of recovery suggest a primarily demyelinating lesion.

Symptoms and Signs
Focal mononeuropathies may affect any peripheral nerve. Sudden palsies of the radial, ulnar, median, sciatic, peroneal, and tibial nerves may occur singly or multiply. There is initial pain in the affected area followed by weakness of the muscles innervated by the nerve, loss of the deep-tendon reflexes of the involved

muscles, and numbness in the cutaneous distribution of the nerve. Gradual and usually complete recovery follows over several to many months.

Cranial nerves may be involved, particularly in elderly diabetics. The oculomotor, abducens, and facial nerves are most commonly involved, in that order. In the elderly patient, oculomotor or abducens mononeuropathy may be the first sign of diabetes, often with no concomitant polyneuropathy. There is usually pain in and behind the eye at the onset of the oculomotor palsy. Most frequently, the pupilloconstrictor fibers are spared and only ophthalmoplegia and ptosis are produced with the eye at rest pointing down and out (see Chapter 1). The sudden onset of head and eye pain with oculomotor palsy immediately raises the question of a ruptured aneurysm of the posterior communicating artery at the junction of the internal carotid artery. In the diabetic patient, if the pupil is spared, the odds heavily favor a diabetic etiology. When the pupil is affected, most neurologists perform carotid arteriography to exclude aneurysm, even in the diabetic patient. In diabetic cranial mononeuropathies, there is spontaneous recovery of cranial nerve function, usually within several weeks to several months after onset.

A common and often misdiagnosed mononeuropathy syndrome is proximal lower extremity motor neuropathy (diabetic amyotrophy). The syndrome occurs most often in overweight, middle-aged and elderly men with type II diabetes. Over several weeks, they develop severe bilateral thigh pain followed by weight loss and bilateral but asymmetric weakness of proximal leg muscles. The quadriceps muscles become atrophic; weakness is principally in the muscles innervated by the femoral nerves (iliopsoas, quadriceps, adductors) and, to a lesser extent, in other proximal leg muscles. Patellar deep-tendon reflexes are absent. Ankle reflexes are not involved but may be absent if the concomitant polyneuropathy is sufficiently severe. Sensory loss is usually inconspicuous, but reduced anterior thigh sensation is occasionally present. The disorder runs a course of four to eight months, during which the pain resolves and muscle bulk and strength returns for the most part. The disorder probably represents multiple proximal lumbosacral plexus infarctions, principally affecting the femoral nerves. A metabolic contribution to the etiology is also suggested by the fact that most cases occur during a period of poor glucose control.

A related disorder is diabetic polyradiculopathy. The lumbosacral nerve roots are affected in 80% of cases, cervical nerve roots in 15%, and thoracic nerve roots in 5%. A subacute onset of radicular pain simulates nerve root compression by herniated disc. Examination discloses weakness in several adjacent nerve roots, some dermatonal sensory loss, and deep-tendon reflex loss appropriate to the lost nerve roots. There is gradual recovery of function and loss of pain over many months. Many patients undergo myelography for suspected mechanical root compression. The disorder is believed to result from multiple infarctions of adjacent spinal nerve roots.

Entrapment neuropathies are more common in the diabetic than in the general population. The most common entrapments are of the median nerve at the wrist (carpal tunnel syndrome), the ulnar nerve at the elbow (cubital tunnel syndrome), the peroneal nerve at the head of the fibula, and the tibial nerve at the ankle (tarsal tunnel syndrome). Peripheral nerves of diabetics seem to be more susceptible to chronic compression than those of nondiabetics despite experimental evidence that their nerves are more resistant to compression ischemia by tourniquets.

LABORATORY TESTS

Electroneurography (ENG) and electromyography (EMG) both have an important role in the diagnosis of diabetic mononeuropathies. EMG reveals evidence of denervation only in those muscles affected by the neuropathy. It permits the identification of the precise nerves and levels involved. ENG demonstrates slowing of nerve conduction across the involved nerve segments in both vascular mononeuropathies and entrapment mononeuropathies.

Muscle biopsy discloses evidence of denervation and adds little information to EMG and ENG findings. The cerebrospinal fluid protein level is often elevated. Serum creatine kinase is usually normal, even in the presence of severe atrophy.

DIAGNOSIS

Isolated palsies of the median, ulnar, radial, sciatic, peroneal, and tibial nerves are easy to diagnose by their characteristic motor and sensory findings. Diabetic amyotrophy and polyradiculopathy are often mistaken for lumbar and sacral nerve root entrapment by herniated disc because of the prominent leg pain, muscle weakness and atrophy, and reflex loss. The major clinical point of differential diagnosis is that the diabetic condition involves multiple nerve roots and/or peripheral nerves, whereas herniated discs usually compress a single nerve root, usually L_5 or S_1. Multiple root or nerve involvement in the diabetic condition may be documented by EMG, but in confusing cases, lumbar myelography or a CT scan is necessary to exclude mechanical nerve root compression. Entrapment neuropathies should be confirmed by ENG. The differential diagnosis of diabetic oculomotor nerve palsy and ruptured aneurysm has been discussed.

MANAGEMENT

All the diabetic mononeuropathy syndromes except the entrapment neuropathies recover spontaneously. In amyotrophy, there is some evidence that improvement in glucose control speeds recovery. Foot braces in peroneal palsy and wrist supports in radial nerve palsies improve function while the nerve is recovering. Physical therapy is often beneficial in the patient with amyotrophy to prevent contractures, to aid ambulation, and to strengthen the quadriceps muscles. Pain control is similar to that in polyneuropathy, but narcotics may be necessary temporarily for cases of amyotrophy and polyradiculopathy. Entrapment neuropathy syndromes are first treated medically with nighttime wrist splints for carpal tunnel syndrome and elbow foam rubber sleeves for cubital tunnel syndrome (see Chapter 11). Surgical release is definitive but should be necessary in only about one-third of the cases.

COMPLICATIONS

Contractures can complicate delayed recovery of mononeuropathy syndromes and are prevented by daily range-of-motion exercises. Unnecessary laboratory investigations as a result of misdiagnosis are common in this group of disorders.

WHEN TO CONSULT

In any diabetic mononeuropathy syndrome, it is advisable to consult a neurologist for clinical and electrical identification of the exact nerves involved. Usually the prognosis is good, which greatly aids the patient in coping with the temporary pain and disability. A physical therapist can recommend range-of-motion exercises, muscle-strengthening exercises, and orthotic supports.

Bibliography

Bastron JA, Thomas JE: Diabetic polyradiculopathy. Clinical and electromyographic findings in 105 patients. *Mayo Clin Proc* 1981; 56:725-732. (Defines the clinical and electrical features of this syndrome.)

Brown MJ, Asbury AK: Diabetic neuropathy. *Ann Neurol* 1984; 15:2-12. (Current, authoritative, thorough summary of the range of diabetic neuropathies from the group of investigators at the University of Pennsylvania.)

Chokroverty S, Ryees MG, Rubino FA, et al: The syndrome of diabetic amyotrophy. *Ann Neurol* 1977; 2:181-194. (Thoroughly reviews the literature on the pathogenesis and clinical features of diabetic amyotrophy. Concludes that metabolic disturbances, not vascular insufficiency, may be the most important pathogenic factor.)

Davis JL, Lewis SB, Gerich JE, et al: Peripheral diabetic neuropathy treated with amitriptyline and fluphenazine. *JAMA* 1977; 238:2291-2292. (Shows analgesic benefit of low-dose amitriptyline and fluphenazine in dysesthesias and other pains of diabetic polyneuropathy.)

Dyck PJ, Thomas PK, Lambert EH et al (eds): *Diabetic Neuropathy.* Philadelphia, Saunders, 1987. (Current, authoritative, and very complete; recommended.)

Editorial: Pain perception in diabetic neuropathy. *Lancet* 1985; 1:83-85. (Reviews the various theories of pain production in diabetic neuropathies, particularly the role of hyperglycemia.)

Judzeqitsch RG, Jaspan JB, Polonsky KS, et al: Aldose reductase inhibition improves nerve conduction velocity in diabetic patients. *N Engl J Med* 1983; 308:119-125. (Shows the modest benefit of sorbinil, an inhibitor of the polyol-pathway enzyme aldose reductase on nerve conduction velocities in stable diabetic patients. Reviews the literature on such therapies.)

Schaumburg HH, Spencer PS, Thomas PK: *Disorders of Peripheral Nerves.* Philadelphia, F.A. Davis, 1983, pp 41-55. (Chapter 4 provides a succinct account of the clinical and pathologic features of diabetic neuropathies.)

Service EJ, Daube JR, O'Brien PC, et al: Effect of blood glucose control on peripheral nerve function in diabetic patients. *Mayo Clin Proc* 1983; 58:283-289. (Discusses and compares the effects of tight and loose glucose control on clinical and electrical evidence of diabetic polyneuropathy. This study did not find much correlation, but it reviews the literature.)

Thomas PK, Eliasson SG: Diabetic neuropathy, in: Dyck PJ, Thomas PK, Lambert EH, et al (eds): *Peripheral Neuropathy* (ed 2). Philadelphia, Saunders, 1984, vol 2, pp 1773-1810. (Very thorough, current, authoritative reference source with 376 references.)

Neurological Complications of Systemic Cancer

Cancer is the second leading cause of death in the United States. More than 700,000 new cases are diagnosed yearly, and more than 400,000 people die of cancer each year. It is estimated that 10% to 15% of patients who have systemic cancer develop some type of neurological complication. Many patients who develop neurological dysfunction are not known to have systemic cancer when they become symptomatic; thus, a neurological syndrome may be the first manifestation of an occult neoplasm.

Cancer can involve the nervous system in several ways. The tumor may metastasize to the brain, spinal cord, or meninges, or it may produce non-metastatic effects on the nervous system. These nonmetastatic effects include paraneoplastic disorders and complications of therapy (chemotherapy, radiation therapy) on the nervous system. A knowledge of common neurological complications of cancer allows the practitioner to recognize and treat them, which in turn can preserve neurological function. This chapter examines common neurological complications of systemic cancer. Epidural spinal cord compression caused by metastatic malignancy is discussed in Chapter 40.

BRAIN METASTASIS

CLINICAL SIGNIFICANCE

Metastasis to the brain is the most common neurological complication of systemic cancer, and metastatic tumor is the most common form of brain tumor. The incidence of primary malignant intracranial tumors is approximately 4.2 per 100,000; that of metastatic brain tumors is estimated to be 8.5 per 100,000. Almost 25% of patients dying of cancer have an intracranial or dural tumor. At autopsy, approximately 15% of patients with cancer have intracranial metastases, almost two-thirds of whom have shown corresponding symptoms during life. In some patients, the cause of death is closely related to the intracranial disease.

ETIOLOGY

Most metastases reach the brain by the hematogenous route, most commonly by way of the arterial circulation. In some cases, spread occurs via Batson's venous plexus or via direct extension through intracranial foramina. Although brain metastases may appear anywhere in the brain, supratentorial structures are invaded twice as frequently as those of the posterior fossa. Metastases occur equally in both hemispheres: approximately 10% to 15% in the cerebellum, 5% in the brain stem, and 5% to 10% in the pituitary gland. Seventy-five percent of metastases are multiple.

The incidence of brain metastasis varies with the type of underlying tumor. Lung cancer is now the most common source of brain metastasis; 30% to 40% of patients with lung cancer have brain metastases at autopsy. Multiple metastases are more common with melanoma and carcinoma of the lung, but any tumor may give rise to multiple metastases. Breast cancer, testicular cancer, and renal cancer commonly metastasize to the brain, whereas tumors of the colon, pancreas, and the prostate rarely spread to the brain. At some time during the course of tumor growth, 6% to 20% of patients with breast cancer have brain metastases, as do 50% of patients with melanoma and approximately 13% of patients with renal cell carcinoma. In the vast majority of patients (80% to 90%) the interval between the identification of the primary cancer and of the brain metastasis is at least 12 months, although in lung cancer the spread to the brain is often evident within three months.

SYMPTOMS AND SIGNS

Headache, focal weakness, and mental status changes are frequent presenting symptoms of metastatic brain disease. Seizures are the presenting symptom in 15% to 20% of patients. Hemiparesis, hemisensory loss, and mental dullness are the most common presenting signs. Papilledema occurs in one-quarter of patients with brain metastasis. The symptoms and signs clearly depend upon the anatomic location of the tumor and whether it is solitary or multiple. Symptoms usually develop and progress over a period of several weeks, but many patients have symptoms for one or two months before they are evaluated medically.

Occasionally, rapid onset occurs, mimicking a stroke. When this happens, there is usually hemorrhage into the tumor. This hemorrhagic process is more common with melanoma, renal cell carcinoma, choriocarcinoma, testicular carcinoma, and bronchogenic tumors, occurring in 5% to 10% of patients. A hemorrhage into a tumor should be considered in all patients who have atypical hemorrhagic strokes. Twenty percent of patients may present with metastatic brain tumor as the first source of symptoms of a previously unknown tumor. Such brain metastases from an occult source usually arise from the lung, but the gastrointestinal tract and the kidney are also sources.

LABORATORY TESTS AND DIAGNOSIS

Computed tomography (CT) of the head is the diagnostic procedure of choice, accurately identifying 90% to 95% of supratentorial and 80% of infratentorial metastases. A CT scan should be performed before and after the injection of intravenous contrast material; a double dose of contrast should be given to increase the sensitivity of the CT for detecting metastatic lesions, especially multiple ones. The typical metastatic tumor is spherical in shape and is surrounded by edema. It may enhance diffusely or have a ring-like appearance (a ring of contrast enhancement with a lucent center). Some tumors, particularly melanoma and carcinoma of the colon, are dense prior to injection of contrast. A radiopaque lesion seen on a nonenhanced CT scan often indicates the presence of a hemorrhage. Tumors of the cerebellum, meninges, and, rarely, the brain stem may cause obstructive hydrocephalus.

The differential diagnosis of solitary or multiple lesions includes brain abscess, primary brain tumor (approximately 4% of gliomas are multicentric), and brain hemorrhage. Meningiomas occur with a much higher frequency in women with breast cancer, so a solitary enhancing brain mass in this setting could be caused by a meningioma, not a metastatic tumor. In the patient with known cancer, a brain lesion is most likely to be of metastatic origin. In the patient without known malignancy, a search should be undertaken for a site of the primary tumor. Tests include chest x-ray, liver and bone scans, mammograms, CBC, urinalysis, liver function, and sputum cytology. Less commonly, intravenous pyelogram (IVP) or barium enema are helpful. A CT scan of the abdomen is the most effective test for detecting an occult malignancy. In approximately 20% of patients with brain metastasis, no involvement of other organs is found. Single lesions in the absence of known systemic cancer should be biopsied to determine the exact diagnosis. Lumbar puncture and cerebrospinal fluid analysis are not usually helpful for determining the presence or the type of intracranial metastasis, and may be hazardous in the presence of increased intracranial pressure or if the lesion is in the posterior fossa. Radionuclide brain scanning may be of some benefit in a community hospital where a CT scan is not available.

Management

There are three treatment modalities that can be directed against brain metastases: radiation therapy, chemotherapy, and surgery. The median survival for patients with metastatic tumors is less than six months; only 10% live one year. Untreated patients with CNS metastasis survive one month; with the use of corticosteroids, two months.

Appropriate anticonvulsants can be given for patients who develop seizures. Because there is a high incidence of seizures with testicular cancer and metastatic melanoma, prophylactic use of anticonvulsants is warranted. Most patients with metastatic brain disease have evidence of brain edema, which should be treated with corticosteroid medication. Dexamethasone, 4 to 16 mg four times daily, or methylprednisolone, 24 to 32 mg four times a day, controls edema in most patients. Sixty to eighty percent of patients treated with corticosteroids manifest clinical improvement. Phenytoin increases the metabolism of dexamethasone, so that the dosage requirements for the latter drug may be higher if there is concurrent use of phenytoin. This interaction does not occur with methylprednisolone. Methylprednisolone is the preferred corticosteroid because it does not interact with anticonvulsants and because it has a shorter onset of action than dexamethasone.

Radiation therapy is the mainstay of the treatment of brain metastasis. Standard treatment is 3000 rads in ten fractions over a two week period. The state of the patient prior to therapy in part determines the length of survival; in general, 60% of patients with metastatic disease who are treated with radiation therapy improve; they have a median survival of three to six months. Patients who are ambulatory tend to survive longer than those who are not. Survival also depends on the type of brain metastasis; choriocarcinoma, testicular carcinoma, and cancer of the breast are radiosensitive, whereas carcinomas of the lung and kidney tend to be radioresistant.

Surgical therapy is generally undertaken only for the patient with a solitary metastasis, although many surgically treated patients do only slightly better than those treated with radiation alone. Excellent long-term results have been reported, however, in patients undergoing surgical excision of a single brain metastasis. If such patients are free of or have well-controlled extracerebral tumor, the median survival is six to seven months. Fewer than 25% survive for one year; however, over 75% of such treated patients are neurologically improved, albeit transiently.

Although *chemotherapy* remains one of the hopes for the future in the treatment of brain metastasis, it has proved to be of little benefit at the present because most metastatic tumors of the brain do not respond to currently available drugs. Intra-arterial chemotherapy of brain metastases with BCNU or cisplatin, a newer mode of delivering chemotherapeutic drugs to the brain, is of benefit. Some brain metastases seemingly disappear following treatment with systemic chemotherapy directed against the primary tumor.

The cause of death in most patients with brain metastases is disseminated systemic cancer, although 20% of patients with a solitary metasasis and one-third of patients with multiple metastases die from primary neurological causes.

WHEN TO CONSULT

When a patient develops a new onset of seizures or focal neurological disturbances, neurological consultation may be indicated. If a CT scan is performed and a tumor is evident, a neurologist may be able to help differentiate clinically as to whether a primary or a metastatic tumor is present, although the primary care physician can perform a diagnostic evaluation without the aid of a neurologist.

LEPTOMENINGEAL CARCINOMATOSIS

CLINICAL SIGNIFICANCE AND ETIOLOGY

Metastasis from a tumor that seeds the leptomeninges is an important and common complication of systemic cancer. Although once considered to be rare, leptomeningeal carcinomatosis is now recognized as a cause of neurological disability and death. There is evidence that the incidence of this type of metastasis is increasing. Prior to CNS prophylaxis, the incidence of leptomeningeal leukemia in children was greater than 50%. Its incidence in childhood leukemias is still high; in children with acute lymphocytic leukemia it has been reported to be as high as 33%. In certain non-Hodgkin's lymphomas (diffuse undifferentiated,

Burkitt's lymphoma) the incidence has been reported to be as high as 30%. Of the solid tumors, leptomeningeal carcinomatosis most commonly occurs as a result of melanoma, oat cell carcinoma of the lung, and breast cancer. Approximately three-quarters of patients with leptomeningeal carcinomatosis have adenocarcinoma. However, any tumor is capable of seeding the leptomeninges with or without CNS metastases. In general, the more widespread the tumor, the greater the likelihood that leptomeningeal carcinomatosis will occur clinically.

It is unclear precisely how the tumor cells reach the leptomeninges. Several mechanisms have been proposed, including rupture of parenchymal brain tumors into the subarachnoid space, hematogenous metastases to the choroid plexus with rupture into the CSF, growth of paravertebral tumor along nerve routes and into the subarachnoid space at the spinal cord level, and growth of subdural tumor through the arachnoid membrane. Although all of these mechanisms probably occur in some patients, the most likely explanation is hematogenous spread of the tumor to the arachnoid.

SYMPTOMS AND SIGNS

Patients with leptomeningeal carcinomatosis develop symptoms and signs at more than one level of the nervous system. The nervous system is thus classified into three areas when dealing with leptomeningeal carcinomatosis: brain, cranial nerves, and spinal areas. Approximately 18% to 20% of patients with leptomeningeal carcinomatosis have signs and symptoms limited to one area of the neuraxis; 50% to 55% have them limited to two areas; 25% have them in all three areas. As the disease progresses, so does the extent of the symptoms and signs. Common cerebral symptoms and signs are listed in Table 32-1.

Almost 50% of patients present with cerebral symptoms, with headache the most frequent complaint. The headache may be diffuse, bifrontal, or at the base of the skull, and it often radiates into the neck. It is often associated with lightheadedness and nausea or vomiting.

A change in the mental status of the patient is one of the most common cerebral complaints, occurring in almost one-third of patients with leptomeningeal carcinomatosis. Patients with mental status changes often complain of lethargy, memory loss, or confusion. Approximately 25% complain of ataxia of gait (often related to hydrocephalus), nausea, and vomiting. Almost two-thirds of patients with cerebral symptoms have evidence of cognitive dysfunction on examination. Generalized or focal seizures are an uncommon mode of presentation (10%), although they develop with increased frequency as the disease progresses. Papilledema, diabetes insipidus, and hemiparesis are uncommon signs on presentation.

Table 32-1 also lists the common cranial nerve symptoms and signs resulting from leptomeningeal carcinomatosis. Cranial nerve symptoms and signs are the initial complaint in more than one-third of patients. Diplopia is the most common complaint, followed by hearing loss, facial numbness (especially in the chin area), and decreased visual acuity. Weakness of the extraocular muscles (cranial nerves III, IV, VI) is the most common cranial nerve sign, followed by facial weakness (cranial nerve VII, producing weakness similar to Bell's palsy), reduced hearing (cranial nerve VIII), visual loss (cranial nerve II, usually monocular), facial

TABLE 32-1 SYMPTOMS AND SIGNS OF LEPTOMENINGEAL CARCINOMATOSIS

Symptom	Frequency (%)	Sign	Cranial Nerve #	Frequency (%)
Cerebral				
Headache	66	Mental status changes	—	62
Mental status changes	33	Seizures	—	11
Gait ataxia	27	generalized (60%)	—	6
Nausea and vomiting	22	focal (40%)	—	4
Loss of consciousness	4	Papilledema	—	11
Language disorders	4	Diabetes insipidus	—	4
Dizziness	4	Hemiparesis	—	2
Cranial Nerve				
Diplopia	36	Oculomotor paresis	(III,IV,VI)	36
Hearing loss	14	Facial weakness	(VII)	30
Visual loss	10	Hearing loss	(VIII)	18
Facial numbness	10	Optic neuropathy	(II)	10
Decreased taste	6	Trigeminal neuropathy	(V)	10
Tinnitus	4	Hypoglossal neuropathy	(XII)	10
Dysphagia	4	Decreased gag reflex	(IX,X)	6
Spinal				
Weakness	46	Reflex asymmetry	—	86
Paresthesias	42	Weakness	—	73
Pain (back/neck)	31	Sensory loss	—	32
Radicular pain	26	+ Straight leg raising	—	15
Autonomic dysfunction	16	Decreased rectal tone	—	14
		Nuchal rigidity	—	9

Adapted from Wasserstrom WR, Glass JP, Posner JB: Diagnosis and treatment of leptomeningeal metastasis from solid tumors: Experience with 90 patients. *Cancer* 1982; 49:760. Used with permission.

numbness (cranial nerve V), tongue weakness (cranial nerve XII), and decreased gag reflex (cranial nerves IX, X).

Spinal symptoms include those that indicate involvement of the spinal cord and its nerve roots or the spinal leptomeninges. The most common presenting signs and symptoms are listed in Table 32-1. Weakness and paresthesias (usually of the legs) occurs in more than one-third of patients as the initial symptom. Pain in the back or neck or radicular pain occurs in about one-third of patients as the first symptom; bowel and bladder dysfunction occurs in 15% of patients. More than two-thirds of patients have signs of spinal involvement on the initial examination, with asymmetry of the deep-tendon reflexes most noticeable. There is often generalized or focal weakness (usually of the lower motor neuron type) and sensory loss. True nuchal rigidity is uncommon. As the disease progresses so does the extent and severity of the symptoms and signs.

LABORATORY TESTS

The most important diagnostic test for leptomeningeal carcinomatosis is the examination of CSF. Some abnormalities of CSF occur in almost all patients with leptomeningeal carcinomatosis, but serial examination of the CSF may be necessary before studies are positive. Often on the initial examination, CSF abnormalities are not striking. The CSF pressure is elevated in more than half of the cases. Cerebrospinal fluid pleocytosis (more than 5 cells/mm³) is also seen in

50% of cases; most of these cells are mononuclear leukocytes; poly-morphonuclear leukocytes (PMNs) have been reported only occasionally. Cell counts range from 0 to 1800 cells/mm³.

The protein concentration is elevated in more than two-thirds of patients, with a level at times above 2 g/dL. In one-third of patients, the glucose concentration is reduced. More than half of the patients have malignant cells in CSF on the first lumbar puncture. The yield increases to more than 90% when additional lumbar punctures are performed. In some patients with cerebral and/or cranial nerve symptoms and signs, CSF cytology is positive in the ventricular or cisternal fluid but not in the lumbar fluid. Cytocentrifugation increases the yield of malignant cells in the CSF and is the preferred method for concentrating CSF for cytologic examination.

The CSF may be examined for biochemical markers of metastatic disease; these markers may be of diagnostic value in the absence of malignant cells in CSF, and may allow monitoring of therapy. Beta-glucuronidase levels (above 80 mU/L) strongly suggest the presence of leptomeningeal disease, particularly in patients with carcinoma of the breast or lung cancer. Carcinoembryonic antigen (CEA) is also elevated in leptomeningeal carcinomatosis, again more commonly in patients with breast or lung carcinoma. A CSF CEA concentration above 1 mg/mL without a serum CEA level above 100 mg/mL is considered pathologic.

Abnormal lactate dehydrogenase (LDH) isoenzyme patterns (with an LDH isoenzyme 5:1 ratio greater than 15%) also commonly occurs in leptomeningeal carcinomatosis. Human chorionic gonadotropin (HCG) levels may be increased in cases of leptomeningeal carcinomatosis from embryonal cell carcinoma, and Beta-2 microglobulin levels may be elevated in cases caused by myeloproliferative disorders (leukemia, lymphoma). Oligoclonal bands may be found in the CSF in leptomeningeal carcinomatosis and may aid in the diagnosis.

The CT scan is also helpful in the diagnosis of leptomeningeal carcinomatosis, although there is no truly diagnostic CT abnormality. Findings on CT are present in 25% to 75% of patients. Enhancement of CSF-containing spaces is present in one-third of patients. Multiple superficial enhancing cortical nodules may be one of the earliest CT abnormalities; the patient with lymphoma, lung carcinoma, or melanoma with this CT appearance should be evaluated for meningeal involve-ment by the tumor. Ventriculomegaly occurs in two-thirds of patients and is often associated with sulcal or cisternal obliteration. These findings may be present on the first CT, or may develop as leptomeningeal carcinomatosis develops clinically.

Myelography may be necessary, particularly in the patient who has equivocal symptoms or signs and in whom CSF findings are nonspecific. There is a strong tendency for malignant cells to adhere to neural tissue or to the leptomeninges, accounting for the occasional patient with negative CSF cytology. In such patients, myelography may disclose irregular filling of the subarachnoid spaces secondary to thickening and nodularity of nerve roots, particularly of the cauda equina.

Cerebral angiography can reveal narrowing of the arteries at the base of the brain in a vasculitis-like pattern. Electroneurography and electromyography may be of diagnostic benefit, particularly in patients with spinal symptoms and signs. Reduced motor nerve conduction velocities and abnormally prolonged F-wave latencies in the legs without sensory nerve disturbances are common findings. Electromyographic (EMG) evidence of denervation at multiple nerve root levels, particularly in the erector spinae, is a characteristic finding.

DIAGNOSIS

In general, the diagnosis is made when there are multifocal levels of nervous system involvement in a patient with cancer (in the absence of other metastases that can explain the symptoms and signs) associated with abnormal CSF (usually cytologic or biochemical markers). On rare occasions, the diagnosis may be accepted on clinical criteria alone, eg, in the cancer patient with multiple levels of neurological dysfunction and an absence of other clinical or radiologic explanation for the neurological findings. A CSF protein level greater than 100 mg/dL or a depressed glucose level supports the diagnosis of leptomeningeal carcinomatosis in the patient with suggestive clinical symptoms and signs. If the clinical evidence is less supportive, then a positive cytologic or myelographic finding, the enhancement of CSF cisterns, or the presence of superficial cortical nodules on CT will help make the diagnosis. Thus, in the vast majority of patients with leptomeningeal carcinomatosis, there are specific laboratory tests that, when coupled with the clinical status of the patient, will allow the diagnosis to be made. The more widespread the systemic involvement, the more likely will be leptomeningeal involvement. In some patients, however (particularly small cell carcinoma patients in remission), the leptomeninges represent the only site of metastasis. Leptomeningeal carcinomatosis should be considered in the differential diagnosis when a chronic meningitis picture is seen in the CSF.

MANAGEMENT

The treatment of leptomeningeal carcinomatosis is radiation therapy and chemotherapy. There are two goals of therapy: to prolong the survival of the patient and to stabilize or ameliorate the neurological symptoms and signs. Untreated, leptomeningeal carcinomatosis leads to progressive neurological dysfunction and results in death from neurological causes within four to six weeks. Optimal treatment must reach the tumor cells within the CNS and must not produce significant toxicity.

The protocol at Memorial–Sloan Kettering Cancer Center in New York consists of radiation therapy (2400 rads in eight doses over 10 to 14 days) directed to the site(s) of major clinical involvement (see Wasserstrom WR, Glass JP, Posner JB, 1982). Few chemotherapeutic drugs used to treat solid tumors cross the blood brain barrier; thus, chemotherapy is usually given intrathecally, either by repeated lumbar puncture or intraventricularly through a catheter inserted into the lateral ventricle (Ommaya or Rickham reservoir). The use of a subcutaneous reservoir with a ventricular cannula virtually assures that (1) the chemotherapeutic agent enters the CNS; (2) the drug follows the pathways of CSF flow, reaching all of the CSF spaces; (3) patient comfort and compliance is maintained. In contrast to the need for multiple lumbar punctures, the injection of a chemotherapeutic agent through a small scalp vein needle is essentially without pain.

Methotrexate (MTX) is the drug used most often for intrathecal administration. The dosage is 7 mg/m², instilled twice a week for five treatments. Citrovorum factor is often given in a dosage of 9 mg every 12 hours on the day of treatment and for three days following. If there is cytologic or clinical improvement, then therapy is given once weekly (as an outpatient); if improvement continues, treatment can be given every third or fourth week thereafter. At each treatment, CSF is withdrawn for cell count, cytology, culture, and biochemical analysis. Other drugs that may be used include cytosine arabinoside (30 mg/m^2), thiotepa, and fibroblast interferon. Approximately 20% to 25% of patients so treated will improve. A similar number of patients will progress in the face of therapy, and 40% to 50% will stabilize.

Even with treatment, the median survival of patients with leptomeningeal carcinomatosis is six months. Patients with carcinoma of the breast respond better to therapy and tend to have a longer survival, whereas those with lung carcinoma or melanoma do the worst. Patients with widespread systemic disease with neurological manifestations live an average of three months. In the absence of systemic disease, however, median survival following therapy is approximately eight months, with a 20% one-year survival in all patients and a 30% survival in those who responded initially to therapy.

The side effects of therapy tend to be minor. Focal radiation therapy is fairly well tolerated by most patients. The placement of an Ommaya reservoir is usually well tolerated. The infection rate in patients with an Ommaya reservoir is less than 4%, and reservoir malfunction is uncommon. Placement of a reservoir should be postponed if a patient has infectious meningitis unless it is also being used to treat meningitis. Thrombocytopenia or the threat of disseminated intravascular coagulation (DIC) or other clotting abnormalities puts the patient at risk for delayed wound healing or perioperative hemorrhage.

An acute meningoencephalitis can follow a few hours after the instillation of MTX. This encephalitis is characterized by headache, fever, a stiff neck (occasionally), disorientation, and confusion. Examination of CSF may remain the same or be associated with an increased cell count and protein level, but CSF cultures are negative; symptoms usually resolve within 24 to 72 hours of their onset. The MTX leukoencephalopathy can develop particularly in patients who earlier have received whole brain radiation. This leukoencephalopathy is evident on CT scan, and clinically there is a change in the patient's cognitive functions; the latter occurs after prolonged use of MTX even in the absence of CT changes.

WHEN TO CONSULT

For the patient with known systemic malignancy who develops focal or multifocal levels of nervous system dysfunction, a neurological consultation is in order. This is particularly true if a CT scan has been performed and was without evidence of mass lesions. Prompt diagnosis and treatment is essential if the quality of life of patients with leptomeningeal carcinomatosis is to be prolonged. Because leptomeningeal carcinomatosis is rarely the initial manifestation of an occult malignancy, atypical spinal fluid findings may need clinical and neurological correlation. A neurologist may help in determining the nature of these changes. A neurologist is also trained in the instillation of intrathecal agents and will not only help with diagnosis but also with therapy. For the patient with documented leptomeningeal carcinomatosis who is a candidate for aggressive treatment, a neurosurgical consultation is also in order to place a Rickham or Ommaya reservoir.

REMOTE EFFECTS OF CANCER ON THE NERVOUS SYSTEM

The paraneoplastic disorders, or remote effects of cancer, encompass a wide range of conditions associated either directly or indirectly with malignant disease but *not* caused by metastatic invasion of the nervous system. These paraneoplastic disorders occur with an increased frequency in patients with cancer. Common paraneoplastic disorders are listed in Table 32-2.

CLINICAL SIGNIFICANCE

Nervous system paraneoplastic syndromes are uncommon, but are important for a number of reasons:

1. Some of the paraneoplastic syndromes are so characteristic that their presence should initiate a search for occult cancer. Such symptoms often appear before the cancer has been diagnosed and when it is still potentially "curable."

2. The identification and subsequent treatment of the underlying tumor in some patients with paraneoplastic syndromes leads to amelioration of the neurological problem.

3. The nervous system symptoms may be more disabling than the neoplasm that caused them.

The precise incidence of the paraneoplastic nervous system disorders is unknown, but estimates are that they appear in approximately 5% of patients with a tumor. It has recently been shown that patients with oat cell carcinoma of the lung associated with paraneoplastic syndromes tend to have a more benign clinical course, with prolonged survival, than those without paraneoplastic syndromes.

TABLE 32-2. PARANEOPLASTIC DISORDERS OF THE NERVOUS SYSTEM

Brain
    Subacute cerebellar degeneration and opsoclonia
    Dementia–limbic encephalitis

Spinal Cord
    Subacute necrotic myelopathy
    Subacute motor neuronopathy

Peripheral nerve
    Subacute sensory neuropathy
    Sensorimotor neuropathy
        Acute (resembles Guillain–Barré syndrome)
        Chronic
        Relapsing

Muscle
    Dermatomyositis
    Polymyositis
    Eaton–Lambert syndrome (myasthenic)

ETIOLOGY

Paraneoplastic syndromes are most frequently associated with carcinoma of the lung (primarily small cell) and ovarian and gastric carcinomas. The cause of paraneoplastic syndromes is not known. Nutritional factors are unlikely, and a viral etiology, although attractive, has not been proven. Progressive multifocal leukoencephalopathy, a white-matter degeneration of the CNS that usually occurs in patients with lymphoproliferative neoplasms, was once believed to be a paraneoplastic disorder. Subsequent studies revealed that it is caused by a Jakob–Creutzfeldt (JC) virus.

An autoimmune etiology is also possible. Some patients have specific circulating antibodies, which probably arise as a reaction to an antigen shared between the cancer and the nervous system. It is possible that the tumor promotes the development of antibodies that attack the nervous system. The secretion of a neurotoxin as a cause of these syndromes has never been proven; nor does there appear to be any evidence of an opportunistic infection.

Subacute Cerebellar Degeneration

SYMPTOMS AND SIGNS

As with other paraneoplastic disorders, subacute cerebellar degeneration may precede or follow the diagnosis of the underlying neoplasm. The interval between discovery of the tumor and the cerebellar disorder has ranged from three months to two years. When neurological symptoms precede the tumor, the interval between the two events is between two months and three years. Clinically, patients exhibit a progressive cerebellar disorder that has developed acutely or subacutely over a period of weeks. Symptoms include vertigo, ataxia of the arms, trunk and legs, dysarthria, and occasionally diplopia. The limbs are usually involved asymmetrically at first, but involvement eventually becomes symmetrical. The ataxia tends to be progressive and severe, so that the patient is not able to stand or walk, and sitting in a chair without support is difficult. Dysarthria can be severe. Nystagmus is present in about 50% of cases; myoclonus is occasionally present. Dementia is common. Occasionally, cerebellar degeneration is associated with uncontrollable opsoclonus (rapid and arrhythmic conjugate oscillations of the eyes in all directions); this occurs with especially high frequency in children with neuroblastoma and in adults with oat cell carcinoma of the lung. Its presence should prompt a diagnostic search for an underlying neoplasm.

The CSF may show a mononuclear pleocytosis; a CT scan may demonstrate pancerebellar degeneration and atrophy. Recently, an antibody to the cytoplasm of the Purkinje cells of the cerebellum has been demonstrated in the sera of some patients with paraneoplastic cerebellar degeneration. Pathologically, there is diffuse loss of cerebellar Purkinje cells and associated perivascular inflammation.

MANAGEMENT

Recovery from severe cerebellar ataxia is unusual; however, the disorder may arrest, while the patient is still ambulatory. Survival generally depends on the nature of the underlying malignancy. Treatment of the underlying tumor occasionally produces improvement or resolution of the cerebellar disorder. Plasmapheresis has been reported to transiently improve this cerebellar syndrome.

Dementia–Limbic Encephalitis

SYMPTOMS AND SIGNS

Paraneoplastic limbic dementia is a subacute encephalopathic process that commonly presents as a confusional state associated with a persistent defect in recent memory. Other mental disturbances include anxiety, depression, hallucinations, and dementia. Generalized seizures may also occur. The course is usually subacute and may be progressive, although there is a tendency to arrest in some cases.

LABORATORY TESTS

The CSF may show pleocytosis and increased protein levels, and the EEG often demonstrates slowing or sharp waves. The CT scan is usually normal. No virus has ever been isolated. On neuropathological examination there are degenerative changes in the hippocampal and amygdaloid nuclei, often associated with perivascular lymphocytic infiltration.

MANAGEMENT

Although there is no effective therapy for limbic encephalitis, several reports have noted complete resolution of the dementia following treatment of the underlying neoplasm.

Necrotizing Myelopathy

SYMPTOMS AND SIGNS

Subacute necrotizing myelopathy is probably the rarest and most obscure of the nervous system paraneoplastic disorders. There tends to be a rapidly ascending sensory and motor loss, usually to a thoracic spinal cord level, associated with autonomic dysfunction. The patient usually becomes incontinent and paraplegic within a few days, and neurological symptoms often precede the discovery of the neoplasm. Back pain and nerve route pain may also be present. The differential diagnosis comprises other spinal cord disorders, including epidural compression from tumor, acute demyelination, transverse myelitis, and vascular disorders.

LABORATORY TESTS

Myelography is usually normal and survival is measured in weeks to months. Pathologically, there is massive necrosis of the thoracic spinal cord.

MANAGEMENT

There is no effective treatment for this progressive myelopathy. General supportive measures are all that can be provided for the patient.

Subacute Motor Neuronopathy

SYMPTOMS AND SIGNS

Subacute motor neuronopathy usually affects patients with Hodgkin's disease or other lymphomas. The course of the illness is subacute, with the development of symmetrical and painless lower motor neuron weakness of the arms and legs, usually in the absence of sensory changes. The lower limbs tend to be involved more severely.

LABORATORY TESTS AND DIAGNOSIS

Cerebrospinal fluid examination is usually normal, although the protein level may be elevated. Electromyography and nerve conduction studies reveal chronic partial denervation associated with spontaneous fibrillations and mild slowing of both motor and sensory nerve conduction velocities. Pathologically, there is anterior horn cell degeneration and motor root demyelination. The pathogenesis is unclear, but the differential diagnosis includes lumbosacral plexus invasion from tumor, Guillain-Barré syndrome, and leptomeningeal carcinomatosis. Many patients improve spontaneously, regardless of the course of their underlying lymphoma.

Peripheral Neuropathy

Peripheral neuropathy associated with carcinoma is probably the most common paraneoplastic nervous system disorder, having an incidence of 2.4% of cancer patients. Most cases occur in patients with carcinoma of the lung (small cell), stomach, or colon. There are three main peripheral nervous system disorders that manifest as paraneoplastic disturbances. *Sensory* neuropathy was the first to be distinguished as a complication of carcinoma, but the *sensorimotor* type is more common (60% of cases of paraneoplastic peripheral neuropathy).

Subacute Sensory Neuropathy

SYMPTOMS AND SIGNS

There is numbness with dyesthesias and paresthesias of the extremities, which begin distally and spread proximally but rarely involve the face. Gait ataxia may develop, and aching pains may be present in the limbs. True weakness is uncommon. On examination, deep-tendon reflexes are depressed or absent and there is sensory loss of all modalities in the extremities. Position and vibratory sensation are most involved, leading to sensory ataxia. Muscle weakness and wasting are unusual, except in late stages of the disease. Sphincter disturbances are uncommon. Diplopia, nystagmus, and anisocoria can also be present. Memory loss and dementia are uncommon.

The usual interval between the onset of symptoms and the discovery of the primary tumor is six to 15 months. The onset tends to be subacute, with progression over a few months. Rarely, an acute onset occurs. It is uncommon for the neuropathy to develop after the diagnosis of malignancy is made. The median survival is 14 months. This type of neuropathy is not common in males.

LABORATORY TESTS

The CSF may be normal, but usually there is modest leukocytosis and an elevated protein level. Few patients reported have had circulating antibodies (IgG polyclonal) detected against the nuclei of neurons. Electromyography and nerve conduction studies reveal distal denervation with fibrillations and absent sensory action potentials. Motor nerve conduction velocities are only minimally slow. Pathologically, there is degeneration of the posterior columns of the spinal cord and the dorsal nerve roots, with sparing of the anterior and lateral spinal cord areas. There is profound loss of nerve cells in the dorsal root ganglia; inflammatory changes (ganglioradiculitis) are also evident in these regions.

MANAGEMENT

There is no specific treatment, and therapy directed against the primary tumor usually does not help the neuropathy. The management of painful neuropathies is discussed in Chapter 31.

Sensorimotor Neuropathy

Sensorimotor neuropathy is the most common paraneoplastic peripheral neuropathy. Approximately 60% of affected patients are males. The site of primary carcinoma is frequently the lung, but it can be in the stomach, breast, uterus, kidney, or other organs. Subtypes of sensorimotor neuropathy include subacute, acute, chronic, and relapsing varieties.

Subacute. The clinical manifestations are usually those of a distal neuropathy (Chapter 31) with numbness, sensory impairment, weakness, and decreased reflexes. Proximal weakness rarely occurs; occasionally, trigeminal sensory loss is evident (giving rise to a "numb chin"). This type of neuropathy may precede the diagnosis of tumor by as many as five years, or may follow it. The neuropathy may be progressive, but it can regress spontaneously.

Spinal fluid protein concentration is elevated. Electrodiagnostic studies reveal evidence of distal denervation with motor nerve conduction velocities only minimally slowed, which is consistent with axonal degeneration.

Acute. In some cases, an acute polyneuropathy complicates cancer (most commonly Hodgkins' disease). It is indistinguishable from Guillain-Barré syndrome (Chapter 31) clinically and pathologically.

Relapsing. In an occasional case, a neuropathy runs a remitting or relapsing course. It may precede the discovery of the neoplasm by two to eight years or become manifest a few years after the tumor is discovered. An association with cancer of the lung is uncommon (in comparison to other forms of neuropathy associated with malignant disease). Neoplasms often associated with this form of neuropathy arise in the breast, stomach, cervix, uterus, and testicle. In most cases, there are two or more episodes of neuropathy, although in some patients a single episode occurs without relapse.

The CSF protein concentration is often elevated, reaching its zenith during the relapse and decreasing when remission occurs. Motor nerve conduction velocities may be slowed, and distal denervation may be evident.

The patient who relapses may improve with steroid therapy. Removal of the offending tumor may result in a remission, particularly in the patient with seminoma.

NEUROMUSCULAR SYNDROMES
Polymyositis and Dermatomyositis

CLINICAL SIGNIFICANCE AND ETIOLOGY
The syndrome of polymyositis is discussed in Chapter 29. In the patient older than 40 years of age who develops polymyositis, the incidence of malignancy has been reported to be as high as 40%, with an average incidence of approximately 15% to 20%. Both polymyositis and dermatomyositis are associated with malignant disease, but in general dermatomyositis is one of the least common paraneoplastic neurological disorders. Carcinomas associated with dermatomyositis are usually found in the breast, lung, or gastrointestinal tract.

SYMPTOMS AND SIGNS
The clinical features of these diseases do not differ from those in patients without malignancy. A rash is the first complaint in 50% of patients, and proximal weakness is present from the onset in more than 80% of patients.

LABORATORY TESTS, DIAGNOSIS AND MANAGEMENT
The creatine kinase (CK) level is often elevated in patients with polymyositis. The characteristic EMG and muscle biopsy changes are discussed in Chapter 29. The diagnosis and management of the malignancy-associated disease is no different than that of the nonmalignant form. Prognosis is usually guarded because of the underlying malignancy. Spontaneous remission may occur; treatment of the underlying tumor does not seem to have a beneficial effect on the muscle disease.

Eaton–Lambert Syndrome

CLINICAL SIGNIFICANCE AND ETIOLOGY
Eaton–Lambert (myasthenic) syndrome is encountered almost exclusively in adults with neoplastic disease. It is frequently associated with small cell carcinoma of the lung, although it has been reported to occur in cases of carcinoma at other sites, including the breast, stomach, rectum, and prostate. Men are affected more than women, and most patients are middle aged or elderly. The cause of this syndrome is not completely known, although it is probably the result of an antibody directed against nerve terminals. The clinical manifestations are the result of an inadequate release of acetylcholine from presynaptic nerve terminals.

SYMPTOMS AND SIGNS
Patients complain of muscular fatigability and often have symptoms of proximal muscle weakness. Common complaints include dryness of the mouth, ptosis, diplopia, impotence, and paresthesias. Physical examination frequently demonstrates mild proximal weakness, usually without atrophy. Deep-tendon reflexes are depressed or absent, particularly in the areas affected clinically. Facilitation of both the deep-tendon reflexes and strength can occur (ie, a temporary increase in muscle strength or reflexes following repetitive stimulation or maximal persistent muscle contraction). Occasionally, Eaton–Lambert syndrome is accompanied by another paraneoplastic disorder.

LABORATORY TESTS AND DIAGNOSIS

The diagnosis is usually made by electrophysiological studies. After repetitive stimulation of a nerve at high rates, there is a marked increment in the amplitude of the muscle-evoked potential (the opposite of myasthenia gravis) as high as 20 times the original value. This incremental response results from the increased release of acetylcholine that occurs at higher rates of nerve stimulation (similar to that seen in cases of botulism).

MANAGEMENT

Drugs that facilitate the release of acetylcholine are used to treat Eaton–Lambert syndrome. Guanidine hydrochloride (20 mg/kg/day) increases the amount of acetylcholine liberated at the motor endplate. Toxic manifestations of this drug include nausea, vomiting, skin rashes, and tremor. With prolonged treatment, bone marrow depression may occur. Prednisone, 40 to 60 mg/day, produces relief in some patients. Plasmapheresis has been reported to be of benefit. Treatment of the underlying neoplasm may reverse the clinical and electrophysiological manifestations of this disease.

COMPLICATIONS OF THERAPY

As is the case with both metastatic and nonmetastatic complications of cancer, the physician must separate the side effects of therapy for the malignancy from the metastatic disease of the nervous system. In discussing the side effects of therapy, this section focuses on disturbances produced by radiation therapy and chemotherapy.

Radiation Injuries of the Nervous System

Radiation-induced damage to the brain or spinal cord depends on several factors: the fractional and total doses of radiation; the volume of tissue and type of tissue irradiated; and the total treatment time. High doses of radiation damage nervous system tissue, but it is not understood why therapeutic or suboptimal doses of radiation produce delayed radiation injury. The incidence of radiation damage in the population of patients with tumor is not known.

Whole-Brain Radiation

The *acute* transient side effects of whole-brain radiation usually arise early in the course of radiation therapy. These acute syndromes usually are characterized by an increase in the preexisting neurological disturbance in addition to headache, fever, photophobia, ageusia, xerostomia, acute parotitis, conjunctivitis, and serous otitis media. All of these side effects are transient; those of cerebral origin are probably the result of increased brain swelling.

Subacute side effects usually occur within a few weeks after the completion of radiation therapy. In adults, drowsiness, headache, nausea, and ataxia appear, and preexisting neurological symptoms can be aggravated. This subacute syndrome is seen in children treated for leukemia, usually receiving prophylactic brain radiation for acute lymphocytic leukemia. Lethargy, somnolence, headache, and occasionally nausea and vomiting occur in the child about six to eight weeks following therapy. In the child and the adult corticosteroids often produce improvement, which would likely also occur without therapy. The pathogenesis of this temporary process in children is not known; edema seems an unlikely cause, but transient demyelination has been suggested. The EEG shows slow activity bilaterally. A CT scan may demonstrate bilateral areas of low attenuation, at times associated with peripheral enhancement.

The most common type of radiation-induced damage is the *chronic,* or late-delayed variety. These chronic side effects usually begin one year or longer following cessation of therapy, and occur in patients irradiated for both intra-cranial and extracranial tumors. The damage is usually associated with more than 6000 rads and occurs six months to three years following therapy. Patients with metastatic disease of the CNS usually do not survive long enough to develop this complication.

Radiation necrosis presents with the clinical picture of a cerebral mass lesion with focal deficits, such as seizures, hemiparesis, and aphasia. A CT scan demonstrates a mass lesion, usually of low density, with associated edema; contrast enhancement and angiography demonstrate that the mass is avascular. Positron-emission tomography (PET) scanning shows decreased metabolism, which is more suggestive of radiation necrosis and does not imply recurrent tumor. The mass can be located in the area of the original tumor; thus, the differential diagnosis is often between radiation necrosis and a recurrent tumor. Occasionally, biopsy and decompression of the lesion are necessary because these procedures are both diagnostic and therapeutic. In general, corticosteroids control the edema and associated mass lesion. The etiology is not clear, but there is probably a vascular component.

Hypothalamic–Pituitary Damage

Abnormalities of hypothalamic–pituitary function can follow brain radiation in both children and adults. Growth hormone deficiency is most common. Children receiving more than 2900 rads demonstrate an inadequate growth hormone response to insulin hypoglycemia; these children respond with an increased growth velocity when given growth hormone. Apparently, as many as 15% of children who receive cranial radiation and who live long enough have growth deficiency. In children and adults treated for brain tumors with radiation therapy, deficiencies of thyroid stimulating hormone (TSH) and adrenocorticotropic hormone (ACTH) may also develop. In some adults, gonadotropin deficiencies also occur. These hormonal deficiencies can be corrected by exogenous hormone therapy; they are becoming more common as patients survive longer.

Cerebral Arteries

Cerebral arterial occlusions resulting from radiation damage are uncommon. Irregularity and narrowing of cortical arteries is seen with cranial irradiation. Patients treated with radiation to extracranial sites (eg, the neck) can also develop premature vascular damage to the carotid and vertebral arteries. The damage presents with stroke-like syndromes or vessel rupture. Pathologically, there is thickening and fibrosis of the vessel wall and premature atheroma.

Spinal Cord

The incidence of radiation myelopathy is 1% to 2%. It tends to occur in areas exposed to radiation, and the process affects white matter more than gray matter. The longer the segment of cord irradiated, the greater the risk of radiation necrosis. The dorsal cord is most susceptible. Necrosis may be patchy or confluent. Vascular lesions are also seen, with fibrinoid necrosis or hyaline fibrosis of the vessel wall. Radiation myelopathy occurs in three forms: (1) an early transient form, (2) a delayed progressive radiation myelopathy, and (3) an asymmetrical lower extremity paralysis of a primary lower motor neuron type.

The *early transient* form usually appears 6 to 12 weeks after treatment. The symptoms, usually mild, often consist of a sensation of electrical-like paresthesias that radiate down the spine or the limbs, usually on neck flexion (Lhermitte's sign). There are usually no objective neurological signs, and the symptoms commonly disappear in three to six months. Treatment is not necessary.

Delayed progressive radiation myelopathy can follow spinal radiation by several months or several years (range, three months to six years). In a minority of patients, the appearance of Lhermitte's sign is the first indication of progressive myelopathy. Early symptoms are more often sensory than motor, but neurological deficits typical of a transverse myelopathy ensue.

Brown–Séquard syndrome (hemicord syndrome with ipsilateral motor signs and contralateral loss of pain and temperature sensation) is not uncommon, but quadriplegia, paraplegia, or a hemiplegic pattern may occur, depending on the area of damage. Often, when there are signs of unilateral cord involvement, signs of bilateral dysfunction eventually develop. This type of myelopathy is usually progressive over several months. Some patients stabilize and, rarely, some improve.

Because the differential diagnosis is primarily that of metastatic disease, all patients must undergo myelography to rule out cord compression. Myelography is usually normal; occasionally, there are areas of cord enlargement with complete block to the flow of the myelographic dye. Although there is no specific treatment for radiation myelopathy, some patients improve following the administration of corticosteroids (methylprednisolone or dexamethasone), which is directed against presumed cord edema.

There is also a rare syndrome of *flaccid paralysis of the lower extremities* following spinal cord radiation. This type of problem tends to follow abdominal or pelvic radiation. Symptoms are those of a progressive lower motor neuron disorder, with weakness, muscular atrophy, reduced or absent deep-tendon reflexes, and preserved sensory and sphincter function. Myelography is negative, but the CSF protein level can be elevated. Electrophysiological studies show normal motor and sensory nerve conduction velocities with evidence of denervation (sharp waves, fibrillations) in the affected muscles. This process tends to stop progressing with time, but the patient may remain disabled. There is no effective therapy.

Chemotherapy

With the increasing use of chemotherapeutic agents in the treatment of malignant diseases, neurotoxic side effects are being documented with greater frequency. A comprehensive review of the neurotoxicity of antineoplastic drugs is beyond the scope of this chapter. For a more detailed discussion the reader is referred to Weiss et al (1974) and Kaplan and Wiernik (1982). A summary of the common neurotoxic effects and the implicated drugs is given in Table 32-3. Instead of reviewing the major groups listed in Table 32-3, the following discussion focuses on commonly used antineoplastic agents that cause significant neurotoxicity.

Methotrexate

Methotrexate (MTX), a folic acid antagonist often used to treat childhood leukemias and sarcomas, CNS lymphoma, tumors of the neck and head, primary brain tumors, and meningeal carcinomatosis. The drug is effective when given orally, intrathecally, or intravenously. A number of nervous system complications of MTX have been reported, related to the route of administration.

Acute Effects. Approximately 30% of patients who receive intrathecal MTX develop signs of meningeal irritation, usually beginning two to four hours after the injection and lasting 12 to 72 hours. Headache, nuchal rigidity, fever, vomiting, and lethargy are common, and CSF pleocytosis is often present. This syndrome tends to be self-limited and requires no treatment. Because it may be confused with infectious or leukemic meningitis, bacterial and fungal cultures and smears are necessary, as is cytologic examination of the CSF if symptoms persist. In addition, CSF pleocytosis may be seen following intrathecal MTX in patients without clinical symptoms. The concomitant use of brain radiation appears to decrease the frequency of this reaction.

A transient or permanent paraparesis related to intrathecal MTX (or Ara-C or thiotepa) has rarely been reported to occur. Leg pain, sensory loss, paraplegia, and sphincter disturbances usually develop between 30 minutes and 48 hours following the intrathecal injection. Improvement may begin within 48 hours or be delayed as long as two to five months. The recovery may be complete or partial, but the deficit may be permanent. The syndrome is the result of direct toxicity or demyelination. Myelography is usually normal. There is no known treatment.

Chronic Effects. A syndrome of confusion and dementia with somnolence, irritability, ataxia, tremor, or seizures has appeared following prolonged therapy with intrathecal MTX for the prophylaxis of childhood leukemias or for the treatment of primary brain tumors. These patients usually have not received oral citrovorum rescue. Occasionally, this syndrome progresses to spasticity, quadriparesis, visual disturbances, other focal CNS findings, coma, or death. It is also known as disseminated necrotizing leukoencephalopathy because the consistent characteristics of the lesions are demyelination with coagulative necrosis of white matter and axonal damage, but no inflammatory lesions. These changes have been reported in approximately 6% of the brains of autopsied patients with acute lymphocytic leukemia.

TABLE 32-3 NEUROTOXICITY OF ANTINEOPLASTIC DRUGS

Encephalopathy

Methotrexate
L-Asparaginase (early or delayed)
Procarbazine
Vinca alkaloids (vincristine, vinblastine)
5-FU
5-Azacytidine
Corticosteroids
Tamoxifen
BCNU*
Cisplatin*
Cytosine arabinoside (Ara-C)
Metronidazole
Interferon
Cyclosporine

Meningeal Irritation/Arachnoiditis (all from intrathecal routes)

Methotrexate
Ara-C
Thiotepa

Cerebellar Syndromes

5-FU
Ara-C (high dose)
BCNU
Methotrexate
Cyclosporine
Interferon

Myelopathy

Methotrexate
Ara-C
Vincristine (inadvertent intrathecal instillation)
Thiotepa

Peripheral Neuropathy

Vinca alkaloids[†]
Cisplatin
Procarbazine[†]
Ara-C
5-Azacytidine
VP-16 (etoposide)
Misonidazole

Cranial Neuropathy

Vinca alkaloids
Cisplatin
5-FU

*Intra-arterial route.
†Also causes autonomic neuropathy.

Although the syndrome occurs with systemic MTX therapy, it increases in frequency when intravenous and intrathecal MTX and irradiation are combined. This type of delayed encephalopathy has become identified with increasing frequency. Computed tomography findings include areas of diminished density (nonenhancing) adjacent to the frontal horns and the occipital horns, with ventricular and subarachnoid dilatation. The risk of developing this disorder

461

apparently increases directly with higher radiation doses (greater than 2000 rads). It is more common with combined radiation therapy and intrathecal MTX, particularly when x-ray therapy is given preceding the intrathecal MTX.

The leukoencephalopathy usually begins within the first year following radiation therapy, but it may begin as early as two weeks following the irradiation or as late as one or two years later. Seizures are frequently seen. The myelin basic protein level may be elevated in the spinal fluid. Methotrexate leukoencephalopathy is often fatal, but some patients survive for months or years with chronic deficits. Some patients recover completely, but partial improvement is more common. If the patient with this syndrome is still receiving MTX by any route, it should be discontinued.

A stroke-like syndrome has been observed in patients with osteogenic sarcoma who are receiving high-dose MTX. It appears early in the course of chemotherapy (within the first to third day of treatment) and does not occur with subsequent doses. Aphasia, hemiparesis, and seizures are the major clinical manifestations. The symptoms abate in a few days.

Vinca Alkaloids

CLINICAL SIGNIFICANCE
Vincristine (VCR) and vinblastine are the most commonly prescribed vinca alkaloids. Vincristine and other vinca alkaloids are toxic primarily to the neuron and to the axon in a dose-limiting fashion. Patients who are in poor nutritional states and those who are bedridden are more likely to develop VCR neurotoxicity. Patients with altered liver function can develop severe neurotoxicity because VCR is metabolized primarily in the liver. Those with prior disorders of the peripheral nervous system (eg, preexisting neuropathy from diabetic or hereditary disorders) may develop rapid weakness after only several doses. Irradiation of peripheral nerves may also augment neurotoxicity. Finally, vinca alkaloids and other chemotherapeutic agents may lead to synergistic neurotoxicity. Adults develop this neurotoxicity about three times as frequently as do children.

SYMPTOMS AND SIGNS
Vincristine usually produces a symmetrical polyneuropathy. The earliest and most consistent sign is loss of the ankle jerk, a finding often asymptomatic in most patients. Paresthesias of the feet or hands are the most common complaint (55% of patients). Muscular pain is also a frequent early complaint. With continued administration of the drug, progressive sensory impairment, weakness, and muscle pain develop. Objective sensory deficits are usually minimal and include decreased pin sensation in a distal distribution. Objective weakness may be more prominent than sensory loss. The dorsiflexors of the foot are most affected and tend not to be severely impaired initially. Weakness of dorsiflexion of the wrist and weakness of the intrinsic hand muscles may also develop. As the condition progresses, general areflexia can develop. VCR neuropathy tends to be dose-related, but is more apparent or severe in those patients who are more susceptible to its toxic effects. It takes one to three months for the reflex abnormalities to disappear following a single dose of VCR, but paresthesias usually disappear

within a few weeks after therapy is stopped. Sensory loss tends to be persistent, and often is only partially reversible.

Alimentary tract dysfunction, manifested as constipation and colicky abdominal pain, occurs in one-third of patients receiving VCR; this is the most common autonomic neuropathic manifestation of VCR neurotoxicity. These symptoms may be the earliest manifestations of VCR toxicity. Reversible paralytic ileus may develop. The most common presentation of autonomic dysfunction is urinary retention secondary to bladder atony. Impotence has also been reported, and orthostatic hypotension also may occur, at times in the absence of overt peripheral neuropathy.

Vinca alkaloids may also affect cranial nerves. Oculomotor nerve dysfunction is usually manifested as bilateral ptosis without other signs; diplopia with ophthalmoplegia has been reported. Optic neuropathy, bilateral facial nerve palsies, and reversible paresis of the recurrent laryngeal nerves have been reported. Severe jaw pain occasionally occurs within a few hours after the first dose of VCR; the pain usually resolves spontaneously within a few days and does not recur with subsequent doses. This symptom is probably related to trigeminal nerve toxicity. All the cranial nerve findings have a tendency to be bilateral; they are usually reversible when the vinca alkaloid is discontinued.

Seizures have been associated with VCR treatment, but occur in fewer than 1% or 2% of the patients treated. Many seizures are probably the result of hyponatremia secondary to the syndrome of inappropriate antidiuretic hormone secretion (SIADH). Likewise, mental changes, including delirium and coma, have been reported in patients receiving VCR, but they may also be the result of SIADH. Hyponatremia can be quite severe; it usually develops within the first ten days of vinca alkaloid therapy and resolves within one or two weeks.

Vinblastine has similar neurotoxic side effects as VCR but requires higher doses to produce them.

LABORATORY TESTS

Electrophysiological tests may document the neuropathy. The changes are compatible with axonal neuropathy, with normal or minimally slowed motor nerve conduction velocities, with distal denervation potentials evident on EMG. Nerve biopsy, when performed, reveals evidence of primary axonal degeneration.

Cisplatin

Cis-diamminodiachloroplatinum (cisplatin) is an alkylating-like drug used primarily to treat testicular, ovarian, head, and neck cancers, CNS lymphomas and recurrent glioblastoma.

SYMPTOMS AND SIGNS

A major dose-limiting toxicity of cisplatin is ototoxicity. Deafness is infrequent and is dose-related. Tinnitus is common and can occur alone or associated with hearing loss; it is usually reversible, but the hearing loss may not be. Vestibular toxicity may also develop. Toxicity tends to be cumulative. Limiting the single or cumulative dose of the drug helps minimize ototoxicity. A baseline audiogram should be performed prior to treatment; serial studies need only be performed if the patient becomes symptomatic.

The peripheral neuropathy caused by cisplatin has been recognized only recently, as higher doses of cisplatin have been utilized. A progressive sensory polyneuropathy occurs in almost all patients who receive a total cumulative dose of 300 mg/M^2 or more. Sensory symptoms develop in a stocking-and-glove distribution, with paresthesias and dysesthesias in the legs that grow worse as treatment continues. Vibratory sensation is involved more than position sense, and light-touch and pin sensation are involved only minimally. No significant motor abnormalities are evident, but deep-tendon reflexes usually disappear, starting at the ankles. Many patients have difficulty walking because of proprioceptive abnormalities. Symptoms tend to increase as treatment continues.

LABORATORY TESTS

Audiometric abnormalities are manifested as high-frequency, pure tone hearing loss, which occur in 24% of patients receiving the drug. Electrophysiological studies demonstrate normal motor nerve conduction velocities, but abnormalities of sensory nerve function are present in all symptomatic patients. The EMG tends to be normal, without evidence of denervation. These findings most suggest a sensory polyneuropathy.

MANAGEMENT

Symptoms become worse as the dose is increased. If significant neuropathy develops, it may be necessary to change therapy.

Cytosine Arabinoside

Cytosine arabinoside (Ara-C), an inhibitor of DNA synthesis, is used widely to treat acute nonlymphocytic leukemia.

SYMPTOMS AND SIGNS

An acute meningeal syndrome or transient paraplegia can occur following intrathecal Ara-C administration. These complications are similar to those from intrathecal MTX discussed above. A few cases of peripheral neuropathy caused by Ara-C have been described, with distal paresthesias occurring in a stocking-and-glove distribution and without objective sensory loss. Subsequent courses of Ara-C exacerbated the symptoms, which were not completely reversible.

Several neurological complications occur with high-dose Ara-C (as high as thirty times the usual dose) in patients with leukemia or lymphoma. A potentially severe cerebellar syndrome can develop during this high-dose therapy with an incidence of approximately 17% of patients. Ataxia of gait and limb movements, dysarthria, and nystagmus develop five to seven days following the first dose, gradually becoming worse over the next few days. Patients then stabilize for two to six days; recovery, albeit incomplete, occurs over the next one to three weeks. The syndrome is irreversible. Other patients receiving high-dose Ara-C may develop a mild, reversible syndrome over the same time course as the irreversible disorder. Nystagmus alone, dysarthria, ataxic gait (without limb ataxia), or reversible encephalopathies may develop.

LABORATORY TESTS

Neuropathologic abnormalities include cerebellar degeneration with loss of Purkinje cells. A CT scan helps exclude mass lesions of the cerebellum.

MANAGEMENT

There is no therapy. The drug should be discontinued if the patient develops progressive or severe ataxia.

5-Fluorouracil

5-Fluorouracil (5-FU) is a pyrimidine analog used widely to treat gastrointestinal tumors or in combination chemotherapy for breast carcinoma.

SYMPTOMS AND SIGNS

Most neurotoxicity from 5-FU affects the cerebellum. Gait ataxia, dysmetria, limb ataxia, dysarthria, nystagmus, and dizziness may develop. The cerebellar syndrome is more common in patients undergoing intensive therapy. It tends to recur two weeks to six months into therapy and is related in part to the peak plasma level of the drug. It is not all caused by cumulative toxicity. A variety of other neurological disturbances occur during therapy with 5-FU. Rarely, patients develop an acute encephalopathy, from which they recover in three to four weeks after therapy is stopped. A reversible parkinsonian syndrome has been reported in one patient; transient blurred vision and diplopia have also been reported.

LABORATORY TESTS AND DIAGNOSIS

The cerebellar syndrome resulting from 5-FU toxicity is of clinical importance because it can be confused with other effects of carcinoma on the cerebellum, including metastatic lesions, leptomeningeal carcinomatosis, and paraneoplastic disorders. The fact that the syndrome resolves quickly and that the CT scan and lumbar puncture are normal solves this problem in most patients.

MANAGEMENT

The cerebellar syndrome is reversible in one to six weeks after 5-FU is stopped or the dosage reduced.

L-Asparaginase

Acute or delayed encephalopathy occurs in 21% to 60% of patients treated with L-asparaginase. *Acutely,* drowsiness, lethargy, somnolence, confusion, depression, or personality changes are common. Stupor, coma, and seizures are rare. Mild abnormalities are seen on the first day of treatment; most cases clear within a few days to a week after the drug is discontinued. The frequency and severity of this toxicity appears to be greater with higher doses. Most patients can continue therapy despite mild drowsiness or confusion. The EEG is often diffusely slowed and returns to normal after the medication is stopped.

A *delayed* form of cerebral dysfunction can also occur. It usually develops within a week after L-asparaginase is given and lasts several weeks. Clinically it resembles the acute form. The cause of the acute syndrome may be an accumulation of toxic metabolic products such as ammonia. The delayed syn-

465

drome is probably caused by primary deficiency of brain protein synthesis, which results from L-asparaginase depletion.

Bibliography

Cairncross JG, Kim JH, Posner JB: Radiation therapy for brain metastases. *Ann Neurol* 1980; 7:529-541. (Review of the Sloan Kettering series of patients with CNS metastases; good discussion.)

Gilbert HA, Kagan AR (eds): *Radiation Damage to the Nervous System: A Delayed Therapeutic Hazard.* New York, Raven Press, 1980. (Detailed monograph covering all aspects of radiation damage to the nervous system.)

Henson RA, Urich H: *Cancer of the Nervous System: The Neurological Manifestations of Systemic Malignant Disease.* London, Blackwell Scientific Publications, 1982. (The only comprehensive textbook that deals with neuro-oncology of metastatic disease.)

Kaplan RS, Wiernik PH: Neurotoxicity of antineoplastic drugs. *Semin Oncol* 1982; 9:103-130. (Review of neurotoxicities of the newer antineoplastic drugs. This article and Weiss HD, Walker MD, Wiernik PH (1974) both should be read for a very comprehensive review.)

Posner JB: Neurological complications of systemic cancer. *Med Clin N Am* 1979; 63:783-800. (Easily accessible overview of nervous complications of cancer.)

Walker MD (ed): *Oncology of the Nervous System.* Boston, Martinus Nijhoff, 1983. (Up-to-date monograph that reviews pertinent aspects of neuro-oncology, including excellent review of brain metastases.)

Wasserstrom WR, Glass JP, Posner JB: Diagnosis and treatment of leptomeningeal metastasis from solid tumors: Experience with 90 patients. *Cancer* 1982; 49:759-772. (Comprehensive discussion of all aspects of leptomeningeal carcinomatosis, based on the Sloan-Kettering experience.)

Weiss HD, Walker MD, Wiernik PH: Neurotoxicity of commonly used antineoplastic agents. *N Engl J Med* 1974; 291:75-81, 127-33. (Classic reference on neurotoxicity of chemotherapy.)

33

Neurological Complications of Alcohol and Alcoholism

Nervous system disease frequently complicates alcoholism. Acutely ill alcoholic patients often present with a complex and confusing array of signs, including confusion, stupor, tremor, hallucinations, nystagmus, and ataxia. The clinician is tempted to make a single Oslerian diagnosis to account for all the symptoms and signs, but these patients usually have several coexisting disorders, which alcoholism has induced by several different mechanisms. Thus, the acutely confused alcoholic patient simultaneously may have portosystemic encephalopathy, Wernicke–Korsakoff syndrome, alcohol-nutritional polyneuropathy, and an acute alcohol withdrawal syndrome. Only by understanding the pathophysiology and clinical features of each individual syndrome can the clinician hope to properly assess and manage the whole patient.

The four major mechanisms by which the nervous system is damaged in chronic alcoholism form the basis of the classification of alcoholic diseases of the nervous system (Table 33-1). They are:

1. The direct toxic effect of an increasing blood alcohol concentration progressively producing behavioral disinhibition, stupor, coma, and apnea. (Alcohol refers to ethyl alcohol.)

2. The effect of decreasing a blood alcohol concentration producing the early and late syndromes of alcohol withdrawal.

3. The state of chronic malnutrition that frequently complicates advanced alcoholism producing the B-vitamin-deficiency diseases. With the exception of patients with chronic diseases, in the Western world, the B-vitamin deficiency diseases are restricted to the alcoholic population.

4. The concomitant chronic alcoholic liver disease that produces acute and chronic portosystemic encephalopathy.

Other mechanisms are operant in specific disorders, including electrolyte imbalance, hypoglycemia, trauma, and direct alcohol neurotoxic effects.

TABLE 33-1 CLASSIFICATION OF THE NEUROLOGICAL
COMPLICATIONS OF ALCOHOLISM AND MALNUTRITION

Increasing Blood Alcohol Concentration (Intoxication)
Alcohol intoxication
Pathologic intoxication
Blackouts
Coma

Decreasing Blood Alcohol Concentration (Withdrawal)
Early withdrawal syndrome
Seizures
Delirium tremens
Protracted abstinence

Malnutrition (Vitamin Deficiency)
Wernicke–Korsakoff syndrome
Polyneuropathy
Optic neuropathy
Cerebellar degeneration
Pellagra

Liver Disease
Portosystemic encephalopathy
Chronic hepatocerebral degeneration

Miscellaneous and Uncertain Pathogeneses
Central pontine myelinolysis
Marchiafava–Bignami syndrome
Dementia
Myopathy
Fetal alcohol syndrome
Peripheral-nerve pressure palsies
Premature stroke

Reproduced from Victor M: Neurologic disorders due to alcoholism and malnutrition, in Baker AB, Joynt RJ: *Clinical Neurology,* vol 4. Philadelphia, Harper & Row, 1986, p 2. Used with permission.

DISORDERS ASSOCIATED WITH INCREASING BLOOD ALCOHOL LEVELS (INTOXICATION)
Pathogenesis

Alcohol consumption produces a dose-related depression of central nervous system function. The degree of CNS depression is directly related to the brain alcohol concentration, which is in turn directly related to the blood alcohol concentration (BAC) and to the rate and duration of alcohol consumption. In the nonhabituated person, there is a fairly predictable dose–response relationship. Impairment of the performance of highly skilled tasks requiring considerable perceptual ability is accompanied by mild euphoria at blood alcohol concentrations around 30 mg/dL. Limb and truncal ataxia and dysmetria appear at blood levels of 50 to 100 mg/dL; legal intoxication is often defined as a blood level higher than 100 mg/dL; at 100 to 200 mg/dL, progressive lethargy and confusion appear. Stupor progressing to coma appears at 200 to 300 mg/dL; death from apnea occurs at levels of 400 to 500 mg/dL and higher.

The habituated subject shows a blunted dose–response curve. Blood alcohol concentrations of 150 to 200 mg/dL, which always produce signs of gross intoxication in naive subjects, may be tolerated with few or no symptoms by habituated patients. The mechanism of habituation is not fully understood.

Mild-to-Moderate Alcoholic Intoxication

Mild-to-moderate alcoholic intoxication produces two coexistent but distinct neurological syndromes: generalized cerebellar dysfunction and behavioral disinhibition. The cerebellar syndrome features limb and truncal ataxia, dysmetria, dysarthria, and nystagmus. The behavioral disinhibition syndrome is characterized by wide and poorly modulated swings in emotion, talkativeness, and more generalized aggressive behavior—as if the ego's restraints on the id were removed. These states present more of a social than a medical problem in the form of disorderly behavior, injuries, and crime. Specific medical therapies to speed the sobering process are usually unnecessary and are probably ineffective.

Alcoholic Stupor and Coma

With rising blood alcohol levels, more medically urgent situations arise. Alcohol is a poor general anesthetic because the dose necessary for coma is dangerously near that which produces apnea. Stupor and coma resulting from alcohol ingestion are seen not infrequently in emergency rooms and represent a true medical emergency. The key considerations when such patients appear are (1) the need for ventilatory assistance; (2) the need to search for underlying serious illnesses frequently coexisting with, but masked by, alcoholic stupor and coma. The latter include other depressant drug poisonings, gastrointestinal hemorrhage, pancreatitis, hepatitis, hypoglycemia, pneumonia, meningitis, and subdural hematoma.

The management of these patients includes intensive care unit surveillance, intake and output measurements, careful hydration, and vasopressors if necessary. Specific therapies include parenteral vitamins and glucose, gastric lavage if it can be performed within two hours of ingestion, and ventilatory support. Hemodialysis is usually unnecessary unless huge amounts of alcohol (BAC>600 mg/dL) or other dialyzable depressant drugs have been ingested, or unless severe acidosis (pH<7.0) is present. Progressive wakefulness occurs when the alcohol in the system has been metabolized and/or excreted. Therapies designed to hasten alcohol excretion (eg, fructose) generally have not been useful.

An important consideration in the emergency room management of an alcoholic patient is the administration of parenteral thiamine-containing multivitamins prior to glucose infusion. Many malnourished alcoholic patients have only a trace amount of thiamine remaining. Infusion of glucose solution may deplete the last trace of thiamine and precipitate acute Wernicke–Korsakoff syndrome, because the thiamine is expended in the metabolism of the infused glucose. This unfortunate iatrogenic situation may be obviated by following the dictum, "Vitamins first."

Alcoholic Blackouts/Blankouts

"Alcoholic blackouts" refer not to a loss of consciousness but rather to a temporary disturbance in new memory recording that may occur during wakefulness in the course of continued, usually heavy alcohol consumption. There is a permanent, short-duration amnesia for this episode. Former beliefs that blackouts are virtually pathognomic for and diagnostic of alcoholism have not been substantiated, because blackouts may occasionally occur in nonalcoholics. However, they are typically associated with heavy drinking, particularly over long periods of time, and most often are seen in alcoholics. The mechanism of alcoholic blackouts is not understood.

Pathologic Intoxication

This vague and controversial state refers to the sudden production of aggressive, violent behavior in a susceptible individual after ingestion of even very small quantities of alcohol, following which the patient has no memory of the episode. Unlike the preceding syndromes, pathologic intoxication is not a dose-related phenomenon. Its mechanism is unclear but two theories have been proposed: (1) there is a preexisting, marginally compensated personality disorder characterized by poor impulse control. The ingestion of a small amount of alcohol is sufficient to release the marginal control; or (2) these cases represent a paradoxical reaction of excitement analogous to the paradoxical excitatory reaction produced occasionally by barbiturates.

DISORDERS ASSOCIATED WITH DECREASING BLOOD ALCOHOL LEVELS (WITHDRAWAL)
Pathogenesis

If alcohol, per se, can be said to be the culprit in the previous set of disorders, the body's own compensatory physiologic adaptation to the continued presence of alcohol can be said to be the cause of this group of disorders. Viewed in a simplified way, tolerance to a given dosage of alcohol is characterized not only by increased hepatic metabolism but, more importantly, by the development of a poorly understood network of nervous system adaptations that counteract the effects of alcohol. Thus, the continued presence of an exogenous depressant drug induces endogenous physiologic and/or pharmacologic excitative mechanisms to "neutralize" its effect. When the exogenous agent is removed or decreased in dosage, the unopposed endogenous stimulative compensatory effects remain and produce the symptoms and signs of withdrawal.

Alcohol withdrawal syndromes may be classified as minor (tremulousness, hallucinosis, seizures) and major (delirium tremens) withdrawal syndromes, or they may be classified as early (tremulousness, hallucinosis, seizures) and late (delirium tremens, late seizures, protracted abstinence) withdrawal syndromes. It is common for the separate syndromes to overlap temporally, to merge into each other, and for a given patient to manifest several syndromes during the course of alcohol withdrawal. The early withdrawal syndrome usually occurs from 6 to 72 hours after withdrawal; the late syndrome, from three to six days after withdrawal.

Tremulousness

Generalized tremor is probably the most common and earliest alcohol withdrawal symptom or sign. The tremor is principally an action tremor and is worsened by anxiety, intention, and sleeplessness. It is the most conspicuous sign of the generalized state of hyperarousal characterizing early withdrawal. Other symptoms present at this time include anorexia, insomnia, nausea, and irritability. Signs include tachycardia, facial and conjunctival hyperemia, an exaggerated startle response, and nystagmus. The amplitude of the tremor is reduced by benzodiazepine therapy.

Hallucinosis

Visual and auditory hallucinations, occuring in early withdrawal, are often frightening to the patient. They begin within the first 24 hours of relative or complete abstinence and usually last several days. They have no particular characteristics and cannot be separated from hallucinations that accompany any kind of delirium.

Conversely, the separate entity of "auditory hallucinosis" is a singular experience of the patient withdrawing from alcohol. There is a distinct paranoid theme to the hallucinations associated with this condition, with voices heard that are threatening or maligning the patient. Fortunately over several days the frightened patient gradually realizes that the voices are not real. Benzodiazepine therapy helps to calm and orient affected patients. Parenteral haloperidol may be helpful if the reaction to the hallucinations is severe.

An unfortunate 10% or so of patients with acute auditory hallucinosis develop the chronic variety and have symptoms of a major thought disorder, including paranoid delusions and disturbed associations. Although chronic auditory hallucinosis resembles paranoid schizophrenia, there are important differences. First, hallucinosis is an alcohol-induced syndrome. Second, the patient is older than the patient developing schizophrenia. Third, there is usually no family history of schizophrenia. Finally, there is not a preexisting schizoid personality type.

Seizures

So-called "rum fits" are a common and serious withdrawal phenomenon. They occur either singly or in small clusters and are usually generalized major motor seizures. They occur most frequently between 24 and 48 hours after relative or absolute abstinence. The progression to status epilepticus (occurring in 2% to 3%) should alert the physician to the possibility of underlying meningitis or subdural hematoma. Purely focal seizures, in particular epilepsia partialis continua, should also suggest an underlying structural abnormality.

Victor (1986) has shown that the time of greatest propensity for seizures correlates with the time of greatest likelihood for a photoconvulsive electroencephalographic (EEG) response. This in turn correlates with hyperventilation, alkalemia, and hypomagnesemia. Thus, the use of magnesium sulfate in the treatment of alcohol withdrawal may have a rational basis, at least for withdrawal seizures.

Alcohol withdrawal seizures are probably distinct from other seizure disorders, including idiopathic and post-traumatic varieties. Aside from the presence of photoparoxysmal responses, interictal EEGs are usually otherwise normal during alcohol withdrawal. Most patients experiencing alcohol withdrawal seizures never have recurrent seizures except during subsequent episodes of acute withdrawal. But the situation is somewhat confused because patients with other forms of epilepsy may have a decreased seizure threshold during alcohol withdrawal.

The management of withdrawal seizures is controversial. Usually the seizures are not treated. The patient is susceptible to them only for a few hours during the withdrawal period. By the time the physician sees the patient after the seizure, the period of susceptibility has elapsed. Phenytoin is recommended only for those patients with a past seizure history (because the diagnosis of pure withdrawal seizure may be in doubt) or for status epilepticus. Loading and maintenance phenytoin doses should be calculated and administered in the customary manner (see Chapter 15). The medication should be discontinued at the time of discharge only if it is clear that the seizure was a pure withdrawal seizure. Patient education about the cause and prevention of seizures is mandatory. Older literature showing that 40% of patients experiencing withdrawal seizures go on to delirium tremens is almost certainly an overestimate.

Delirium tremens

The most feared and serious withdrawal syndrome is delirium tremens (DT). DT produces the quintessence of delirium: global confusion and gross disorientation; vivid hallucinations and paranoid delusions; excess motor activity with restlessness, tremor, agitation and hyperreflexia; and marked hyperautonomia with fever, tachycardia, hyperhidrosis, mydriasis, and tachypnea. In inadequately treated cases, an 8% to 25% mortality results principally from dehydration and shock. In treated cases there remains a 1% to 2% mortality from coexistent pneumonia, meningitis, GI bleeding, or acute alcoholic liver disease. Unlike the withdrawal syndromes discussed previously that occur within the first two days, DT frequently occurs three to five days following abstinence or relative abstinence. Usually, DT is short-lived, and the marked excess of motor, psychomotor, and autonomic activity terminates in a consuming sleep with permanent retrograde amnesia for the episode.

Delirium tremens is a true medical emergency and demands immediate intervention and careful monitoring. There are five principles of DT therapy:

1. *Sedation.* In the initial withdrawal period, benzodiazepines should be given; their judicious use probably aborts a full-blown DT. If DT should occur, benzodiazepines should be carefully increased in dosage with frequent monitoring of the patient to maintain light sedation. Often very large doses are required

even for light sedation, thus no standing orders should be given. The patient must be seen frequently and incremental benzodiazepine doses ordered accordingly. Paraldehyde, barbiturates, and phenothiazines have been used for this purpose in the past, but they have been replaced generally by the benzodiazepines, which have high efficacy, superior anticonvulsant activity, lower toxicity, and lower habituation potential. Recently, beta blockers have also been used successfully.

2. *Fluid and Electrolyte Balance.* The hyperhidrosis, tachycardia, tachypnea, and increased glomerular filtration rate of DT patients cause a tremendous fluid loss, which quickly produces hypotension and shock. These patients frequently require 6 to 10 L/day of intravenous crystalloid solutions, and adequate hydration alone may produce therapeutic benefit. Hypomagnesemia may be treated with parenteral magnesium sulfate.

3. *Search for Underlying Illnesses.* Most of the deaths that occur in treated cases of DT are caused by unsuspected or inadequately treated pneumonia, meningitis, hypoglycemia, subdural hematoma, or fulminant liver failure. The symptoms and signs of DT may mask the classic signs of infection or head injury, and adequate physical examination for these disorders may be virtually impossible. Appropriate body fluids, x-rays, and scans should be obtained.

4. *Vitamin Therapy.* Precipitation of acute Wernicke–Korsakoff syndrome has been discussed, and DT patients should always be considered to be vitamin deficient. Parenteral administration is advisable because of malabsorption and impaired intestinal transport of vitamins.

5. *Nursing Considerations.* The physician should order gentle, firm restraints, positioning of patient on his side or prone but not supine to lessen chances of aspiration, and a well-lighted room with a minimum of personnel and patient movement. The presence of a friend, family member, or (if one of these is not available) a member of the hospital staff is helpful to orient, calm, and reassure the patient, to reinforce reality, and to gently explain what is being done in the hospital. Given the nature of delirium, explanation often must be given repeatedly.

Other Late Withdrawal Syndromes

The use of benzodiazepine in the early withdrawal period may delay the onset of certain withdrawal symptoms until the benzodiazepines are tapered and discontinued. Late withdrawal seizures (at the time the benzodiazepine is tapered two to three weeks after alcohol withdrawal) have features identical to early withdrawal seizures. Similarly, tremor, agitation, and hallucinosis may occur as later signs. These are usually treated by a reintroduction and slower tapering of the benzodiazepine.

Another syndrome occurring late in the withdrawal period is that of "protracted abstinence." For many weeks after withdrawal, the patient may complain of disordered sleep, depression, anxiety, tremor, alcohol craving, and memory disturbance. There may be prolonged EEG abnormalities that suggest hyper-arousal. Several months may be needed for this prolonged state of hypervigilance to clear; its amelioration by alcohol may be one reason many patients resume drinking after discharge from an alcohol detoxification program.

NUTRITIONAL NERVOUS SYSTEM DISORDERS OCCURRING IN ALCOHOLISM
Pathophysiology

Alcoholics are particularly prone to the development of nutritional diseases of the nervous system via numerous mechanisms. First, alcohol provides caloric intake and displaces food from the diet, thereby acting as an anorectic agent. Second, alcohol impairs absorption, intestinal transport, and storage of B-vitamins, particularly thiamine. Third, alcohol causes an increased demand for B-vitamins, which are required for its own metabolism.

Because the nutritional diseases of alcoholism are not primarily caused by the pharmacologic properties of alcohol, it is no surprise that the same disorders may be seen as in malnourished nonalcoholics. In fact, all of these diseases have been reported in malnourished populations of the Third World and in those western patients with chronic debilitating illnesses who are chronically malnourished. These diseases require months or years of malnutrition to develop, frequently feature multiple vitamin deficiencies, and produce the unusual clinical picture of simultaneous central and peripheral nervous system dysfunction. All patients with chronic alcoholism entering the hospital for any reason should be suspected of vitamin deficiency and should be treated with multivitamins and with B-vitamin supplementation and folate.

Wernicke–Korsakoff Syndrome

First described 100 years ago, the essential features of this and other alcoholic nutritional disorders were given their modern definitions by the work of Victor, Adams, and Collins (1971). The affected patient has the triad of ophthalmoplegia, truncal ataxia, and amnestic psychosis. The eye signs, the most conspicuous features of the disorder, include (in order of decreasing frequency) gaze-paretic horizontal nystagmus on lateral gaze, abducens nerve palsies, gaze-paretic vertical nystagmus on upward gaze, and horizontal and vertical conjugate gaze palsies. The truncal ataxia is identical to that seen in alcoholic cerebellar degeneration. It primarily affects gait and station, produces some incoordination of the legs, and usually does not affect the arms. The amnestic psychosis is a state of global confusion featuring the complete inability to record new memories, diminished spontaneity and initiative, and the frequent presence of confabulation in the acute phase. Additional frequent findings in these patients include alcoholic polyneuropathy, impaired vestibular function, orthostatic hypotension, tachycardia (from beriberi heart disease), and, rarely, stupor or coma.

The pathology of Wernicke–Korsakoff syndrome is now mostly understood. The petechial hemorrhages and the symmetric zones of necrosis seen in the periventricular and periaqueductal gray matter of the brain stem readily account for the ocular signs and vestibular dysfunction. The atrophy of the folia of the anterior superior cerebellar vermis accounts for the truncal ataxia. Necrosis of the medial dorsal thalamic nuclei, hypothalamus, and mamillary bodies probably accounts for the amnestic psychosis.

That thiamine deficiency is responsible for the Wernicke–Korsakoff syndrome has been shown clinically and experimentally. Recently it was proposed that there is also a genetic predisposition to the development of the syndrome as a result of a congenital deficiency of the enzyme transketolase. This important finding awaits corroboration by other investigators.

After the administration of thiamine, the ocular signs are the first to reverse, and mental changes the last. This reflects the fact that eye signs may become flagrant when only a metabolic shortage of thiamine has occurred, before any structural damage has been produced. Conversely, the amnestic psychosis usually does not appear until considerable diencephalic structural damage has already occurred. Why these particular neural structures are most sensitive to thiamine deficiency is not known.

When Wernicke–Korsakoff syndrome is suspected, the patient should immediately receive thiamine, 50 mg intravenously and 50 mg intramuscularly, and parenteral multivitamins as well, prior to the administration of glucose. Daily parenteral vitamin therapy should be continued until an adequate diet is guaranteed. Strict bed rest is necessary to prevent fatal complications from beriberi heart disease, the only signs of which may be tachycardia and exertional dyspnea. Treatment also includes carefully counseling the patient at discharge regarding the importance of an adequate dietary intake and the use of daily multivitamins with B-vitamin supplementation and folate. Reversal of eye signs is usually complete, but ataxia, vestibular dysfunction, and memory disturbances are often permanent.

Alcoholic Polyneuropathy

Disturbance of peripheral nerve function is a frequent finding in chronic alcoholism. The classic polyneuropathy of alcoholism begins with pain and burning paresthesias of the soles of the feet and ascends up the legs. By the time the mid-calf is involved, the hands become symptomatic. Mild weakness that affects the hands and feet may progress to complete wrist and foot drops in the severely affected patient. The disease is diagnosed more often before this stage, usually when only the feet are symptomatic. Loss of ankle jerks is an early sign and "stocking-and-glove" impairment of touch, pain, vibration, and position sensations can usually be elicited. Dysautonomia is seen, with excess sweating of the hands and feet. In occasional patients, there is clear involvement of the vagus and sympathetic nerves, which produces hoarseness, dysphagia, hypotension and hypothermia. Atrophy, fasciculations, and weakness of hands and feet are later signs. Slowing of nerve conduction velocity can often be demonstrated.

The primary pathologic process in alcoholic polyneuropathy is axonal degeneration, with secondary segmental breakdown of myelin. Although some investigators still embrace a toxic etiology, most of the evidence points toward a purely nutritional cause. There is a marked clinical and pathologic similarity between this neuropathy and beriberi neuropathy.

Treatment of this condition includes abstinence from alcohol, multivitamins with B-vitamin supplementation and folate, adequate dietary intake, and physical and occupational therapy for hands and feet. Phenytoin or carbamazepine may be useful to treat the dysesthesias. Vitamins should be continued after hospital discharge. Recovery is usually incomplete.

Nutritional Optic Neuropathy

A subacute symmetric bilateral optic neuropathy occurs in some alcoholic patients; an identical syndrome has been described in heavy tobacco users. This syndrome, formerly called "alcohol–tobacco amblyopia," has been shown to be caused by a B-vitamin deficiency rather than to toxic effects of alcohol or tobacco smoke. The patients note gradual bilateral blurring of vision, and eye examination reveals poor acuity, dyschromatopsia, bilateral centrocecal scotomata, and optic disc pallor or atrophy. Treatment includes multivitamin supplementation and the reestablishment of an adequate diet. Recovery is typically gradual and incomplete.

Alcoholic Cerebellar Degeneration

The acute or subacute onset of truncal ataxia occurs commonly in the alcoholic population. This disturbance is most common in middle-aged men and is most likely nutritional in origin. Clinical and pathological findings are identical to those of cerebellar involvement in Wernicke–Korsakoff syndrome. Thus, ataxia of station and gait exceeds ataxia of limbs, although some degree of leg incoordination is usually present. When ataxia is severe, walking is impossible. Even in advanced cases, dysarthria and nystagmus are not prominent. As in Wernicke–Korsakoff syndrome, most patients with cerebellar degeneration also have polyneuropathy and cutaneous signs of malnutrition.

Pathologically, there is Purkinje cell dropout of the anterior superior cerebellar vermis. Gross atrophy of the folia of this region is obvious on sagittal section. The site of pathologic involvement correlates well with the clinical signs, because midline cerebellar degeneration produces truncal and gait ataxia. The general sparing of the cerebellar hemispheres results in the absence of appendicular ataxia.

As with other nutritional disorders, adequate diet and multivitamins are the mainstays of therapy. As is true in Wernicke–Korsakoff syndrome, the recovery of midline cerebellar function is typically incomplete after treatment.

Pellagra

This disorder of niacin deficiency today is seen very rarely even in the malnourished alcoholic population, principally because of the fortification of breads and cereals with niacin. The classical clinical triad of dermatitis, diarrhea, and dementia is still valid because the nervous system, gut, and skin bear the brunt of the disease.

The mental symptoms consist of varying degrees of confusion, hallucinations, insomnia, anxiety, and depression. These signs are often mistakenly ascribed to alcohol withdrawal. Polyneuropathy is present in about one-third of patients. The rare patient has a partial transverse myelopathy with spastic paraplegia and a thoracic sensory level.

The principal pathologic change in the brain is "central neuritis," a neuronal swelling and degeneration seen in many motor nuclei throughout the brain stem and in the cortical gray matter.

Treatment with nicotinic acid improves the skin and gastrointestinal symptoms and some of the mental symptoms. The central neuritis is not improved, which suggests that concomitant deficiencies in B-vitamins other than niacin must be necessary for pellagra to develop.

Other Nutritional Disorders

The identical nature of beriberi to the malnutritional component of alcoholic polyneuropathy has been mentioned. Rare instances of scurvy are encountered. It is worth reiterating that malnutrition predisposes to multiple vitamin-deficiency disorders and that once one is suspected, *all* should be treated with dietary measures—multivitamins with B-vitamin supplementation and folate.

NERVOUS SYSTEM DISORDERS IN ALCOHOLICS CAUSED BY CIRRHOSIS
Portosystemic Encephalopathy

Acute and chronic encephalopathies caused by alcoholic cirrhosis and alcoholic hepatitis are often seen in hospitalized alcoholic patients. The term portosystemic encephalopathy (PSE) describes the neurobehavioral syndrome that results from the action of specific toxins on the brain in patients with parenchymatous liver disease. Acute and chronic PSE often complicate the course of patients suffering from other neurological complications of alcoholism (eg, Wernicke–Korsakoff syndrome and polyneuropathy) and can confuse the clinical picture. Clinicians should always suspect PSE in the patient admitted for toxic, withdrawal, or nutritional complications of alcoholism.

When PSE occurs in chronic liver disease, the clinical signs of longstanding liver disease are present. These include cutaneous changes (spider angiomata, palmar erythema), hyperestrogenic changes (testicular atrophy, gynecomastia), ascites, edema, hepatosplenomegaly, icterus, and Dupuytren's contractures. Less frequently in the alcoholic, PSE complicates acute liver disease without a preexisting chronic component, in which case many of the aforementioned features are absent.

Whether PSE arises from acute or chronic liver disease, it has specific neurological signs. The earliest is a subtle disturbance of mood, memory, and attention. With progression, lethargy occurs, proceeding to stupor and coma in severe cases. Fetor hepaticus, a characteristic musty odor to the breath because of increased mercaptans, is often present. Asterixis, a flapping tremor of outstretched hands and other body parts caused by sudden lapses in muscle tone is characteristic of PSE but may be seen in any metabolic encephalopathy. Hyperventilation producing respiratory alkalosis is often seen, roughly paralleling in magnitude the severity of PSE.

Laboratory findings in PSE include an elevated serum ammonia level and elevated cerebrospinal fluid glutamine and alpha-ketoglutaramate levels. Hypoglycemia, hypokalemia, and liver function test abnormalities are also commonly present. The electroencephalogram reveals slowing and increased voltage of the background rhythm, which are sensitive but not specific findings for PSE.

Pathologic findings in PSE are remarkably scanty. Of the few patients who die from PSE caused by fulminant liver failure, cerebral edema sufficient to produce cerebral herniation is present in one-third to one-half. Cerebral edema is not a feature of the more common chronic variety of alcohol-induced PSE, however. Histologically, there is proliferation of so-called Alzheimer type II astrocytes in the gray matter, basal ganglia, and brain stem nuclei.

The pathogenesis of PSE is most likely multifactorial, and is thought to be caused by (1) alterations in synaptic transmission from disturbed neurotransmitter balance; (2) disturbances in neural membranes; and (3) neuronal metabolic abnormalities of energy production. Four groups of toxins have been identified that can produce these effects: ammonia, short-chain fatty acids, mercaptans, and amino acids acting as false neurotransmitters. Of this group, ammonia remains the most important putative toxin.

Treatment in PSE is directed toward reducing the production and action of ammonia and other nitrogenous toxins. Treatment modalities include:

1. *Avoid excess protein intake.* Dietary protein in the gut forms ammonia and other toxins. Initially all protein should be excluded from the diet, then gradually reintroduced in small amounts. In PSE from chronic liver disease, a level of protein intake can usually be identified above which patients experience symptoms of PSE. It is important when restricting protein to ensure adequate caloric intake (at least 1600 calories/day) to prevent catabolism of endogenous proteins. The quality of protein intake is also important. Vegetable protein, which contains' less methionine and fewer aromatic amino acids than animal protein, is tolerated better. Branched-chain amino acids seem to be tolerated best of all.

2. *Avoid sedatives, opiates, and diuretics.* Sedatives and opiates further depress the central nervous system. Diuretics exacerbate alkalosis and hypokalemia and produce hypovolemia, which exacerbates prerenal azotemia (generating excess ammonia by increasing enterohepatic circulation of urea). If sedation is absolutely necessary, oxazepam is preferred because it has a short duration of action and does not depend greatly on hepatic metabolism.

3. *Prevent gastrointestinal bleeding.* Blood in the gut forms excess ammonia and produces hypovolemia, which exacerbates prerenal azotemia. Aspirin and other mucosal irritants should be avoided. Stool softeners and antitussives should be employed to prevent Valsalva maneuver, which might trigger GI bleeding.

4. *Eliminate constipation.* Colonic bacteria have a greater opportunity to convert nitrogenous fecal material into ammonia and other absorbable toxins. Initially, cleansing enemas should be given, followed by stool softeners and laxatives.

5. *Treat infections.* Infections result in tissue breakdown and endogenous

production of ammonia. Fever and dehydration also exacerbate prerenal azotemia. Infections must be vigorously searched for and treated in these patients.

6. *Prevent excessive diuresis.* Excessive diuresis produces hypokalemia, alkalosis, hypovolemia, and prerenal azotemia. The physician should not order diuretics and should replace K^+ and H^+ as necessary.

7. *Use nonabsorbable antibiotics.* These reduce intestinal flora, thereby reducing production of ammonia and other nitrogenous toxins. Neomycin, 2 to 4 grams by mouth daily, is the usual route, but 1% neomycin by colonic enema is an alternative route. The chief complications of neomycin are ototoxicity, nephrotoxicity, and severe diarrhea.

8. *Use lactulose.* This sugar is converted to lactic acid and acetic acid in the colon and has several beneficial effects. The lower pH discourages ammonia absorption and favors the growth of poor ammonia-producing bacteria, such as *Lactobacillus acidophilus,* over good ammonia-producing bacteria, such as *Escherichia coli.* Lactulose also produces diarrhea, reducing the opportunity for colonic flora to act on intestinal contents to produce toxins. Furthermore, lactulose has been shown to increase the incorporation of fecal nitrogen into bacterial proteins. Lactulose is just as effective as neomycin, and is preferred when long-term use is desired or when there is a preexisting hearing loss or nephropathy.

9. *Other therapies are not proven to be effective.* L-Dopa and bromocriptine are currently experimental; their role in the management of PSE has not been adequately studied. Colonic bypass reduces symptoms of PSE but has an unacceptably high mortality.

Severe Chronic PSE (Hepatocerebral Degeneration)

Rarely, the patient with long-standing portosystemic shunting develops a progressive, irreversible neurologic syndrome characterized by choreoathetosis, tremor, grimacing, asterixis, dysarthria, gait impairment, and dementia. Because of the simultaneous involvement of the liver and basal ganglia, the disease was labeled "non-Wilsonian chronic hepatocerebral degeneration." Rather than having a specific disease entity, these patients probably are at the endpoint of a spectrum of chronic PSE, which requires years of sustained portosystemic shunting and chronic toxic effects on the brain.

Pathologic features include Alzheimer type II astrocytes, cortical laminar and pseudolaminar necrosis, and microcavitations in the corpus striatum. The lesions have the highest frequency in areas of the brain located between major arterial blood supplies (watershed areas). The clinical features are irreversible and do not respond to the treatment of PSE described above. PSE treatment should be begun, however, to reverse any acute PSE that may also be present.

ALCOHOLIC NERVOUS SYSTEM DISORDERS OF UNPROVEN PATHOGENESIS
Central Pontine Myelinolysis

This rare condition was first described in alcoholics but has been seen subsequently in chronic renal disease, lymphoma, and other chronic disorders, particularly those complicated by severe hyponatremia. The patient suffers an acute fulminating quadriplegia and bulbar palsy, often progressing to the "locked-in syndrome." Postmortem examination discloses a large demyelinating plaque occupying the base and tegmentum of the pons. Pathophysiologic hypotheses include selective damage to brain stem oligodendroglia from the combination of malnutrition and hyponatremia or from the too-rapid correction of the latter. Most patients die quickly, but rare spontaneous recoveries have been recorded.

The pontine zone of demyelination can usually be detected by a CT scan. Brain stem auditory evoked responses reveal findings of an intrinsic pontine lesion. There is no specific therapy other than the prevention of severe electrolyte disturbances and the cautious correction of hyponatremia.

Marchiafava–Bignami Syndrome

This is another rare fulminant focal demyelinating disorder first described in alcoholism but subsequently noted in other chronic illnesses. The patient suffers confusion progressing to coma, and a variable combination of seizures, quadriparesis, ataxia, and incontinence, often progressing to death. Postmortem examination discloses a large zone of demyelination occupying the corpus callosum. Its cause is unknown, but speculations include ingested toxins and vitamin deficiency. In a few early cases, abnormalities showing of interhemispheric disconnection have been detected in neuropsychological tests.

Alcoholic Dementia

Chronic alcoholics often develop dementia by the sixth decade. "Alcoholic deteriorated state" is the old term for this syndrome. Symptoms and signs are those of a mixed cortical–subcortical dementia with cognitive dysfunction, paratonia, regressive reflexes, and later incontinence. A CT scan often reveals cortical atrophy and *ex vacuo* hydocephalus. Neuropsychological batteries disclose high organic impairment ratings.

The syndrome of dementia in alcoholism has no specific pathology and is not a specific disease entity. Dementing illnesses may be produced from any or all of the following pathogeneses: repeated bouts of alcohol withdrawal, repeated seizures, repeated attacks of hypoglycemia, repeated head trauma with cortical contusions or subdural hematomas, chronic malnutrition, toxins in ingested drinks, toxic effect of alcohol, and portosystemic encephalopathy. There is no specific treatment, and the dementia is usually irreversible. Correctable illnesses that can produce the syndrome of dementia in these patients must be excluded; they include hypothyroidism, vitamin B_{12} deficiency, subdural hematomas, neurosyphilis, and chronic meningitis.

Alcoholic Myopathies

Alcoholics are susceptible to acute and chronic primary muscle diseases of unknown cause. In acute myopathy of alcoholism, there is a sudden onset of myalgias, muscle tenderness, acute rhabdomyolysis, marked elevation of muscle enzymes, and myoglobinuria that leads to acute renal failure. Occasionally, severe hypokalemia is an accompaniment. Muscle biopsy shows a noninflammatory acute destruction of muscle fibers. The illness is monophasic and of brief duration. Gradual recovery occurs over several weeks.

Chronic myopathy has a subacute onset, with a less spectacular rise in muscle enzymes. It clinically resembles chronic polymyositis, although biopsy fails to reveal an inflammatory etiology. Recovery is slower and less complete than in acute myopathy. Because proximal muscle weakness is common in alcoholic polyneuropathy, some have questioned the existence of chronic alcoholic myopathy as a separate illness.

Etiologies suggested for these disorders include chronic malnutrition, toxic effect of alcohol, fluid and electrolyte disturbances, and seizures. There is no specific treatment other than bed rest, abstinence from alcohol, adequate nutrition, multivitamins, and physical therapy.

Fetal Alcohol Syndrome

About one-third of infants whose mothers drink more than 6 ounces of absolute alcohol daily are born with a symptom complex called fetal alcohol syndrome. Growth and development are retarded, and the children are below the third percentile for height, weight, and head circumference. They have facial and major organ system dysmorphogenesis, with characteristic facies and various organ malformations. The teratogenicity of alcohol is exerted in the first trimester of pregnancy. Fetal alcohol syndrome occurs with an incidence of 1/1600 to 1/1000 live births in the United States. Clarren has estimated that 75% of mothers are dead within five years after bearing an infant with fetal alcohol syndrome.

Central nervous system involvement in fetal alcohol syndrome is manifest at birth by irritability, hyperacusis, poor sucking, and tremulousness. Older children are hyperactive, with attention-deficit disorder and impaired fine coordination. The average full-scale IQ of affected children is 60 to 75. The few postmortem examinations on affected patients have disclosed small brains with abnormal histologic formation of cerebral neurons.

Other Disorders

The alcoholic is susceptible to a variety of other disorders of the nervous system. The increased susceptibility to bacterial meningitis, subdural hematoma, and hypoglycemia have been discussed. Head trauma producing the postconcussion syndrome and posttraumatic seizure disorders have a high incidence in alcoholics.

There is a much heightened susceptibility to peripheral nerve palsies. The most common compression neuropathies occur in the radial, ulnar, median, and peroneal nerves. The increased incidence of peripheral nerve palsies is caused by several factors: greater incidence of trauma; less adipose tissue protecting the nerves; and, most importantly, preexisting axonal degeneration secondary to alcoholic polyneuropathy.

Recently it was shown that during alcohol intoxication, there is a higher incidence of cerebral infarction and subarachnoid hemorrhage, particularly in young adults. Alcohol intoxication affects the antifibrinolytic system to predispose the person to intra-arterial thrombosis. Consequently, alcoholism is now regarded as a risk factor for stroke.

Bibliography

Clarren, SK: Recognition of fetal alcohol syndrome. *JAMA* 1981;245:2436-2439. (Describes the clinical features of the fetal alcohol syndrome.)

Fraser CL, Arieff AI: Hepatic encephalopathy. *N Engl J Med* 1985; 313:865-873. (Current, but reviews pathophysiology more thoroughly than diagnosis and treatment.)

Hoyumpa AM, Desmond PV, Avant GR, et al: Hepatic encephalopathy. *Gastroenterology* 1979; 76:184-195. (A thorough review of the pathogenesis, clinical features, and treatment of portosystemic encephalopathy.)

Kraus ML, Gottlieb LD, Horwitz RI, et al: Randomized clinical trial of atenotol in patients with alcohol withdrawl. *N Engl J med* 1985;313:905-909. (Shows the value of beta blockers in the management of the early withdrawl syndrome.)

Lishman WA: Cerebral disorder in alcoholism: Syndromes of impairment. *Brain* 1981; 104: 1-20. (A study of the mental effects of chronic alcoholism, including neuropsychological and radiographic findings.)

Sellers EM, Kalant H: Alcohol intoxication and withdrawal. *N Engl J Med* 1976; 294:757-762. (A good discussion of the clinical pharmacology of alcohol.)

Thompson WL: Management of alcohol withdrawal syndromes. *Arch Intern Med* 1978; 138:278-283. (A practical bedside guide to treating alcohol withdrawal.)

Victor M: Neurologic disorders due to alcoholism and malnutrition, in Baker AB, Joynt RJ (eds): *Clinical Neurology,* vol 4. Philadelphia, Harper & Row, 1986. (The definitive work on the subject by the world's expert; 94 pages of detailed descriptions and 556 references.)

Victor M, Adams RD: The effect of alcohol on the nervous system. *Res Publ Assoc Nerv Ment Dis* 1953; 32:526-673. (The first modern study of CNS complications of alcoholism; the classic report of a series of patients in Boston City Hospital.)

Victor M, Adams RD, Collins GH: *The Wernicke–Korsakoff Syndrome. A Clinical and Pathological Study of 245 Patients, 82 with Post-Mortem Examinations.* Philadelphia, FA Davis, 1971. (A classic study of all nutritional nervous system complications of alcoholism, with excellent clinical–pathologic correlations.)

West LJ, Maxwell DS, Noble EP, et al: Alcoholism. *Ann Intern Med* 1984; 100:405-416. (A current overview of alcoholism in general, with up-to-date references.)

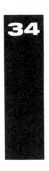

34

Neurological Complications of Pregnancy

Some neurological diseases can be affected by pregnancy; others can result from pregnancy. The physician has a twofold duty when treating pregnant patients: to consider the health and welfare of the mother and that of the fetus. The approach to neurological conditions that may be affected or arise because of pregnancy, therefore, needs to be modified because of the risk of harm to the fetus.

The pregnant woman with possible neurological disease may need to undergo neurodiagnostic procedures. Fear of fetal damage may inhibit the physician from ordering certain tests, and may motivate the mother not to have diagnostic procedures performed. Most neurodiagnostic tests can be performed without risk to the mother or fetus, including electroencephalography, electromyography, nerve conduction studies, and evoked potentials. Lumbar puncture can be safely performed as long as there is no evidence of increased intracranial pressure from a mass lesion.

Radiographic studies of the nervous system pose a greater problem. The report of the National Council on Radiation Protection (1977) concludes, however, that if a radiologic examination is in the best interest of the mother's health, and if the examination is carried out with adequate equipment and careful technique, then the potential benefit to the health of the patient outweighs possible fetal harm from radiation. In fewer than 0.1% of radiographic examinations (fluoroscopy excluded) carried out with good technique and equipment is the fetus subject to a radiation dose of 1 rad or more. Doses less than 5 rads probably do not result in any specific malformations. X-rays of the head, cervical spine, arms, and legs can be done with relative safety. X-ray examination of the pelvis and lumbar spine deliver a high dose of radiation to the fetus and should be avoided. Computed tomography (CT) scans of the head can be performed safely. Because contrast material does not produce fetal thyroid abnormalities, cerebral angiography can be performed without additional risk to the fetus. The abdomen should always be shielded during radiographic procedures. Lumbar myelography results in the greatest fetal radiation dose of all procedures. Thus, lumbar myelography should be avoided, although cervical myelography can be performed with adequate shielding. Pregnancy is a relative contraindication for the use of magnetic imaging resonance (MRI), primarily for legal reasons. There is no known biological risk to the fetus or mother, and many obstetric MRI studies have been performed. In summary, pregnancy does not contraindicate most neurodiagnostic procedures. Lumbar and thoracic myelography produce a high dose of fetal exposure to radiation so should be avoided.

EPILEPSY

Seizure disorders are the most common serious neurological condition encountered by the obstetrician. The effect of seizures on pregnancy can be quite unpredictable for the individual patient. In general, the chance of increased frequency of seizures during pregnancy is correlated best with the frequency before pregnancy. In one cumulative series, seizures during pregnancy occurred more frequently in 50% of patients but remained unchanged in 42%, only 8% had fewer seizures. Maternal age and the age of onset of seizures were not relevant. Altered phenytoin absorption and metabolism result in lower blood levels of this drug and result in an increased frequency of seizures in women who take this commonly prescribed medication.

Idiopathic epilepsy may occur randomly during pregnancy; not all first-time seizures in the pregnant woman are caused by eclampsia. Evaluation should be performed to exclude space-occupying lesions, toxic and metabolic disturbances, infections, or eclampsia. Fewer than 25% of women have a seizure for the first time when pregnant that is not related to toxemia. The appearance of so-called gestational fits during one pregnancy does not mean that they will occur during subsequent pregnancies, or at other times.

Mental retardation, microcephaly, stillbirth, and nonfebrile seizure disorders occur with greater frequency in the offspring of women with seizure disorders. The risk of any unfavorable outcome is doubled in women with seizures.

There is no difference between epileptic women and controls in the incidence of toxemia, abruptio placentae, or hyperemesis gravidarum. Induction of labor and intervention during delivery are reported more often in patients with coexisting seizure disorders.

A decline in plasma levels of anticonvulsant drugs occurs during pregnancy, even when the maintenance dose is constant. In one reported series, 37% of women reported increased seizures during pregnancy or puerperium, but 68% of these women were not complying with their prescribed treatment regimen. Phenytoin (Dilantin), carbamazepine (Tegretol), and phenobarbital are cleared more rapidly from the plasma during pregnancy; accelerated metabolism of the drugs may be the cause.

Anticonvulsants are readily transferred across the placenta. Phenytoin concentrations are identical in the cord and maternal serum at term, and phenobarbital concentrations are identical to those of the mother's plasma. The half-life of phenytoin in the plasma of the newborn ranges from 55 to 69 hours, whereas elimination of phenobarbital takes as long as seven days in the newborn. Infants born of epileptic mothers on phenobarbital may experience withdrawal symptoms, such as tremor, hyperexcitability, restlessness, and sleep difficulties, but they do not develop seizures as part of the withdrawal syndrome. The half-life of carbamazepine is shorter (8 to 28 hours), which is not different from that in the adult.

Anticonvulsant Teratogenicity

It has been suggested that the incidence of congenital malformations among infants exposed to anticonvulsants in utero is greater than that of the general population, in which the incidence varies from 1% to 6%. The most common anomalies are cleft palate and lip, and cardiac defects. Risk of such teratogenesis may be a function of anticonvulsant drugs themselves, the occurrence of frequent convulsions during pregnancy, and complications of pregnancy, as well as the social class and habits of the mother.

The risk of bearing a child with a malformation is approximately 1.25 times greater in a woman with epilepsy than in one without seizures. The incidence of malformations in one series was 1.8% in mothers who remained free of epilepsy who were unmedicated during pregnancy, 2.6% in mothers with seizures who did not take antiepileptic medications, and 11.5% in mothers free of seizures who took medication.

Fetal hydantoin syndrome, characterized by craniofacial abnormalities, mental retardation, deficient growth, and limb defects, is purportedly a consequence of phenytoin, but similar groups of anomalies have been reported in children of epileptic mothers who were not treated with anticonvulsants or who were treated with drugs other than phenytoin. Thus, this syndrome is not specific for phenytoin and may have nothing to do with the anticonvulsants. An undisputed trimethadione syndrome does exist, and this drug should be avoided in the pregnant woman. Valproic acid (Depakene) is teratogenic in animals, causing cleft palates and renal defects; in humans there is a possible association with valproic acid and neural tube defects. This drug should be avoided, if possible, during pregnancy. Amniocentesis is advised before the 20th week of gestation to determine if there is an increase in alpha-fetoprotein levels, which may be associated with neural tube defects.

What should be recommended to the woman with a seizure disorder who requires daily medication? Clearly, there is a greater than 90% chance that she will have a normal child; but the chance of mental retardation or congenital malformations is twice that of a mother without seizures who does not take anticonvulsant medication. There is no reason to withdraw medication or to switch to other medication (such as to phenobarbital from phenytoin).

TREATMENT
When treating the patient with a seizure disorder, it is preferable to use a single drug (monotherapy). Phenytoin or carbamazepine is preferred, and plasma levels should be maintained, as always, in the therapeutic range. This requires more frequent attention to the plasma drug level because marked changes occur in the availability and metabolism of anticonvulsants during pregnancy, resulting in a net decline if dosages are kept constant.

The effective daily dosage of phenytoin is 300 to 400 mg per day, best given in divided doses. Blood drug levels should be measured early in pregnancy and maintained between 10 and 20 μg/mL. Levels should be determined every four to six weeks—sooner if the patient is symptomatic. The dosage should be raised or lowered to maintain therapeutic blood levels and seizure control. Sometimes, 1000 mg of phenytoin is required to maintain adequate serum concentrations during pregnancy. Increased dosages may be required after delivery, but toxicity from elevated doses probably would result within weeks of delivery. Thus, levels should be determined weekly during the postpartum period, with necessary adjustments (reduction) in dosage based on these levels.

Carbamazepine is effective for the control of primarily generalized seizures or complex partial (temporal lobe) seizures. The dosage range is 400 to 1200 mg per day. Because it has a shorter half-life than phenytoin, carbamazepine should be given two to three times per day. Many physicians outside of neurology are afraid to use carbamazepine because of the fatal hematologic abnormalities that have been reported with its use. Such a profound hematological change occurs rarely, perhaps no more often than with phenytoin. Nevertheless hematological parameters should be followed and the drug discontinued if there is evidence of major bone marrow depression. Patients who have had adverse hematologic reactions to other drugs are at a greater risk if treated with carbamazepine, so it is best avoided in this group.

True absence seizures, such as petit mal, are rare in the adult. They may be seen in the pregnant patient, although they should be differentiated from complex partial seizures. Ethosuximide (Zarontin), 250 mg three or four times a day, or clonazepam (Clonopin), 1 mg three to four times a day are the drugs of choice.

What should be done about the patient who has repeated seizures during monotherapy with anticonvulsants, when plasma levels indicate good compliance? It is important that plasma trough levels be obtained, usually by testing the blood in a fasting state before the first dose of the day. Increasing the dosages of the medication to the high-therapeutic range should be done, although a fine line usually exists between high therapeutic and toxic levels. Any environmental problems should be corrected, such as lack of sleep, extreme anxiety, or stress. If seizures continue, a second drug should be added. It is ideal to gradually withdraw the first drug after therapeutic levels of the second have been attained, and the withdrawal should be gradual. If seizures continue, then it is easiest to give two drugs and reach the therapeutic concentrations of both.

Grand mal status epilepticus, which rarely occurs in the pregnant woman, requires hospitalization. It is usually the result of poor compliance or to subtherapeutic levels of medication because of an inadequate maintenance dosage. Treatment for grand mal status epilepticus is outlined in Chapter 39. There is no evidence that drugs used intravenously to treat status epilepticus have adverse effects on the fetus.

Hemorrhagic Disease of the Newborn

Decreased levels of vitamin K-dependent clotting factors may develop in the newborn who is exposed to barbiturates or phenytoin. The deficiency is manifested during the first day of life as bleeding. This drug-induced vitamin deficiency occurs sooner than the normal physiologic deficiency, which is usually manifested between the second and fifth days, and can be treated with injections of vitamin K in the mother before delivery. One milligram of vitamin K should be given to the newborn immediately; clotting studies should be performed two hours later. If clotting levels continue to be abnormal, additional vitamin K can be given and clotting studies monitored.

In summary, the epileptic woman who wishes to become pregnant should be aware of changes in medication requirements that may arise from the pregnancy, as well as the possible teratogenic effects of anticonvulsant medication. Special attention should be paid to the plasma levels of the anticonvulsant, both during pregnancy and postpartum. The fetus exposed to anticonvulsants should be examined and treated for any possible bleeding disorders.

HEADACHE

Vascular headaches (including migraine, hypertensive, and toxic-vascular types) and muscle contraction–tension headaches are encountered often in the pregnant woman. Migraine is largely a disease of women of childbearing age. It can begin during pregnancy, usually in the first trimester, but more common is a dramatic improvement of migraine during pregnancy, occurring in 50% to 80% of the women studied who had migraine previously. Patients with menstrual migraine tended to have greater relief of headache during pregnancy. It is unclear whether there is an increased frequency of pre-eclampsia in women with migraine. Any type of migraine (classic, common, complicated) may occur during pregnancy or in the puerperium, and migraine has been noted to develop during breast-feeding. Ophthalmoplegic migraine is so rare that the sudden appearance of a third nerve palsy in a pregnant woman is likely to be caused by an expanding intracranial aneurysm, and not caused by migraine.

The most common nonmigrainous vascular headache is that produced by fever, but other common causes are CO_2 retention and nitrites in food.

Sudden extreme elevations of blood pressure, producing encephalopathy, may occur with toxemia of pregnancy, or in patients with malignant hypertension. Hypertensive encephalopathy consists of severe headache (which is often continuous and pounding), nausea and vomiting, convulsions, stupor, and coma. Papilledema and retinal hemorrhages are present as a sign of increased intracranial pressure. Hypertensive headaches, usually described as dull and aching with intermittent throbbing, often are present on awakening in the morning and are usually associated with diastolic blood pressure greater than 110 mm Hg.

Muscle contraction–tension headache is the most common headache of pregnancy. It is characterized by dull, aching pain, which frequently is persistent and circumcerebral in location. Headache typically occurs as the day goes on and is worst in the evening. It may become persistent and quite severe, often to the point of incapacitation.

Proper therapy for headache depends on the correct diagnosis of the cause. Clearly, the vast majority of head pain is caused by muscle contraction–tension or vascular causes. Rarely will it occur as a result of brain tumor, subarachnoid or intracerebral hemorrhage, or cortical vein thrombosis.

Migraine

Treatment of acute migraine consists of avoiding known precipitating factors (such as red wine, alcohol, cheese, nitrites, monosodium glutamate, chocolate). Eating habits should be regulated and stress and emotional factors addressed. If migraine occurs despite environmental modifications, analgesics and sedatives can be used to provide relief. Ergot alkaloids are best avoided in the pregnant patient. Though the most commonly used antimigraine ergot preparation, ergotamine tartrate, does not have oxytoxic effects on the uterus when used orally, it does when given parenterally. True chronic migraine occurs rarely in pregnancy. Propranolol, 40 to 160 mg daily in divided doses, can be used with caution during pregnancy. It can cross the placenta; infants born to mothers taking 180 to 240 mg daily have been depressed at birth, with bradycardia and postnatal hypoglycemia. Chlorpromazine can be used to reduce nausea and vomiting; acetaminophen or codeine can be used to control pain. Rarely, amitriptyline (75 to 100 mg at bedtime) is needed to control seemingly intractable pain. Biofeedback and relaxation techniques may also be beneficial in the selected patient with chronic migraine who prefers not to take medication.

Muscle Contraction

Intermittent muscle contraction headache is best relieved with mild analgesics such as acetaminophen; more potent prescription medications should be avoided. Physical therapy, including massage and heat to the neck, may be helpful. Occasionally, the injection of trigger points with local anesthetic agents or corticosteroids will help reduce pain.

Chronic muscle contraction headache should be treated by environmental modifications, heat, massage, and if these measures give no response, biofeedback. The use of benzodiazepines (valium, librium) should be avoided in the pregnant woman or breast-feeding mother. There may be an increased risk of orofacial cleft in the newborn if these drugs are taken in the first trimester, and the newborn metabolizes benzodiazepines poorly. Also, diazepam and its active metabolite are excreted in breast milk. The use of tricyclic antidepressants may be necessary in the patient with severe muscle contraction headache; and amitriptyline is the agent of choice (75 to 100 mg daily). Narcotics should almost never be used, and frequent analgesic intake should be avoided. Patients with intractable head pain may need psychiatric referral and counseling.

In summary, it is best to avoid ergot alkaloids in the pregnant woman; the use of chronic analgesics or narcotic agents should also be avoided. Medications, such as propranolol or amitriptyline, can be used in the selected patient, but attempts to control pain by environmental modifications or with biofeedback or psychotherapy are preferred.

NEUROPATHY

Neuropathic processes may complicate pregnancy. They are best classified into two categories: (1) *mononeuropathies,* which afflict single nerves, usually caused by compression; and (2) *polyneuropathies,* which affect multiple nerves, usually as a result of metabolic or autoimmune dysfunction affecting the peripheral nervous system.

Mononeuropathy

Many mononeuropathies are caused by trauma or the fluid retention and weight gain that accompanies pregnancy.

Cranial Nerve

Bell's Palsy. Idiopathic facial paralysis, better known as Bell's palsy, may occur during pregnancy or in the puerperium. The onset of symptoms is usually acute; signs and symptoms of paralysis may develop within a few hours. Both the upper and lower face are involved, taste may be decreased (from involvement of the chorda tympani nerve), and sometimes the patient hears sounds louder on the involved side (because of paralysis of the stapedius muscle). Although patients usually complain of vague facial numbness and postauricular pain, there is no objective loss of facial sensation. If pain is a predominant symptom, then associated conditions such as otitis media or geniculate ganglion herpes zoster (Ramsay Hunt syndrome) may be the cause of the facial paralysis.

One study of Bell's palsy revealed that 20% of the patients surveyed were pregnant or in puerperium; there was also a higher-than-normal incidence of toxemia in this series. Overall, the incidence of Bell's palsy in women of all ages and those of childbearing age has been reported to be 17/100,000; the frequency in pregnancy and the first two portpartum weeks rose to 57/100,000. Three quarters of these cases occurred in the third trimester and in the first two postpartum weeks, with an incidence of 118/100,000.

Most cases of Bell's palsy are self-limited with recovery over two to six weeks. If the eye on the affected side cannot be closed, it should be patched; if it is dry, artificial tears can be used three to four times a day. Because the vast majority of cases of Bell's palsy are self-limited, it is difficult to recommend treatment with corticosteroids, which is frequently advocated in the acute case (within 72 hours of the onset) of idiopathic facial paralysis. The successful use of prednisone, 40 to 60 mg per day, for seven to ten days following the onset of Bell's palsy, has been reported in pregnant women, without apparent ill effects to the infant. Surgical decompression is not helpful and should not be performed. Bell's palsy does not affect the course of pregnancy.

Upper Extremity

Median Nerve. The most common mononeuropathy of pregnancy is carpal tunnel syndrome, related to median nerve compression at the wrist. Pain and paresthesias in the distribution of the median nerve in the hand are the most common symptoms, often with a significant nocturnal component. Sensory loss may result and motor weakness may result. As many as 20% of pregnant women complain of hand pains, but few actually are suffering from median nerve compression. Of pregnancy-related carpal tunnel syndromes, 85% clear spontaneously, usually in the postpartum period. Thus, treatment should be conservative, including the use of a lightweight plastic splint applied to the wrist in a neutral or slightly flexed position. Local injections of steroids into the carpal tunnel may be necessary in the more painful cases. Because the vast majority of cases abate in the postpartum period, surgical therapy is not recommended, unless there is significant pain, motor or sensory loss, and no response to conservative measures. As always, the diagnosis of carpal tunnel syndrome should be confirmed by electrodiagnostic testing; it should be reserved for the pregnant patient with atypical symptoms or signs, one in whom the diagnosis is in question, and in one for whom surgery is being contemplated because of the failure of medical therapy.

Ulnar Nerve. Neuropathy of the ulnar nerve usually is the result of elbow trauma, which may not be easily recognized. Numbness and paresthesias occur in the fourth and fifth digits, and weakness of the intrinsic hand muscles may develop. The avoidance of certain precipitating factors, such as repeated pressure on the elbow or repeated flexion and extension of the arm, should be attempted. It is rarely necessary to perform surgery, and, as with median nerve compression, the symptoms usually abate in the immediate postpartum period. Much less common is distal ulnar nerve compression at the wrist. It has the same prognosis as other nerve compression syndromes and can be treated with splinting and, rarely, steroid injection (Chapter 9). The diagnosis of the ulnar neuropathies can be made with electrophysiologic tests, but they are not usually necessary in the typical case.

Brachial Plexus. Brachial plexus neuropathy occurs in as many as 5% of pregnant women. The brachial plexus and the subclavian artery are compressed by the clavicle and first rib in pregnancy, when the increased weight of the breasts and the abdomen may lead to sagging of the shoulders and the appearance of symptoms. The presence of a cervical rib or hypertrophic scalenius anticus muscle may predispose the pregnant woman to brachial plexopathy. The symptoms of "brachialgia" include pain, often referred to the ulnar side of the forearm and hand, and paresthesias in the same distribution. True weakness is uncommon, but blanching or coldness of the fingers may occur. These symptoms are usually worse at nighttime or when driving a car or elevating the arm. This syndrome tends to be self-limited, and can be successfully treated with physical medicine measures. The syndrome usually resolves after delivery, and surgical therapy is not indicated during pregnancy. Quite rare are cases of recurrent familial brachial plexopathy (perhaps a brachial plexus neuritis), which may also be associated with involvement of the lower cranial nerves or lumbosacral plexus. Of the women with familial brachial plexopathy, 65% have recurrent attacks when pregnant or postpartum.

Lower Extremity

Meralgia Paresthetica. Pain and paresthesias in the lateral thigh often are caused by compression of the lateral femoral cutaneous nerve. The clinical syndrome is known as meralgia paresthetica. The lateral femoral cutaneous nerve is a purely sensory nerve that arises from the second and third lumbar nerve roots, running inferior to the iliacus muscle to exit the pelvis from under the inguinal ligament. Weight gain and the exaggeration of the lumbar lordosis that occur during pregnancy predispose the nerve to trauma and compression.

Clinically there are variable areas of numbness in the lateral thigh without weakness or reflex loss. During pregnancy the symptoms of meralgia paresthetica usually begin about the 30th week of gestation. There is no predilection for either side, although the syndrome may be bilateral. Age and parity are not factors, although meralgia paresthetica may recur in subsequent pregnancies. Normally the complaint is a minor one, and symptoms can be expected to resolve within three months. The best therapy is patient reassurance combined with the avoidance of tight fitting garments and with the attempt to limit further weight gain. Infiltration of local anesthetic into the nerve as it passes the inguinal ligament or surgical decompression of a section of the nerve should not be necessary and should be avoided.

Obturator Nerve. The obturator nerve arises from the third and fourth lumbar roots and passes along the pelvic wall below the psoas major muscle, emerging near the pelvic brim, where it exits through the obturator canal. The obturator nerve supplies sensation to the upper inner thigh and innervates the large adductors of the thigh and the gracilis muscle. Pain in the groin and upper thigh may be the initial symptoms of obturator neuropathy; weakness of thigh adduction with sensory loss over the upper medial aspect of the thigh may be clinically evident. Obturator neuropathy is rare and may be caused by compression by the fetal head before or during labor and delivery. Usually it is self-limited and responds to physical therapy.

Femoral Nerve. The femoral nerve arises from the second through fourth lumbar nerve roots. Within the pelvis it courses along the lateral border of the psoas muscle before entering the thigh deep to the inguinal ligament and in close association with femoral blood vessels.

The symptoms and signs of a femoral nerve lesion are weakness of the quadriceps muscles, sensory disturbances over the anterior thigh and medial calf, and reduction in the patellar reflex. If the proximal femoral nerve has been damaged, the hip flexors (iliopsoas) will also be weak. The femoral nerve may be injured during cesarean section; it rarely may follow a normal vaginal delivery. The lesion usually is unilateral, but cases of bilateral involvement have been reported. Typically, a day or two following surgery or delivery, the patient notices weakness and numbness of the leg and difficulty in walking up stairs or getting up from a sitting position. Motor involvement is usually more predominant than sensory loss. The prognosis is excellent; recovery usually begins within a few weeks, although it may take a few months to be complete.

Peroneal Nerve. The common peroneal nerve is subject to several forms of damage as it winds around the fibular head in the lateral upper calf. Physical findings of a lesion include foot drop as a result of weakness of the dorsiflexors of the foot; eversion is also weak, but inversion is preserved because the muscles that invert the foot are supplied by the posterior tibial nerve, another branch of the sciatic nerve. Sensory loss is occasionally noted, most often in an area between the first and second toes. Tinel's sign can be elicited by tapping over the fibular head.

Compression on the lateral fibular head is often caused by crossing the legs; in the pregnant woman it may be caused by pressure on the nerve from prolonged labor and from pressure by knee stirrups. The condition is usually noted one or two days postpartum; the prognosis for recovery is usually good. In the patient troubled by foot drop, a short, plastic leg brace is necessary. This condition must be differentiated from postpartum foot drop caused by proximal involvement of the lumbosacral plexus (see below).

Lumbosacral Plexopathy. Compression of the lumbosacral plexus in the pelvis occurs in short women carrying a relatively large baby. Prolonged labor and midforceps rotation after a transverse arrest are common. Foot drop occurs, often unilaterally and on the same side as the infant's brow during the descent through the pelvis. The foot drop is first noted when the woman becomes ambulatory. Weakness of ankle eversion, dorsiflexion, and sensory loss along the lateral aspect of the leg and across the dorsum of the foot are evident. Compressive neuropathy of the peroneal nerve at the fibular head is not associated with sensory loss above the site of compression.

This form of postpartum foot drop can be differentiated from other forms by electromyographic examination and nerve conduction studies. A poorer prognosis is associated with an unexcitable peroneal nerve distally and axonal degeneration of the involved muscles. Prognosis is good when nerve conduction velocity is normal a week after the injury; recovery usually occurs within three months. If the nerve is unexcitable with secondary denervation, then the prognosis is poor; recovery is prolonged and often incomplete. A short, plastic leg brace should be used to improve ambulation and to help prevent shortening of the heel cords. In subsequent pregnancies, the physician must attempt to prevent further nerve injury. Low forceps can be used with caution, but midforceps should probably be avoided. Cesarean section may be necessary for the woman with unsuccessful labor or who has a large infant.

Polyneuropathy
Guillain-Barré Syndrome

A thorough discussion of Guillain–Barré syndrome (GBS) is in Chapter 28. This section discusses only GBS as it develops in the pregnant patient. The syndrome rarely has been reported in pregnancy. When it does, it may occur at any time during gestation, although in a recent study the majority of cases occurred in the third trimester. Pregnancy, delivery, and the fetus do not seem to be affected by the disease, and there does not appear to be an increased rate of spontaneous abortion. Many cases of GBS during pregnancy have followed a mild viral syndrome. Recovery may be prolonged, but frequently is complete. A recurrent form of GBS can occur in subsequent pregnancies, but this is extremely uncommon. Recovery in the recurrent variety is slow and often incomplete, but corticosteroids may be of benefit. It is unclear as to whether there is a cause-and-effect relationship between the pregnancy and GBS, but frequently improvement occurs rapidly after childbirth or termination of the pregnancy. Guillain–Barré syndrome is, however, not usually an indication for the termination of pregnancy. Most deliveries can be accomplished vaginally; if there is respiratory weakness or profound generalized weakness, cesarean section is advised.

Porphyria

Acute intermittent porphyria is an inborn error of heme metabolism, transmitted as an autosomal dominant, which affects women more than men. Recurrent abdominal pain is the most common manifestation, and recurrent psychiatric disturbances and neuropathy are seen frequently. An axonal neuropathy with autonomic manifestations may develop, at times mimicking Guillain–Barré syndrome. The ingestion of certain medications will provoke a porphyric attack, including barbiturates, anticonvulsants, estrogens, oral contraceptives, and steroids. Seizures may occur, and in some patients are a result of hyponatremia from the inappropriate secretion of antidiuretic hormone. An increase in urinary excretion of porphobilinogen and δ-aminolevulinic acid is the hallmark of the disease; the Watson–Schwartz test shows the typical red-wine appearance.

Pregnancy has a deleterious effect on porphyria: approximately 75% of women have an exacerbation of porphyric complaints during pregnancy, but only 16% go into remission. In one series, 36% of women had their initial attack when pregnant. Subsequent to pregnancy, one-third of the patients had remissions and one-third had exacerbations, but maternal death in the puerperium occurred in one-fifth. When porphyria is activated by pregnancy, fetal loss is high (approximately 40%), and the spontaneous abortion rate is twice normal. Maternal mortality in pregnancies with symptomatic porphyria is approximately 22% with almost half the deaths occurring during the first attack of porphyria. There does not appear to be any benefit from spontaneous or therapeutic abortion early in the pregnancy; some physicians feel that abortion is contraindicated in the acute stages of an exacerbation of porphyria. Fetal malformations do not arise from the maternal porphyric episode.

The treatment of an acute porphyric attack is a medical emergency. The patient should be admitted to the intensive care unit, and should receive careful attention to autonomic functions, such as breathing and blood pressure. Respiratory failure may develop, necessitating endotracheal intubation and ventilatory support. Hypertension can be controlled with propranolol, but seizures are difficult to control because almost all anticonvulsants induce the production of δ-aminolevulinic acid, which worsens the porphyric episode. Carbamazepine (Tegretol) is the preferred anticonvulsant (conventional) because it induces δ-aminolevulinic acid the least, but bromide therapy, at least initially, may be the safest way to treat recurrent, frequent seizures. The infusion of hematin will provide negative feedback control and will dramatically induce remission of central nervous system manifestations. It should probably be the first line therapy in the patient with a severe porphyric crisis.

Nutritional Polyneuropathy

A distal polyneuropathy from vitamin B deficiency may occur in the pregnant woman who has poor nutritional intake, profound alcoholic intake, or severe hyperemesis gravidarum. It is more prevalent in areas of the world where continuous malnutrition exists. It may occur as a mild sensorimotor neuropathy with an acute onset that coincides with the development of Wernicke–Korsakoff syndrome, or as a more subacute neuropathy that may include encephalopathy as a late manifestation. The cause of the syndrome is most likely acute thiamine deprivation superimposed on chronic vitamin B deficiency. See Chapter 33 for a discussion of neurological complications of alcohol and alcoholism, including various vitamin deficiency states.

LUMBAR RADICULOPATHY

Extremity pain arising from herniation of a lumbosacral intervertebral disc usually occurs at the L5-S1 interspace. The pain arising from the pressure on the first sacral nerve root radiates down the leg in a distribution corresponding to the sciatic nerve (see Chapter 9). The pain is felt primarily in the buttock, but also in the posterior thigh, calf, and lateral foot. There may be associated muscle spasm, and any movement, particularly those which increase intra-abdominal pressure (coughing, straining), will increase the pain. Disc rupture appears to be rare in pregnancy; the incidence is 1 per 10,000 pregnancies.

Examination reveals loss of the normal lumbar lordosis, and restriction in movement of the spine. Straight leg raising is often positive; the ankle reflex may be reduced or absent. Weakness of plantar or dorsiflexion of the foot may result, in addition to weakness of other L5-S1 root innervated muscles. Sensory loss usually is present over the lateral foot, heel, and back of the calf, although objective sensory findings may be minimal. Rarely, in the pregnant patient, tumors or vascular malformations cause such a root disturbance. Chronic low-back pain without secondary nerve root compression is a common finding in the multiparous woman with an excessive weight gain. Pain is usually localized to the lower back and tends not to be radicular but is aggravated by movement. Approximately 50% of pregnant women develop some degree of lumbosacral pain. In one-third of them the pain is disabling; in half, it may radiate into the legs. The sacroiliac joints are the source of backache in pregnancy. Hormonal relaxation of these joints and the symphysis pubis develops during pregnancy.

The diagnosis of back pain or the radicular syndrome is based on the history and examination. Electromyography helps localize the root lesion and, if positive, adds confirmatory evidence that secondary axonal degeneration caused by the compression on the involved nerve has occurred. Myelography or CT of the involved spinal area is rarely necessary and should be avoided because of the radiation dose to the fetus.

Treatment should be conservative, with bed rest and, if necessary, pelvic traction. Potent analgesic medications and chronic ingestion of analgesics should be avoided. Occasionally, conservative measures do not relieve pain, or the deficit is progressive. In these circumstances, removal of the offending disc can be performed without adverse affects on the pregnancy, although such surgery should be performed after the first trimester. A cesarean section should be performed to avoid the increased CSF pressure and subsequent nerve injury associated with a vaginal delivery. Following delivery, the patient should be instructed on how to strengthen the abdominal and pelvic muscles to help avoid a chronic postpartum back pain syndrome.

MULTIPLE SCLEROSIS

Multiple sclerosis, a demyelinative disease of the central nervous system of unknown etiology, is characterized by relapses and exacerbations. It tends to be a disease affecting women in their child-bearing years (see Chapter 23). Multiple sclerosis usually has no effect on pregnancy, the duration of the three stages of labor is normal, and there need be no change in the management of labor and delivery. There is no increased risk for toxemia. If multiple sclerosis is complicated by a neurogenic bladder, the enlarging uterus may interfere with bladder function. The incidence of urinary tract infections in the pregnant woman with multiple sclerosis and a neurogenic bladder is increased.

Because multiple sclerosis is characterized by exacerbations and remissions, it is not easy to know if pregnancy truly affects the course of the disease; however, most series consistently report that relapses are more common during the first three months postpartum. Multiple sclerosis is usually not a reason to have an abortion. There is no specific therapy for active MS. Some neurologists recommend a short course of prednisone or ACTH, but there is no major indication for long-term or maintenance therapy with corticosteroids.

MYASTHENIA GRAVIS

Myasthenia gravis is a disease of the neuromuscular junction that affects females more than males (see Chapter 29), usually beginning in the third decade of life. Fewer than 1% of the total cases of myasthenia gravis are congenital. Familial myasthenia gravis represents 3% to 4% of all cases and is more common in children. Remission of myasthenia gravis has been described during pregnancy, although in some patients the disease is exacerbated, more so in early pregnancy. Exacerbations may occur within the first six weeks postpartum. Approximately one-third of patients experience a remission during pregnancy, one-third suffer an exacerbation, and one-third remain unchanged. Exacerbations and remissions are often abrupt in onset, so the patient must be evaluated monthly.

During labor, anticholinesterase drugs should be administered parenterally. Spinal or caudal anesthesia is preferred because curare and ether cause marked exacerbation of myasthenia. After delivery, it is best to avoid breast-feeding because anticholinesterase drugs may be excreted in the milk. Medication taken by the mother may need to be adjusted after the first week portpartum, particularly if the dosage was lowered or raised during pregnancy. If it is not adjusted, cholinergic or myasthenic crises may result.

Approximately 12% of babies born to mothers with myasthenia gravis develop neonatal myasthenia. There does not appear to be any relationship to the duration or severity of the maternal disease, or to the maternal dosage of anticholinesterase agents. Neonatal myasthenia gravis usually appears within the first 96 hours after delivery and may persist for weeks. Signs include poor sucking, difficulty swallowing, and respiratory distress. The condition is transient, usually lasting 24 to 36 hours. Treatment is symptomatic to prevent aspiration and to maintain respiration. A short course of anticholinesterase drugs may be necessary. Pyridostigmine (Mestinon) 4 to 10 mg or neostigmine 1 to 2 mg orally is the preferred drug.

CEREBROVASCULAR DISEASE

The incidence of stroke in pregnancy is approximately 1 per 20,000 births, with most occurring in patients under 35 years of age. Ischemic stroke is more common during the first trimester, but as many cases appear in the immediate postpartum period as in the six months prior to delivery. The signs and symptoms depend on the site of the lesion. The onset is usually sudden; a progressive course is more suggestive of tumor, brain abscess, or intracerebral hemorrhage.

Most nonhemorrhagic strokes during pregnancy and the first few postpartum weeks are caused by arterial occlusions and involve the carotid artery distribution. Middle cerebral artery occlusions occur twice as often during pregnancy as at other times. Thrombosis is the most common cause of arterial occlusive disease. Cardiac emboli or vasculitis are other causes of arterial occlusions, and a search for these causes must be performed (see Chapter 20).

There are several unusual sources of brain emboli in the pregnant woman. Amniotic fluid emboli can occur during or just after childbirth. The most susceptible patient is the multiparous woman over the age of 30. Labor is frequently prolonged. Sudden dyspnea with cyanosis and shock are the most characteristic symptoms. Ten percent of patients have a sudden onset of seizures, usually within 10 minutes of the onset of dyspnea and shock. The etiology of the seizures is likely dyspnea and shock. Paradoxical cerebral amniotic fluid emboli may also occur.

Paradoxical emboli from the right heart to the left heart through a patent foramen ovale is another rare cause of stroke. An anatomically patent foramen ovale is present in more than 30% of the population. Pulmonary hypertension secondary to a pulmonary embolus or multiple emboli can raise right-sided pressure opening the foramen ovale, allowing emboli to enter the systemic circulation, and producing brain infarction. Air emboli can cause death during pregnancy or in the early puerperium. Clinically, there is a sudden appearance of anxiety, tachycardia, dyspnea, and cyanosis, which lead to shock. Sudden death may also occur, but is the result of cardiac disease rather than brain pathology.

The evaluation of ischemic stroke should include evaluation of blood clotting factors as well as a blood count and platelet count. A sedimentation rate and an antinuclear antibody assay (ANA) should be performed in an attempt to diagnose a connective tissue disease. Blood cultures may be necessary to exclude infective endocarditis; an echocardiogram of the heart is indicated to look for mitral valve prolapse, atrial myxoma, or a patent foramen ovale. In selected patients, heart catheterization may be necessary to find a cause for possible paradoxical emboli.

Treatment depends on the underlying pathology. Vital signs must be carefully monitored, and fluid balance should be assured. In cases of ischemic stroke where there is marked hypertension, sodium nitroprusside can be used as an antihypertensive agent. Cerebral edema may occur, but there is no convincing evidence for the value of corticosteroids. Antiosmotic agents (mannitol) should be reserved for cerebral herniation.

Subarachnoid Hemorrhage

Subarachnoid hemorrhage from a ruptured intracranial aneurysm occurs with the greatest frequency between the ages of 35 and 65 (Chapter 37). In one review of maternal deaths at a university hospital, 12% were caused by ruptured aneurysms. More than half of the patients with ruptured aneurysms had one or more pregnancies without complications. When rupture of an aneurysm occurs during pregnancy, the risk to the mother's life is two to three times greater than when it occurs in the nonpregnant person. Approximately half of the subarachnoid hemorrhages of pregnancy are caused by an aneurysm, the remainder, by arteriovenous malformations (AVM). AVMs are seen in younger women (ages 20 to 25) and usually 15 to 20 weeks into the pregnancy. Aneurysmal hemorrhage tends to occur in the older patient (ages 30 to 35) and will present by 30 to 40 weeks gestation, rarely during labor or the puerperium. Fetal prognosis is related to that of the mother in the case of aneurysmal rupture, but it is poor with rupture of an AVM. Normal term delivery can be anticipated in the aneurysm patient who has bled and who has been treated surgically. There is no appreciable fetal risk when the operation is performed under hypothermic conditions. The only apparent indication for elective cesarean section and tubal ligation is the presence of an untreated AVM. If the patient with a known AVM does become pregnant, some complications may be expected, and delivery by cesarean section is indicated. If an aneurysm or AVM are surgically inoperable, a cesarean section should be performed routinely at 38 weeks' gestation.

Cortical Venous Thrombosis

During adult life, aseptic venous thrombosis is associated with malignancy, trauma, and oral contraceptives. Intracranial venous thrombosis has been recognized as a cause of brain infarction during pregnancy and the puerperium; cases arise from infectious or noninfectious processes. Since the introduction of antibiotics, most cases of intracranial venous thrombosis during pregnancy or the puerperium have not been associated with infection.

Saggital sinus thrombosis has an incidence of approximately 1 per 600,000 pregnancies. Approximately 5% of venous infarctions related to child bearing occur during pregnancy. The vast majority of the remainder occur after the first postpartum week, usually during the second or third week. In contrast, more than 80% of arterial occlusions occur during pregnancy or within the first postpartum week. The patient with intracranial venous thrombosis often presents with either intracranial hypertension or paraplegia, often following generalized seizures. Headache may be severe and is often accompanied by nausea and vomiting. Weakness and sensory loss may be bilateral or unilateral and tends to selectively involve the legs, more so distally. Seizures are much more common with venous disease than with arterial disease. They may be generalized or focal, and can be the presenting symptoms. The seizures often coincide with severe headache. The seizures may be persistent, which may indicate an enlargement of the clot. If the clot reaches the superior saggital sinus, intracranial hypertension may develop. Consciousness is disrupted more frequently with venous thrombosis.

A careful examination should be performed to exclude the presence of pelvic or extremity phlebothrombosis, or local infection of the sinuses, ear, or face. A CT scan, with and without intravenous contrast, should be performed. It will exclude other causes of intracranial pathology, but it may be normal in the presence of cortical venous or superior saggital sinus thrombosis. With superior saggital sinus thrombosis, CT may reveal hemispheric edema, hemorrhagic infarction, and occasionally thrombosed veins or venous sinuses. Lumbar puncture may be necessary to exclude subarachnoid hemorrhage or meningitis, but CT should be done prior to the lumbar puncture. Usually, the spinal fluid is normal, but increased pressure and protein may be present in addition to a few red blood cells. If the clinical suspicion is not confirmed by other tests, carotid angiography will be necessary with careful attention paid to the venous phase. Digital subtraction angiography may be sufficient to visualize the venous sinuses. Magnetic resonance imaging (MRI) is also of value in detecting intracranial venous thrombosis, but it is best avoided during pregnancy.

Anticonvulsants are often needed to control the seizures; if focal, they may be difficult to treat. Parenteral phenytoin is the best anticonvulsant. In the case of status epilepticus, lorazepam, 4 mg intravenously, will terminate a high percentage of nonfocal seizures. There is much controversy regarding the use of anti-coagulants. If the diagnosis is made early and the CT scan and spinal fluid analysis provide no evidence of subarachnoid bleeding, then the early administration of heparin to retard clot propagation must be considered. Anticoagulation in the early puerperium also increases the risk of uterine bleeding. Mannitol may be necessary if cerebral edema is present, but steroids are without proven benefit. Hyperventilation can safely be used to control intracranial hypertension.

BRAIN TUMORS

Primary brain tumors are uncommon during childbearing years; metastatic brain disease is even less likely. There are no brain tumors specifically related to pregnancy, but meningiomas and neurofibromas may enlarge during pregnancy. The pituitary gland grows during pregnancy, but change in the growth pattern of a pituitary adenoma has not been reported.

The initial symptoms usually occur during the second and third trimesters. Headache is the most common complaint, and focal signs related to the location of the tumor are found. Therapeutic abortion may be necessary, but it depends on the location, size, and type of tumor. Usually a brain tumor is not an indication for cesarean section unless there is danger of obstructing CSF pathways (eg, colloid cyst of the third ventricle). Biopsy can be performed and radiation given, but adequate shielding of the fetus is necessary. Chemotherapy should be withheld because of fetal toxicity.

Choriocarcinoma is a highly invasive tumor that is unusual in western countries, but occurs more frequently in the tropics and the Orient. Most choriocarcinomas present in the first few months following a molar pregnancy, although a few present after a full-term pregnancy. Metastatic CNS disease is the most common neurological manifestation of choriocarcinoma. Because choriocarcinoma is a vascular neoplasm, the presenting manifestation is often that of a stroke or multiple strokes, usually caused by a hemorrhagic lesion. Solitary mass lesions can also be the mode of presentation; headache, seizures, and focal signs are not uncommon. Chorionic gonadotropin levels may be elevated in the CSF and serum. Brain radiation and chemotherapy (methotrexate) may be curative.

Pituitary tumors may develop during pregnancy, but they can usually be followed symptomatically. If visual symptoms develop, surgical intervention may be necessary. Surgery can be performed at any time, but induction of labor is recommended if gestation has reached the 36th week. A pituitary tumor may shrink after parturition. Radiation therapy, surgery, or bromocriptine therapy may be used effectively in the postpartum period. Patients with pituitary tumors should have periodic visual field examinations because the only sign of enlargement may be a developing visual field deficit.

Pseudotumor Cerebri

Pseudotumor cerebri is defined by headache, papilledema, and increased intracranial pressure in the absence of focal neurological abnormalities (Chapter 21). Pseudotumor cerebri is more prevalent in women, especially the young obese woman of childbearing age. Many neurologists believe it is provoked or exacerbated by pregnancy. Although headache may be intractable, therapy is usually instituted to prevent visual loss, the most feared complication.

Diagnostic criteria include papilledema, increased CSF pressure, normal CSF content, and the absence of other neurological diseases. Lumbar puncture, which is both therapeutic and diagnostic, is not contraindicated but should always be preceded by a CT scan to exclude a mass lesion or hydrocephalus.

Treatment of the pregnant patient with pseudotumor cerebri is as varied as that of the nonpregnant person. Pseudotumor cerebri is not a reason for a therapeutic abortion. Almost all treatment protocols for the nonpregnant patient can be used during pregnancy except for caloric restriction, which may lead to adverse ketotic effects on the fetus. There is no contraindication to repeated lumbar puncture. The use of corticosteroids has been associated with birth defects in laboratory animals; this association has not been shown in humans. Acetazolamide may be used after 20 weeks' gestation. Glycerol should be avoided because it has the potential to decrease placental blood flow associated with diminished maternal blood volume. Diuretics are controversial for the same reason as glycerol. There are no obstetrical contraindications to surgical decompression (lumboperitoneal shunt, or optic sheath decompression). Visual acuity and visual fields must be monitored closely.

The recurrence rate of pseudotumor cerebri in nonpregnant patients varies in studies between 2% and 43% (most often 6% to 10%); in one series, the recurrence rate in pregnancy was 20%. In general, pregnancy occurs in cases of pseudotumor cerebri at about the same rate of pregnancy in the general population. Pseudotumor cerebri may occur in any trimester, although it usually appears during the first half of pregnancy. Patients have the same spontaneous abortion rate as the general population; visual outcome for the pregnant patient is the same as for the nonpregnant person. Therapeutic abortion to limit progression of the disease is not indicated. Subsequent pregnancy does not increase the risk of recurrence of pseudotumor cerebri.

MOVEMENT DISORDERS
Chorea Gravidarum

Chorea that occurs during pregnancy is termed chorea gravidarum. Chorea, the abrupt, nonrhythmical movement of the face or limbs, is often exaggerated by emotional stress but disappears during sleep. Usually, these movements are random, jerking, and purposeless. Facial grimacing and difficulty in swallowing and speaking may also occur. Many patients with chorea gravidarum have had rheumatic fever. Most have the onset of symptoms in the first trimester; the problem can recur during subsequent pregnancies. Twenty-five percent of women who have chorea in childhood notice a recurrence during pregnancy.

Without treatment, chorea gravidarum usually disappears in one-third of patients before they give birth. In those patients in which it persists until the puerperium, symptoms usually disappear within a few days of childbirth. Treatment for chorea gravidarum is sedation and rest. Chlorpromazine or haloperidol benefit some patients; phenothiazines cross the placenta, but they rarely are associated with fetal or neonatal complications. The fetus is not affected by the disease, and the risk of spontaneous abortion is normal. Twenty percent of women will have recurrent chorea with subsequent pregnancies.

The differential diagnosis includes rheumatic fever, Wilson's disease, systemic lupus erythematosus, and Huntington's disease. Cases of chorea have been associated with polycythemia, hyperthyroidism, hyperglycemia, and idiopathic hypoparathyroidism. Phenothiazines to control nausea and vomiting may also produce a movement disorder, but it is usually dystonic, not choreic.

Wilson's Disease

Wilson's disease (hepatolenticular degeneration) is the result of an inborn error of copper metabolism that leads to an accumulation of copper in many organs, primarily the brain and liver. It is transmitted as an autosomal recessive trait. Symptoms usually begin in the second decade of life. Cirrhosis often results, and Kayser-Fleischer corneal rings and CNS dysfunction are evident. Impaired higher cortical functions often result, as well as a movement disorder that varies from a flapping tremor to akinesia (parkinsonian-like). Dysarthria, dysphagia, and pseudobulbar palsy are also common. Before D-penicillamine treatment was introduced in 1956, most affected women suffered infertility and amenorrhea, or had severe cirrhosis and died. Most women with Wilson's disease who became pregnant suffered spontaneous abortion in the third or fourth month of gestation. With treatment, this disorder tends to be fatal no longer. One series of infants born to mothers with Wilson's disease who had been treated with penicillamine (1 g daily), reported that all infants were unaffected at birth and remained asymptomatic.

Bibliography

Birk K, Rudick R: Pregnancy and multiple sclerosis, *Arch Neurol* 1986;43:719-726. (Excellent up-to-date review of the effects of pregnancy on multiple sclerosis.)

Dalessio DJ: Neurologic diseases, in Burrow GN, Ferris TF (eds): *Medical Complications During Pregnancy,* ed 2. Philadelphia, Saunders, 1982, pp 435-473. (Comprehensive synopsis of neurological illnesses that complicate pregnancy.)

Dalessio DJ: Seizure disorders and pregnancy. *N Engl J Med* 1985; 312:559-563. (Current review of seizure disorders in pregnancy; also covers anticonvulsant teratogenicity.)

Digre KB, Varner MW, Corbett JJ: Pseudotumor cerebri and pregnancy. *Neurology (Cleve)* 1984; 34:721-729. (Best current review of this topic.)

Donaldson JO: *Neurology of Pregnancy.* Philadelphia, Saunders, 1978. (Comprehensive review of neurological disorders during pregnancy.)

Goldstein PJ (ed): *Neurological Disorders of Pregnancy.* Mt. Kisco, NY, Futura, 1986. (Current review of various neurological disorders of pregnancy . Each chapter is well-referenced.)

Hanson JW, Smith DW: The fetal hydantoin syndrome. *J Pediatr* 1975; 87:285-290. (One of the first reviews of the effects of phenytoin on the fetus.)

LaBan MM, Perrin JCS, Latimee FR: Pregnancy and the herniated lumbar disc. *Arch Phys Med Rehabil* 1983; 64:319-321. (Reviews the modern management of herniated discs during pregnancy.)

Roelvink NCA, Kamphorst W, Van Alphen HAM, et al: Pregnancy-related primary brain and spinal tumors. *Arch Neurol* 1987;44:209-215. (Comprehensive review of the literature on primary brain and spinal tumors in pregnancy.)

Wiebers DO: Ischemic cerebrovascular complications of pregnancy. *Arch Neurol* 1985; 42:1106-1113. (Discusses diagnosis and management of all types of cerebrovascular disease during pregnancy; well referenced.)

Neurological Complications of Medications

The reported incidence of clinically significant adverse drug reactions is 10% to 28%. Approximately 5% of hospital admissions are drug-induced disorders, but the morbidity certainly must exceed that figure. Fatal drug reactions represent as many as 0.31% of all hospital admissions.

There are two types of adverse drug reactions: augmented and idiosyncratic. An augmented reaction occurs when the reaction to the drug is an exaggeration of the expected response. Such a reaction is usually dose-dependent and predictable on the basis of known pharmacology. The mortality is low but morbidity is high. An idiosyncratic reaction is not expected from the type of drug prescribed in the usual therapeutic dosage. Such a reaction is unpredictable, and although overall the morbidity is low, the mortality tends to be high.

This chapter reviews major neurological complications of commonly prescribed medications. The majority of these reactions are of the idiosyncratic type. The neurotoxicity of cancer chemotherapy is discussed in Chapter 32, and the reader is referred to Silverstein (1982) and Davies (1981) for more detail of the drug-induced neurological syndromes. A discussion of the side effects of commonly prescribed neurological medications are found in the appropriate chapters of this book.

Adverse drug reactions may affect the nervous system at different levels, including the brain, cranial nerves, peripheral nerves, neuromuscular junction, and the muscles (Tables 35-1 to 35-8).

CARDIOVASCULAR DRUGS
Cardiac Glycosides

Neurological complications are second in frequency to gastrointestinal symptoms as manifestations of digitalis toxicity. Delirium may result from toxicity, with confusion that can progress to coma. Restlessness, agitation, visual hallucinations, convulsions, and psychotic episodes have also been associated with digitalis

TABLE 35-1 DRUG-INDUCED CNS DISORDERS

Type of Reaction	Drugs
Delirium	ACTH Alcohol (withdrawal, intoxication) Amantadine Anticholinergics Antihistamines Antituberculous drugs Barbiturates Beta-blockers Bromides Bromocriptine Benzodiazepines Cardiac glycosides Corticosteroids Cycloserine Gluthemide L-Dopa Meprobamate Penicillin Phenothiazines Tricyclic and tetracyclic antidepressants
Dementia	Amphetamines Corticosteroids Isoniazid Lithium Phenytoin Procainamide Primidone Quinidine Sedative-hypnotics
Extrapyramidal Syndromes	Antidepressants (Amitriptyline, Amoxapine, Imipramine, Desipramine) Phenothiazines (Chlorpromazine, Fluphenazine, Perphenazine, Prochlorperazine, Promazine) Butyrophenones (Haloperidol) Diphenhydramine L-Dopa Lithium Metoclopramide Phenytoin Reserpine Tetrabenazine Thiothixene
Headache	Amphetamines Bromides Calcium-channel blockers Digitalis Dipyridamole Ergotamine (withdrawal) Nitrates Nonsteroidal anti-inflammatory agents (Indomethacin, Ibuprofen, Naproxen) Methysergide (withdrawal) Oral contraceptives
Seizures	Alcohol (withdrawal) Amantadine Baclofen Benzodiazepines (withdrawal) Beta-blockers (Atenolol)

TABLE 35-1 continued

Type of Reaction	Drugs
Seizures	Butyrophenones
	Corticosteroids
	Digitalis
	Insulin
	Isoniazid
	Ketamine
	Lidocaine and Tocainide
	Lithium
	Metrizamide
	Nalidixic acid
	Penicillins
	Phenothiazines
	Tricyclic and tetracyclic antidepressants
	Vincristine
	X-ray contrast

toxicity. Visual abnormalities include blurring with a yellowish halo over objects, photophobia, scotomata, and red–green color blindness. Resolution of these abnormalities may take as long as two weeks after the digitalis has been stopped. Seizures associated with paroxysmal EEG abnormalities also have been reported; when digitalis was discontinued, the EEG returned to normal. Transient chorea has also been reported as a manifestation of digitalis toxicity, as have short- and long-term memory deficits and learning impairment. Impairment in learning may occur in the absence of toxicity. Because trigeminal neuralgia is a reversible manifestation of digitalis toxicity, the patient who develops trigeminal neuralgia while on digitalis should have the blood level of the medication measured.

Vasodilators

Headache is the most common neurological complication of the various nitrates used to treat angina pectoris. Such headache commonly occurs at therapeutic dosages. The pain is throbbing and similar to that of common migraine. Most patients note that the headache subsides after they have been taking the medication for several weeks. If persistent, it usually disappears with a reduction in dosage. Isosorbide dinitrate has been reported to cause typical cluster headache, which ceases when the medication is stopped. Acute Wernicke's encephalopathy has developed in some patients after the intravenous infusion of high-dose nitroglycerin, secondary to the metabolism of the ethanol and propylene glycol diluents.

Transient visual disturbances may accompany therapy with nitrates, usually as a result of transient postural hypotension. However, transient myopia has been reported that was reversed with a cycloplegic agent implicating drug-induced ciliary spasm. Dipyridamole, although released as a coronary vasodilator, is prescribed most often as an antiplatelet drug. Throbbing head pain is a common complication of this medication, and at least 25% of patients cannot tolerate it because of the cephalgia.

Perihexilene has been associated with a sensorimotor peripheral neuropathy. These patients have a high level of the drug in their system most likely the result of slow drug metabolism. Distal paresthesias are common, and may progress from the lower extremity to the upper extremity; weakness may follow. The process is slowly progressive and associated with slowing of nerve conduction velocities. Improvement usually begins within a few weeks after the medication has been stopped. Baseline nerve conduction velocities should be measured and repeated yearly in any patient who is placed on this medication.

Anti-arrhythmic Drugs
Procainamide

Procainamide may produce a lupus-like syndrome in which confusion and disorientation can develop. Lightheadedness and syncope are also caused by this medication, usually as a result of orthostatic hypotension. A reversible dementia syndrome has been reported. Procainamide may also exacerbate myasthenia gravis.

Quinidine

Headache and auditory and visual disturbances are often seen during the early stages of quinidine therapy. Quinidine toxicity produces nausea and vomiting, cramps, tinnitus, vertigo, and blurred vision. Speech disorders, confusion, excitement, somnolence, and coma, which alternate with delirium, have also been reported. Generalized convulsions may occur. Also associated with quinidine is a slowly progressive chronic dementia, which is reversible after the quinidine is stopped. Quinidine may cause a myopathy associated with proximal weakness and elevated creatine kinase levels. It may also exacerbate myasthenia gravis.

Beta-Blockers

The beta-blockers are known to cause a variety of neuropsychiatric disturbances. The lipophilic drugs (eg, propranolol, metoprolol) carry a greater risk than do the hydrophilic drugs (eg, timolol, atenolol) for producing neuropsychiatric morbidity. The hydrophilic drugs may, however, also produce toxic CNS reactions.

Insomnia and hallucinations are common side effects experienced by patients receiving beta-blocking drugs, and there is a high incidence of depression and acute toxic confusional states. In one report, propranolol produced a psychotic reaction that relapsed when hydrophilic beta-blockers were substituted (atenolol, timolol). Propranolol-induced depression cleared in one patient when atenolol was substituted.

The beta-blocking drugs may cause postural hypotension with syncope and giddiness. Topical application of timolol eye drops for glaucoma has caused depression and psychosis. The beta-blockers all may exacerbate myasthenia gravis, including agents applied to the eye.

Amiodarone

Amiodarone is highly effective for treating ventricular and supraventricular arrhythmias. A reversible neurological syndrome consisting of tremor, ataxia, and peripheral neuropathy may develop in as many as 50% of patients treated with this medication. These neurological disturbances usually improve or resolve within two days to four weeks after the medication is discontinued or when the dosage is reduced.

The tremor is indistinguishable from essential tremor (Chapter 12); a preexisting tremor may also be exacerbated. The patient may have gait or limb ataxia with frequent falls or staggering. The neuropathy usually presents after four months of therapy. Its manifestations are distal lower extremity paresthesias associated with absent deep-tendon reflexes and decreased vibratory sensation. A myeloneuropathy with combined features of a distal neuropathy and myelopathy has been reported during therapy with amiodarone; it is reversible after the drug is discontinued. The majority of patients who develop neurological complications are taking at least 800 mg daily.

Lidocaine and Tocainide

Lidocaine is used parenterally for the control of ventricular arrhythmias. Tocainide, a cogener of lidocaine, is a recently released oral anti-arrhythmic agent.

The major adverse effects of lidocaine are on the central nervous system. At plasma levels of 5 μg/mL, drowsiness, agitation, and paresthesias (often perioral) develop. With higher serum concentrations, disorientation, myoclonus, decreased hearing, respiratory arrest, and convulsions may occur. The more severe manifestations are life threatening, but the mild ones are not dangerous and can be treated by decreasing the drug infusion rate.

Unlike lidocaine, tocainide does not undergo rapid first-pass hepatic metabolism enabling it to be used orally. Lightheadedness, dizziness, tremors, and anorexia are common adverse reactions. With toxicity, visual hallucinations, confusion, agitation, myoclonus, tremor, asterixis, and ataxia can result. Seizures have also been reported. As is the case with toxicity from lidocaine, reducing the dosage of the drug or discontinuing therapy will result in a resolution of the neurological symptoms.

Calcium-Channel Blockers

The calcium-channel blockers are used to treat cardiac arrhythmias and angina pectoris. Nifedipine, verapamil, and diltiazem are the preparations approved for use in the United States. Adverse reactions are less common with verapamil, the drug in this class that has been used primarily for cardiac arrhythmias. Nifedipine can produce excessive vasodilatation; dizziness, syncope, digital dysesthesias, flushing, nausea, vomiting, sedation and headaches are side effects that occur in 20% of patients. The symptoms usually abate with time or after the dosage of the drug has been reduced. Nightmares, visual hallucinations, gingival hyperplasia, myoclonus, dysosmia, dysgeusia, and myalgias with muscular weakness have also been reported to complicate therapy with nifedipine.

A small percentage of patients receiving verapamil develop headache, flushing, dizziness, and constipation. Few neurological complications have been reported during therapy with diltiazem; minor headache is the most common. Dysosmia, dysgeusia, and hyperactivity with mania or akathisia have been reported in a few patients.

Disopyramide

Major adverse neurological reactions that result from treatment with disopyramide (Norpace) are the result of its anticholinergic effects. Toxic psychosis, confusion, urinary retention, and precipitation of glaucoma may all develop in the susceptible patient. Lightheadedness and syncope may develop secondary to hypotension. Hypoglycemia can also occur. Severe toxicity produces seizures and coma.

Thrombolytic Drugs
Streptokinase

Streptokinase is a fibrinolytic drug that is used for intracoronary and intravenous thrombolysis in the patient with an acute myocardial infarction. It is also used to treat other types of arterial and venous thrombosis and for pulmonary embolism. Bleeding complications, which often require transfusions, are common, occurring in 4% to 7% of patients with intracoronary infusions. Intracranial hemorrhage is the most common neurological complication, occurring with an incidence of approximately 2.2%. In patients treated with streptokinase for brachial–carotid arterial thrombosis, thromboembolic nonhemorrhagic stroke sometimes develops probably because streptokinase-lysed clot fragments embolize from these vessels. The Guillain–Barré syndrome has been reported to occur within 10 to 14 days following intracoronary thrombolysis.

Antihypertensive Drugs
Reserpine

Reserpine is a dopamine-depleting drug that may cause depression and parkinsonism; depression is a much more frequent side effect. Seizures have been reported, as has a vasospastic type of migraine. These reactions usually occur after at least four weeks of therapy; they commonly resolve within a few weeks after the drug is stopped. Because of its ability to produce depression, reserpine should not be prescribed for the depressed patient.

Methyldopa

Methyldopa may cause many neurological effects, including orthostatic hypotension (with lightheadedness and syncope), depression, sedation, headache, nightmares, and hallucinations. Methyldopa dementia has also been reported, and is reversible once the drug is stopped. A parkinsonian-like syndrome may also develop, with rigidity and bradykinesia but without predominant tremor.

Clonidine

Clonidine may cause confusion in patients of any age. Lethargy, agitation, and seizures have also been reported.

Prazosin

Prazosin (Minipress) produces a first-dose phenomenon 30 to 90 minutes after the first dose in 1% of patients. Manifestations include dizziness, headache, weakness, and blurred vision. Syncope may develop, and transient coma has been reported. Subsequent doses of prazosin do not produce this dramatic syndrome, but they may produce vertigo, lightheadedness, headache, irritability, weakness, and depression.

Hydralazine

Dizziness, headache, and peripheral neuropathy may result from hydralazine, although the neuropathy is uncommon when daily dosage is less than 200 mg. Distal numbness and paresthesias result, probably the result of pyridoxine deficiency.

Nitroprusside

Nausea, drowsiness, hypotension, and the exacerbation of migraine may all complicate therapy with nitroprusside. With continued administration of nitroprusside, cyanide accumulates and toxicity may result. The infusion of sodium thiosulphate helps prevent cyanide toxicity. One patient was reported who was treated with sodium nitroprusside for hypertension; at autopsy lesions were found in the basal ganglia characteristic of cyanide poisoning.

Captopril

Captopril is an angiotensin-converting enzyme inhibitor that produces minor neurological disturbances, including vertigo, lightheadedness, headache, and a disturbance of the sense of taste (Table 35-2). A steep fall in blood pressure may occur following the first dose of captopril in the severely hypertensive patient being treated with multiple drugs (including diuretics). With prolonged therapy orthostatic hypotension can develop, which may lead to lightheadedness and syncope.

ANTIMICROBIAL DRUGS

Antibiotics are among the most widely prescribed medications. Consequently, a variety of neurotoxic side effects have become apparent. This discussion is presented according to the level of neuraxis involvement.

CNS Toxicities
Penicillin

Penicillin (including synthetic preparations) has a direct convulsive effect when applied intrathecally or directly to the cerebral cortex. Intrathecal administration

TABLE 35-2 DRUGS THAT PRODUCE DISORDERS OF TASTE AND SMELL

CLASS	DRUG
Anesthetics (local)	Benzocaine Cocaine Procaine hydrochloride Tetracaine
Anticonvulsants	Carbamazepine Phenytoin
Antidepressants	Imipramine
Antidiabetics	Phenformin
Antihistamines	Chlorpheniramine
Antihypertensives	Captopril Diazoxide Ethacrynic acid
Antimicrobials	Amphotericin B Ampicillin Cefamandole Griseofulvin Ethambutol Lincomycin Metronidazole Neomycin Sulfasalazine Streptomycin Tetracyclines
Antineoplastic	Azathioprine Carmustine Doxorubicin Methotrexate Vincristine
Antirheumatic and Anti-inflammatory	Allopurinol Aspirin Colchicine D-penicillamine Gold salts Phenylbutazone
Antithyroid	Carbimazole Methimazole Methylthiouracil Propylthiouracil
Opiates	Codeine Hydromorphone Morphine
Psychopharmacologic	Lithium Psilocybin Trifluoperazine
Miscellaneous	Amphetamines Baclofen Clofibrate Diltiazem Disulfiram L-Dopa

Adapted from Schiffman SS: Taste and smell in disease. *N Engl J Med* 1983; 308:1277. Used with permission.

of penicillin (3000 to 5000 U) has been associated with irritability, convulsions, vomiting, and meningeal irritation. Intravenous (IV) doses produce similar side effects, except they occur at much higher dosages (Table 35-1). Daily IV dosages from 25,000 to 50,000,000 U may be associated with hyperreflexia, seizures, and generalized myoclonus. The patient with renal dysfunction often is predisposed the most to these neurotoxic reactions.

Convulsions have been reported following high IV doses of ampicillin, carbenicillin, and cloxacillin. These seizures may result from a reduction of the centrally active inhibitory neurotransmitter gamma-aminobutyric acid (GABA). There is also a relationship between the neurotoxicity of the various penicillins and their hydrophobic character. As partition coefficients increase, neurotoxicity increases in the following order: carbenicillin, ticarcillin, methicillin, oxacillin, cloxacillin, and dicloxacillin.

Sulfonamides

Whether the sulfonamides produce CNS toxicity is unclear. Use of the early sulpha drugs was associated with CNS abnormalities, including fatigue, lassitude, depression, ataxia, psychosis, and auditory or visual hallucinations. However, controlled clinical trials with these drugs have failed to reproduce these neurological disturbances.

Cephalosporins

High cephalosporin levels are associated with CNS toxicity that produces reversible encephalopathy, hallucinations, and nystagmus. Renal failure promotes drug accumulation by extending its half-life and by extending its free concentration in the plasma. Intrathecal use of cephaloridine has produced convulsions, and cefazolin has produced convulsions in patients with renal failure.

Tetracycline

There are no known CNS toxic effects of tetracycline in the adult. In infants tetracycline has been associated with bulging fontanelles 12 hours to four days following therapy (probable pseudotumor cerebri). There are no associated neurological findings, and the bulging resolves upon the discontinuation of the drug.

Chloramphenicol

A vague psychiatric disturbance may occur following prolonged use of chloramphenicol. The drug can interact with the metabolism of phenytoin and can produce subacute phenytoin toxicity with its attendant clinical manifestations. Careful monitoring of the phenytoin level is recommended.

Aminoglycosides

The type of neurotoxicity produced by the aminoglycosides depends upon the route of administration. Central nervous system toxicity is commonly associated with intrathecal administration. In animals, ataxia and apnea have developed following intrathecal injection of gentamicin. In a clinical series, the death rate for infants with meningitis treated with intrathecal gentamicin was 3½ times greater than for those treated with IV medication. Intravenous kanamycin has been associated with bulging fontanelles, psychosis, and blurred vision; IV gentamicin, with encephalopathy and psychosis. In all cases, toxic levels were the most likely cause of the CNS disturbances.

Metronidazole

Ataxia, seizures, and encephalopathy have been associated with the use of metronidazole. A cerebellar syndrome of ataxia and dysarthria may develop following high-dose therapy. Paresthesias associated with encephalopathy and major motor convulsions also have occurred during therapy with high doses.

Isoniazid

Isoniazid (INH) has a stimulatory effect on the CNS. Myoclonus and vertigo have been reported in patients receiving 4 mg/kg/day. Patients with an overdose (6 to 8 g) have either exaggerated or absent deep-tendon reflexes and generalized or focal tonic–clonic convulsions. Isoniazid induces seizures by lowering the GABA level. Pyridoxine (vitamin B_6, 1 gram for each gram of INH injested) should be administered. Memory impairment, encephalopathy, and toxic psychosis have been reported in patients not receiving pyridoxine.

Cranial Nerve Toxicities

Antibiotic neurotoxicity most commonly affects cranial nerve VIII (Table 35-3).

Aminoglycosides

The cochlear toxicity that results from therapy with aminoglycosides may be unilateral or bilateral; it can occur during the administration of the drug or days to months after therapy has been stopped. Vestibular abnormalities can also occur.

Tinnitus with decreased auditory acuity sometimes develops first. Tinnitus may be so great that audiometric analysis is not possible. Neomycin, kanamycin, and amikacin are associated with a higher incidence of cochlear toxicity than are gentamicin and streptomycin. Because of its great ototoxic potential, neomycin should not be used parenterally. Vestibular damage usually presents as vertigo, dizziness, nystagmus, and ataxia. It may occur with cochlear injury or months after the completion of therapy. Gentamicin, streptomycin, and dihydrostreptomycin have the greatest association with vestibular toxicity. Tobramycin has a low incidence of ototoxicity. High daily doses of the aminoglycosides, prolonged treatment, renal insufficiency, previous cochlear dysfunction, and concurrent or previous therapy with ototoxic drugs are all risk factors for aminoglycoside ototoxicity. Loop diuretics potentiate the ototoxic effects. The aminoglycosides destroy the hair cells of the inner ear.

TABLE 35-3 DRUG-INDUCED CRANIAL NERVE DISORDERS

TYPE OF DISTURBANCE	DRUG
Optic Neuropathy	Barbiturates
	Chloramphenicol
	Chlorpromazine
	Clioquinol
	Diabinese
	Digitalis
	Ergotamine
	Ibuprofen
	Indomethacin
	Isoniazid
	MAO inhibitors
	Oral contraceptives
	D-penicillamine
	Phenacetin
	Phenytoin
	Quinidine
	Streptomycin
	Thallium
	Thioridazine
Impaired Color Vision	Barbiturates
	Digitalis
	Ethambutol
	Methaqualone
	MAO inhibitors
	Nalidixic acid
	Streptomycin
	Sulfonamides
	Thiazides
	Vitamin A
Refractive Changes	Acetazolamide
	ACTH
	Anticholinergics
	Antidiabetics
	Antihistamines
	Chlorthiazide
	Corticosteroids
	Diuretics
	Fenfluramine
	Hydrochlorthiazide
	Insulin
	Oral contraceptives
	Phenytoin
	Sulfonamides
	Tetracycline
	Thiamine
	Tricyclic and tetracyclic antidepressants
Mydriasis	Amitriptyline
	Anticholinergics
	Antihistamines
	Beta-blockers
	Chlorpropamide
	Fenfluramine
	Indomethacin
	MAO inhibitors
	Oral contraceptives
	Phenylpropanolamine
	Protriptyline
	Salicylates

TABLE 35-3 continued

TYPE OF DISTURBANCE	DRUG
	Transdermal scopolamine
	Tricyclic antidepressants
Ocular Palsies	Barbiturates
	Carbamazepine
	Cardiac glycosides
	Diazepam
	Gold salts
	Imipramine
	Nitrofurantoin
	Oral contraceptives
	Phenobarbital
	Phenytoin
	Reserpine
	Vincristine
	Vitamin A
Vestibulotoxicity or Ototoxicity	Aspirin
	Chloramphenicol
	Chloroquine
	Cimetidine
	Colistin
	Gentamicin
	Kanamycin
	Neomycin
	Phenylbutazone
	Polymyxin B
	Streptomycin
	Vancomycin
	Viomycin

Erythromycin

Oral erythromycin stearate and its parenteral lactobionate form have been associated with reversible ototoxicity. Intraperitoneal instillation of erythromycin has also been associated with temporary deafness. Usually the hearing loss is above 4000 cycles/second and is associated with low-pitched tinnitus. Nystagmus is absent, and audiometric improvement often begins a few days after the medication is stopped. In most cases, there is associated renal insufficiency and/or excessively high drug levels.

Tetracycline

Mincocycline given in standard doses usually produces vestibular dysfunction (nausea, vomiting, and ataxia) 48 to 72 hours after the initial dose. Dysfunction ceases within 48 hours after therapy is stopped. In one case, acute transitory myopia developed after an injection of tetracycline.

Sulfonamides

Optic neuritis has been reported as a rare side effect of sulfanilamide. This drug can produce vertigo and tinnitus.

Chloramphenicol

Optic neuritis may develop in patients receiving extremely high doses of chloramphenicol. The initial symptoms include blurred vision and haloes around objects, followed by decreased visual acuity and impaired red–green color discrimination. A central scotoma is present, and visual fields are constricted. Funduscopic changes may result and include papilledema, flame hemorrhages, hyperemia, and exudates. Vision usually returns to normal following the discontinuation of therapy.

Vancomycin

Ototoxicity may occur with the use of vancomycin, usually at toxic levels. Persons older than 65, those who are receiving other potentially neurotoxic drugs, or those with underlying renal insufficiency are at greater risk for developing vancomycin ototoxicity.

Isoniazid and Ethambutol

Optic neuritis, often in combination with peripheral neuropathy, has been associated with INH. Ethambutol is associated with two types of ocular toxicity. (1) Central toxicity is associated with reduced visual acuity, central scotomata, and impaired color perception; (2) periaxial toxicity is associated with slight loss of visual acuity, normal color discrimination and partial visual field defects (scotomata, visual field constriction). Toxicity is usually noted in patients receiving doses higher than 35 mg/kg/day for 180 days. The patient who receives ethambutol at doses greater than 15 mg/kg/day should have a complete eye examination before therapy is started; visual acuity should be checked monthly thereafter. If blurred vision or the inability to see green develops, therapy should be stopped and the patient should consult an ophthalmologist.

Peripheral Nerve Toxicity

The antibiotics that produce a disturbance of the peripheral nervous system are listed in Table 35-4.

Penicillin

Prolonged intrathecal use of penicillin has been associated with pain in the distal lower extremities, bladder dysfunction, myelopathy, radiculitis, paralysis, and nausea and vomiting. Parenteral administration has not been linked to peripheral nerve toxicity unless the medication is inadvertently injected into a peripheral nerve.

Nitrofurantoin

Ten to fifteen percent of patients who receive nitrofurantoin experience significant adverse reactions; neurotoxicity accounts for approximately 2% of them. Polyneuropathy is the most common neurotoxic side effect. It is primarily sensory, of sudden onset, more distal in location, and it affects the lower extremities more

TABLE 35-4 DRUG-INDUCED PERIPHERAL NEUROPATHY

Antimicrobial Drugs
  Amphotericin B
  Chloramphenicol
  Clioquinol
  Dapsone
  Ethambutol
  Isoniazid
  Metronidazole
  Nitrofurantoin
  Penicillins
  Polymyxin B and colistin
  Sulfonamides

Cardiovascular Drugs
  Amiodarone
  Clofibrate
  Disopyramide
  Hydralazine
  Nifedipine
  Perhexilene
  Propranolol
  Streptokinase

Antirheumatic Drugs
  Chloroquine
  Colchicine
  D-Penicillamine
  Gold
  Indomethacin
  Phenylbutazone

Psychotropics
  Amitriptyline
  Imipramine
  Lithium
  Phenelzine

Other Drugs
  Anticoagulants
  Chlorpropamide
  Disulfiram
  Ergotamine
  Glue (N-hexane)
  Glutethimide
  Methaqualone
  Phenytoin
  Pyridoxine (overdose)
  Thalidomide
  Tolbutamide

Adapted from Mastaglia FL, Argov Z: Drug-induced neuromuscular disorders in man, in Walton J (ed): *Disorders of Voluntary Muscle.* New York, Churchill Livingstone, 1981, pp 873-906; and from Snavely SR, Hodges GR: The neurotoxicity of antibacterial agents. *Ann Intern Med* 1984;101:93; used with permission.

than the upper extremities. It typically ascends bilaterally and symmetrically with paresthesias and numbness. Vibratory and position sense are affected more than pain and temperature sensations. Motor weakness usually follows the sensory deficit, with weakness, atrophy and fasciculations. Patients who develop this neurotoxicity are usually elderly women. Eighty percent of cases develop after less than 45 days of therapy; 35% of patients experience total recovery after nitrofurantoin withdrawal, 50% have partial recovery, and 15% do not improve. Recovery usually takes days to several months, but usually occurs in four to eight weeks. In the absence of clinical toxicity, nerve conduction velocities are slowed—even after only a few weeks of therapy.

Chloramphenicol

Paresthesias, numbness, and burning may be caused by chloramphenicol. They frequently accompany optic neuritis after prolonged use of the drug.

Sulfonamides

Peripheral nerve dysfunction rarely complicates therapy with sulfonamides. The first sulfonamide preparations produced a neuropathy with motor weakness (without loss of sensation), reduced or absent deep-tendon reflexes, pain, tenderness, and paresthesias.

Metronidazole

Metronidazole produces a sensory neuropathy characterized by burning, paresthesias, and hyperesthesia of the toes, feet, and calves, occurring in a stocking-and-glove distribution. Finger paresthesias may also develop. Weakness and depression of the deep-tendon reflexes, unaccompanied by muscle wasting, are evident on examination. A total dose of greater than 50 g in a month or longer places the patient at risk. The toxicity usually resolves over three to four weeks (or longer) after therapy has been stopped.

Isoniazid

The typical symptoms of INH neuropathy are paresthesias of the feet, which often spread proximally if therapy is continued. Ataxia, weakness, and myalgias often accompany the neuropathy. Distal sensory modalities are reduced and deep-tendon reflexes are depressed, but they may revert to normal if therapy is stopped. This neuropathy can be prevented by the addition of pyridoxine (vitamin B_6), 10 mg/day. Children are not as susceptible as adults to the development of neuropathy.

Neuromuscular Blockade

Drugs that produce blockade of the neuromuscular junction are listed in Table 35-5. In general, symptoms are similar to those of myasthenia gravis (Chapter 29) and Eaton–Lambert syndrome (Chapter 32).

Aminoglycosides

The aminoglycosides that produce neuromuscular blockade are listed in Table 35-5. Clinical manifestations of neuromuscular blockade include flaccid paralysis, impaired respirations, and dilated pupils. All modes of therapy except the intrathecal route have been associated with this condition. Underlying renal insufficiency, neuromuscular disease, hypocalcemia, ether anesthesia, and treatment with succinylcholine, d-turbocurarine or gallimine all increase the risk for this drug-induced neuromuscular blockade. This complication should be suspected when there is a prolonged neuromuscular block after aminoglycosides despite the use of anticholinesterases. Neomycin and streptomycin inhibit the presynaptic release of acetylcholine and decrease the postsynaptic response to acetylcholine (similar to botulism and Eaton–Lambert syndrome). Tobramycin exhibits predominantly presynaptic effects, whereas netilmicin acts postsynaptically. Netilmicin and neomycin are the most potent neuromuscular blockers, and kanamycin the least potent.

Both calcium gluconate and neostigmine are effective in reversing aminoglycoside-induced apnea and muscle weakness. Ventilatory support and repeated doses of calcium may be needed until recovery from the neuromuscular blockade occurs.

TABLE 35-5   DRUG-INDUCED NEUROMUSCULAR BLOCKADE

SYNDROME	DRUGS IMPLICATED
Myasthenic	Beta-blockers Colistins D-penicillamine Gentamicin Kanamycin Neomycin Phenytoin Polymyxin B Streptomycin Trimethadione
Unmasking or aggravation of myasthenia gravis	ACTH Beta-blockers Chlorpromazine Kanamycin Colistin Corticosteroids Lithium Methoxyflurane Phenytoin Procainamide Quinidine Streptomycin Tetracycline Thyroid hormone
Antibiotic-induced respiratory arrest	Clindamycin Colistin Kanamycin Lincomycin Neomycin Streptomycin
Potentiation of muscle relaxants	Chloroquine Diazepam Ether Ketamine Lidocaine Lithium Phenelzine Procaine Promazine Propranolol Quinidine

Adapted from Mastaglia FL, Argov Z (1981). Used with permission.

Tetracyclines

Tetracycline can produce a weak neuromuscular blockade. Tetracycline and oxytetracycline potentiate the neuromuscular blockade produced by d-turbocurarine and magnesium. Mincocycline also produces mild neuromuscular blockade.

Polymyxin B and Colistin

Polymyxin B produces a nondepolarizing neuromuscular blockade. Prolonged respiratory paralysis may occur after IV or intraperitoneal administration. The block can be prolonged if large doses of medication are given. Therapy is supportive, although calcium chloride partially antagonizes the block. Colistin has been reported to cause neuromuscular blockade manifested as hypotonia and respiratory depression. Therapy is supportive, because little or no reversal of the blockade occurs after the use of calcium or neostigmine.

Lincomycin and Clindamycin

Lincomycin is a weak neuromuscular blocker which produces a nondepolarizing competitive blockade. It potentiates the action of pancuronium and d-tubocurarine. Clindamycin, a derivative of lincomycin, is associated with neuromuscular blockade similar to that produced by lincomycin. Both lincomycin and clindamycin produce neuromuscular blockade through a postsynaptic action, although clindamycin has a marked presynaptic stimulating effect at high doses.

GASTROINTESTINAL DRUGS
H$_2$ Blocking Agents

The H$_2$ blockers produce reversible competitive antagonism of histamine on H$_2$ receptors and inhibit gastric acid secretion. Cimetidine and ranitidine are the most commonly used H$_2$ blockers.

Cimetidine binds to the cytochrome P-450 system of the liver and diminishes the action of certain microsomal enzyme systems. Thus, the following drugs can accumulate to toxic levels when they are being given concurrently with cimetidine: phenytoin, phenobarbital, theophylline, diazepam, propranolol, and imipramine. Ranitidine does not bind as greatly with the cytochrome P-450 system, hence it does not reduce the metabolism of other medications.

Common side effects of both drugs include headache, dizziness, malaise, myalgia, nausea, loss of libido, and impotence. Gynecomastia may result from treatment with cimetidine because it binds to androgen receptors. Sexual dysfunction is the result of elevation of the serum prolactin level. Ranitidine does not have antiandrogenic activity; it does not cause gynecomastia or sexual dysfunction.

Cimetidine can cause various CNS disturbances that probably result from the blocking of H$_2$ receptors in the brain. Elderly patients and those with impaired renal function are more likely to develop CNS toxicity. Confusion, lethargy, agitation, disorientation, chorea, myoclonus, hallucinations, and seizures all have been reported with cimetidine therapy. Mania may be exacerbated by cimetidine, and respiratory depression has also occurred. A pure motor neuropathy has also been attributed to cimetidine. Ranitidine is associated with less CNS toxicity because it does not cross the blood–brain barrier as well as cimetidine does. Headache and confusion are the most frequently observed CNS complications of therapy with ranitidine.

Anti-emetics
Phenothiazines

The phenothiazines are utilized widely to control nausea and vomiting and to control intractable hiccups. The neurological toxicity of these drugs is discussed below in the section on psychiatric medications.

Metoclopramide

Metoclopramide produces antidopaminergic and anticholinergic effects. It improves gastric motility and is often used to treat nausea and vomiting associated with delayed gastric emptying. Its major use is for prophylaxis of nausea and vomiting associated with cancer chemotherapy, especially from *cis*-platinum.

Extrapyramidal reactions can occur that are similar to those produced by other dopamine blocking drugs. These reactions include dyskinesias, parkinsonism, tardive dyskinesia/dystonia, and neuroleptic malignant syndrome (discussed in the section on psychiatric drugs). Depression may also result. Parkinsonian symptoms may develop acutely or subacutely, are most often bilateral, are often accompanied by orofacial dyskinesias and postural tremor. Parkinsonism may develop after short-term (few months) to long-term (two years) therapy. Symptoms usually subside rapidly after the drug is stopped, but it usually takes several months for the parkinsonism to clear. A few cases have been reported in which the extrapyramidal syndrome persisted for one or two years. Overall, extrapyramidal reactions are less common with metoclopramide than those that occur with the phenothiazines or butyrophenones. Metoclopramide overdose produces irritability, somnolence, agitation, and convulsions.

Anticholinergic Drugs

Anticholinergic drugs are used to treat peptic ulcer disease and to reduce gastric motility. Atropine is the prototype anticholinergic. Other anticholinergics (often used for nongastrointestinal conditions) include benztropine, trihexyphenidyl, and biperidin. Topical anticholinergic drugs (eg, transderm scopolamine) are used to prevent motion sickness. The anticholinergic effects of different drugs are additive and may produce both central and peripheral effects.

Mental disturbances occur in approximately 20% of patients treated with standard doses of anticholinergics. These side effects occur more frequently in the elderly and in patients with mental impairment. The syndrome of *central* anticholinergic toxicity features forgetfulness, impairment of recent memory, drowsiness, agitation, and confusion. It may be episodic and can be accompanied by dysarthria, ataxia, and complex visual hallucinations. Paranoia with delirium can develop, possibly triggered in part by the visual hallucinations. With higher doses, coma may develop with associated anhydrosis and fever. Tremor and choreiform movements may also occur with central anticholinergic toxicity. Reduction of the dosage of the medication will usually reverse the neurological syndrome. Severe intoxication can be reversed by IV physostigmine (1 to 2.mg).

The *peripheral* anticholinergic side effects include blurred vision (often near vision), constipation, and dryness of the mouth. The mydriasis and cycloplegia that results can exacerbate glaucoma. Urinary retention may be precipitated in the elderly man with prostatic hypertrophy. Transdermal scopolamine, used to treat motion sickness, produces predominantly peripheral anticholinergic side effects. However, confusion and psychosis have been associated with this transdermal preparation. Mydriasis is usually bilateral, but unilateral mydriasis can result if the patient touches the patch and then touches the eye, allowing minute amounts of scopolamine to be absorbed intraocularly. This can be recurrent if another patch is applied during the ensuing 24 to 48 hours. If 1% pilocarpine applied to the eye fails to produce pupillary constriction (in the absence of glaucoma or trauma to the eye), the mydriasis is drug-induced and is not a "neurosurgical emergency."

Miscellaneous Agents
Antacids

Antacids can produce neurological complications, usually the result of electrolyte abnormalities. In chronic renal failure, magnesium trisilicate and magnesium hydroxide may produce hypermagnesemia with associated depression of CNS function and muscle weakness. Chronic renal failure patients on hemodialysis are prone to developing hypophosphatemia from aluminum hydroxide. Tremor, malaise, weakness, and neuropathy may develop. Dialysis encephalopathy may also result, likely from an accumulation of aluminum.

Laxatives

The abuser of laxatives may develop muscle weakness from hypokalemia. Hypomagnesemia, hyponatremia, and hypocalcemia can also develop.

Sulfasalazine

Sulfasalazine is a sulfa derivative used to treat ulcerative colitis. Adverse neurological reactions occur in 5% to 55% of patients. These reactions are either dose related or are the result of hypersensitivity reactions. Hypersensitivity neurological reactions include peripheral neuropathy, which is most marked in the lower extremities and is associated with paresthesias, numbness, hyporeflexia, and impairment of proprioception. The dose-dependent reactions usually occur during the first 8 to 12 weeks of therapy with doses of sulfasalazine exceeding 4 g daily. Nausea, vomiting, fever, headache, and arthralgias are common symptoms that typically subside as the medication is stopped or the dosage is decreased.

PSYCHIATRIC DRUGS
Antidepressants

The tricyclic antidepressants are the most commonly prescribed drugs for the treatment of depression. Tetracyclic antidepressant medications have been released recently for the treatment of affective disorders. The tetracyclics are reported to have less toxicity overall than do the tricyclics, but they also produce adverse side effects. These antidepressant drugs are sedatives, not stimulants. They have both central and peripheral anticholinergic actions, which lead to their most common side effects. Amitriptyline has the strongest anticholinergic activity; desipramine, the weakest. They exert their antidepressant effect by blocking the amine pump in the presynaptic nerve endings.

Peripheral and central anticholinergic toxicities have been discussed previously. Confusion can develop in the susceptible individual; as with other side effects, it may be dose related. Sexual dysfunction includes erectile dysfunction, ejaculatory problems, and changes in libido. Delay in achieving orgasm has been reported in women. Orthostatic hypotension is present in most patients receiving tricyclic antidepressants; it can be asymptomatic or can lead to postural light-headedness and/or syncope.

Approximately 10% of patients receiving tricyclic antidepressants develop abnormal movements. Tremor similar to essential tremor is most common; it can be suppressed with propranolol. Generalized myoclonus has been reported as a rare complication of the tricyclics (amitriptyline) when taken in both nontoxic and toxic amounts. Oral (buccal–lingual) dyskinesias have occured during treatment with imipramine and amitriptyline. Generalized choreoathetosis has been reported as a manifestation of toxicity. Withdrawal of the drug or a reduction in the dosage usually stops these movements. Amoxapine is a newer tricyclic antidepressant initially reported to have less cardiovascular and CNS toxicity than other tricyclics. Unlike other tricyclic drugs, it has a higher propensity to produce extrapyramidal syndromes. Akinesia, cogwheel rigidity, and weakness have been reported in patients receiving therapeutic amounts of the drug. Tardive dyskinesia, usually reversible, has occured from four days to four months after the amoxapine was stopped.

Severe tinnitus has been reported to complicate therapy with imipramine. The tinnitus may be severe enough to produce hearing disability; it diminishes or disappears with dose reduction.

Many psychiatric medications lower the seizure threshold (Table 35-6). The incidence of tricyclic-induced seizures is approximately 2.2% Imipramine and amitriptyline are the most highly epileptogenic; the least epileptogenic tricyclic is doxepin. Maprotoline, a tetracyclic, has a strong tendency to induce seizures; in

TABLE 35-6 PSYCHOTROPIC DRUGS THAT LOWER
SEIZURE THRESHOLD

SEIZURE POTENTIAL	NEUROLEPTICS	ANTIDEPRESSANTS	OTHER DRUGS
High	Chlorpromazine Promazine	Maprotoline	
Moderate	Perphenazine Thiothixene Haloperidol	Amitriptyline Protriptyline	Lithium
Low	Fluphenazine Mesoridazine Thioridazine Molindone	Imipramine Desipramine Doxepin Nomifensine	Meprobamate Hydroxyzine Glutethimide

Adapted from Mendez MF, Cummings JL, Benson DF: Epilepsy: Psychiatric aspects and use of psychotropics. *Psychosomatics* 1984; 25:886. Used with permission.

one series, the incidence was 15.6%. The higher epileptogenic potential of maprotoline may be due to its strong lipophilic activity producing higher brain concentrations. Predisposing brain damage or coexistent seizure disorders may all increase the epileptogenic potential of the antidepressants and psychotropic medications.

Neuroleptic Agents

Antipsychotic drugs (phenothiazines, butyrophenones), also known as neuroleptic agents, are useful in treating the psychotic patient. These drugs exert their effects primarily by blocking dopamine receptors, although they also block histamine, α-adrenergic, muscarinic, and serotonergic receptors. Most of the side effects of these drugs result from a blockade of these receptors. The different types of adverse neurological reactions produced by neuroleptics are listed in Table 35-7.

Many neuroleptic drugs can lower the seizure threshold (Table 35-7) and can induce paroxysmal EEG discharges. The aliphatic phenothiazines with low potency (eg, chlorpramazine) are more likely to produce seizures, whereas more potent neuroleptics (fluphenazine, thiothixene) are less likely to do so. Approximately 1.5% of patients who take chlorpromazine develop seizures. The incidence is dose-related. Patients taking less than 800 mg have an incidence of

TABLE 35-7 NEUROLOGICAL SIDE EFFECTS OF NEUROLEPTIC DRUGS

Reaction	Clinical Features	Time of Greatest Risk	Treatment
Acute Dystonia	Spasm of muscles of neck, face, tongue, back	1-5 days	Anticholinergics (benztropine), diphenhydramine
Akathisia	Motor restlessness; *not* anxiety	5-60 days	Reduce dose or change drug; diazepam, propranolol
Parkinsonism	Rigidity, bradykinesia tremor, abnormal gait	5-30 days (acute)	Stop neuroleptic; antiparkinsonian drugs; anticholinergics; amantadine
Neuroleptic malignant syndrome	Catatonia, dyskinesias, rigidity, stupor, fever, autonomic instability	days to weeks	Stop neuroleptic; dantrolene sodium; bromocriptine
Tardive dyskinesia	Orofacial dyskinesia; extremity and truncal choreoathetosis	months to years	Prevention; reserpine; tetrabenazine
Rabbit syndrome	Perioral tremor	months to years	Antiparkinsonian drugs Anticholinergics

Adapted from Goodman AG, Goodman LS, Rall TW, et al (eds): *Goodman and Gilman's The Pharmacological Basis of Therapeutics*, ed 7. New York, MacMillan, 1985, p 406. Used with permission.

seizures of 0.5%, whereas those who take more than 1000 mg have an incidence as high as 10%. The butyrophenones (haloperidol) have variable and unpredictable effects on seizure activity. Lithium has been reported to cause seizures, which usually occur at toxic levels. Part of the increased seizure incidence with the use of lithium could result from associated electrolyte disturbances. Overt seizures are more likely to occur in patients with a history of seizures or in those who are predisposed to seizures.

In the patient with epilepsy who requires psychotropic medication, the psychotropic should be started at low dosages and increased slowly. In certain cases, it may be best to have the patient hospitalized. Seizures are more likely to occur within the first 10 days after starting or increasing the dosage of the drug, especially in the patient with a known seizure disorder or one at risk for seizure development. Risk factors include brain injury, dementia, focal neurological abnormalities, mental retardation, advanced age, systemic medical illness, history of electroconvulsive therapy, drug use or alcohol withdrawal, family history of seizures, and a history of seizures. Late-occurring seizures usually are the result of high dosages. The risk of seizures is increased by multiple drug therapy. Psychotropics with lower potency should be used (eg, thioridazine). An EEG should be performed before starting the medication; it should be repeated when the patient has been on the psychotropic for several weeks. Anticonvulsant drug levels should be obtained periodically, as there is anticonvulsant–psychotropic drug interaction. Many of the psychotropics reduce the hepatic metabolism of phenytoin and phenobarbital, and toxic levels may result.

Early-Onset Adverse Reactions

Dystonia. Acute dystonic reactions occur in about 12% of patients receiving neuroleptic agents. Dystonias include torticollis, grimacing, and extremity dyskinesias. Dystonia may involve the laryngeal and pharyngeal muscles, producing dysphonia, gagging, and severe respiratory distress. Oculogyric crisis may occur, with upward or lateral deviation of the eyes associated with blepharospasm. Dystonias commonly occur between the ages of 5 and 45, and occur twice as often in men. Most cases occur within the first four days after the onset of drug therapy. Fluphenazine, perphenazine, haloperidol, and thiothixene (high dopamine-receptor antagonists) most frequently produce these reactions. Intravenous or intramuscular administration of anticholinergic drugs (benztropine, biperiden) or diphenhydramine produces a rapid reversal of this syndrome. Diazepam is also effective in reducing the dystonia. Switching to a less potent antidopaminergic drug (chlorpromazine, thioridazine, mesoridazine) may be necessary, although these reactions become less frequent with time.

Akathisia. Akathisia is a state of motor restlessness characterized by a subjective feeling of tension associated with the inability to tolerate inactivity. Patients feel jittery and are unable to stand or sit still. This condition occurs early during treatment with neuroleptics; it resembles anxiety. The incidence of akathisia varies from 20% to 45%, and in one study 59% of patients with akathisia experienced other extrapyramidal disturbances. Patients of all ages are affected, although the elderly may be more predisposed to developing this complication, as are patients who have a long record of hospitalization, those who have not responded well to neuroleptics, and those who were treated with fluphenazine. Women are affected twice as frequently as men.

More than 85% of patients develop symptoms within seven days after reaching the maximum dosage of the neuroleptic. Such patients may be misdiagnosed as having agitation related to their psychosis, and they may be treated with higher doses of the neuroleptic. The high-potency antipsychotics are most likely to produce akathisia; switching to lower-potency drugs (eg, chlorpromazine, thioridazine) may be helpful. Tolerance to this side effect may occur. Reducing the dosage of the neuroleptic, giving diazepam or a short-acting barbiturate, or propranolol, 10 mg tid, may reduce akathisia. Antiparkinsonian drugs usually do not produce a reliable effect.

Parkinsonism. The incidence of early-onset neuroleptic-induced parkinsonism is approximately 13%. Women are affected twice as often as men, and persons of all ages are affected. Most cases develop within 72 hours of the start of neuroleptic therapy. Patients receiving high-potency neuroleptics (fluphenazine, haloperidol, thiothixene, perphenazine) have the highest incidence of parkinsonism. The anticholinergic drugs (benztropine, trihexyphenidyl, diphenhydramine, biperiden) are effective in treating this syndrome. Amantadine also may be of benefit, although it has a slower onset of action and is not as effective for controlling rigidity. Drug-induced parkinsonism usually takes 10 to 60 days to clear after the offending medication has been discontinued. Parkinsonism can occur as a late-onset side effect of neuroleptic medication, but it is often difficult to determine if the movement disorder is idiopathic or caused by the neuroleptic.

Variable-Onset Adverse Reactions

Neuroleptic Malignant Syndrome. Neuroleptic malignant syndrome (NMS) is a life-threatening side effect of neuroleptic therapy. It was first described and named in 1968, and it has an incidence of 0.5% to 1% in all patients exposed to neuroleptics. It affects all ages and both sexes, although young men are affected more frequently. Predisposing factors include physical exhaustion, dehydration, concurrent organic brain syndrome, and the use of long-acting depot neuroleptics (eg, fluphenazine decanoate). Hyperthermia, muscle hypertonicity, instability of the autonomic nervous system, and altered levels of consciousness are the core features of NMS. It typically develops over 24 to 72 hours. It will last five to ten days after oral drugs are discontinued, and two to three times longer when depot drugs have been used.

The autonomic features may appear before other symptoms. Typical autonomic abnormalities include pallor, diaphoresis, tachycardia, blood pressure instability, and cardiac arrhythmias. Muscle tone of the "lead-pipe" type is markedly increased. This increased muscle tone may reduce compliance of the chest wall and produce respiratory problems severe enough to necessitate respiratory support.

Akinesia or dyskinesias may be present. Agitation may be evident, and the level of consciousness often fluctuates from an alert state to mutism or stupor. The temperature may rise to 41° C or higher. Leukocytosis, myoglobinuria, markedly elevated creatine kinase levels, and elevated transaminase and alkaline phosphatase levels usually occur. Mortality ranges from 10% to 20%.

The first therapeutic measure is to stop the neuroleptic. Dantrolene sodium, 0.25 mg/kg body weight qid should be given, and, if the patient is able to swallow, bromocriptine mesylate (a dopamine agonist), 5 mg po tid, should be given. Anticholinergics and other dopamine agonists have been utilized without much success. Recently, sodium nitroprusside was used successfully to treat NMS. The more rapid the diagnosis is made and appropriate therapy started, the greater the chance for recovery.

Late-Onset Adverse Reactions

Tardive Dyskinesia. Tardive dyskinesia is a series of abnormal movements that are associated with chronic exposure to neuroleptic agents. Prochlorperazine and metoclopramide, used on a long-term basis for nausea and vomiting, have also produced tardive dyskinesia. The movements are choreiform, involving the tongue, mouth, and lips. Choreoathetoid movements of the fingers, hands, arms, and feet may be present, and truncal and diaphragmatic hyperkinesias may also result, the latter resulting in grunting and difficult breathing. Symptoms fluctuate; they disappear during sleep and increase with anxiety. Cognitive impairment may also occur. Almost one-third of patients who have received long-term therapy with neuroleptics develop tardive dyskinesias. Women over the age of 50 have the highest incidence of this disorder.

There is no effective treatment. Anticholinergic drugs exacerbate the symptoms. Increasing the dose of the neuroleptic reduces the dyskinesias, but produces further damage to the dopamine receptors. Switching the neuroleptic to thioridazine (which has the lowest incidence of drug-induced parkinsonism of the available neuroleptics) may also benefit the patient who requires neuroleptic medications. Cholinergic agonist drugs such as deanol and anticholinesterase agents such as physostigmine do not produce sustained clinical benefits. Dopamine-depleting drugs, such as tetrabenazine and reserpine, are useful, but reserpine should not be used if the patient is depressed. Lithium and propranolol are of benefit occasionally. The best way to treat tardive dyskinesia is to prevent its occurrence. Continuous treatment with neuroleptics is preferred to intermittent treatment.

Tardive Dystonia. Tardive dystonia is related to tardive dyskinesia and may coexist with it. It is characterized by slow, often sustained, involuntary twisting movements of the face, neck, trunk, or limbs. It can be focal or generalized, and it occurs in patients of all ages. Tardive dystonia usually develops after more than 3½ years of exposure to neuroleptics. Increasing the dose of the neuroleptic does reduce the intensity of the dystonia, but, as in tardive dyskinesia, further damage to the dopamine receptor may result. One-third of patients treated with anticholinergics improve, as do two-thirds of those treated with tetrabenazine.

Rabbit Syndrome. Rabbit syndrome is a perioral tremor similar to that which may develop in patients with Parkinson's disease. It tends to occur as a late manifestation of neuroleptic therapy. It responds well to treatment with anti-parkinsonian drugs (eg, anticholinergics).

ANTI-INFLAMMATORY DRUGS
Nonsteroidal Agents

Nonsteroidal anti-inflammatory drugs (NSAIDs) produce minor neurological complications.

Indomethacin

The most frequent neurological side effect of indomethacin is headache. It is usually located frontally, is throbbing, and occurs in 25% to 50% of patients who take the drug chronically. Headache is a puzzling complication. Indomethacin is effective for the treatment of certain types of vascular headache, yet it paradoxically produces a vascular type of head pain, probably caused by extracranial vasodilation. Dizziness, vertigo, lightheadedness and mental confusion are infrequent complications. Severe depression, psychosis, hallucinations, and suicide have also been reported.

Sulindac

Sulindac is closely related to indomethacin, although it is less toxic. Ten percent of patients develop CNS side effects, including drowsiness, headache, and dizziness. Recurrent aseptic meningitis has also been reported to occur during treatment with sulindac in a patient without connective tissue disease.

Tolmetin

Tolmetin is an anti-inflammatory and antipyretic that is more potent than aspirin. Side effects on the CNS are few and include nervousness, anxiety, insomnia, drowsiness, and visual disturbances. Tinnitus, deafness, and vertigo occur less commonly than with aspirin. A case of aseptic meningitis has been reported in a patient with systemic lupus erythematosus (SLE).

Ibuprofen

Ibuprofen produces relatively minor neurological side effects, including headache, hallucinations, confusion, dizziness, and blurred vision. A number of cases of aseptic meningitis have been reported in association with mixed connective tissue disease or SLE.

Naproxen

Drowsiness, headache, ototoxicity, and depression have been reported infrequently as neurological side efects of naproxen.

Fenoprofen

Fenoprofen (Nalfon) produces minor neurological symptoms, including tinnitus, deafness, lassitude, confusion, and anorexia.

Corticosteroids

A variety of neurological complications may result from treatment with corticosteroids. Toxic effects that are usually observed result from either the withdrawal of the drug, or from the continued use of large dosages. Most neurological reactions occur during the continuous use of the steroid preparation.

Pseudotumor cerebri (Chapter 21) may follow the reduction or withdrawal of corticosteroid therapy. The characteristic corticosteroid withdrawal syndrome consists of fever, myalgia, malaise, and arthralgias ("pseudo-rheumatism"). Neurological syndromes that result from large doses of corticosteroids include behavioral abnormalities (psychosis), myopathy, seizures, and dementia. Intractable hiccups have been associated with both high-dose methylprednisolone (IV) and dexamethasone therapy.

Psychosis

Psychiatric reactions occur in as many as 5% of steroid-treated patients. Most show affective and/or psychotic symptoms. Depression, mania, delirium and psychosis can occur. More than one-third of patients develop depression; 20% develop mania. Only 12% develop psychosis alone, but more than 50% of the other psychiatric disturbances are associated with psychosis. These disturbances typically occur early in the course of therapy: 43% of patients develop symptoms during the first week, and 93%, during the first six weeks. The risk for psychiatric disturbances is highest in women, in patients with SLE, and in those receiving high-dose steroids. Seventy-seven percent of patients are receiving more than the equivalent of 40 mg of prednisone daily at the time of their psychosis. Higher dosages do not cause an earlier onset of symptoms, however. Occasionally, withdrawal of the steroid produces the psychiatric syndrome, although this is uncommon. With alternate-day therapy, mental changes may be cyclical, with psychiatric disturbances occurring predominantly on each day of treatment. Suicidal tendencies are not rare; it has been estimated that the suicide rate in steroid psychosis is 3%.

Steroid psychosis almost always responds to reduction of the dosage or withdrawal of therapy. Withdrawal should be done slowly to avoid steroid withdrawal syndrome. Lithium prophylaxis, 300 mg tid, often effectively controls steroid-induced mania. Tricyclic antidepressants have been reported to exacerbate the clinical state of the patient, whereas phenothiazines (chlorpromazine, thioridazine) have been beneficial in controlling this toxic psychosis.

The vast majority of patients improve when the steroid is discontinued and do not show mental status changes of a primary affective or thought disorder. An occasional patient has persistent or recurrent psychiatric problems, most likely resulting from preexisting psychopathology.

Seizures

Steroids lower the seizure threshold and produce EEG abnormalities such as spike and wave discharges. Often, the patient is receiving steroids for a connective tissue disorder such as SLE, which may be associated with seizures secondary to

CNS vasculitis. In some patients, seizures are the result of an anaphylactoid reaction to the steroid preparation, especially IV methylprednisolone. Seizures should be treated with an appropriate anticonvulsant.

Dementia

Dementia occasionally occurs without psychosis. The patient demonstrates a dementia-like decline in mental function that often mimics early Alzheimer's disease. He complains of disturbances in memory retention, attention, and

TABLE 35-8   DRUG-INDUCED MUSCLE DISORDERS

DISORDER	DRUGS IMPLICATED
Focal myopathy	IM injections of various drugs
Muscle Fibrosis or Contractures	Pentazocine Antibiotics Heroin
Acute or Subacute Painful Proximal Myopathy	Clofibrate Alcohol Epsilon-aminocaproic acid Emetine Heroin Vincristine Danazol Cimetidine Lithium Cytotoxics Diuretics Licorice Amphotericin B D-Penicillamine Procainamide Levodopa
Chronic Painless Proximal Myopathy	Corticosteroids Alcohol Perhexilene Chloroquine Diuretics Amphotericin B
Acute Rhabdomyolysis	Amphetamine Barbiturates Diazepam Isoniazid Heroin Methadone Amphotericin B Phencyclidine
Malignant Hyperthermia	Halothane Chloroform Ketamine Enflurane Cyclopropane Diethyl ether Psychotropics

Adapted from Mastaglia FL, Argov Z (1981). Used with permission.

concentration, which are sometimes associated with significant intellectual loss. Affected patients are usually taking high doses of corticosteroid, equivalent to 60 to 120 mg of prednisone. This syndrome may reverse when therapy is discontinued. It has been suggested that this syndrome is a prodrome to steroid psychosis.

Myopathy

Myopathy is a well-known complication of corticosteroid therapy (Table 35-8) occurring particularly in patients treated with fluorinated steroids (triamcinolone, betamethasone, and dexamethasone). It has also complicated therapy with prednisone, cortisone, prednisolone, and methylprednisolone. Myopathy can occur soon after treatment is begun, and is more likely to occur in patients receiving large doses of medication for prolonged periods. It may complicate topical steroid therapy. The appearance of myopathy is often insidious. Myalgia is a common initial symptom. In the typical case, there is symmetrical weakness of the proximal limb muscles, which spreads from the proximal pelvic girdle to the proximal shoulder muscles. If therapy is continued without a reduction of dosage, the distal muscles become involved and the weakness becomes generalized.

Deep-tendon reflexes are usually preserved. Serum muscle enzyme levels are normal, but urinary creatine excretion is usually increased. The EMG is suggestive of a myopathic process, and muscle biopsy (usually not indicated) reveals an atrophic process that typically involves type-II fibers. The only effective therapy is to reduce or discontinue the steroid preparation.

Bibliography

Black JL, Richelson E, Richardson JW: Antipsychotic agents: A clinical update. *Mayo Clin Proc* 1985; 60:777-789. (A must for physicians who prescribe antipsychotic drugs; good review of the neurotoxicity of these drugs.)

Davies DM (ed): *Textbook of Adverse Drug Reactions,* ed. 2. New York, Oxford University Press, 1981. (Reviews, by organ system, various drug-induced toxicities. The chapter on neurological side effects is concise and complete.)

Dukes MNG, Beeley L (eds): *Side Effects of Drugs: Annual 9.* Amsterdam, Elsevier, 1985. (Annual review of drug toxicities, based on classes of medication; most current review of this topic.)

Goodman AG, Goodman LS, Rall TW, et al (eds): *Goodman and Gilman's The Pharmacological Basis of Therapeutics,* ed. 7. New York, Macmillan, 1985. (Current edition of the "Bible" of pharmacology. Excellent, brief discussions of most medications, including their side effects.)

Jabbari B, Bryan GE, Marsh EE, et al: Incidence of seizures with tricyclic and tetracyclic antidepressants. *Arch Neurol* 1985; 42:480-481. (Maprotoline has the highest epileptic potential of all the antidepressants.)

Mastaglia FL, Argov Z: Drug-induced neuromuscular disorders in man, in Walton J (ed): *Disorders of Voluntary Muscle,* ed. 4. New York, Churchill Livingstone, 1981, pp 873-906. (Comprehensive review of neuromuscular effects of medications.)

Mendez MF, Cummings JL, Benson DF: Epilepsy: Psychiatric aspects and use of psychotropics. *Psychosomatics* 1984; 25:883-894. (Best review of the effect of antidepressants and neuroleptics on seizure frequency; provides guidelines for management.)

Mitchell DM, Collins JV: Do corticosteroids really alter mood? *Postgrad Med* 1984; 60:467-470. (Reviews numerous reports on psychosis allegedly caused by steroids.)

Schiffman SS: Taste and smell in disease. *N Engl J Med* 1983; 308:1275-1279. (State-of-the-art review of disorders that affect taste and smell. Provides information about drug causes.)

Silverstein A (ed): *Neurological Complications of Therapy. Selected Topics.* Mount Kisco, NY, Futura, 1982. (Reviews the neurological complications of various therapies, including medications.)

Snavely SR, Hodges GR: The neurotoxicity of antibacterial agents. *Ann Intern Med* 1984; 101:92-104. (Well-referenced, current review of antibiotic neurotoxicity.)

FOUR

Emergencies

Coma

Evaluation of the patient in coma forms the cornerstone of the treatment of neurological emergencies. The physician must proceed quickly and in an orderly, efficient manner to identify and treat the cause of coma. While diagnostic studies are being undertaken, measures must be followed to protect the brain from further damage. This chapter emphasizes the correlation between examination findings and the cause of coma to permit the clinician to differentiate various structural causes from metabolic causes. The emergency management of the comatose patient is defined, and brain death and the persistent vegetative state are discussed briefly. Traumatic coma and the use of the Glasgow Coma Scale are discussed in Chapter 38.

DEFINITION

Consciousness is the awareness of self and environment; it is believed to require two anatomico-physiologic systems for its normal operation. The ascending reticular activating system (ARAS) in the brain stem tegmentum subserves the arousal system and permits wakefulness. The cerebral hemispheres to which the ARAS projects subserve the content of consciousness and provide memory, behavior, abstraction, perception, and language. Damage to either the ARAS or to both hemispheres impairs consciousness and leads to pathological states of unconsciousness.

Pathological states of unconsciousness form a spectrum from subtle confusional states to deep coma. Coma is defined operationally by Plum and Posner (1980) as "a state of unarousable psychologic unresponsiveness in which the subjects lie with eyes closed." Vigorous external stimulation (eg, pain) does not produce psychologic responsiveness. In "light" coma, stimulation elicits a variety of reflex responses, such as limb posturing, grimacing, or mydriasis. In "deep" coma, reflex responses are minimal or absent. Stupor is a state of sleep-like psychologic unresponsiveness from which the patient may be aroused briefly to psychologic responsiveness by vigorous stimulation. Less severe states of altered consciousness are termed obtundation, lethargy, or drowsiness.

Stupor and coma require dysfunction of the ARAS, the cerebral hemispheres, or both structures. The ARAS may be damaged directly or indirectly. Direct damage may occur by a brain stem tegmental infarction or hemorrhage. Indirect ARAS dysfunction may be produced by an expanding hemispheric mass lesion that produces cerebral herniation and communicates the increased pressure to the brain stem, resulting in ischemia to the ARAS. Lesions that selectively damage both hemispheres while sparing the brain stem are less common, but have been seen in bilateral hemispheric strokes, in hypoxic–ischemic damage during cardiac arrest, and in encephalitis. More common is a metabolic encephalopathy that concurrently depresses the functions of both hemispheres and the brain stem.

EMERGENCY MANAGEMENT

While assessing the cause and course of coma, the physician must guarantee that no acute harm befalls the comatose patient. Plum and Posner (1980) have identified 12 principles of emergency management of comatose patients:

1. *Assure oxygenation.* The airway must be protected and the patient must have an adequate respiratory rate and tidal volume. Obtaining arterial blood gases is a crucial step to ascertain oxygenation and ventilation. Intubation and ventilatory assistance should be performed in patients with dangerous hypoxemia or hypercapnia.

2. *Maintain circulation.* Adequate cerebral perfusion pressure depends upon an adequate pulse and blood pressure. Mean arterial blood pressure should be kept at 90 to 100 torr with volume replacement and vasopressors, if necessary. Life-threatening cardiac arrhythmias should be monitored closely and treated promptly.

3. *Administer glucose.* The acutely comatose patient should be considered hypoglycemic until proved otherwise. After venous blood samples are obtained for glucose, electrolytes, calcium, complete blood count, renal and hepatic function tests, coagulation status, and toxicology, the patient should be given 50 mL of 50% glucose intravenously (IV). If laboratory results later show that the patient was hypoglycemic, valuable time has been saved by not waiting for the report of the glucose determination. If the patient was actually hyperglycemic, the 25 grams of glucose would not have significantly worsened the hyperglycemia. In states of hypoglycemia, much additional glucose is needed subsequently, and frequent blood glucose determinations are necessary.

4. *Lower raised intracranial pressure.* In states of intracranial hypertension, the intracranial pressure may be lowered by ventilating the patient to a pCO_2 of 20 to 25 torr. If incipient cerebral herniation is occurring, 20% mannitol is given IV bolus at 1.5 to 2.0 g/kg. If the herniation is not reversed within ten minutes, furosemide, 40 to 80 mg IV, should be given. If the raised intracranial pressure is the result of cerebral edema from brain tumor or brain abscess, dexamethasone, 10 mg IV, should be administered.

5. *Stop seizures.* Frequent seizures must be terminated. Management of status epilepticus is discussed in Chapter 39.

6. *Search for and treat infections.* Adequate cultures of body fluids for infectious agents and treatment of infections should be performed in the febrile comatose patient. The risks and benefits of lumbar puncture in this setting are discussed in Chapter 22.

7. *Restore acid–base balance.* Arterial blood gas acid–base imbalances should be corrected. When severe metabolic acidosis from diabetic ketoacidosis is corrected with intravenous sodium bicarbonate, there is often a "paradoxical" worsening as the cerebrospinal fluid pH drops initially before rising to more normal values.

8. *Normalize body temperature.* Severe hypothermia (<34°C) and severe hyperthermia (>41°C) should be treated promptly because the brain cannot function at extremes of temperature.

9. *Give thiamine and multivitamins.* The acutely comatose patient also must be considered to be thiamine deficient until proved otherwise. Acute Wernicke–Korsakoff syndrome may produce coma, and acute niacin deficiency may cause stupor. An ampule of multivitamins should be added to the first bottle of intravenous fluids, and supplemental thiamine, 100 mg IV, should be administered.

10. *Give narcotic antagonists.* Because narcotic drug overdose is prominent in the differential diagnosis of the acutely comatose patient, narcotic antagonists should be administered when the exam suggests a metabolic/toxic encephalopathy. Naloxone, 0.4 mg IV, should be administered as a trial dose. If arousal occurs, the dose can be repeated at five-minute intervals. In narcotic addicts, acute withdrawal will be precipitated, which requires specific management.

11. *Control agitation.* The patient should be protected from harming himself. It is not safe to administer depressant drugs until the cause of the coma has been identified and treated and respiratory support assured. Small doses of haloperidol may help quiet an agitated patient who is recovering from coma.

12. *Protect the eyes.* After the eyes of a comatose patient have been carefully examined for pupillary reflexes, funduscopic findings, corneal reflexes, and vestibulo-ocular reflexes, they should be lubricated with artificial tears and taped closed with a corneal bandage to protect them from corneal ulcerations.

HISTORY

Obtaining an adequate history is particularly important for the assessment of the comatose patient. Because the patient is unable to provide information, the clinician must interview family members, friends, or co-workers who have knowledge of the illness or injury that induced the coma. Reports of the ambulance crew are also useful to delineate the course of the 30 minutes before arrival at the hospital.

The clinician needs to know if the *onset* of coma was sudden or gradual. Sudden onset suggests a cerebrovascular catastrophe, whereas gradual onset suggests a metabolic encephalopathy. The *evolution* of coma should be investigated. Progressive deepening of coma suggests a worsening metabolic encephalopathy or cerebral herniation from a structural lesion.

The possibility of preceding *head trauma* must be ascertained. In the patient who falls and strikes his head, it is critical to try to determine whether he lost consciousness first, thereby causing the fall, or if he tripped and the coma is the result of the head injury itself.

The patient's *prior illnesses* and *medications* should be ascertained. The diabetic patient may have hypoglycemia, ketoacidosis, or hyperosmolar coma. Overdoses of prescribed medications are a common cause of coma. In such cases, friends or relatives should be dispatched to count the remaining pills in the patient's medication bottles to determine how many pills may have been ingested. The presence of preexisting hepatic or renal failure is important to ascertain. Whether the patient was depressed or suicidal should always be investigated.

EXAMINATION

Examination of the comatose patient includes a careful assessment for evidence of head trauma (see Chapter 37) and major organ system trauma, examination of the optic fundi, cardiopulmonary examination, and testing for the presence of meningeal signs (see Chapter 22), and vital signs. The five critical areas of assessment of the neurological exam, which when tested can provide information as to the level and type of coma, are (1) level of consciousness; (2) respiratory rate and pattern; (3) pupillary size and reactivity; (4) vestibulo-ocular reflexes; and (5) motor function.

It is useful to consider the concept of "functional levels" of the brain in analyzing examination findings in states of stupor and coma. In cases of coma caused by progressive metabolic encephalopathy or progressive central transtentorial cerebral herniation from a supratentorial mass lesion, the patient shows a pattern of examination findings called "rostrocaudal deterioration." Here, progressive impairment of brain function proceeds as if sequential sections were made through the brain: first at diencephalic, then midbrain, pontine, and finally medullary levels. Because each functional level has characteristic examination findings, the clinician can assess the comatose patient to be functioning at "a diencephalic level" or at "a midbrain level," for example, based on the examination findings. The identification of the functional level assists our assessment of the cause and progression of the patient's coma.

Level of Consciousness

The clinician should determine whether the patient is comatose, stuporous, asleep, drowsy, or lethargic. The patient's name is called loudly into his ear. If there is no response, the physician opens the patient's eyes and repeats the name-calling. If no response ensues, the clinician asks the patient to move his eyes up and down in the vertical plane if he can hear the clinician. (This tests for the presence of the locked-in syndrome to be discussed under "Differential Diagnosis.") If still there is no response, the physician applies noxious stimuli to the patient to assess reflex response. The tip of a cotton-tipped applicator can be introduced into the patient's nose to touch the nasal septum and tickle the nasal hairs. This seemingly innocuous procedure is regarded by the body as a very noxious stimulus, probably because we all have an inborn primitive reflex mechanism to protect our airway. Other acceptable noxious stimuli are the production of bone pain by applying pressure with the knuckles on the patient's sternum and the discomfort induced by ice-water caloric testing.

The patient who is drowsy or in light stupor is said to be functioning at the upper diencephalic level, whereas the deeply stuporous patient is at the lower diencephalic functional level. Patients in light coma are functioning at the upper midbrain level, while those in deep coma are at the lower midbrain, pontine, or medullary level.

Respiratory Rate and Pattern

The patient's respirations should be observed for 30 to 60 seconds to determine respiratory rate and pattern. Patients normally breathe 10 to 20 times per minute with a regular rate. At the upper diencephalic functional level, yawning and sighing occur. If the patient is awake enough to cooperate at this level, posthyperventilation apnea may be seen. The clinician asks the patient to take five deep breaths then continues with the examination while surreptitiously observing the patient. Normally, there is less than 10 seconds of apnea following five deep breaths. In the upper diencephalic level of function (most often seen in early metabolic encephalopathy), posthyperventilation apnea can be shown to be present because a 10 to 30 second apneic phase follows the five deep breaths.

Cheyne–Stokes respiration (CSR) is a periodic type of breathing seen in patients at the lower diencephalic level. The amplitude of breathing in CSR follows a sinusoidal curve, with periods of progressively deep breathing that reach a crescendo at hyperpnea alternating with periods of progressively shallower breathing that reach a decrescendo at apnea. The apnea periods usually last 5 to 30 seconds. CSR is often seen in early metabolic encephalopathy, particularly during sleep.

Central neurogenic hyperventilation is a regular form of rapid, deep breathing associated with lesions of the rostral brain stem tegmentum (midbrain functional level). Because this form of breathing combines tachypnea and hyperpnea, the patient develops severe respiratory alkalosis. The arterial blood gas findings permit differentiation of the two major causes of hyperventilation in comatose patients: central neurogenic hyperventilation and compensatory hyperventilation in states of metabolic acidosis. Blood gases in the former type disclose a pure respiratory alkalosis (eg, pH = 7.70; pCO_2 = 20), whereas blood gases in the latter type disclose a partially compensated metabolic acidosis (eg, pH = 7.25; pCO_2 = 20).

Apneustic breathing is characterized by a prolonged pause during inspiration and is sometimes seen in pontine lesions. Ataxic breathing is an irregular, inadequate, agonal form of breathing seen in advanced medullary failure.

Pupillary Size and Reactivity

As described in Chapter 1, pupillary size and reactivity depends upon age, ambient light, and the integrity of the sympathetic pupillodilating fibers and parasympathetic pupilloconstricting fibers. Pupils should be tested in dim light for size and with a bright flashlight for reactivity.

In the diencephalic functional level (eg, early metabolic encephalopathy), pupils are small (2.0 to 3.0 mm) and reactive to light. At the midbrain level, the pupil dilates and becomes light unreactive because the Edinger–Westphal midbrain parasympathetic oculomotor nucleus has been damaged. At midbrain, pontine, or medullary functional levels, after the central sympathetics are also damaged, the pupil returns to midposition and remains unreactive to light.

In pure lesions of the pontine tegmentum, such as pontine infarcts or hemorrhages, the pupils are "pinpoint" (less than 1.0 mm) and reactive. To appreciate light reactivity in such cases requires a magnifying glass or an ophthalmoscope turned to +10 diopters. Pinpoint pupils are caused by sympathetic denervation and concomitant parasympathetic stimulation, presumably an irritative effect of the pontine lesion on the adjacent midbrain Edinger–Westphal nucleus. Pinpoint pupils are seen only in lesions of the pons in which the midbrain is intact. In patients who herniate down to the pontine level, the pupils are midposition and unreactive.

Vestibulo-Ocular Reflex

The vestibulo ocular reflex (VOR) is a brain stem reflex yoking eye movements to the vestibular system, thus allowing the eyes to make rapid compensatory conjugate movements for sudden changes in head position. Cranial nerve VIII is the afferent limb; cranial nerves III and VI and the median longitudinal fasciculus (MLF) connecting them are the efferent limb. Stimulation of one vestibular system reflexively drives the eyes to the contralateral side. The reflex is clinically useful for evaluating the comatose patient because specific brain lesions produce specific abnormalities of the reflex (see Table 36-1).

The VOR is tested clinically by two procedures: oculocephalic (doll's eyes) maneuver and by caloric stimulation. In the oculocephalic maneuver, the patient's head is rotated suddenly to the right or left. In the normal person, this movement

TABLE 36-1 VESTIBULO-OCULAR REFLEX TESTING IN COMATOSE PATIENTS

Test	Normal	Diencephalic Level	Midbrain Pontine Level	Medullary Level
Oculocephalic reflexes ("doll's eyes")	Normally inhibited	Disinhibited; full	Eye abduction only	No eye movement (absent)
Ice-water caloric testing	Sustained nystagmus	Conjugate tonic deviation	Tonic eye abduction only	No eye movement (absent)

elicits a brief conjugate movement of the eyes in the direction opposite to the head movement. The cortical gaze centers then "check" the brain stem reflex movement by directing the eyes in the direction of head movement.

In the patient with a diencephalic level of function (eg, early metabolic coma), the cortical gaze center is not functioning, so the VOR is not "checked." As the clinician rotates the patient's head, there are wide, uninhibited conjugate eye movements in the direction opposite to head movement. This has been called "disinhibited" or "hyperactive" doll's eyes. In the patient at a medullary level with a damaged brain stem, the reflex is lost, so the eyes turn with the head without reflex movement. Occasionally, with midbrain or pontine lesions, the MLFs are damaged but cranial nerve VI is intact. In such a case, only the lateral rectus muscles contract on reflex movement, and only abduction eye movements result.

Caloric stimulation permits a stronger and more enduring vestibular stimulus. The patient is lying supine with the head 30° from the horizontal, to orient the lateral semicircular canal in the true vertical position. Water is injected by a syringe and 16- to 20-gauge catheter into the external auditory canal. Warm water sets up convection currents in the semicircular canals toward the ampulla, thereby stimulating the labyrinth and reflexly driving the eyes contralaterally. Cool water sets up reverse currents, suppressing the labyrinth and allowing the unsuppressed contralateral labyrinth to drive the eyes toward the side of the cool water injection. In practice, cool or ice water is used because hot water may damage the eardrum. At least 20 mL is injected in the comatose patient.

After cool water has been injected, currents are created in the labyrinth for several minutes. In the normal person, the eyes tonically deviate to the irrigated side, but the cortical gaze centers "check" the tonic deviation with a quick, saccadic movement in the opposite direction. Sustained horizontal nystagmus is thus created, with the tonic reflex movement contributing the slow component and the cortical saccadic response contributing the fast component. It is sustained until the evoked labyrinthine currents cease.

Caloric testing in the patient at a diencephalic level produces tonic deviation of the eyes toward the cold without nystagmus. In the midbrain-pontine level, only abduction eye movements are elicited because of involvement of the MLF. At the medullary functional level, no eye movements can be evoked.

Motor Function

The motor responses to verbal and noxious stimuli are observed. Patients functioning at an upper diencephalic level frequently show diffusely increased tone (paratonia) and have positive forced grasp reflexes. At a lower diencephalic level, the patient rests quietly unless stimulated in a noxious manner at which time "posturing" of limbs occurs.

Posturing at this level has been termed "decorticate rigidity." It consists of extension at all lower-extremity joints but flexion of all upper-extremity joints. In patients with lesions of the midbrain and pons, noxious stimulation frequently produces "decerebrate rigidity," a kind of posturing with total leg extension and extension of the arms at the elbows but flexion at the wrists and fingers. Patients at a medullary level merely show quadriflaccidity without posturing when stimulated noxiously.

LABORATORY INVESTIGATION

The acutely comatose patient needs urgent evaluation of complete blood count, coagulation status, electrolytes, calcium, renal and hepatic function, arterial blood gases, electrocardiogram, and chest x-ray. Serum and urine should be submitted for toxicology screening tests. If structural disease remains part of the differential diagnosis following history, examination, and blood tests, an emergency computed tomography (CT) brain scan is desirable. Cerebrospinal fluid may be examined to exclude bacterial meninigits if a CT scan excludes a brain mass lesion or, in the absence of CT availability, only if the patient is febrile or has meningeal signs and the neurological exam is nonlateralizing. In patients with lateralizing findings, particularly those of incipient cerebral herniation, lumbar puncture is contraindicated unless a CT scan shows no ventricular displacement. Evoked potential and EEG studies are of value in coma differential diagnosis but are not usually available on an emergency basis.

DIFFERENTIAL DIAGNOSIS

The differential diagnosis of states producing coma is listed in Table 36-2. The first four categories are discussed in detail later.

Psychogenic pseudocoma is seen occasionally; the patient feigns unconsciousness but is actually conscious. He or she lies motionless, except for regular breathing, with eyes closed. The pupils are normal in size and reactivity to light. Limbs may be flaccid or have "increased" tone. Ice-water caloric testing is diagnostic, producing brisk nystagmus with nausea and vomiting, the expected response with normal consciousness. The seemingly unconscious patient often sits up and attempts to terminate the test. The EEG shows normal patterns of wakefulness. If the examiner lifts the hand of the patient and lets it fall toward the face, there will often be enough voluntary guarding movement to prevent the hand from striking the face. In cases in which it is uncertain whether the patient's stupor is organic or functional, the intravenous injection of sodium amobarbital (Amytal interview) may permit the experienced clinician to distinguish etiologies; the organic patient only becomes more encephalopathic, but the functional patient may improve or remain stable.

TABLE 36-2 STATES THAT PRODUCE COMA OR APPARENT COMA

PATHOPHYSIOLOGIC MECHANISM	COMMON EXAMPLE
Supratentorial mass lesion	Hemisphere tumor
Subtentorial mass lesion	Cerebellar hemorrhage
Brain stem destructive lesion	Pontine infarction
Metabolic/toxic encephalopathy	Barbiturate overdose
Psychogenic pseudocoma	Conversion reaction
De-efferentation pseudocoma	Locked-in syndrome

The most important form of pseudocoma to identify is the *locked-in syndrome*. In this disturbance, a large, usually vascular lesion in the base and tegmentum of the pons produces supranuclear de-efferentation of all movements, except vertical eye movements, but spares consciousness. Voluntary vertical eye movements are preserved because their neural circuits are entirely rostral to the pontine lesion. Consciousness remains because the lesion spares the ARAS. The patient has quadriplegia, bulbar and facial palsy, no horizontal eye movements (either voluntarily or to VOR caloric testing), pinpoint pupils, and muteness. On cursory examination, the patient appears comatose because reflex eye movements and limb movements are absent and the patient is unresponsive. Such a patient may be identified by asking: "Move your eyes up and down if you can hear me." This is the patient's only preserved voluntary movement and can serve as a basis for communication; ie, move eyes up for "yes" and down for "no." The EEG is normal, as expected, for such a normally conscious but profoundly paralyzed patient.

SUPRATENTORIAL MASS LESIONS

Mass lesions of the brain produce coma because their locally increased intracranial pressure produces shifts of intracranial contents (herniation) resulting in pressure-induced ischemia of the brain stem ARAS. Cerebral herniation tends to occur only in states of focally increased intracranial pressure with ventricular shifts. In pseudotumor cerebri, despite the high intracranial pressures, herniation does not occur because the pressure is generalized and there is no ventricular shift.

Two types of herniation are commonly seen from supratentorial mass lesions: central transtentorial and uncal transtentorial herniation. In both types, structures normally rostral to the tentorium cerebelli (the tough connective tissue sheath between the cerebellum and hemispheres) are pushed through the tentorial incisura into the posterior fossa. This shift compresses the brain stem, producing signs of herniation that include coma as the ARAS is first made ischemic, then infarcted. In the central pattern of transtentorial herniation, the diencephalon is gradually pushed into the posterior fossa. This pattern occurs in patients with slowly enlarging neoplasms, particularly those near the midline. In the uncal pattern of herniation, the uncus of the temporal lobe is pushed into the tentorial incisura, compressing the ipsilateral cranial nerve III and posterior cerebral artery and displacing and compressing the midbrain. Uncal herniation is seen in laterally lying supratentorial mass lesions and in acutely expanding supratentorial lesions of any location. The usual acute herniation syndrome is uncal herniation.

Patients with herniation from supratentorial mass lesions have hemiplegia from their primary lesion and, initially, stupor without brain stem signs. With progressive herniation, they show a rostrocaudal pattern of deterioration of function, as if serial sections were being made first through the diencephalon, then the midbrain, the pons, and finally the medulla. The major difference between central and uncal herniation schemes is the early involvement of ipsilateral cranial nerve III in uncal herniation, with unreactive mydriasis often occurring while the patient remains partially conscious. The findings at each stage of central and uncal transtentorial herniation are listed in Table 36-3.

TABLE 36-3 PATTERNS OF TRANSTENTORIAL HERNIATION FROM SUPRATENTORIAL MASS LESIONS

FUNCTIONAL LEVEL	CONSCIOUSNESS	RESPIRATION	PUPILS	VESTIBULO-OCULAR REFLEX	MOTOR
Central Herniation					
High diencephalic	Light stupor	Eupnea with yawns & sighs	Small and reactive	Depression of checking component	Paratonia; grasp reflexes
Low diencephalic	Deep stupor	Cheyne–Stokes respiration (CSR)	Small and reactive	Loss of checking component	Decorticate posturing
Midbrain	Coma	Central neurogenic hyperventilation (CNH)	Midposition fixed (MPF)	Loss of medial rectus function	Decerebrate posturing
Upper pons	Coma	CNH	MPF	Loss of medial rectus function	Decerebrate posturing
Lower pons	Coma	Ataxic	MPF	Absent	Flaccid
Medulla	Coma	Apnea	MPF	Absent	Flaccid
Uncal Herniation					
Early nerve III	Unreliable	Normal	Ipsilateral dilated	Normal	Contralateral hemiparesis
Late nerve III	Coma	CSR or CNH	Ipsilateral dilated and contra-lateral MPF	Medial rectus dysfunction	Ipsilateral hemiparesis and contralateral decerebrate posturing
Midbrain/upper pons	Coma	CNH or ataxic	MPF	Absent	Bilateral decerebrate posturing

SUBTENTORIAL LESIONS

Posterior fossa lesions can produce coma by direct destruction of the brain stem ARAS or by its direct compression. Lesions that destroy the ARAS include pontine and midbrain hemorrhage, infarction, and neoplasms. Lesions that directly compress the ARAS include cerebellar hemorrhage, infarction, and neoplasms. Expanding posterior fossa masses produce different patterns of herniation than do expanding supratentorial masses. Subtentorial masses can create upward transtentorial herniation in which the midbrain is pushed rostrally through the tentorial incisura. Equally common is downward herniation of the cerebellar tonsils through the foramen magnum, which acutely compresses the medulla and produces sudden respiratory arrest.

Clinically, lesions that acutely destroy the ARAS induce an abrupt loss of consciousness. In the usual case of a pontine stroke, the pupils are pinpoint and reactive. Severe bilateral pyramidal involvement is revealed by quadriplegia. All reflex horizontal eye movements are usually lost. Focal cranial nerve dysfunction, such as facial diplegia, belies the pontine location of the lesion.

In lesions that compress the ARAS, focal signs of cerebellar or brain stem dysfunction usually precede loss of consciousness. In the usual instance of massive cerebellar hemorrhage, the patient suffers a sudden onset of headache, vomiting, vertigo, and dysarthria. Ipsilateral gaze paresis, facial paresis, and ataxia are often present, then from minutes to hours later, the patient slips into irreversible coma and dies.

METABOLIC DISTURBANCES

The major differential diagnosis in the comatose patient is between structural and metabolic causes. Metabolic causes account for about two-thirds of coma cases seen in the emergency room. Table 36-4 lists the extensive differential diagnosis of the etiologies of metabolic coma.

The examination of the patient in metabolic coma reveals findings useful for diagnosis. There is often a gradual onset of loss of consciousness preceded by a confusional state. Early there are disturbances of attention and vigilance; later, orientation, cognition, and memory are impaired; finally, drowsiness and stupor are produced.

Respirations in the patient with metabolic coma may be increased or decreased. Cheyne–Stokes respirations are common. Table 36-5 lists the differential diagnosis of states of hypoventilation and hyperventilation in metabolic coma by findings on arterial blood gases.

Pupillary reflexes to light are the most important single test for differentiating metabolic from structural coma because pupillary reflexes are preserved until very late in the course of metabolic coma. By the time deep coma has ensued in the patient with a supratentorial or subtentorial mass lesion, the pupils are midposition and fixed to light. The patient with a metabolic disorder may be in a deep coma but has small pupils that have retained their reactivity to light.

TABLE 36-4 CAUSES OF METABOLIC COMA

Lack of Metabolites

Hypoxia
    Low PO_2
    Anemia
    Carbon monoxide poisoning
Ischemia, decreased cerebral blood flow
    Decreased cardiac output
        Cardiac arrhythmias
        Myocardial infarction
        Congestive heart failure
    Decreased peripheral resistance
        Syncope (see Chapter 7)
        Hypovolemia
    Increased peripheral resistance
        Hyperviscosity
        Hypertensive encephalopathy
    Multiple small-vessel occlusions
        Disseminated intravascular coagulation
        Thrombotic thrombocytopenic purpura
        Fat embolism
Hypoglycemia
Cofactor Deficiency
    Thiamine
    Niacin

Organ System Dysfunction

    Portosystemic encephalopathy
    Uremic encephalopathy
    Hypercapneic encephalopathy
    Endocrine hypofunction and hyperfunction
        Pituitary
        Thyroid
        Adrenal

Exogenous Poisons and Drug Intoxications

Acid–Base and Ionic Abnormalities

    Water and sodium (hyper- and hyponatremia)
    Acidosis and alkalosis
    Magnesium, calcium, or phosphorus abnormalities

Hypothermia/Hyperthermia

Infection and Inflammation

    Meningitis
    Encephalitis
    Vasculitis
    Subarachnoid hemorrhage

Causes of Acute Delirium (see Chapter 14)

Seizures

Concussion

Degenerative CNS Diseases

Adapted from Plum F, Posner JB: *The Diagnosis of Stupor and Coma* (ed 3). Philadelphia, F.A. Davis, 1980, pp 178-180. Used with permission.

TABLE 36-5 ARTERIAL BLOOD GASES IN METABOLIC COMA

Hyperventilation

Metabolic acidosis
  Anion gap
      diabetic ketoacidosis
      diabetic hyperosmolar coma
      uremia
      lactic acidosis
      acidic exogenous poisons
      childhood salicylate intoxication
  No anion gap
      diarrhea
      renal tubular acidosis
Respiratory alkalosis
  Gram-negative sepsis
  Portosystemic encephalopathy
  Pneumonia, pulmonary edema
Mixed metabolic acidosis and respiratory alkalosis
  Salicylate intoxication

Hypoventilation

Respiratory acidosis
  Depressant drug poisoning
  Pulmonary disease with CO_2 retention
  Neuromuscular disorders
Metabolic alkalosis
  Diuretic therapy
  Gastric HCl depletion by vomiting or drainage
  Cushing's syndrome
  Hyperaldosteronism

Adapted from Plum F, Posner JB: *The Diagnosis of Stupor and Coma* (ed 3). Philadelphia, F.A. Davis, 1980, p 186. Used with permission.

The VOR is less useful in differential diagnosis. Because metabolic disorders tend to render the hemispheric cortex dysfunctional sooner than the brain stem, the patient in early metabolic coma retains tonic, full horizontal eye movements to caloric stimulation, mimicking the lower diencephalic stage of rostrocaudal deterioration.

There are several specific motor findings in metabolic coma. Early, paratonia and forced grasp reflexes are present. With more severe involvement, tremor, asterixis, and multifocal myoclonus are seen. The tremor in metabolic encephalopathy is a coarse action tremor, worst in the outstretched hands. Asterixis (Chapter 1) frequently coexists with the tremor when the hands are outstretched. Multifocal myoclonus (Chapter 1) is particularly common in encephalopathies from CO_2 retention, uremia, and after hypoxic–ischemic hemispheric damage from cardiac arrest.

In general, metabolic encephalopathies (as opposed to structural causes of coma) are marked by examinations that lack major lateralizing findings. However, severe metabolite and electrolyte imbalances, particularly acute hyponatremia and hypoglycemia, may induce lateralizing findings, such as aphasia, hemiparesis, and gaze paresis.

BRAIN DEATH

There is now a consensus among professionals in medicine, law, philosophy, and religion that irreversible cessation of functioning of the entire brain defines death. Over three-fourths of the states in the United States have special statutory provisions to formalize the concept of "brain death." It is desirable that only physicians who have experience in determining brain death be called upon to declare death by showing permanent absence of all brain function.

The most authoritative battery of tests to determine brain death is described in the Report of the Medical Consultants on the Diagnosis of Death (1981). These tests are designed to show (1) total absence of all clinically measurable brain functions; and (2) the irreversibility of the absence of brain functions. The tests certify the presence of apnea, unresponsivity, and brain stem areflexia. They require the exclusion of depressant drug effects, hypothermia, and severe metabolic encephalopathy in addition to serial examinations over time to prove irreversibility. Confirmatory tests, including EEG, evoked potentials, cerebral arteriography, and radionuclide angiography are useful in specific instances. See Bernat (1987) for futher discussion.

PERSISTENT VEGETATIVE STATE

Many patients suffer profound, but not total, irreversible brain damage from trauma or diffuse hypoxic–ischemic insult during cardiac arrest. Such a patient recovers from the trauma or cardiac arrest with severe damage to both hemi-spheres but with a largely intact brain stem. The patient breathes spontaneously, has sleep–wake cycles, and moves his eyes fully but purposelessly, but has no behavioral response to stimuli. He requires a tracheostomy, feeding gastrostomy, and total skilled nursing care. With adequate care, the patient can continue a vegetative existence for many years, being referred to as in a "persistent vegetative state." Karen Ann Quinlan was the best known example of such a patient. The ethical and legal aspects of the care of such patients are described by Bernat (1987). It is critical that the clinician differentiate patients in persistent vegetative states from those with brain death. The former are alive, the latter are dead.

Bibliography

Bernat JL: Ethics in neurology, in Baker AB, Joynt RJ (eds): *Clinical Neurology.* Philadelphia, Harper & Row, 1987. (Contains up-to-date information on brain death and the persistent vegetative state, with discussions of ethical and legal aspects.)

Fisher CM: The neurological examination of the comatose patient. *Acta Neurol Scandinav* 1969; 45 (suppl):1-56. (An authoritative and excellent discussion supplementing the ideas of Plum and Posner.)

Levy DE, Caronna JJ, Singer, et al: Predicting outcome from hypoxic-ischemic coma. *JAMA* 1985; 253:1420-1426. (Provides tables with which clinicians may predict recovery in patients after cardiac arrest.)

Plum F, Posner JB: *The Diagnosis of Stupor and Coma* (ed 3). Philadelphia, F.A. Davis, 1980. (The single best reference available on all aspects of coma; the majority of this chapter was abstracted from it. Plum and Posner contains a wealth of clinical neurologic "pearls" in its 373 pages. It should be read and studied by all physicians who are charged with the care of comatose patients.)

Report of the Medical Consultants on the Diagnosis of Death to the President's Commission for the Study of Ethical Problems in Medicine and Biomedical and Behavioral Research. *JAMA* 1981; 246:2184-2186. (Prevents the most widely accepted battery of bedside test to determine brain death.)

Ropper AH: Lateral displacement of the brain and level of consciousness in patients with an acute hemispheral mass. *N Engl J Med* 1986; 314:953-958. (Points out that solely lateral shifts of the brain stem may produce coma in the absence of transtentorial herniation.)

Sigsbee B, Plum F: The unresponsive patient: Early diagnosis and management. *Med Clin North Am* 1979; 63:813-834. (A brief review of the concepts put forward in Plum and Posner.)

Weber LE: Medical and surgical coma in the emergency room. *Semin Neurol* 1983; 3:33-45. (Contains practical tips on emergency management.)

37

Intracranial Hemorrhage

This chapter will consider the common kinds of intracranial hemorrhage including subarachnoid hemorrhage (SAH) from ruptured aneurysm or arteriovenous malformation (AVM) and intracerebral hemorrhages associated with hypertension, anticoagulation, and senescence. The diagnosis and management of ischemic cerebrovascular disease is discussed in Chapter 20.

SUBARACHNOID HEMORRHAGE
Aneurysm

CLINICAL SIGNIFICANCE AND ETIOLOGY

An aneurysm is a pathological outpouching of an arterial wall. Most intracranial aneurysms are the result of congenital defects in the media of the vessel wall, compounded by hemodynamic damage to the internal elastic lamina. Infectious (mycotic) and traumatic aneurysms also occur in fewer than 5% of all aneurysm patients. An increased incidence of intracranial aneurysms is associated with polycystic kidney disease, Ehlers–Danlos syndrome, and coarctation of the aorta.

Approximately 95% of aneurysms occur close to the circle of Willis. They point in the direction that the proximal stream of blood flow would normally take. Aneurysms are multiple in 15% to 22% of patients; 47% of multiple aneurysms occur on the opposite side, 21% on the same side, and 29% at the midline and one side. Multiple aneurysms are more common in females (74%). In 87% of multiple aneurysms, the largest aneurysm is the one that ruptures first.

The incidence of SAH varies from 6 to 9 per 100,000 persons; 77% of these cases are aneurysmal. Ninety percent of aneurysms are asymptomatic until rupture. It is estimated that approximately 2% of the entire population may be harboring an intracranial aneurysm. The likelihood of rupture varies directly with the aneurysm's size. Aneurysms under 3 mm do not usually rupture; those of 7 mm may produce signs of mass effect without rupture.

Aneurysm can manifest as several clinical syndromes. The most common presentation is that of rupture into the subarachnoid space with SAH. Aneurysms may also produce transient ischemic attacks (TIA) or ischemic stroke as a result of partial thromboembolism of the aneurysm wall. Aneurysms greater than 7 mm can produce symptoms by compressing adjacent neural structures. A common presentation is ipsilateral third cranial nerve palsy (with ptosis, mydriasis, or diplopia) caused by compression of the third cranial nerve by an expanding intracranial aneurysm involving the posterior communicating artery. A giant aneurysm (greater than 2.5 cm in diameter) may occur at any location and produce symptoms due to mass effect.

Several conditions predispose to rupture of aneurysms. Physical activity and exertion are associated with rupture, although one-third of aneurysms rupture during sleep. Smoking and alcohol intoxication have been linked to increased incidence of rupture.

SYMPTOMS AND SIGNS

The neurological syndrome produced by SAH consists of severe headache, nausea, vomiting, photophobia, and nuchal rigidity. Headache may only occur in one-third to one-half of patients at first. It is usually abrupt in onset and is frequently described as the worst of the patient's life. Nausea and vomiting occur in half of patients; nuchal rigidity is evident in two thirds. Depression of consciousness is common, and coma may develop if the SAH extends to the ventricular system. The patient may also complain of back and leg pain as blood accumulates in the spinal subarachnoid space. Approximately 10% to 15% of patients with SAH have a seizure at the onset of the hemorrhage. Seizures are often tonic–clonic, although they may be focal. They tend not to recur.

Table 37-1 lists the clinical classification of SAH, which can be used in part for prognosis and also for the timing of surgery. Findings on examination depend in part on the location of the ruptured aneurysm. Nuchal rigidity (with positive Kernig's or Brudzinski's sign) is present in the vast majority of patients. Subhyaloid hemorrhage and/or papilledema may be evident on funduscopic examination. Focal deficits may result from parenchymal extension of the hemorrhage, or they may be due to a postictal state. Third-nerve palsy is likely the result of a posterior communicating artery aneurysm, but may be due to uncal herniation from a large temporal lobe hematoma or subdural hematoma. A unilateral visual field deficit can result from an aneurysm at the internal carotid artery-ophthalmic artery junction; a chiasmal syndrome (bilateral visual impair-

TABLE 37-1 CLINICAL CLASSIFICATION OF SUBARACHNOID HEMORRHAGE

GRADE	
1	Asymptomatic or with slight headache and nuchal rigidity
2	Moderate to severe headache; nuchal rigidity; no neurological deficits other than cranial nerve palsy
3	Confusion or drowsiness; mild neurological deficit
4	Stupor with major neurological deficit
5	Deep coma (moribund); decerebrate posturing

ment), from an anterior communicating artery aneurysm. Middle cerebral artery aneurysms may rupture into the brain parenchyma, producing motor, sensory, or speech disturbances.

LABORATORY TESTS

Computed tomography (CT) is the first diagnostic procedure of choice. It should be performed both without and with infusion of an intravenous contrast agent. In a large majority of cases, SAH is evident; the addition of contrast may demonstrate the aneurysm. A CT scan is positive in approximately 90% of cases within the first 24 hours after hemorrhage, and in 50% by the end of the first week. As with other intracranial hemorrhages, anemia may cause the hemorrhage to appear isodense rather than hyperdense.

The site of the aneurysm can sometimes be determined by the anatomic distribution of the intracranial hemorrhage. Anterior communicating artery aneurysms often rupture into the hemispheric fissure, septum pellucidum, and adjacent frontal lobe. A middle cerebral artery aneurysm may rupture into the adjacent temporal and parietal lobes and into the sylvian fissure. Rupture of an internal carotid artery aneurysm may produce a hematoma in the area of the basal ganglia and the frontal and medial temporal lobes. A basilar artery aneurysm may rupture into the interpeduncular cistern and brain stem. In general, posterior fossa aneurysms do not frequently bleed into the supratentorial subarachnoid spaces or the lateral ventricles.

If SAH is clinically evident and CT is negative, CSF analysis is necessary to look for signs of subarachnoid bleeding. When CT is available, it is usually unnecessary to perform a lumbar puncture first. When CT is not available, a skull x-ray should be taken; when clinical evidence of a posterior fossa hemorrhage (primarily cerebellar) is not found and the pineal gland is midline, a lumbar puncture can be performed. If SAH is strongly suspected, however, it is preferable to transfer the patient to a medical center where CT and neurosurgical services are available instead of performing lumbar puncture.

Laboratory tests, including CBC, electrolytes, blood chemistry profile, BUN, glucose, and coagulation studies, should be performed. Transfemoral angiography should be performed in all patients with SAH. Because aneurysms may be multiple, four-vessel angiography is mandatory. It is positive in 90% to 95% of patients with aneurysmal SAH. If negative, it should be repeated in four to six weeks, depending on the clinical condition of the patient. Many neurosurgeons advocate early angiography, although the conservative approach is to wait 10 to 14 days, at which time most patients are candidates for surgery. Recent evidence shows that early surgery may be preferred in some patients, making early angiography necessary too.

MANAGEMENT

Subarachnoid hemorrhage from any cause is a medical emergency. Approximately 10% of patients die at the time of the hemorrhage. One-third to one-half die or become ill subsequently from complications or from surgical intervention.

The patient should be placed in an intensive care unit, with frequent monitoring of neurological and vital signs. Absolute bed rest is essential. The room should have dim lighting to reduce photophobia. The number of visitors should be limited. Blood pressure should be controlled in the range of 140/90 mm Hg, preferably with sodium nitroprusside. Fluids should be restricted to 1,200 to 1,500 mL/day. If an initial seizure has occurred anticonvulsant drugs are indicated. Although phenytoin (Dilantin) is effective, phenobarbital is used more often because it has the dual effect of reducing the number of additional seizures and of producing sedation. A stool softener should be given to minimize straining with bowel movements.

Vasospasm, a serious complication of SAH, occurs in approximately 40% of patients—most often between days 4 and 17, with a peak incidence at days 6 and 7, and rarely occurring before the third day after the SAH. Vasospasm is the leading cause of morbidity following aneurysmal SAH; it is second only to the initial bleed as the cause of death. Spasm occurs in more than 80% of patients and produces ischemic symptoms in roughly one-third of them. The nature of symptoms depends on the arterial distribution involved, but are those of ischemia of the involved hemisphere or brain area.

No therapy can prevent vasospasm. Many drug regimens have been tried, including isoproterenol and lidocaine, kanamycin and reserpine; methylprednisolone and ibuprofen; aminophylline, and sodium nitroprusside. Recently, however, the investigational calcium-channel blocker nimodopine has been reported to significantly reduce the incidence of symptomatic vasospasm. This drug will likely be approved for clinical use in the near future, and will probably be used in the initial treatment of all patients with aneurysmal SAH.

Positive fluid balance may improve the rheological characteristics of blood. Hypervolemic hypertensive therapy has also been used to attempt to overcome vasospasm. The main danger of this kind of treatment is rerupture of the aneurysm. In an attempt to reduce brain edema, most neurosurgeons limit the total daily fluid intake.

Rebleeding of the aneurysm is the most important complication and is a major cause of death and disability. The incidence of rebleeding peaks during the first 24 to 48 hours after hemorrhage. The cumulative rate during the first two weeks after the initial SAH is approximately 20%. Any procedure that will decrease the transmural pressure on the aneurysm wall will decrease the likelihood of rebleeding. Therapy, with the antifibrinolytic drug epsilon aminocaproic acid (EACA) directed at preventing lysis of the clot in the aneurysm wall, reduces the incidence of subsequent rebleeding. It is administered intravenously for 14 to 16 days in an initial dose of 48 g per day for 2 days, then reduced to 36 g per day for 14 days. At the end of 14 to 16 days, the medication is switched from the intravenous to the oral route. It is tapered over the ensuing week. Numerous complications may result from EACA, including venous and arterial thromboses and necrotizing myopathy. Evidence suggests, however, that EACA, or similar drugs, diminish the rebleeding rate.

Brain edema may develop in the patient with a large SAH. This complication can be treated by fluid restriction, although some neurosurgeons advocate dexamethasone, 12 to 24 mg daily in four divided doses. However the combination of fluid restriction and steroid drugs may produce a hyperosmolar state. Hydrocephalus occurs shortly after SAH in 10% to 15% of patients. It is usually noncommunicating, although a ventricular clot may obstruct CSF outflow. The use of EACA has been associated with a rise in the incidence of hydrocephalus.

The hydrocephalus may be asymptomatic initially, but gradual depression of the patient's level of consciousness and cognitive functions may occur with time.

Five percent to 10% of patients with post-SAH hydrocephalus will ultimately require a subarachnoid shunt. The syndrome of inappropriate secretion of antidiuretic hormone (SIADH) may complicate SAH resulting from hypothalamic dysfunction. Careful monitoring of fluid intake and serum electrolyte levels is necessary. If hypo-osmolarity develops, cerebral edema will occur and may worsen the neurological deficit.

Surgical clipping of the aneurysm is the definitive procedure for most patients. Larger aneurysms occasionally must be bypassed and, depending on their size and location, coated with a gluelike substance that reduces the risk of further hemorrhage. To avoid the period of vasospasm, it is customary to delay surgery for at least ten days to two weeks following the SAH. Although surgical management of the patient with aneurysmal SAH has progressed greatly over the past 30 years, the overall morbidity or mortality has not dropped significantly. Under the common practice of delaying surgery, fewer than 40% of patients have a favorable outcome.

Recently, there has been a resurgence in performing early surgery. In some series a favorable outcome has been reported in 70% of patients. Recent reports have shown that surgery in patients older than 60 years can be performed with the same surgical morbidity as in younger patients, and that acceptable surgical results can be achieved in grade 1 patients. Advantages of early surgery are a reduction of rebleeding and avoidance of vasospasm, as it allows the neurosurgeon to open the cisterns of the brain and to irrigate and remove blood clots that are surrounding major arteries. Furthermore, if the aneurysm has been clipped and spasm then develops, hypertensive and hypervolemic therapy can be used without the risk of rupture. When there is a coexistent intracerebral or subdural hemorrhage, early evacuation of the clot and clipping of the aneurysm may be lifesaving, even though morbidity and mortality are greater in this group.

WHEN TO CONSULT

Neurological or neurosurgical consultation should be obtained immediately in all cases of suspected intracranial hemorrhage or SAH.

Arteriovenous Malformations

CLINICAL SIGNIFICANCE

Arteriovenous malformations (AVM) are congenital malformations of blood vessels in which one or more communications between otherwise normal arterial and venous channels are preserved. These congenital lesions develop between the fourth and eighth weeks of embryonic life. Seventy percent to 90% are supratentorial, usually involving the cerebral hemisphere in the middle cerebral artery distribution. AVM occurs approximately one seventh as often as do intracranial aneurysms (approximately 0.14/100,000 persons). Most lesions become symptomatic by age 40.

Symptoms and Signs

In adults, the first symptom of AVM is usually a seizure or hemorrhage. Each occurs with equal frequency: hemorrhage ranges from 42% to 64%; seizures, from 28% to 67%. The average age for the onset of seizures is 25 years; for hemorrhage, 30 years. Patients with large AVMs are twice as likely to present with seizures, while patients with smaller lesions are more likely to present with SAH. Headache is usually present before hemorrhage or seizures in one-third of patients. AVMs can also mimic tumors or multiple sclerosis. Intellectual deterioration tends to accompany large AVMs, especially in older patients. In children, the initial event is seven times more likely to be a hemorrhage than a seizure.

Seizures may be focal or generalized. In almost 20% of patients they are severe and refractory to treatment. Headache may be nonspecific, or may mimic classic migraine. The clinical course is usually slowly progressive. Mortality from the initial bleed is approximately 10%; from the second bleed, 13%; from the third, 20%. The risk of hemorrhage after the initial bleed is approximately 3.5% to 4% per year; the risk of hemorrhage in a patient who presented with seizures is approximately 1% to 2.3% per year. In one series of 35 patients with AVMs who had epilepsy alone, researchers found that over a 15-year follow-up 17% of patients died and 20% suffered disability due to the hemorrhage. Patients who had one hemorrhage had a 25% risk of a recurrence within the next year. Pregnancy was more likely to produce hemorrhage, often between the 15th and 20th weeks of gestation.

On examination, signs are similar to those of SAH caused by intracranial aneurysmal rupture. Nuchal rigidity may be prominent; focal neurological signs are more common with AVMs because of their frequent supratentorial location. Massive hemorrhage and death are unusual.

Laboratory Tests

CT can visualize the AVM and may detect multiple lesions. It does not demonstrate significant anatomic detail, and approximately 80% of scans will enhance following intravenous contrast injection. Cerbral angiography is the definitive study. Bilateral carotid and vertebral views are necessary because shunting is common between these arterial distributions. Angiography can also reveal intracranial aneurysms that coexist with AVMs in about 1% of cases. Magnetic resonance imaging may also demonstrate an AVM, especially if it is primarily of venous origin.

Management

AVMs are treated medically or surgically. Medical therapy includes the treatment of seizures and headaches, both of which usually can be controlled. Bragg peak proton beam therapy can be given for AVMs that are located deep in the brain that are surgically difficult to reach. Conventional radiation therapy of 4000 to 6000 rads delivered over four to five weeks is an alternative. It takes two years for Bragg peak therapy or for convential radiation therapy to be effective. The result is apparently a proliferation of the intima of the vascular malformation with resultant occlusion. SAH can be treated in a fashion similar to that produced by an aneurysm. Vasospasm does not occur, however, and antifibrinolytic therapy is not required.

Based on the natural history of AVMs and the risk of bleeding as opposed to the risk of surgery, the neurosurgeon must determine whether surgery is indicated. In older patients with seizures without neurological signs and hemorrhage, medical therapy offers a better outcome. Surgery itself does not always control seizures. In younger patients, the risk of morbidity and mortality with surgery is low, especially with lesions that have not bled. Deep lesions are inoperable, but there are alternatives to surgery that can reduce the risk of hemorrhage even though they do not remove the mass lesion. Embolization with pellets of various types can reduce the size of an AVM, and can also be used before surgical removal. These pellets are usually silicone spheres (0.5 to 3.0 mm in diameter) designed to occlude feeding arteries. If used before surgery, the operation is delayed for three to six weeks. Sclerosing-gluelike agents (bucrylate) are also used to occlude AVMs. This kind of interventional neuroradiological procedure is performed in only a few institutions.

WHEN TO CONSULT
In all patients with an SAH or a mass lesion that could be caused by an AVM, neurological or neurosurgical consultation is indicated for help with diagnosis and management.

HYPERTENSIVE INTRACRANIAL HEMORRHAGE

CLINICAL SIGNIFICANCE AND ETIOLOGY
Hypertensive brain hemorrhage accounts for 16% to 20% of strokes. A fatal outcome occurs in 50% of patients with large hematomas and in 21% of patients with smaller hematomas. The common pathogenesis is hypertension-induced degeneration of the media of the small penetrating arteries of the circle of Willis and/or the formation of microaneurysms from the small penetrating branches. A sudden rise in arterial blood pressure can lead to rupture of the vessel wall, producing a hematoma.

Hypertensive hemorrhage occurs within the brain and displaces adjacent tissue as the hematoma grows. Rupture or leakage into the ventricular system often occurs, and the CSF is bloody in more than 90% of cases. Hemorrhages are considered as massive if they are several centimeters in diameter, small if they are 1 to 2 cm. Hypertensive hemorrhages show a predilection for certain anatomic sites: (1) the putamen and adjacent internal capsule (basal ganglia) in 40% of cases; (2) lobar (subcortical white matter at the junction of white and grey matter), 25%; (3) thalamus, 20%; (4) cerebellum, 10%; (5) pons, 5%.

Cerebellar Hemorrhage

CLINICAL SIGNIFICANCE
The most lethal and potentially treatable hypertensive hemorrhage occurs in the cerebellum. This type of hemorrhage is often fatal because it compresses adjacent brain stem structures.

Symptoms and Signs

In most cases, the onset is sudden, with nausea, vomiting, vertigo, inability to stand or walk (ataxia), and suboccipital headache. Initial loss of consciousness is uncommon, although subsequently consciousness becomes impaired, often precipitously.

Examination often reveals evidence of limb or gait ataxia, peripheral facial nerve palsy, and paresis of conjugate gaze. These signs are usually ipsilateral to the side of the hematoma, and three-fourths of patients demonstrate two of these three signs. Ocular bobbing, dysarthria, and dysphagia may also develop. Weakness may be evident, but it must be differentiated from ataxia. In continuing hemorrhage, signs of brain stem compression may appear suddenly, followed by sudden death.

Laboratory Tests

A CT scan should be performed without delay; it often reveals hemorrhage into the lateral or midline cerebellum (vermis). Obstructive hydrocephalus is often present. Lumbar puncture should *not* be performed on the patient with a possible cerebellar hemorrhage because it can precipitate sudden cerebellar herniation and death.

Management

The sudden onset of cerebellar syndrome in the hypertensive patient should alert the physician to the possibility of a cerebellar hemorrhage. Because abrupt brain stem compression may occur without warning, expeditious diagnosis and prompt therapy improve the prognosis. Immediate evacuation of the hematoma is recommended. If the patient has an altered level of consciousness or is deteriorating, medical management is necessary with hyperventilation, intravenous mannitol and furosemide, while the patient is being prepared for surgery. Bedside ventriculostomy can be performed by the neurosurgeon to decompress the ventricles and perhaps allow the patient to survive the trip to the operating room. Overall, the higher the preoperative level of consciousness, the more favorable the prognosis. Almost all comatose patients die or have severe residual disability; thus the importance of early diagnosis is evident. Surgical intervention has low morbidity, and rehemorrhage is unusual. A satisfactory outcome is possible if surgery precedes the coma.

When to Consult

Whenever a cerebellar hemorrhage is suspected—even before CT scan—an immediate neurosurgical consultation should be obtained.

Putamenal Hemorrhage

Clinical Significance

Most hypertensive hemorrhages occur in the posterior half of the putamen (basal ganglia). The hemorrhage may remain localized to the putamen, it may expand and extend laterally and superiorly, or it may dissect medially across the internal capsule and into the ventricular system.

Symptoms and Signs

The majority of putamenal hemorrhages occur when the patient is active. Hemiparesis develops within five to 30 minutes, sometimes accompanied by hemisensory loss or aphasia if the dominant hemisphere is involved. When the nondominant hemisphere is involved, the patient may have no awareness of the deficit (cortical neglect). Approximately 60% of patients have a gradual to slow course, but an abrupt syndrome develops with symptoms maximal at onset in one-third of them. Headache is present in 70% of patients and vomiting in 40%. Papilledema and subretinal (subhyaloid) hemorrhages may be present. The eyes tend to deviate toward the side of the hemorrhage and away from the hemiparesis. Hemiparesis is associated with hyperreflexia and Babinski's sign, although the limbs may be flaccid. If the hematoma is large or is expanding, signs of upper brain stem compression appear, including a depressed level of consciousness, irregular respiration, small-to-fixed pupils, and bilateral Babinski's sign.

Laboratory Tests

A CT scan precisely localizes the hematoma and demonstrates any associated mass effect or ventricular hemorrhage. Neither angiography nor CSF analysis is necessary.

Management

The majority of putamenal hemorrhages are treated medically with dehydrating agents (mannitol, furosemide) and blood pressure control. Antifibrinolytic therapy is not necessary. Rarely, especially in the young patient with signs of an expanding mass, surgery will be necessary to evacuate the clot. Clot evacuation has been performed more with nondominant lesions, but may be lifesaving in all cases. The value of surgery has not been established in the stable patient. Prognosis appears related to the size of the hemorrhage and to the clinical course. Mortality is approximately 40%, but in patients with small hemorrhages and preserved consciousness it ranges from 13% to 20%. Sudden coma with flaccidity is almost universally fatal.

Thalamic Hemorrhage

Symptoms and Signs

Approximately 20% of hypertensive hemorrhages occur in the thalamus. Onset is sudden, with contralateral sensory loss and hemiplegia (with spread to the adjacent internal capsule). If the hemorrhage extends far enough laterally, horizontal gaze palsy develops. A variety of eye signs may manifest, depending on the site and size of the hematoma. The classical ocular picture is downward and medial deviation of the eyes, as if they were looking at the nose. Vertical gaze restrictions are common. The pupils may be unequal and unreactive to light. Ipsilateral miosis and ptosis may also be present as a consequence of involvement of descending sympathetic fibers. Fluent aphasia with literal paraphasias may be present when lesions occupy the dominant thalamus. Neglect may occur with nondominant lesions. Nuchal rigidity is common because most thalamic hematomas extend into the ventricular system.

LABORATORY TESTS
The diagnosis is made by CT, which documents the site of hemorrhage and determines the presence of subarachnoid or intraventricular blood. Cerebral spinal fluid is almost always bloody, but lumbar puncture is not necessary.

MANAGEMENT
Medical therapy with mannitol aims to reduce blood pressure and control the size of the mass lesion. Obstructive hydrocephalus can be treated with draining ventriculostomy. Usually thalamic hematomas, with or without ventral extensions, are not surgically decompressed, although Japanese surgeons are aggressive with surgical treatment of these (and putamenal) hematomas; they report a more favorable outcome with surgical treatment. Surgery might be indicated in the patient who has deteriorated in the face of appropriate medical therapy. Mortality is high for thalamic hemorrhage—greater than the 40% to 50% rate for all intracranial hemorrhages.

Pontine Hemorrhage

SYMPTOMS AND SIGNS
Approximately 10% of hypertensive intracerebral hemorrhages are located within the pons. Large pontine hemorrhages are usually marked by the sudden onset of coma, quadriplegia, decerebrate rigidity, small pinpoint pupils, hyperthermia, ocular bobbing, and ophthalmoplegia. Smaller hemorrhages, which can now be recognized by CT, may mimic small pontine infarctions. They feature preserved consciousness with evidence of contralateral motor and sensory involvement, bilateral corticospinal tract signs, and cranial nerve palsies (predominantly cranial nerves VI and VII). The "locked-in" syndrome (total paralysis except for limited eye movement) may also result from pontine hemorrhage.

LABORATORY TESTS
A CT scan is diagnostic, revealing the hematoma. The scan may demonstrate acute obstructive hydrocephalus caused by compression of the fourth ventricle by a large hematoma. Lumbar puncture is not indicated, but, if performed, usually reveals hemorrhagic CSF.

MANAGEMENT
Medical therapy includes control of blood pressure and care of respiratory function. Many patients need ventilators. Dehydrating agents (mannitol, furosemide) can be given but usually do little to change the outcome. Evacuation of pontine hemorrhage has not improved the outcome, although associated hydrocephalus can be treated with ventricular drainage. The majority of large pontine hemorrhages (greater than 1.0 cm) are fatal, but the outcome may be favorable in the patient with a partial pontine hemorrhage.

Lobar Hemorrhage

SYMPTOMS AND SIGNS

A lobar hemorrhage occurs at the junction of gray and white matter. Clinical manifestations depend on its anatomic localization. Progressive headache, nausea, vomiting, and drowsiness are common. Four clinical syndromes have been defined, based on the site of the hemorrhage: (1) *occipital,* the most common site, producing pain around the ipsilateral eye and homonymous hemianopia; (2) *temporal,* marked by pain anterior to the ear and homonymous hemianopia or quadrantanopsia; (3) *frontal,* with contralateral hemiplegia primarily of the arm, and ipsilateral frontal headache; and (4) *parietal,* producing anterior temporal headache and contralateral hemisensory deficit. A good clinical outcome is common for them all.

LABORATORY TESTS

A CT scan is the diagnostic procedure of choice. It should be performed immediately when diagnosis of intracranial hemorrhage is suspected. The site of the hemorrhage is easily identified, and subarachnoid or intraventricular blood, mass effect, or ventricular dilation are evident if present. Small hemorrhages (less than 1.5 cm) may be difficult to visualize. The need for CSF analysis is usually obviated by the CT scan, but in cases of hypertensive hemorrhage, the CSF is often bloody and under increased pressure.

DIAGNOSIS

The differential diagnosis is that of other intracranial lesions, including brain infarction, extracerebral hematoma, tumor (with bleeding), or other causes of intracranial hemorrhage (aneurysms or AVMs). A CT scan will document the hemorrhage and often will correlate well with the clinical syndrome.

MANAGEMENT

The general medical management of intracranial hemorrhage is supportive. Patients with large intracerebral hemorrhages need treatment with mannitol and furosemide, in addition to a restricted fluid intake. Hyperventilation to a PCO_2 of 25 also helps reduce intracranial hypertension. Corticosteroids are not indicated. A paradoxical effect from mannitol may be noted three or four days after therapy begins: the mannitol may "leak" into the hemorrhage, causing a paradoxical increase in size of the clot as a result of osmotic effects.

Supratentorial hemorrhages that occupy more than 12% of the supratentorial space are potentially fatal and should be removed. Hemorrhages occupying 4% to 8% of the space need evacuation only if clinical deterioration occurs. Those occupying less than 4% of space rarely need surgery.

INTRACEREBRAL HEMORRHAGE: NONHYPERTENSIVE TYPES

About one-third of all intracerebral hemorrhages and about 55% of lobar hemorrhages are nonhypertensive. Two common causes of nonhypertensive intracerebral hemorrhages are anticoagulants and cerebral amyloid angiopathy.

Anticoagulant-Induced Hemorrhage

CLINICAL SIGNIFICANCE

Approximately 8% of patients receiving oral anticoagulants (primarily warfarin) develop bleeding complications, 0.5% to 1.5% of which occur intracranially. The common intracranial sites of bleeding are the subdural spaces, the brain parenchyma, and the subarachnoid space. Hemorrhage into these areas as the result of oral anticoagulants has high mortality and morbidity. The risk of intracerebral hemorrhage is increased 8- to 11-fold by the use of anticoagulants.

ETIOLOGY

Eighty percent of patients with intracranial hemorrhage from oral anticoagulants have excessively prolonged prothrombin times at the onset of the hemorrhage. Although a prolonged prothrombin time at 1½ to 2½ times the control value is recommended by some experts, a prothrombin time in the range of 1½ times the control value offers good protective anticoagulation and few hemorrhagic complications. The duration of anticoagulant therapy or history of preceding head trauma are not associated with an increased risk of intracranial hemorrhage.

SYMPTOMS AND SIGNS

The clinical manifestations depend on the anatomic location of the hemorrhage. The course of anticoagulant-induced intracranial hemorrhage is that of gradual, slow progression over 24 to 72 hours. This slow course is present in almost 60% of patients, in contrast to the typical, more rapid course of hypertensive hemorrhage. A cerebellar location for anticoagulant-induced hemorrhage is much more common than other locations, again in contrast to hypertensive hemorrhage.

LABORATORY TESTS AND DIAGNOSIS

The prothrombin time usually is elevated to at least 2½ times the control value, although anticoagulation in the therapeutic range is also associated with an increased incidence of intracranial hemorrhage, particularly subdural hematomas in the elderly. CT demonstrates the hematoma, which may slowly enlarge in size as noted on repeated CT. The hematoma may appear isodense if the hemoglobin level is less than 10 g/dl. Lumbar puncture is usually not indicated—and is probably contraindicated because it increases the risk of spinal epidural and subdural hemorrhage. An iatrogenic etiology must be assumed in the anticoagulated patient who develops an intracranial hemorrhage.

MANAGEMENT

When the diagnosis of anticoagulant-induced hemorrhage is made, clotting abnormalities should be corrected immediately with vitamin K and fresh frozen plasma. Secondary mass effect and edema from the hematoma can be treated with dehydrating agents such as mannitol and furosemide. Hyperventilation may be necessary. Surgical evacuation of the hematoma can be performed, especially if the clot is within the cerebellum. Yet, despite the use of vitamin K, fresh frozen plasma, dehydrating agents, and surgery, mortality for anticoagulant-induced hemorrhage is approximately 65%.

Kase et al (1985) made the following observations and recommendations about anticoagulant-induced intracranial hemorrhage: (1) in the patient who is taking oral anticoagulants, the onset of a focal neurological sign (especially if slowly progressive) suggests the possibility of intracranial hemorrhage; (2) lack of systemic bleeding does not lessen the diagnostic possibility of a central nervous system hemorrhage in the patient taking warfarin; (3) the period of high risk is within the first year of anticoagulation, making close monitoring of the prothrombin time essential during this period; and (4) an excessively prolonged prothrombin time correlates best with the occurrence of intracranial hemorrhage.

Physicians should maintain the prothrombin times of anticoagulated patients at 1½ times the control value to prevent iatrogenic intracranial hemorrhages.

WHEN TO CONSULT

The patient with an acute onset of focal or generalized neurological signs, who is taking oral anticoagulants, should undergo an emergency neurosurgical or neurological consultation. A stat CT scan and a prothrombin time should be performed.

PATIENT EDUCATION

Any patient receiving oral anticoagulants should be instructed to inform the physician if he develops any neurological symptoms. Patient compliance in obtaining frequent prothrombin time measurements should be stressed, and the patient should be instructed to avoid preparations that contain aspirin.

Cerebral Amyloid Angiopathy

CLINICAL SIGNIFICANCE AND ETIOLOGY

Cerebral amyloid angiopathy, an increasingly reported disease, is marked by deposits of amyloid in the media and adventitia of small- and medium-sized arteries of the cerebral hemispheres. This amyloid deposition tends to occur in the superficial layers of the cortex and is virtually nonexistent in the deeper areas of the cortex where hypertensive hemorrhages often occur. The disease is restricted to the CNS with no systemic amyloid deposition. Cerebral amyloid angiopathy is the cause of lobar intracerebral hemorrhage (often recurrent) in the elderly. Its incidence is approximately 8% during the seventh decade of life.

SYMPTOMS AND SIGNS

The intracranial hemorrhage that results from cerebral amyloid angiopathy usually occurs in a superficial or lobar location. Many of these hemorrhages occur in the posterior cerebral hemispheres, primarily the occipital and parietal areas. Head trauma has preceded the onset of these hemorrhages in only a few patients. Otherwise the symptoms and signs are those resulting from the location of the hemorrhage (see lobar hemorrhage). These hemorrhages may be recurrent or may complicate neurosurgical procedures.

Laboratory Tests

Basic screening laboratory tests, including coagulation profiles, are normal. A CT scan detects the location of the hemorrhage. The distinguishing feature of hemorrhage due to amyloid angiopathy is its superficial location; it often communicates with the cortical surface. Pathologically, cerebral amyloid angiopathy is characterized by deposits of congo red-positive material in the media and adventitia of cortical vessels. The vascular wall may be thickened, and stenotic and pseudoaneurysms may form.

Management

Treatment does not differ from that of intracranial hematomas at other sites. If possible, surgical evacuation should be avoided because hemostasis tends to be poor, resulting in increased bleeding or recurrent hemorrhage.

When to Consult

Indications for consultation are similar to those for other intracranial hemorrhages.

Bibliography

Allen GS, Ahn HS, Preziosi TJ, et al: Cerebral arterial spasm: A controlled trial of nimodopine in patients with subarachnoid hemorrhage. *N Engl J Med* 308:619-624, 1983. (The use of calcium blockers will likely reduce the incidence of symptomatic vasospasm.)

Ausman JI, Diaz FG, Malik GM, et al: Current management of cerebral aneurysms: Is it based on facts or myths? *Surg Neurol* 24:625-635, 1985. (Discusses 18 misconceptions or "myths" surrounding treatment of aneurysmal subarachnoid hemorrhage. Current and well referenced.)

Gilbert JJ, Vinters HV: Cerebral amyloid angiopathy: Incidence and complications in the aging brain. Parts I and II. *Stroke* 14:915-923, 924-928, 1983. (Review of amyloid angiopathy, with good bibliography.)

Heros RC, Kistler JP: Intracranial arterial aneurysm: an update. *Stroke* 18:1-5, 1983. (Overview of aneurysm therapy.)

Heros RC, Tu Y-K: Is surgical therapy needed for unruptured arteriovenous malformations? *Neurology* 1987;37:279-286. (Current review of AVMs. The authors conclude that because of the high morbidity and mortality from each hemorrhage, the patient with an unruptured AVM should be considered for surgical resection.)

Kase CS, Robinson RK, Stein RW, et al: Anticoagulant-related intracerebral hemorrhage. *Neurology* 35:943-948, 1985. (Reviews 24 patients with anticoagulant induced hemorrhage. Good discussion of the problem with guidelines for treatment.)

Kassell NJ, Torner JC, Adams HP: Antifibrinolytic therapy in the acute period following aneurysmal subarachnoid hemorrhage; preliminary observations from the Cooperative Aneurysm Study. *J Neurosurg* 61:225-230, 1984. (Antifibrinolytic drugs reduced the incidence of rebleeding.)

Ott KH, Kase CS, Ojemann RG, et al: Cerebellar hemorrhage: Diagnosis and treatment. A review of 56 cases. *Arch Neurol* 31:160-167, 1974. (Reviews the Massachusetts General Hospital experience with diagnosis and treatment of cerebellar hemorrhage in the pre-CT era.)

Ropper AH, Davis KR: Lobar cerebral hemorrhage: Acute clinical syndromes in 26 cases. *Ann Neurol* 8:141-147, 1980. (Reviews the four clinical syndromes of hypertensive lobar hemorrhage.)

Silverstein A: Neurological complications of anticoagulation therapy. *Arch Intern Med* 139:217-220, 1979. (Reviews the hemorrhagic nervous system complications from anticoagulant medications.)

Stein BM, Wolpert SM: Arteriovenous malformations of the brain. I and II: Current concepts and treatment. *Arch Neurol* 37:1-5, 69-75, 1980. (Comprehensive review of all aspects of AVMs.)

Brain and Spinal Cord Trauma

HEAD TRAUMA

CLINICAL SIGNIFICANCE

Trauma is the leading cause of death in the United States for persons between the ages of 1 and 44 years. In approximately three-fourths of trauma-related deaths, head injuries contribute to the patient's demise, although approximately 20% of patients with cranial injuries also sustain severe noncerebral injuries. In San Diego County, California, the incidence of head injuries is 300/100,000 with mortality of 24/100,000. The death rate of males exceeds that of females, and 65% of fatalities occur at the scene of the accident or en route to a medical facility. Thus, of the severe injuries that lead to death only one-third are evaluated by a physician.

Because the craniocerebral trauma patient may have a lesion that is reversible with prompt diagnosis and definitive therapy, it is important for the physician who has initial contact with the patient to have a basic understanding of the different types of head trauma, and the best diagnostic and therapeutic approach to such a patient.

Most head injuries are caused by one of two mechanisms: contact or acceleration. Contact injury is from forces that occur during impact. It occurs locally or near the site of impact, or it may occur in a location remote from the impact. With local impact, linear and depressed skull fractures commonly result as well as epidural and coup type contusions beneath the site of the impact. Remote contact injuries result from mechanical distortion of the skull or from shock-wave formation. The shock wave originates at the site of impact and travels rapidly in all directions from it. Injuries caused by acceleration result in compressive and sheer strains with shift of the brain mass relative to the skull and dura, resulting in lesions such as subdural hematomas (SDH) or cerebral contusions.

Closed-head injuries are those in which there is no injury to the skull or only a linear skull fracture. Concussion is the transient impairment of neurological function from a head injury, in the absence of structural damage of the brain. The contusion is a lesion in the brain characterized by hemorrhage, necrosis, or tissue tears; it can usually be visualized by CT scan. The patient suffering from a concussion usually has briefly lost consciousness.

EMERGENCY EVALUATION AND MANAGEMENT

The evaluation of the head-injured patient requires a systematic approach that defines the problems requiring urgent diagnostic or therapeutic intervention. Thirteen percent of head injury patients arrive in the emergency ward in variable degrees of shock. The ABCs of emergency care should be followed. Thus, the first step is to assess the *airway* and to clear it of any obstructive material. If *breathing* is compromised, nasotracheal or endotracheal intubation should be performed. The neck should be kept in a neutral position because there is a possibility of coexistent spinal trauma.

Almost one-third of head injury patients who are resuscitated at the accident scene have hypoxia on arrival at the emergency ward, 15% have significant arterial hypotension, and 12% have anemia. After the airway is assessed and established, the patient's respiratory status should be evaluated. Alterations of the respiratory pattern may reflect a level of central nervous system (CNS) dysfunction. For example, bilateral hemispheric or diencephalic lesions may cause Cheyne–Stokes respiration. Central neurogenic hyperventilation may result from upper brain stem lesions, and irregular or ataxic breathing is often a result of pontine or medullary lesions (see Chapter 36). The patient may need to be oxygenated at this point to keep the pO_2 within the normal range.

Attention is then directed to the patient's *circulatory status.* Arterial hypotension is common in the head-injured patient, but shock rarely results from head injury alone. Therefore other sites of injury should be assessed for a cause of shock. Multiple peripheral IV lines should be started with Ringer's lactate or saline infusion. A pneumatic antishock garment also may be required at this time if it was not placed at the accident scene. In addition to the determination of the cause of circulatory dysfunction, the systolic blood pressure should be maintained above 100 mm Hg.

A basic and prompt general examination should follow to look for facial or scalp wounds, asymmetry of facial structures, evidence of CSF leakage (from the nose or ear), and spinal injuries. Periorbital ecchymosis (raccoon eyes) may be associated with fracture of the anterior cranial vault. Ecchymosis of the mastoid process (Battle's sign) is associated with basal skull fracture. Abduction and external rotation of the lower extremity may indicate a fracture of the hip or femoral neck, or hemiplegia or paraplegia.

Determination of the patient's level of consciousness is necessary. A wide variety of descriptive terms have been utilized, ranging from coma to obtundation, but they often have different meanings to each examiner. Various definitions and scales for the assessment of mental status have been proposed for the head-injured patient, but the most widely used scale is the Glasgow Coma Scale (GCS) (Table 38-1). It includes measurements of eye opening, motor response, and verbal response. Because comatose patients cannot obey commands, speak, or open their eyes, the GCS has incorporated these three major groups of responses.

TABLE 38-1 GLASGOW COMA SCALE

Eye Opening (E)

4—opens eyes spontaneously
3—opens eyes to voice
2—opens eyes to pain
1—no eye opening

Best Motor Response (M)

6—obeys commands
5—localizes to pain
4—withdraws to pain
3—abnormal flexor response
2—abnormal extensor response
1—no movement

Best Verbal Response (V)

5—appropriate and oriented
4—confused conversation
3—inappropriate words
2—incomprehensible sounds
1—no sounds

Scores from the three sections are added to determine severity of injury. Cutoffs are as follows:

E + M + V = <9 (comatose)
E + M + V = 9–12 (moderate head injury)
E + M + V = 13–15 (minor head injury)

Alterations of the level of consciousness in the head-injured patient may be the result of damage to the reticular activating system in the brain stem or of bilateral cerebral hemispheric dysfunction. Because metabolic abnormalities, such as hypoxia or drug intoxication, may alter the level of consciousness, depression of the level of consciousness does not itself localize the site of the lesion. For the responsive patient, tests of higher cortical function can be performed, including tests of the ability to concentrate and of recent and remote memory. Memory loss is not uncommon and may be either *retrograde* (loss of memory for events prior to the accident) or *anterograde* (loss of memory from the time of injury to the return of consciousness). Anterograde amnesia usually covers a longer period of time than retrograde amnesia.

Motor function should be assessed to determine if motor responses are present and whether they are normal or abnormal. Abnormal flexor (decorticate) posturing is characterized by both adduction of the shoulders and flexion of the elbows, with pronation of the forearm; the lower extremities may be flexed or extended. This type of posturing may be seen with severe metabolic disturbances and indicates rostral brain stem or bilateral supratentorial dysfunction.

Decerebrate posturing, the extensor response to painful stimulation, consists of extension, adduction, and hyperpronation of the arms with extension of the legs; at times opisthotonus may result. Abnormalities from the pons to the upper midbrain have been associated with decerebrate posturing. Flaccidity without a response to noxious stimuli may be the result of severe metabolic–toxic disturbances (such as alcohol or barbiturate intoxication) or of severe pontomedullary dysfunction. If there is no extremity movement, a high cervical spinal cord injury should be considered.

Abnormalities of the pupils may develop following head trauma. The pupillary pathways are resistant to metabolic dysfunction until late stages, so the presence or absence of the pupillary light reaction helps distinguish a metabolic or structural process (see Chapters 1 and 36). Bilaterally small pupils may be a result of drug intoxication or may reflect pontine injury from an intrinsic lesion or from an extra-axial hematoma compressing the brain stem. Unilateral miosis is often associated with ptosis and anhydrosis (Horner's syndrome). Involvement of the lateral medullary areas or the cervical spinal cord are frequent causes of post-traumatic Horner's syndrome, whereas a hypothalamic lesion is an uncommon cause. Unilateral mydriasis is a potentially ominous sign, often resulting from uncal herniation caused by third cranial nerve compression by a supratentorial hematoma. With continued herniation, contralateral hemiparesis invariably results. Oculomotor nerve dysfunction may also result from trauma to the third cranial nerve.

Damage occurring anywhere from the brain stem to the orbit may result in abnormalities of extraocular movements. Damage to the cortical gaze center area in the anterior frontal lobe produces deviation of the eyes toward the lesion and away from any resulting hemiparesis. With unilateral brain stem (pontine) abnormalities, the eyes deviate toward the side of the weakness and away from the site of injury. With severe head injuries, bilateral brain stem involvement is possible. The vestibulo-ocular (cold caloric testing) and/or the oculocephalic (doll's eyes) maneuvers may be utilized to assess extraocular motility as well as the integrity of the brain stem. These tests are discussed in detail in Chapter 36. In the head-injured patient, the oculocephalic response should not be performed until the status of the cervical spinal cord is known. If a cervical fracture is present, performing the oculocephalic response may either cause or exacerbate spinal cord dysfunction. Other cranial nerves should be tested for evidence of facial asymmetry, weakness, and sensory loss. Deep-tendon reflexes are assessed for their absence, exaggeration, or asymmetry, as well as for an extensor plantar response.

The Glasgow Coma Scale, introduced in 1975, incorporates tests of eye opening (**E**), motor response (**M**), and verbal response (**V**). As seen in Table 38-1 these are ranked numerically depending on the type of response. The GCS is determined by adding the best eye opening response (E) to the best motor response (M) to the best verbal response (V). Coma is defined as a score of 8 or less. A score of 9 or more precludes the diagnosis of coma.

The GCS permits determination of neurological outcome from the first few days after head trauma to six months later. In a cooperative study of head injury, a GCS score of 3 or 4 was associated with a 97% incidence of death or persistent vegetative state, whereas a score of 8 resulted in a 25% death or vegetative rate, and a 61% moderate-disability to good-recovery rate. As the GCS rises, mortality declines, so that in most patients with scores of 9 or above, mortality is low. A GCS of 3 to 8 is indicative of a severe injury (coma), 9 to 12 of moderate head injury, and 13 to 15 of mild head injury.

LABORATORY TESTS

Laboratory tests need to be individualized for each patient. Routine blood studies, including a blood chemistry profile, BUN, glucose, and blood clotting parameters

(PT, PTT, fibrinogen, fibrin split products) all should be performed in the patient with a moderate-to-severe head injury.

Skull x-rays are frequently performed in most patients with any type of head injury. Although a linear skull fracture significantly increases the likelihood of an intracranial hematoma, the actual yield of abnormalities on skull films following all types of head trauma is only 2% to 3%. With the advent of CT, there has been some reduction in the mortality of the severely head-injured patient because the rapid demonstration of potentially surgically treatable abnormalities is now possible. The CT scan has replaced angiography as the initial diagnostic procedure and it is the definitive diagnostic procedure in the acute head-injured patient. In centers where CT is not available, angiography may be necessary depending on the clinical syndrome defined. CT is superior to the skull x-ray in evaluating depressed skull fractures because it demonstrates associated mass lesions.

SKULL FRACTURES

Fractures of the skull usually result from impact injuries. They are commonly divided into linear, depressed, and basal types.

Linear Fractures

Approximately 80% of skull fractures are linear. Most *closed* linear fractures are minor and are not associated with significant morbidity. However, a fracture that traverses the middle meningeal groove should alert the physician to the possibility of an epidural hematoma (EDH). An *open* linear fracture usually needs to be carefully inspected for foreign material, but, other than debridement and closure of the wound, no treatment is usually necessary.

Depressed Fractures

If a fracture is depressed to the thickness of the skull, it is classified as depressed. A depressed fracture may be open or closed, with the open depressed fracture being most common. The depressed fracture produces more neurological deficits as a result of the depressed fragment injuring the cerebral cortex. Treatment is surgical, with elevation of the depressed fragment. There is an increased incidence of post-traumatic epilepsy if the dura is lacerated.

Basilar Fractures

Basilar skull fractures are extensions of fractures of the cranial vault. They are usually located in the petrous portion of the temporal bone, the orbit, or the basiocciput. These fractures are often difficult to diagnose by skull x-ray. Clinical symptoms and signs that suggest a basilar skull fracture include CSF atorrhea or rhinorrhea, hemotympanum, Battle's sign (ecchymosis over the mastoid), and periorbital ecchymosis (raccoon eyes). Defects in lower cranial nerves may occur, including peripheral facial nerve palsy and/or vestibulo-auditory dysfunction (especially with petrous fractures).

Otologic examination is necessary to evaluate for bleeding from the ear, hemotympanum, Battle's sign, or deafness. Bleeding from the ear is diagnostic of a basilar skull fracture, but an external laceration may also cause blood to drain into the ear. Facial paralysis occurs in 20% to 25% of patients and may be complete. Partial or delayed facial paralysis has a more favorable prognosis. Dizziness (vertigo) is of vestibular origin and often disappears within three to four weeks. Hearing impairment always occurs to some degree with temporal bone fractures.

Treatment is symptomatic. The role of antibiotics is controversial, although most neurosurgeons do not use them because the risk of developing meningitis is low. Surgery is not necessary unless there is persistent CSF rhinorrhea or otorrhea.

TRAUMATIC INTRACRANIAL HEMATOMAS

Head injury has the potential of producing a variety of hemorrhagic lesions in the substance of the brain and in the epidural or subdural spaces.

Acute Subdural Hematomas

CLINICAL SIGNIFICANCE AND ETIOLOGY

An SDH is classified as acute if it occurs within 24 to 72 hours after the injury. Approximately 10% to 15% of patients with severe head injury develop an acute SDH. The SDH results from acceleration of the brain relative to the skull, which tears the veins that traverse the space between the cortical surfaces and the dural venous sinuses. Because the impact that produces an acute SDH also commonly causes severe parenchymal injury, morbidity and mortality from acute SDH is much higher than that from extradural hematomas (EDH).

SYMPTOMS AND SIGNS

The clinical findings are related to the location and size of the hematoma, and to the rapidity of its development. The patient with a relatively minor injury may have lost consciousness only briefly at the time of the impact. As the hematoma develops and expands, consciousness may be lost. Altered levels of consciousness, anisocoria, and motor defects are the most frequently noted signs in patients with acute SDH. Most mass lesions are found ipsilateral to the site of pupillary dilation and contralateral to the hemiparesis. Occasionally, false localizing ipsilateral hemiparesis is seen caused by midbrain trauma or compression of the opposite cerebral peduncle against the tentorium (Kernohan's notch). Injury to the orbit or globe, direct third nerve injuries, or a cerebral injury on the side opposite the SDH may also cause deviation from the typical pattern described above.

An SDH located in the posterior fossa is rare, and accounts for fewer than 1% of SDHs. Disturbances of consciousness, headache, and vomiting are common signs, and lower cranial nerve palsies occur in fewer than 50% of patients. Symptoms and signs may appear immediately or after more than 24 hours.

LABORATORY TESTS AND DIAGNOSIS

Skull x-rays are usually not helpful; a linear fracture may be present, but it does not predict the site or presence of an SDH. A shift of the pineal gland is identified in fewer than 20% of patients with acute SDH. If the patient is obtunded or deteriorating rapidly, skull x-rays only delay definitive diagnosis and therapy. The preferred diagnostic test for the patient with a suspected SDH is CT; it accurately and reliably documents the hematoma and reveals whether it is intra or extra parenchymal. A high density (blood) area is evident in the subdural area, often associated with compression of the adjacent brain parenchyma and ventricles. The anemic patient (hemoglobin less than 9 mg/dL) may have a hematoma that is isodense to normal brain. If CT is not available, carotid angiography is necessary for diagnosis. There is no role for lumbar puncture, echoencephalography, or radionuclide brain scanning in the diagnosis of SDH.

MANAGEMENT

The acute SDH usually produces increased intracranial pressure. As soon as diagnosis is made or suspected (especially in the deteriorating patient) medical treatment should be started in an attempt to lower intracranial pressure. Intravenous osmotic diuretics, including mannitol and furosemide, should be administered. The patient should be hyperventilated to a pCO_2 of 25 mm Hg, and the head should be elevated. Definitive treatment is prompt surgical evacuation of the clot. In the rapidly deteriorating patient, emergency burr holes may be necessary to evacuate the hematoma and to "buy time." Half of patients with an acute SDH have increased intracranial pressure following surgery, most commonly caused by brain edema. The hematoma may redevelop, or a delayed hematoma may occur in areas of the brain with minor contusions; thus, frequent postoperative CT scans are recommended. Because one-third of patients with an acute SDH develop seizures, anticonvulsants should be given prophylactically.

The mortality of acute SDH is 35% to 50%. Many patients who survive do not return to normal and can no longer function independently. The sooner the diagnosis is made and definitive therapy carried out, the better the prognosis. In one series, patients conscious at the time of surgery had 9% mortality, whereas patients who were comatose had a 40% to 65% mortality. Patients operated upon within 170 minutes of their injury had a more favorable prognosis, but those operated on 390 minutes or more after the trauma expired.

WHEN TO CONSULT

As with any head injury it is best to obtain an immediate consultation; the neurosurgeon is the most experienced specialist for evaluating and treating the patient with an acute head injury.

Subacute and Chronic Subdural Hematomas

CLINICAL SIGNIFICANCE AND ETIOLOGY

An SDH that develops between three days and three weeks following head trauma is termed subacute; one presenting more than three weeks after injury is chronic. Chronic SDH has an incidence of 1 to 2/100,000. Most patients are more than 50 years old, and almost 50% are without a history of antecedent head trauma. Within the first week of the trauma, a small SDH will be covered by an outer membrane beneath the dura; within three weeks, an inner membrane forms between the hematoma and the arachnoid of the brain, enclosing the hematoma. The hematoma may increase in size because of recurrent hemorrhage or the diffusion of albumin across the hematoma membrane. Some chronic SDHs regress spontaneously and require no further treatment.

SYMPTOMS AND SIGNS

The symptoms and signs are variable. Many patients have impaired mental status or hemiparesis. Because chronic SDH tends to occur in the older patient, the symptoms and signs might suggest other diagnoses, including subacute dementia, transient ischemic attacks, stroke, or tumor. Thus, many chronic SDHs are not clinically suspected.

LABORATORY TESTS AND DIAGNOSIS

A CT scan of the head is the procedure of choice. A subacute hematoma remains hyperdense compared with normal brain for only the first week (if the patient is not anemic). During the second to third weeks the SDH becomes isodense compared with normal brain, and after three weeks the majority become hypodense. Because intermittent bleeding of chronic SDHs often occurs, mixed-density lesions can be seen. A bilateral isodense SDH gives rise to the appearance of a "hypernormal" brain on CT scan because of the lack of cortical atrophy and the presence of small ventricles. Magnetic resonance imaging (MRI) is valuable for diagnosing both acute and chronic SDH. Cerebral angiography was formerly the diagnostic procedure of choice but it is now rarely necessary.

MANAGEMENT

Most subacute SDHs should be treated surgically. Medical management can be used in the selected patient with the greatest anesthetic risk and the smallest hematomas. Bed rest and corticosteroids are of benefit in the patient with very minimal neurological signs.

Residual and recurrent hematomas occur in as many as half of cases following surgical evacuation of SDH. Thus, patients who do not improve or who deteriorate following surgery should have a repeat CT. Subdural empyema, meningitis, and brain abscess are uncommon complications of surgical therapy and occur in approximately 1% of patients; seizures occur in 10%. The mortality following treatment of chronic SDH is less than 10%; as many as three-fourths of patients are able to resume normal function.

Extradural Hematomas

CLINICAL SIGNIFICANCE AND ETIOLOGY

The extradural (epidural) hematoma (EDH) is a collection of blood between the inner table of the skull and the dura mater. In contrast to the SDH, an EDH occurs in less than 2% of patients with craniocerebral trauma. An EDH rarely occurs in the first two years of life and in persons over the age of 60 years. An EDH most commonly results from an injury to the middle meningeal artery. Occasionally, an EDH arises from tears in the transverse or superior saggital sinuses. The hematoma is unilateral and is associated with a temporal fracture in 90% of adult cases. An EDH of the posterior fossa is the most common traumatic hematoma confined to the posterior fossa, yet it accounts for fewer than 5% of all intracranial traumatic hematomas.

SYMPTOMS AND SIGNS

The symptoms and signs of EDH depend primarily on the rapidity of the onset of the hematoma. Approximately one-third of patients with EDH are operated on within 12 hours of injury and approximately 75% within 48 hours. A delayed presentation of two to seven days (or longer) is uncommon.

The classical story is that of a mild head injury that leads to transient loss of consciousness, followed by a return of consciousness (lucid interval), until the expanding EDH causes unconsciousness again. This triphasic presentation is seen in only 10% of patients with EDH; however, the lucid interval is *not* pathognomonic for EDH. The signs of an EDH depend on its location and rapidity of growth. Depression of the level of consciousness, ipsilateral pupillary dilation and hemiparesis (contralateral to the pupillary change) are frequently seen.

In the posterior fossa, 40% of EDHs produce symptoms within the first 24 hours. Headache and neck stiffness are usually present and ipsilateral cerebellar signs occur in less than 50% of patients. Corticospinal signs may be evident, resulting from extension of the clot into the occipital lobe, or due to coexistent supratentorial injury. A posterior fossa EDH should be considered when there is depression of the level of consciousness following occipital trauma.

LABORATORY TESTS AND MANAGEMENT

Most EDHs are associated with a skull fracture, especially fractures that cross a vascular groove. A CT scan is the procedure of choice; an acute EDH is seen on CT as a high-density biconvex area between the skull and the brain. The patient with a suspected EDH can be stabilized with IV mannitol or furosemide and hyperventilated to a pCO_2 of 25 mm Hg. Following CT, immediate evacuation of the hematoma is necessary. In the rapidly deteriorating patient with a suspected EDH (or SDH), even performing a CT is an inappropriate expenditure of time. Instead, emergency burr holes should be placed ipsilateral to the side of pupillary dilation.

Mortality from EDH is low for children (5% to 10%) but increases (35% to 50%) in persons over age 40. Delay in diagnosis and treatment is the most common cause of morbidity and mortality. Patients who are alert or only slightly lethargic at the time of surgery have low mortality, whereas those unconscious have a mortality of greater than 50%. Associated intracranial lesions also have a detrimental effect on prognosis. Mortality of posterior fossa EDH ranges from 37% to 69%.

Intracerebral Hematomas

CLINICAL SIGNIFICANCE AND ETIOLOGY

Traumatic intracerebral and intracerebellar hematomas occur in as many as 12% of patients admitted to the hospital with craniocerebral trauma. Most hematomas are located in the deep anterior frontal lobe, the anterior temporal lobe, or the occipital poles. Multiple hemorrhages occur in 20% of patients; 60% of intracerebral hematomas are associated with extracerebral hematomas. Intracerebellar hematomas are uncommon, usually resulting from a direct blow to the occipital area. A posterior fossa SDH usually coexists with a traumatic intracerebellar hematoma.

Symptoms and Signs

The injury that results in a traumatic intracerebral hematoma is usually severe. More than 50% of patients lose consciousness at the time of injury. Symptoms and signs depend on the location of the hematoma and the multiplicity of lesions; they are indistinguishable from those of EDH and SDH. Deterioration in the level of consciousness or neurological status a few days after trauma can occur, often as the result of brain swelling or an increase in the size of the hematoma.

Laboratory Tests

A CT scan is the procedure of choice. It determines the site and number of intracranial hematomas, as well as associated areas of contusion and/or edema.

Management

The treatment of traumatic intracerebral hematoma is usually nonsurgical unless the hematomas are large and produce midline shift, focal deficits, and altered levels of consciousness. Patients with severe injuries who are not considered surgical candidates should have intracranial pressure monitored; serial CT scans should be performed every two to four days following injury. Surgery is indicated if the intracranial pressure is increasing and is refractory to medical management, or if the hemorrhage is enlarging. Mortality ranges from 25% to 50%. Patients conscious at the time of surgery have less than 10% mortality, whereas those who are unconscious have at least 50% mortality.

Cerebral Contusion

Clinical Significance and Etiology

Cerebral contusions are multiple areas of traumatic hemorrhage, infarction, and/or brain necrosis. They are the most common lesions seen on CT following head injury. Contusions occur at the site of impact, whereas the "contre coup" injury (caused by acceleration effects of head trauma) is seen at sites removed from the impact, frequently in the frontal or temporal lobes.

Symptoms and Signs

Clinical manifestations vary according to the size and location of the contusion(s). The associated brain necrosis and hemorrhage, which occurs within a few days following a cerebral contusion may produce progressive neurological deterioration from raised intracranial pressure.

Laboratory Tests and Diagnosis

The diagnosis is established by CT, which documents small, multiple areas of increased density associated with areas of decreased density (edema–necrosis).

MANAGEMENT

Therapy is directed toward the reduction and prevention of increased intracranial pressure. Intravenous osmotic diuretics (furosemide and mannitol), hyperventilation to a pCO_2 of 25 mm Hg, and intracranial pressure monitoring are necessary in these patients. Mortality ranges from 25% to 60%, and outcome depends on the level of consciousness and the presence of other lesions.

Childhood Epidural and Subdural Hematomas

In children as in adults, extracerebral hematomas are more common in the supratentorial regions. Acute SDH occurs five to ten times more frequently than EDH. Approximately 25% of EDHs are of venous origin in children, as are most acute SDHs. Shaking injury with indirect trauma to the head may produce an SDH. It usually occurs in infants, whereas EDH tends to occur in children over the age of 2. EDHs are usually unilateral, whereas three-fourths of SDHs are bilateral. Seizures occur in less than 25% of children with acute EDH but occur in approximately three-fourths of children with acute SDH. EDHs are two to three times more common in the posterior fossa than are acute SDHs and occipital skull fractures. Increased intracranial pressure frequently develops, and uncal herniation may occur. EDH may cause loss of consciousness with vomiting, ataxia, and hydrocephalus. A CT scan is diagnostic.

Although 25% of children with acute EDH die, those who survive have little morbidity. In contrast, mortality is lower with acute SDH but morbidity is greater. The definitive treatment of EDH is craniotomy to remove the clot. An SDH in an infant may be treated with aspiration of the subdural space performed through the anterior fontanelle. Craniotomy is also indicated if the clot cannot be aspirated entirely, or if it reaccumulates.

Minor Closed Head Injury

By definition, the patient with a minor head injury has a GCS of 13 to 15. Of 8 million head injuries that occur annually in the United States, approximately 1.5 to 2 million of them are minor. Patients with minor head injury are slightly younger and are more often female than are those with severe injuries. At highest risk for minor head injury are students. Chronic alcohol abuse or intoxication are less commonly causitive in the patients with minor head injury than in those with major injuries. High-velocity trauma, which results from auto accidents or assaults, is a common cause of *severe* injuries; minor falls and athletic injuries account for a large percentage of *minor* injuries.

The management of the patient with a minor head injury is somewhat controversial. Many emergency room physicians order skull x-rays for the patient who has suffered from any type of head trauma, but only about 5% have a linear skull fracture. Because a skull fracture over the middle meningeal groove may lead to EDH, a skull x-ray in the patient with minor head trauma is probably indicated, although the yield of such a study is low. A CT scan is not indicated in every patient with minor head trauma; it should be reserved for the patient who is intoxicated or who has deteriorated neurologically.

All patients with minor head injury should be supervised for 24 to 48 hours. If there is adequate family and social support and the patient does not live a great distance from the hospital, supervision can be on an outpatient basis. The patient with a minor scalp injury without signs of brain injury usually can be discharged safely and followed as an outpatient. If the scalp wound is extensive or if there has been major blood loss, it is best to admit the patient.

The patient who is not fully oriented at the time of evaluation and who demonstrates defective immediate recall and recent memory should be hospitalized for 24 to 48 hours. A preschool child with minor head trauma should be admitted to the hospital even if the neurological examination is unremarkable. It is common for a child to respond unusually to minor head trauma—eg, with intermittent somnolence, agitation, nausea, vomiting, and visual disturbances (hemianopia, cortical blindness). An appreciation of the severity of the head injury may be delayed for one to two days following the trauma.

Many patients following minor head trauma complain of difficulty with concentration, memory loss, dizziness, and headache. This symptom complex, called postconcussive syndrome, may be the result of nonorganic psychological disease (see Chapter 8), but as many as 50% of such patients studied with neuropsychiatric testing have demonstrated organic cognitive defects. Post-traumatic dizziness is also frequently organic (see Chapter 6).

SPINAL CORD INJURY

CLINICAL SIGNIFICANCE AND ETIOLOGY

Spinal cord injury is a catastrophic event and a leading cause of disability of teenagers and young adults. The incidence of spinal cord trauma is 5/100,000. It is particularly common among young men: nearly two-thirds of spinal cord injuries are sustained by persons between the ages of 15 and 30 years, with males accounting for 80% of cases. Many spinal cord injuries are the result of vehicular accidents, which account for 30% to 45% of all new cases of spinal cord injury each year. Other causes include diving into shallow water, sports injuries, stabbing, gunshot wounds, and birth injuries.

The extent of spinal cord injury is related to the amount of force applied to the spinal cord at the site of impact. Forces are generated by sudden hyperextension, flexion, rotation, or vertebral compression. Vertebrae may be fractured, misaligned, or dislocated, or a bone may splinter and penetrate the spinal cord. The spinal cord can be contused, stretched, compressed, or lacerated. Direct injury to the spinal cord may be caused by stabbing or by a high-velocity missile. When there is associated spinal stenosis or cervical spondylosis, significant spinal cord dysfunction may occur following a seemingly trivial injury.

SYMPTOMS AND SIGNS

Spinal cord concussion is rare. As with brain concussion, there is transient loss of neurological function with complete recovery. The most common sites of injury are at the C5 and C6 areas during fracture–dislocation, and at the T11 and T12 areas.

There are four syndromes of spinal cord injury. The clinical manifestations depend on the region of spinal cord damaged (see Chapter 40), but the majority affect the cervical spinal cord.

Transverse myelopathy is the most severe consequence of spinal cord trauma. All neurological activity below the level of the lesion is lost. There is complete anesthesia and paralysis below the lesion, with associated hypotonia and hyporeflexia (spinal shock). The plantar responses may be absent, but within three to four weeks pyramidal signs usually appear, including spasticity, hyperreflexia, and extensor plantar responses. Mass reflexive lower extremity movements may occur. Rarely, an ostensibly severe injury to the spinal cord spontaneously resolves within 24 to 72 hours because it was a "concussion."

Anterior cord syndrome is also associated with a poor prognosis. Clinically, there is evidence of damage to the anterior two-thirds of the spinal cord. There is complete involvement of the corticospinal and spinothalamic tracts. Functions mediated by the posterior columns usually are unaffected. Thus, there is loss of all motor activity and pain and temperature sensation below the level of the lesion, with preservation of vibratory, touch, and position sensation. Reflex activity below the level of the lesion is usually absent, although Babinski's response may be seen. This syndrome may result from compression of the anterior spinal artery, which supplies the anterior two thirds of the spinal cord.

The *central cord syndrome* involves the cervical spinal cord and is characterized by weakness that is greater in the arms than in the legs. Sensory symptoms and signs are less common, but there may be a burning sensation in the hands. Deep-tendon reflexes are preserved in the lower extremities, but those in the upper extremities (at the level of the lesion) may be absent. Urinary retention may develop. The central spinal cord syndrome is usually associated with x-ray evidence of cervical spondylosis or spinal stenosis. The prognosis is good.

The *Brown–Séquard syndrome* results from damage confined to half of the spinal cord. It is not often seen following blunt trauma, but stab wounds are a common cause. Seen on examination are loss of contralateral pain and temperature sensation below the lesion, with loss of ipsilateral vibratory and position sensation associated with ipsilateral paresis below the lesion.

Injuries of the conus medullaris occur with fracture of the T12-L1 junction, and cauda equina injuries may result from lumbar injuries. These lesions are associated with a combination of upper and lower motor neuron signs, the former caused by conus involvement, the latter by involvement of the cauda equina. Damage confined to the cauda equina produces a flaccid areflexive paralysis with sensory loss that corresponds to the involved spinal roots and bladder and bowel disturbances. If the conus medullaris is also damaged, there is urinary and/or fecal incontinence, erectile dysfunction in the male, and dissociated sensory loss in the saddle area. With pure conus medullaris involvement, deep-tendon reflexes are preserved, but ankle reflexes are often absent. The prognosis for patients with cauda equina lesions is quite good, and for conus lesions it is intermediate.

Vertebral fractures can injure the spinal cord at all levels. The most common site of involvement is the cervical spinal cord; 80% of cases involve the odontoid process or C1–C2 area, and 20% involve the spine below the axis. Most cervical fractures are at C5; and most fracture–dislocations occur at C5-C6. Multiple spinal fractures occur in approximately 5% of cases. The patient may die acutely if the lesion is above the phrenic nerve outflow (C4). The Jefferson fracture involves C1, usually results from a blow to the head, and rarely is associated with neurological deficit. Fracture of the spine at C2 (through the pedicles), is known as hangman's fracture; it produces sudden death or no deficit. Upper cervical spinal cord syndromes are the result of flexion or hyperextension injuries. Hyperflexion injuries usually are associated with x-ray changes; hyperextension injuries usually are associated with spinal column damage *without* malalignment of the vertebrae.

LABORATORY TESTS AND MANAGEMENT

The patient suspected of having a spinal cord injury should be immobilized to prevent further injury to the spinal cord from movement of a fractured or dislocated bone. When cervical spine trauma is possible, the neck should be immobilized before the patient is moved. As with the patient with craniocerebral trauma, associated traumatic lesions outside of the spinal cord should also be considered at cardiac, pulmonary, and intra-abdominal sites. If the patient is quadriplegic or paraplegic, intra-abdominal injury may be difficult to diagnose; unexplained hypotension may be the only sign. If necessary, an adequate airway should be established with a nasotracheal tube or tracheostomy. The patient should be evaluated and treated for shock (if present); external bleeding should be controlled.

Neurological evaluation begins by questioning the patient about spine or neck pain. The level of neurological function is determined by the lowest level of motor contraction or sensory preservation. Deep-tendon reflex evaluation is not reliable during the acute phase of a spinal cord injury. Careful attention should be paid to the examination of the perineal region because sacral sensory sparing may be the only guide to an incomplete lesion for which the prognosis is more favorable. The ability of the patient to void should be tested, as well as the degree of anal sphincter tone. Quadriplegia or paraplegia should be suspected in the unconscious patient who is areflexic, has no response to pain stimulation below the level of injury, or has loss of intercostal respirations with abdominal breathing.

A plain x-ray (anterior-posterior and lateral) is the best initial diagnostic study in patients with suspected spinal cord injury. For possible cervical spine injury, a single lateral film encompassing C1 to T1 is the best initial screening test. Flexion and extension films should be avoided initially until the degree of spinal pathology has been established. Polytomography or CT will help to better delineate fractures of selected areas.

Although 15% to 20% of patients with cervical spinal cord injuries have no overt vertebral injury by x-ray examination two-thirds have spinal abnormalities visualized by CT. A CT scan should be utilized to (1) better delineate suspicious findings on plain x-ray, and (2) visualize associated fractures in patients with known fractures. The role of myelography in acute spinal cord injury is controversial, but intrathecal administration of metrizamide with CT of the involved areas can be performed. Myelography may be useful in the patient with neurological findings that are out of proportion to findings on plain x-ray examination and in the patient with a progressive deficit.

Because hypoxia is a common cause of confusion in the patient with cervical spinal cord injury, arterial blood gas determinations should be performed. Routine laboratory tests, including a CBC, blood chemistry profile, coagulation studies, EKG, and chest x-ray should be performed. Further diagnostic tests will depend upon the sites of potential non-nervous system trauma (eg, paracentesis in abdominal trauma).

Neurological deterioration in the spinal cord injured patient can be the result of ischemic injury of the cord, hypotension, or concurrent injuries. The blood pressure should be normalized with fluids or vasopressors. Hypothermia from loss of sympathetic thermoregulation can be treated with anticholinergic medications. An indwelling urinary catheter during the acute phase of spinal cord injury is usually necessary because of neurogenic bladder. Respirations should be carefully monitored because loss of intercostal functions or phrenic nerve function may result in respiratory insufficiency.

Skin care is important, so the patient should be turned from side to side every two hours. A sheepskin on the bed or an alternating pressure mattress is indicated. Adynamic ileus may develop and persist for weeks necessitating a nasogastric tube. If bowel distension occurs, a rectal tube may be necessary. A high-calorie–high-protein diet should be begun, if necessary, by hyperalimentation. Thrombophlebitis may occur in the patient who is immobilized from a spinal cord injury, so heparin, 5000 units subcutaneously every 12 hours, should be started. Elastic stockings or inflatable compression boots are not of benefit in reducing the incidence of pulmonary embolism. Pain control can be accomplished with codeine. Psychiatric consultation is usually necessary at some time during hospitalization, especially for the patient with quadriplegia or paraplegia.

A number of drugs have been used to attempt to reduce the severity of spinal cord injury. These include megadose corticosteroids, mannitol, and DMSO, but despite their use, there is no evidence to suggest that these treatments are beneficial. Hyperbaric oxygen therapy has been shown to reduce disability in some spinal cord injured patients, but it is available at only a few centers.

Naloxone and thyroid-releasing hormone (TRH), are opiate antagonists that in high doses have been shown experimentally to reduce the severity of spinal cord injuries. Phase 1 clinical trials have shown that naloxone is well tolerated and can produce clinical improvement in the spinal cord-injured patient. The effects from TRH infusions are likely to produce the same results.

The spine may be stabilized by a variety of methods, including bedrest, cervical collar, halo, or neck traction. Dislocation or fracture of the cervical spine is treated with axial traction through skull calipers (Crutchfield tongs). In cases of thoracolumbar fractures, pillows or pads are placed under the lumbar curvature to produce hyperextension of the spine.

Surgical therapy remains somewhat controversial. Compound fractures or cervical and lumbosacral lesions with bony fragments compressing the spinal cord are an indication for surgery. In general, indications for emergency surgery are few. Surgery does not help patients whose paralysis is immediate and complete, and an incomplete lesion may be made worse by early surgery.

The single most important factor determining the outcome for spinal cord injury is the initial severity of the injury. Mortality may be reduced by certain surgical procedures (by reducing the incidence of complications such as pulmonary embolism and infection), but there is little change in neurological function. Delayed deterioration may occur after a period of stabilization and can result from treatable conditions such as post-traumatic syringomyelia or persistent spinal cord compression.

Recovery of useful hand function after central cervical spinal cord injury is less likely to occur than is recovery of ambulation. Only about half of the patients with anterior cord syndrome will be able to ambulate freely.

The goal of patients with spinal cord injury is to ambulate freely and to live a normal life. This is not possible for many patients with cervical spinal cord injuries, but can be accomplished in those who have lower spine injuries. Intense physical therapy is best provided in a rehabilitation unit or performed in a spinal cord injury treatment center. Multiple mechanical assisting devices can be used. Psychological manifestations of the injury should be addressed, and vocational therapy provided in an attempt to help the patient return to gainful employment.

Bibliography

Braakman R, Schouten JA, Dishore MD, et al: Megadose steroids in severe head injury. *J Neurosurg* 1983; 58:326-330. (The use of corticosteroids does not produce any benefit, even in megadoses of dexamethasone, 100 mg/day.)

Bracken MB, Shepard MJ, Hellenbrand GG, et al: Methylprednisolone and neurological function 1 year after spinal cord injury. Results of the National Acute Spinal Cord Injury Study. *J Neurosurg* 1985; 63:704-713. (Multicenter randomized trial that shows no benefit from low, 100 mg, or high, 1000 mg, methylprednisolone on neurological recovery following spinal cord injury.)

Donovan WH, Bedbrook G: Comprehensive management of spinal cord injury. *Ciba Clinical Symposia* 1982; 34 (2):1-36. (Reviews acute care and rehabilitation of the patient with a spinal cord injury.)

Flamm ES, Young W, Collins WF, et al: A Phase 1 trial of naloxone treatment in acute spinal cord injury. *J Neurosurg* 1985; 63:390-397. (Naloxone and other opiate antagonists may be of benefit in reducing the severity of spinal cord injury.)

Friedman WA: Head injuries. *Ciba Clinical Symposia* 1983; 35:1-32. (Briefly covers most aspects of head injuries; many color drawings of the different types of head trauma from pathological and surgical perspective.)

Jennett B, Bond M: Assessment of outcome after severe brain damage: A practical scale. *Lancet* 1975; 1:480-484. (Article in which the Glasgow Coma Scale was originally described.)

Jennett B, Teasdale G: *Management of Head Injuries.* Philadelphia, F.A. Davis, 1981. (Comprehensive, readable monograph that covers all aspects of head injuries.)

Rosman NP, Herskowitz J: Trauma to the brain and sppinal cord, in Swaiman KF, Wright FS (eds): *The Practice of Pediatric Neurology.* St Louis, C.V. Mosby, vol 2, 1982, pp 958-984. (Comprehensive discussion of pediatric brain and spinal cord trauma.)

Vogel HB: Trauma of the head, spine, and peripheral nerves, in Earnest MP (ed): *Neurological Emergencies.* New York, Churchill-Livingstone, 1983, pp 177-217. (Another good overview of the management of head and spinal cord injuries.)

Wilkins RH, Rengachary SS (eds): *Neurosurgery, part VIII. Trauma.* New York, McGraw-Hill, 1985, vol 2, pp 1531-1763. (Current neurosurgery textbook with excellent and comprehensive multi-authored chapters covering all aspects of craniospinal trauma; well referenced and quite readable.)

Yarkony GM, Roth EJ, Hainemann AW, et al: Benefits of rehabilitation for traumatic spinal cord injury. *Arch Neurol* 1987;44:93-96. (Self-care skills and mobility are improved in patients with spinal cord injuries who participate in comprehensive rehabilitation programs.)

Status Epilepticus

Status epilepticus (SE) is an emergency condition in which seizures occur with sufficient frequency or duration to produce more than 30 minutes of seizure activity or loss of consciousness. There are three major types of status epilepticus. *Convulsive, or generalized major motor, status epilepticus* is a true medical emergency in which the patient has recurrent tonic–clonic (grand mal) seizures without regaining consciousness between them. *Nonconvulsive status epilepticus* is a prolonged complex partial seizure or absence seizure in which the patient appears dazed and confused (twilight state). A third type of status is *focal continuous epilepsy,* or epilepsia partialis continua (EPC), in which focal, usually clonic, activity persists unabated while consciousness is maintained. Nonconvulsive status is less of an emergency than convulsive status, whereas EPC is not an emergency at all. Both conditions are discussed further in Chapter 15. This chapter discusses the diagnosis and emergency management of generalized major motor status epilepticus.

CLINICAL SIGNIFICANCE
SE occurs with a prevalence of 4 to 7/1000. Untreated, SE lasting more than a few hours is usually fatal. Even in treated cases, current mortality is 5% to 12%. The causes of morbidity and mortality in SE are the complications of prolonged seizure discharges, prolonged muscle contractions, and inadequate ventilation. These causes include respiratory and metabolic acidosis, cardiac arrhythmias, hypoglycemia, hyperthermia, and cerebral edema. Status epilepticus is a medical emergency because the longer it persists untreated, the worse is the patient's outcome. Retrospective studies have shown that patients who have been successfully treated and have made a complete recovery had an average duration in SE of 90 minutes. Surviving patients with neurological sequelae had an average duration of 10 hours in SE. Patients who died despite treatment averaged 13 hours in SE.

ETIOLOGY

The causes of SE are listed in Table 39-1. Among patients with known seizure disorders, the discontinuation or irregularity of compliance with their prescribed anticonvulsant regimen is overwhelmingly the most likely cause. Alcohol withdrawal is also a common cause in this group. Among patients presenting in SE without a seizure history, the clinician should consider alcohol withdrawal, drug overdose, metabolic disturbance, stroke, tumor, and infection.

SYMPTOMS AND SIGNS

The usual patient in SE has tonic–clonic or generalized tonic seizure activity lasting several minutes, with 5 to 15 minute intervals between seizures during which the patient remains deeply comatose. The tonic and clonic activity is bilateral but is often more pronounced on one side. Head and eye lateral deviation during the ictal phase of the seizure (adversive seizures) usually suggests that the major seizure discharge is from the contralateral hemisphere. Focal hemispheric predominance, however, does not necessarily indicate an underlying structural lesion. Many cases of SE from metabolic or toxic disorders have focal features.

Respiratory embarrassment is a common, serious problem in SE. During the tonic phase of the seizure, there is ventilatory paralysis that leads to hypoxemia and cyanosis. During the clonic phase, respirations are ineffective and do not improve the hypoxemia. During the postictal phase, there is hypoventilation as the patient is comatose. Because the process repeats without intervening time for normal ventilation, the patient in SE becomes progressively hypoxemic.

Adults in generalized major motor SE cannot usually sustain a tonic or tonic–clonic phase lasting longer than a few minutes. The cerebral hypermetabolic state produces cerebral neuronal exhaustion, resulting in the postictal

TABLE 39-1 CAUSES OF STATUS EPILEPTICUS

Inadequate anticonvulsant therapy in the known epileptic
  Discontinuation of drug
  Irregularity of dosage; non-compliance
  Concomitant medication reducing anticonvulsant concentration
Metabolic imbalance
  Hyponatremia
  Hypocalcemia
  Hypomagnesemia (especially in alcoholics)
  Hypoglycemia
Drug overdose
Alcohol and other sedative drug withdrawal
Head trauma
Brain tumor
Cerebrovascular disease
CNS infections
  Meningitis
  Encephalitis
  Brain abscess
Cardiac arrest
Idiopathic

state of depression. Infants and young children have a greater ability to sustain continuous motor activity, often for 30 to 45 minutes. This type of status leads more quickly to acidosis and hyperthermia than does the adult type. In adults, the overt motor manifestation of the seizures tends to decrease with time, but the severity increases and the prognosis becomes worse in direct proportion to the duration of SE.

Fever is a common sign of SE. Most patients in SE have temperatures of 37° to 40°C, most likely the result of continuous massive muscle contractions. Malignant hyperthermia (T > 41°C) is a bad prognostic sign that when present connotes death or severe neurological disability.

LABORATORY TESTS

Peripheral leukocytosis (> 10,000 WBC/mm^3) is a common finding, occurring in about three-fourths of patients in SE. In only about 10% is the WBC greater than 20,000/mm^3.

Arterial blood gases usually show a metabolic acidosis, a respiratory acidosis, or both abnormalities. Metabolic acidosis is caused by lactate production by overactive skeletal muscles that cannot obtain an adequate amount of oxygen. Respiratory acidosis is the result of hypoventilation during and between seizures.

Cerebrospinal fluid white blood cell (WBC) pleocytosis is common in patients in SE, even in the absence of CNS infection. Usually, WBC of 3 to 50 cells/mm^3 are seen. This pleocytosis presumably reflects minor meningeal inflammation during the seizure (postictal pleocytosis). Protein and glucose concentrations in CSF are usually normal.

DIAGNOSIS

The patient with more than 30 minutes of continuous seizures or with seizures of sufficient frequency that consciousness is not regained interictally has status epilepticus by definition. Generalized major motor SE is therefore easy to recognize. The diagnosis of complex partial SE and absence SE that produces confusional states requires EEG confirmation of ictal seizure activity.

MANAGEMENT

The clinician must concurrently terminate the seizures with drug therapy and attempt to correct the underlying cause of the seizures. The most widely accepted protocol for drug therapy of status epilepticus was developed in an international workshop on the management of SE and was first published in 1982 (Delgado-Escueta et al). The protocol is reproduced on Table 39-2.

This protocol is based on the fact that SE treatment is a race against time. The clinician's goal is to terminate seizures after 20 minutes because that is when the first evidence of brain damage begins. If routine anticonvulsant drugs do not terminate the seizures after 60 minutes, the patient should be placed under general anesthesia because diffuse, irreversible neuronal damage begins after this duration of SE.

The patient is given a 25 gram bolus of glucose to treat presumed hypoglycemia as a cause or consequence of the seizures. Thiamine and other B-vitamins are added to the intravenous fluids to prevent precipitation of an acute Wernicke–Korsakoff syndrome.

TABLE 39-2 PROTOCOL FOR THE MANAGEMENT OF TONIC–CLONIC STATUS EPILEPTICUS

TIME FROM START OF TREATMENT (MINUTES)	PROCEDURE
0	1. Assess cardiorespiratory function as the presence of tonic–clonic status is verified. If unsure of diagnosis, observe one tonic–clonic attack and verify the presence of unconsciousness after the end of the tonic–clonic attack. Insert oral airway and administer O_2 if necessary. Insert an indwelling intravenous catheter. Draw venous blood for anticonvulsant levels, glucose, BUN, electrolyte, and complete blood count determinations. Draw arterial blood for immediate determination of pH, PO_2, PCO_2, HCO_3. Monitor respiration, blood pressure, and electrocardiogram. If possible monitor electroencephalogram.
5	2. Start intravenous infusion through indwelling venous catheter with normal saline, containing vitamin B complex. Give a bolus injection of 50 mL 50% glucose.
10	3. Infuse diazepam intravenously no faster than 2 mg/min until seizures stop or to total of 20 mg. Also start infusion of phenytoin no faster than 50 mg/min to a total of 18 mg/kg. If hypotension develops, slow infusion rate. (Phenytoin, 50 mg/ml in propylene glycol, may be placed in a 100 mL volume-control set and diluted with normal saline. The rate of infusion should then be watched carefully.) Alternatively, phenytoin may be injected slowly by intravenous push.
30-40	4. If seizures persist, two options are available: IV phenobarbital or diazepam IV drip. The two drugs should not be given in the same patient, and an endotrachial tube should now be inserted.
	IV phenobarbital option: Start infusion of phenobarbital no faster than 100 mg/min until seizures stop or to a loading dose of 20 mg/kg.
	OR
	Diazepam IV drip option: 100 mg of diazepam is diluted in 500 mg 5% dextrose in water and run in at 40 mL/hr. This ensures diazepam serum levels of 0.2 to 0.8 μg/mL.
50-60	5. If seizures continue, general anesthesia with halothane and neuromuscular-junction blockade is instituted. If an anesthesiologist is not immediately available, start infusion of 4% solution of paraldehyde in normal saline; administer at a rate fast enough to stop seizures. Or 50 to 100 mg of lidocaine may be given by intravenous push. If lidocaine is effective, 50 to 100 mg diluted in 250 mL of 5% dextrose in water should be dripped intravenously at a rate of 1 to 2 mg/min.
80	6. If paraldehyde or lidocaine has not terminated seizures within 20 min from start of infusion, general anesthesia with halothane and neuromuscular-junction blockade must be given.
	7. If status epilepticus reappears when general anesthesia is stopped, a neurologist who is an expert on status epilepticus should be consulted. Advice from a regional epilepsy center should also be sought on the management of intractable status epilepticus.

Reprinted by permission of The New England Journal of Medicine, Delgado-Escueta AV, Wasterlain C, Treiman DM, et al: Management of status epilepticus. *N Engl J Med* 1982; 306:1338.

Diazepam is infused slowly, as directed in Table 39-2, to terminate seizures during the first 15 to 20 minutes of therapy. If diazepam is infused slowly and to a total dosage of no more than 20 mg, blood pressure and respirations should not be affected adversely. The termination of seizures in the first 15 to 20 minutes provides the clinician with sufficient time to infuse phenytoin intravenously, the most important part of the therapy. As soon as phenytoin is infused, 63% of patients will have the SE under control. The advantage of phenytoin is that it does not depress respirations in the dosage range that produces anticonvulsant efficacy.

A branch-point in the protocol is reached at 30 to 40 minutes. If seizures are still uncontrolled, the patient must be given intravenous phenobarbital or diazepam at the dosages listed in Table 39-2. In the dosages necessary to terminate seizures, these agents will surely depress respiration, so the patient must first be intubated and ventilated. After these drugs have been given, 88% of patients with SE will have their seizures arrested.

General anesthesia and neuromuscular blockade are reserved for the few patients who fail these drugs and are still having seizures at 60 minutes. General anesthesia suppresses the cortical seizure focus and reduces the high metabolic demands of the seizing brain. Neuromuscular blockade eliminates muscular contractions even if the seizure focus persists, which improves hyperthermia and acidosis. Recrudescence of seizures after general anesthesia is withdrawn indicates a very poor prognosis. Halothane and enflurane are the preferred general anesthetic agents.

In the recently head-injured patient in SE, or in other clinical instances in which it is essential to maintain and follow the patient's level of consciousness, intravenous phenytoin only should be administered. Complex partial SE should be treated aggressively according to the protocol because temporal lobe damage may occur after prolonged seizures of temporal lobe origin. Absence and petit mal status are not as serious as the other status forms. They should be terminated with intravenous diazepam, then prevented with oral valproic acid and/or ethosuximide.

A new benzodiazepine, lorazepam (Ativan), is being tested for the primary treatment of SE. Preliminary data suggest that its efficacy is similar to that of diazepam or to that of diazepam plus phenytoin. The drug has not yet been approved for this indication, but in the future lorazepam may become the drug of choice to suppress SE. See Leppik et al (1983).

COMPLICATIONS

Mention has been made of the important complications of inadequately treated SE, including hypoxemia, cardiac arrhythmias, acidosis, hyperthermia, cerebral edema, and hypoglycemia. These abnormalities are the major causes of morbidity and mortality in SE. They must be carefully watched for and quickly treated.

Iatrogenic complications from improperly performed intravenous infusions of phenytoin and diazepam are common, unfortunately. Because of the basic pK of phenytoin, the drug requires a very basic pH to go into solution. Phenytoin should not be given intramuscularly. Its very basic pH induces muscle fiber necrosis, pain at the injection site, intramuscular precipitation of phenytoin crystals, and erratic absorption. Pain and irritation are also common when phenytoin is infused intravenously if the phenytoin concentration is too great or if the infusion is not free-flowing. Hypotension, bradycardia, and other cardiac arrhythmias may occur if phenytoin or diazepam is infused too quickly or through a central venous catheter. In the patient who is awake, too rapid infusion may cause ataxia, confusion, dizziness, or drowsiness.

Most neurologists and clinical pharmacologists advocate that the physician slowly inject phenytoin by intravenous push without further dilution. Phenytoin can form microcrystals and precipitate out of solution when mixed with dextrose and water, normal saline, and lactated Ringer's solution. Earnest et al (1983) have shown that phenytoin may be used safely when diluted with normal saline if the concentration does not exceed 6.7 mg/mL (ie, phenytoin 1 g in 130 mL normal saline).

In either event, phenytoin must be given through a peripheral, not a central line. The intravenous line should be properly positioned and free flowing. If phenytoin in saline solution is administered, it should be given "piggy-back" on an existing intravenous line to permit independent and careful control of the phenytoin infusion rate. The phenytoin never should be infused at rates exceeding 50 mg/minute nor at rates exceeding 25 mg/minute in the elderly and in patients with known cardiovascular disease. A loading dose of phenytoin of 18 mg/kg body weight is needed to achieve a 15 to 20 μg/mL therapeutic serum level. Blood pressure, pulse, and ECG pattern should be assessed during the phenytoin infusion. The intravenous line should be checked frequently to assess proper placement. The infusion rate should be slowed if hypotension, bradycardia, or cardiac arrhythmia occurs.

WHEN TO CONSULT

A neurologist, neurosurgeon, or intensivist experienced in the management of SE is desirable to consult if seizures cannot be terminated in 20 to 30 minutes by the above measures. An anesthesiologist should be consulted to provide endotracheal intubation aand respiratory support if an intravenous drip of phenobarbital or diazepam becomes necessary.

PATIENT EDUCATION

The epileptic patient who develops SE by failure to properly follow the recommended anticonvulsive dosage schedule must be carefully counselled to prevent a recurrent episode. The patient must be counselled to report to the physician any new medication prescribed by other physicians because drug interactions may raise or lower the serum anticonvulsant levels and provoke seizures.

Bibliography

Aminoff MJ, Simon RP: Status epilepticus: Causes, clinical features and consequences in 98 patients. *Am J Med* 1980; 69:657-666. (A carefully studied large series. It is particularly good on description of etiologies and examination of findings. Does not discuss treatment, however.)

Ballenger CE, King DW, Gallagher BB: Partial complex status epilepticus. *Neurology* 1983;33:1545-1552. (Discusses the confusional states produce by partial complex status epilepticus.)

Delgado-Escueta AV, Wasterlain C, Treiman DM, et al: Management of status epilepticus. *N Engl J Med* 1982; 306:1337-1340. (The most accessible, authoritative reference, the source of Table 39-2. This paper concentrates on aspects of treatment and should be consulted as a first source.)

Delgado-Escueta AV, Wasterlain C, Treiman DM, et al: *Status Epilepticus: Mechanisms of Brain Damage and Treatment (Advances in Neurology* ser, vol 16). New York, Raven, 1983. (An expansion of Delgado-Escueta et al (1982), containing information on SE pathophysiology and all aspects of treatment.)

Earnest MP, Marx JA, Drury LR: Complications of intravenous phenytoin for acute treatment of seizures: Recommendation for usage. *JAMA* 1983; 249:762-765. (Defines and defends the safety of infusing phenytoin in an intravenous solution of normal saline.)

Guberman A, Cantu-Reyna G, Stuss D, et al: Nonconvulsive generalized status epilepticus: Clinical features, neuropsychological testing, and long-term follow-up. *Neurology* 1986; 36:1284-1291. (Defines nonconvulsive status and shows the similarity to several psychiatric syndromes.)

Leppik IE, Derivan AT, Homan RW, et al: Double-blind study of lorazepam and diazepam in status epilepticus. *JAMA* 1983;249:1452-1454. (Shows the superiority of lorazepam over diazepam in the treatment of status.)

Lockman L: Status epilepticus, in Morselli PL, Pippenger CE, Penry JK (eds): *Antiepileptic Drug Therapy in Pediatrics.* New York, Raven, 1983, pp 173-179. (Discusses status epilepticus occurring in childhood.)

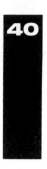

Spinal Cord Compression

Acute spinal cord compression is a neurological emergency in a sense analogous to cerebral herniation from an intracranial mass lesion. Early diagnosis and treatment are both necessary to prevent central nervous system ischemia from evolving into infarction. Chronic spinal cord compression most often results from cervical spondylosis (Chapter 9) and from intradural, extramedullary benign spinal cord tumors (Chapter 27). This chapter stresses the emergency recognition and management of acute spinal cord compression from epidural metastatic carcinoma, epidural abscess, and epidural hematoma. Acute spinal cord compression by spinal trauma is discussed in Chapter 38.

In much of this discussion, compression of the cauda equina is considered along with compression of the spinal cord. The spinal cord ends at the level of vertebral body L1; the intrathecal contents below that level are the lumbar and sacral nerve roots comprising the cauda equina. Although the cauda equina is part of the peripheral nervous system, hence more resistant to compression ischemia, the syndromes of its compression produce signs very similar to the signs of spinal cord compression. Furthermore, the same pathological processes cause compressions of both structures, and the diagnosis and treatment are nearly identical. Therefore, acute compressions of the spinal cord and the cauda equina are considered together.

The disorders described in this chapter arise in the epidural space. They first compress the dura mater, that tough connective-tissue meningeal sheath that provides the first line of protection for the brain and spinal cord. As the process progresses, the next meningeal layer, the arachnoid, becomes compressed, with obliteration of the subarachnoid space and exclusion of the cerebrospinal fluid contained therein. Finally, the cord itself is displaced and becomes compressed against its bony canal and the ligamentum flavum. Cord symptoms are first induced as the focally raised intraspinal pressure exceeds blood perfusion pressure. If the ischemia is not reversed promptly, spinal cord infarction ensues.

Recovery of function cannot be expected if medical or surgical decompression belatedly follows complete spinal cord infarction.

SPINAL CORD COMPRESSION BY EPIDURAL METASTATIC CARCINOMA

CLINICAL SIGNIFICANCE

Aside from trauma, the most common cause of acute epidural spinal cord compression is by metastatic carcinoma. Posner (Gilbert et al, 1978) estimates that this complication now occurs in 5% of patients with systemic cancer. A general hospital can thus expect to encounter one case annually for every 40 to 50 beds. Cord compression usually occurs late in the course of cancer when bony and organ metastases are widespread. As patients with metastatic cancer are kept alive longer, more cases of acute spinal cord compression will be seen. Even in treated cases, the median survival is three to six months. The one-year survival rate is 20% to 30%, although some patients survive for several years. The goal of early diagnosis and therapy is to prevent the patient from spending his final months as a paraplegic.

SYMPTOMS AND SIGNS

The prerequisite for epidural cord compression is the vertebral body metastatic lesion. As the vertebral metastasis grows, it invades the spinal canal and encircles the meninges and cord, traversing the epidural space. Direct hematogenous spread to the epidural space is rare if it occurs at all. Lymphomas and neuroblastomas can spread through the intervertebral foramena and produce acute cord compression with neither vertebral metastasis nor pain.

Most cases of cord compression occur in the thoracic area, particularly from T6 to T12. Of those remaining, the lumbosacral area is more common than the cervical area. The tumor types most likely to produce acute cord compression (in order of decreasing frequency) are: lung, breast, prostate, lymphoma, melanoma, sarcoma, and kidney. The complication has been described, however, in nearly every type of cancer.

Pain is the earliest, most important sign of cord compression, occurring in 95% of cases. The pain is both local and radicular and is often very severe. It is produced by the vertebral metastasis itself and by the mechanical distortion of the spinal cord and nerve roots. Pain precedes the sensory and motor signs of myelopathy for weeks or months. Thoracic radicular pain is often mistaken for intrathoracic and intra-abdominal visceral disease. Spine tenderness on percussion is often present at the site of metastasis.

With progression, the signs of transverse myelopathy evolve. The patient complains of leg weakness, difficulty in walking, and trouble in climbing stairs. Examination discloses a mild spastic paraparesis, particularly of the iliopsoas muscles, in 85% of cases. The patient may complain of numbness, tingling, and paresthesias below the site of compression. Examination discloses sensory abnormalities below the lesion or a frank sensory dermatomal "level" in 70% of patients. Deep-tendon reflexes are hyperactive below the lesion in 65% of patients; extensor plantar responses are present in 50%. In cauda equina compression, deep-tendon reflexes are hypoactive or absent below the lesion with flexor plantar responses because of lower motor neuron involvement.

Decreased rectal tone is present in 60% of cases, and local spine tenderness in 70%. Bowel and bladder dysfunction is seen in 40% of cases overall, but is present earlier and more severely in cases in which the lumbosacral cord segments (conus medullaris) are compressed first, corresponding to vertebral bodies T11, T12, and L1. In cancer patients with back pain, constipation does not necessarily suggest spinal cord involvement; more often it is a side effect of prescribed narcotic analgesics.

LABORATORY TESTS

Plain x-rays of the spine reveal evidence of metastatic carcinoma in 80% of cases, and radionuclide bone scan reveals metastases in the vertebral bodies in 80%. When both tests are performed, one or both are positive for vertebral metastases in 90% of cases. Cerebrospinal fluid analysis reveals an increase in the protein concentration that roughly parallels the severity of cord compression.

The definitive test for epidural spinal cord compression is the myelogram. Partial or complete blockage of myelographic contrast dye at the level of compression is diagnostic. The compression often is seen to extend over several spinal segments. In cases of complete obstruction, a cervical or cisternal puncture is additionally necessary to delineate the superior margin of the lesion.

The computed tomography (CT) scan is also of diagnostic value. It has the advantage of being less invasive than the myelogram and provides data on tumor metastases outside the spinal column. For example, the CT scan may reveal lumbosacral plexus metastasis as well as revealing tumor spread to the lumbar epidural space. The disadvantages of CT are that it is difficult to interpret in the high-thoracic and cervical region. It only investigates "segmentally"; thus, it does not identify other clinically unsuspected regions of cord compression (present in 10% of cases), and it does not provide CSF for cytology examination.

Myelography has three advantages: it can examine the entire spinal canal; it can provide CSF for examination; and it can be performed in hospitals without a CT scanner. Disadvantages of myelography are that it is painful and that it might transiently worsen incipient cord compression. On balance, myelography remains the diagnostic procedure of choice. Generally, a few milliliters of iophendylate (Pantopaque) are injected by lumbar intrathecal injection, and the entire spinal subarachnoid space is quickly screened for total compression. If total compression is not present, more dye is instilled to permit a proper study of the suspected area.

Many centers with magnetic resonance imaging scanners have switched completely to MRI as the first or only diagnostic test to detect acute epidural spinal cord compression. MR can image the entire cord in sagittal section, thereby overcoming the major defiency of CT, namely segmental scanning. Like CT, MR is painless and noninvasive.

DIAGNOSIS

The clinical diagnosis of epidural spinal cord compression by metastatic carcinoma is presumptive; in the early stage it is a difficult diagnosis of which to be certain. Patients suspected clinically of this diagnosis, but who later have negative myelograms, actually suffer from uncomplicated vertebral metastases, carcinomatous meningitis, or a variety of neuropathies and plexopathies. Intramedullary spinal cord metastasis is very rare, occurring with only 1% of the frequency of epidural compression.

Clinical diagnosis is suspected when the patient with known cancer develops new back pain followed in time by symptoms of leg weakness and/or numbness and of bowel or bladder dysfunction. Clinical diagnosis is made when plain vertebral x-rays or bone scan confirm the vertebral metastasis and the examination discloses motor, sensory, or reflex signs suggesting an early myelopathy. Such patients should undergo immediate myelography or MR scanning to confirm the diagnosis.

In some centers, cancer patients with new back pain and radiologic confirmation of vertebral metastasis are sent for myelography, even in the absence of motor, sensory, or reflex signs of myelopathy. In these centers, clinicians are willing to accept many negative myelograms so that they can be certain to detect all those patients with actual cord compression early in their course. The clinician who chooses to wait until some evidence of myelopathy is present should be prepared to perform the myelogram rapidly as soon as these signs appear, for the compression may evolve within hours. See Portenoy et al (1987).

MANAGEMENT

Treatment of epidural cord compression by metastatic carcinoma includes surgery, radiation therapy, and glucocorticoids. When the diagnosis is confirmed, the patient should immediately receive dexamethasone, 10 mg intravenously. He should continue to receive 8 mg orally every 12 hours until the radiation therapy is completed. Posner (Gilbert et al, 1978) has shown that ultra-high-dose dexamethasone (100 mg, then tapered) is preferable in instances in which intractable pain is present because analgesia is superior by this regimen. The neurological outcome is no better with ultra-high-dose dexamethasone than for more conventional doses. Dexamethasone reduces edema at the site of metastasis, helps alleviate pain, and improves neurological function within hours.

Posner has shown that emergency radiation therapy is at least as effective and is much safer than surgical decompression. This equivalence in results persists even for tumors of "known radioresistance." Surgical treatment is simply laminectomy and decompression; removal of the entire metastasis is rarely feasible. Because these patients usually are very ill from multiple metastases, surgery has significant morbidity and mortality. Only in the few centers where vertebrectomy and anterior fusion is performed are surgical results superior to those of radiation therapy.

Radiation therapy consists of 400 rads daily for the first three days, then 200 rads daily to a total dosage of 2000 to 4000 rads. Radiation therapy is usually recommended as the primary therapeutic mode. There are four instances in which decompression laminectomy is indicated:

1. If the patient is not known to have cancer. What otherwise appears to be a metastatic lesion in fact may be an epidural abscess, hematoma, or ruptured disc.

If the lesion is a tumor, the tissue obtained at surgery will be diagnostically valuable. If the patient has known cancer, it is reasonable to assume that the epidural lesion is a metastatic tumor.

2. If the radiation therapist cannot provide emergency service but the neurosurgeon can. This situation will vary from community to community.

3. If the patient deteriorates while on radiation therapy. Unfortunately, such a patient also does not fare very well with surgical decompression.

4. If the patient has had previous radiation therapy to the area, making additional radiation hazardous. A myelopathy induced by radiation itself can occur if the cord has been exposed to more than 4500 rads.

Response rates vary by tumor type. Myeloma, lymphoma, and breast cancer are most radioresponsive; kidney and lung are intermediately responsive; prostate and melanoma are poorly responsive. Studies of conventional surgery plus radiation versus radiation alone show no difference in outcomes. The size of metastasis is also not a factor favoring surgery over radiation. The otherwise uncomplicated patient with known systemic carcinoma but no other complications who develops acute cord compression should be treated urgently with dexamethasone and radiation.

COMPLICATIONS
The most important variable that influences the outcome is the speed with which diagnosis and treatment are accomplished. Therapy is primarily preventive: the neurological status at the initiation of treatment is roughly the same as at the conclusion of therapy. Patients who are allowed to become paraplegic under observation will rarely walk again. Every attempt should be made to diagnose and begin treating the patient before the myelopathy becomes fully developed.

WHEN TO CONSULT
A neurologist or oncologist with experience in diagnosing myelopathies in cancer patients should be consulted when the known cancer patient develops back pain and symptoms of leg weakness or numbness or a new bowel or bladder disturbance. If the experienced referral clinician feels there is at least a reasonable likelihood of cord compression, the patient should urgently undergo myelography or MR scanning.

SPINAL CORD COMPRESSION BY EPIDURAL ABSCESS

CLINICAL SIGNIFICANCE
Spinal epidural abscess is an uncommon but very treatable form of acute spinal cord compression. It is estimated to occur in approximately 1 of every 15,000 hospital admissions, and in fewer than half of cases is the diagnosis made before the patient becomes paraplegic or dies. Unlike patients with acute epidural spinal cord compression by metastatic carcinoma, patients with epidural abscess are potentially curable. Thus, it is crucial to make an early diagnosis and institute treatment promptly.

Symptoms and Signs

Severe back pain is the earliest and most common chief complaint. The pain is local, radicular, and almost always severe enough to justify narcotic analgesia. Severe local spinal tenderness accompanies the pain in almost every case. Fever is also a constant symptom, usually in the range of 39°C. Within several days to a week of the fever and back pain, radicular pain develops. Then, after an interval of a few hours to days, an acute myelopathy with paraplegia occurs. Patients in whom the diagnosis is not made become permanently paraplegic and then afebrile later in their course.

A spinal epidural abscess can arise from hematogenous seeding, adjacent osteomyelitis, or from a contiguous source such as a surgical incision. Of abscesses that occur by hematogenous spread of organisms, the primary infection is usually in the skin or pharynx. Bacteria are the most common pathogens, and *Staphylococcus aureus* is the most common organism. *Pseudomonas aeruginosa* or other Gram-negative organisms should be suspected if the patient is a drug addict. If fever is not conspicuous, *Mycobacterium tuberculosis* with Pott's disease should be considered. Antecedent back injury is a common historical feature in bacterial cases, but its role is uncertain. MR scanning is an excellent way to image the epidural abscess.

As is true with metastatic carcinoma, epidural abscesses usually occur in the thoracic spine; of those elsewhere, the lumbar region is more common than the cervical. The posterior epidural space is involved in 80% of cases, the anterior in 20%.

Laboratory Tests

There is a peripheral leukocytosis in the range of 15,000 to 20,000 in acute cases, but in the long-standing cases, the WBC may revert to normal. Signs of vertebral osteomyelitis by plain spine x-rays are present in about half of the acute patients; the longer the abscess persists, the greater the percentage of positive x-rays. In tuberculous osteomyelitis, plain x-rays are almost always positive. The cerebrospinal fluid is nondiagnostic with findings suggestive of spinal parameningeal inflammation: elevated protein (average 400 to 500 mg/dL), pleocytosis (50 to 100 WBC), and a normal or slightly depressed glucose level.

Myelography is the confirmatory test of choice, revealing the presence, location, and extent of the spinal epidural abscess in nearly all cases. A complete spinal block is present in 80%. It is imperative that the spinal puncture for the myelogram not be introduced in the vicinity of the abscess. The role of CT in this condition is uncertain.

Diagnosis

The combination of fever, severe new back pain, radicular pain, spinal tenderness, and progression to spinal cord dysfunction should immediately raise the question of spinal epidural abscess. Such patients should undergo plain vertebral x-rays, then emergency myelography or MR scan to confirm the diagnosis.

Management

Emergency surgical drainage of the epidural abscess and intravenous antibiotics are the treatment of choice. The pus removed at surgery should be stained and cultured and treatment begun on that basis. An antistaphylococcal drug should always be included in the intitial antibiotic regimen. The abscess must be widely decompressed surgically for it usually extends over four to five vertebral body segments. Antibiotics are continued for four weeks in the absence of osteomyelitis and six to eight weeks in the presence of osteomyelitis. Glucocorticoid therapy is useful preoperatively to reduce edema, but it should not be continued postoperatively because of its immunosuppressant effects.

COMPLICATIONS

Analogous to epidural metastatic carcinoma, the outcome of treatment is directly related to pretreatment neurological status. With early drainage, paraplegia can be prevented in the majority of cases. The usual problem is delay in diagnosis, as when the epidural abscess is misdiagnosed as lumbar strain, herniated disc, epidural metastatic carcinoma, or an intrathoracic or intra-abdominal visceral disorder. In the largest reported series of epidural abscesses, 20% of patients died.

WHEN TO CONSULT

A neurologist or neurosurgeon should be asked to see the patient with fever, new back pain and vertebral tenderness. Even when a consultant is not available, such a patient should undergo immediate myelography. Immediate neurosurgical decompression should follow myelographic demonstration of abscess.

SPINAL CORD COMPRESSION BY EPIDURAL HEMATOMA

CLINICAL SIGNIFICANCE

Unlike patients with epidural spinal cord compression from metastatic carcinoma and epidural abscess, patients with acute spontaneous epidural hematoma have only a very short time interval between their first complaint of back pain and the onset of paraplegia. The causes of acute epidural hematoma are classified in Table 40-1. Autopsy studies have shown that although some patients have epidural arteriovenous malformation or angiomas, the majority have no demonstrable predisposing lesion that can account for the epidural site of hemorrhage. Acute cord compression from epidural hematoma is a neurosurgical emergency analogous to that of epidural abscess.

SYMPTOMS AND SIGNS

The typical patient has a spontaneous onset of local and radicular back or neck pain, followed within minutes or a few hours by paraplegia, sensory dysfunction below the lesion, and bowel or bladder dysfunction. Some patients have a history of antecedent minor trauma to the involved area. The thoracic region is the most common site for epidural hematoma, followed by the lumbar, then cervical areas. Like metastatic carcinomas and abscesses, most hematomas extend over two or three vertebral segments and are located in the posterior epidural space. There is no fever.

LABORATORY TESTS

Plain spinal films and CSF are usually normal. The myelogram is the definitive test, disclosing the location and extent of the hematoma. The myelographic ap-

TABLE 40-1 ETIOLOGY OF SPINAL EPIDURAL HEMATOMA

Coagulopathy
  Thrombocytopenic disorders
  Liver disease, hypoprothrombinemia
  Hemophilias
  Coumadin therapy
Increased venous back pressure
  Valsalva maneuver
      Coughing
      Sneezing
      Straining at stool
  Portal hypertension
Hypertension (rarely)
Iatrogenic
  Lumbar puncture
  Spinal epidural anesthesia
  Dorsal column stimulation
Traumatic
  Vertebral fracture
Idiopathic

pearance is that of total or nearly total epidural compression—the same as for epidural abscess and epidural metastatic carcinoma. MR scanning, where available, is an excellent way to confirm the diagnosis. Coagulation studies, including prothrombin time and platelet count, should be performed in suspected cases.

DIAGNOSIS
The sudden, spontaneous onset of back or neck local and radicular pain followed quickly by progressively severe paraplegia should immediately raise the possibility of epidural hematoma. A myelogram should be performed as the first diagnostic test. Idiopathic transverse myelitis (Chapter 27) may present with pain followed by paraplegia, but will have a normal myelogram. Spinal subdural hematoma produces the same symptoms and signs as epidural hematoma and can also be diagnosed by myelogram or MR scan.

MANAGEMENT
Coagulation disturbances should be looked for and corrected as the neurosurgeon prepares to operate. Surgical removal is not feasible if the coagulopathy cannot be reversed. As is true in other causes of epidural spinal cord compression, the sooner the compression is relieved, the better the prognosis for the return of leg function. Glucocorticoid therapy has no role.

COMPLICATIONS
If surgery is performed within 24 hours from the onset of symptoms, full recovery of function is seen in 42% of patients with incomplete sensorimotor symptoms, in 26% of patients with incomplete sensory but complete motor symptoms, and in 11% of patients with complete sensorimotor lesions. Of the above three groups, incomplete recovery but the ability to walk occurs in 95%, 87%, and 45% of cases, respectively.

593

When to Consult

Patients with any acute myelopathy should be seen immediately by a neurologist or a neurosurgeon. Most should undergo emergency myelography or MR scanning.

Bibliography

Baker AS, Ojemann RG, Swartz MN, et al: Spinal epidural abscess. *N Engl J Med* 1975; 293:463-468. (Excellent report on 39 patients from Massachusetts General Hospital, with a lucid account of their clinical features; a classic paper.)

Bernat JL, Greenberg ER, Barrett J: Suspected epidural compression of the spinal cord and cauda equina by metastatic carcinoma: Clinical diagnosis and survival. *Cancer* 1983; 51:1953-1957. (Compares the fates of two groups of patients, both clinically suspected of cord compression: those shown to have cord compression by myelography and those subsequently shown not to have it.)

Foo D, Rossier AB: Preoperative neurologic status in predicting surgical outcome of spinal epidural hematomas. *Surg Neurol* 1981; 15:389-401. (A detailed review of 158 cases from the literature; the correlation of outcomes and clinical findings discussed in the chapter are from this paper.)

Gilbert RW, Kim JH, Posner JB: Epidural spinal cord compression from metastatic tumor: Diagnosis and treatment. *Ann Neurol* 1978; 3:40-51. (A complete report on 130 cases from Memorial–Sloan Kettering Cancer Center in New York, showing no difference in outcome in neurosurgically treated or radiated patients.)

Kaufman DM, Kaplan JG, Litman N: Infectious agents in spinal epidural abscesses. *Neurology* 1980; 30:844-850. (Points out the key differences between tuberculous and other bacterial epidural abscesses in 27 cases.)

McQuarrie IG: Recovery from paraplegia caused by spontaneous spinal epidural hematoma. *Neurology* 1978; 28:224-228. (Shows that patients who make better postoperative recoveries had a shorter interval between onset of symptoms and operative decompression.)

Portenoy RK, Lipton RB, Foley KM: Back pain in the cancer patient: An algorithmn for evaluation and management. *Neurology* 1987;37:134-138.(Provides decision trees for the management of back pain in the cancer patient. Highly recommended.)

Rodichok LD, Harper GR, Ruckdeschel JC, et al: Early diagnosis of spinal epidural metastases. *Am J Med* 1981; 70:1181-1188. (Shows that in patients with back pain but no neurological abnormalities on exam, the presence of metastases on plain vertebral x-rays predicted cord compression in 82%. The same group confirmed this finding in a prospective series [*Ann Neurology* 1986;20:696-702].)

Rodriguez M, Dinapoli RP: Spinal cord compression with special reference to metastatic epidural tumors. *Mayo Clin Proc* 1980; 55:442-448. (A reasonably thorough review.)

Siegal T, Siegal T: Surgical decompression of anterior and posterior malignant epidural tumors compressing the spinal cord: A prospective study. *Neurosurgery* 1985; 17:424-432. (Shows that surgical outcomes are better with anterior vertebrectomy than with the usual posterior approach to epidural metastatic carcinoma.)

Patient Information Guide for Neurology

Reprinted with permission of the American Academy of Neurology.
Developed by AAN Practice Committee, E. Wayne Massey, MD, Coordinator.

AMERICAN ACADEMY OF NEUROLOGY
2221 University Avenue S.E., Suite 335
Minneapolis, MN 55414

KEY TO SERVICES

This guide lists numerous resources dealing with a wide range of neurologically related disorders. A multitude of services is available through these helping groups. After each address, you will find one or more symbols. These identify some of the many services offered. The key below defines the symbols.

rr.....referrals
We encourage each group to furnish local information to patients and list all qualified local neurologists.

ss.....support groups
Many groups provide the opportunity to share experiences with others.

ll.....local chapters
This guide lists the national organizational office, which will supply local chapter information.

bb.....brochures, pamphlets
The majority of resources listed in the guide have this type of information available free or for sale. Inquire also about slides, cassettes or films.

ee.....special equipment assistance
Specific organizations will help in procuring special equipment as necessary. Information about loans may be available through local chapters.

pp.....periodicals
Many groups publish newsletters and/or magazines.

mm.....medication information
Select organizations have information on less costly and/or generic medications.

cc.....clinics
Select organizations support special clinics for neurological diseases.

Many groups are also involved in research.

ALCOHOLISM

Alcoholics Anonymous
General Service Office
Box 459
Grand Central Station
New York, NY 10017

(212) 686-1100
ss,ll,bb
NOTE: Alcoholics Anonymous is best
able to help at the local level. The best
resource for contacting them is your
phone book. If you cannot track a local
chapter, contact the New York office
which will put you in touch with a near-
by chapter.

ALZHEIMER'S DISEASE

Association for Alzheimer's
and Related Diseases
360 North Michigan Avenue
Chicago, IL 60601

(312) 853-3060
rr,ss,ll,bb

Alzheimer Society of Canada
491 Lawrence Avenue W.
Suite 501

Toronto, Ontario
CANADA M5M 1C7

(416) 789-0503
rr, ss, ll, bb

AMYOTROPHIC LATERAL SCLEROSIS

Amyotrophic Lateral Sclerosis
Society of America
15300 Ventura Boulevard
Suite 315
Sherman Oaks, CA 91403

(818) 990-2151
rr, ss, bb

National ALS Foundation, Inc.
185 Madison Avenue
Room 1001
New York, NY 10016

(212) 679-4016
rr, ll, ee, pp, cc

Les Turner ALS Foundation,
Ltd.
3325 West Main Street
Skokie, IL 60076

(312) 679-3311
rr, ss, ll, bb, pp
NOTE: The Les Turner ALS
Foundation primarily serves the
Chicago area.
See also: Muscular Dystrophy

ATAXIA

National Ataxia Foundation
600 Twelve Oaks Center
15500 Wayzata Boulevard
Wayzata, MN 55391

(612) 473-7666
rr, ll, bb, pp
NOTE: Friedreich's Ataxia is also within
the scope of the National Ataxia
Foundation.

AUTISM

National Society for Children and
  Adults with Autism
1234 Massachusetts Avenue N.W.
Suite 1017
Washington, DC 20005

(202) 783-0125
rr, ll, bb

BENIGN ESSENTIAL BLEPHAROSPASM

Benign Essential Blepharospasm
  Research Foundation, Inc.
755 Howell Street
Beaumont, TX 77706

(409) 892-1339
rr, ss, ll, bb, pp

See also Dystonia

BIRTH DEFECTS

March of Dimes Birth Defects
  Foundation
1275 Mamaroneck Avenue
White Plains, NY 10605

(914) 428-7100
rr, ss, ll, bb, pp

BLINDNESS

American Foundation for the Blind
15 West 16th Street
New York, NY 10011

(212) 620-2000
bb, ee, pp, cc

National Society to Prevent
  Blindness
79 Madison Avenue
New York, NY 10016

(212) 684-3505
ll, bb, pp

CEREBRAL PALSY

United Cerebral Palsy
66 East 34th Street
New York, NY 10016

(212) 481-6300
ll, bb, cc

American Academy of Cerebral Palsy
  and Developmental Medicine
2315 Westwood
P.O. Box 11083
Richmond, VA 23230

(804) 355-0147
rr, bb

DEAFNESS

National Association for Hearing and
  Speech Action
10801 Rockville Pike
Rockville, MD 20852

(301) 897-8682
(800) 638-8255
rr, bb, ee

Better Hearing Institute
1430 K Street NW
Suite 700
Washington, DC 20005

(202) 638-7577
rr, bb, ee

National Hearing Association
721 Enterprise Drive #101
Oak Brook, IL 60521

(312) 323-7200
rr, bb, pp

Alexander Graham Bell Association
for the Deaf, Inc.
3417 Volta Place N.W.
Washington, DC 20007

(202) 337-5220
rr, ss, bb

DOWN SYNDROME

National Down Syndrome Congress
1640 West Roosevelt Road
Chicago, IL 60608

(312) 226-0416
ss, bb, pp

DYSAUTONOMIA

Dysautonomia Foundation, Inc.
370 Lexington Avenue
Suite 1504
New York, NY 10017

(212) 889-5222
rr, ll, bb, pp, cc

DYSTONIA

Dystonia Medical Research
Foundation
9615 Brighton Way
Beverly Hills, CA 90210

(213) 272-9880
rr, ll, bb, pp

EPILEPSY

Epilepsy Foundation of America
4351 Garden City Drive
Landover, MD 20784

(301) 459-3700
rr, bb, pp

Epilepsy-Canada
2099 Alexandre-DeSeve
P.O. Box 1560
Station C
Montreal, PQ
CANADA H2L 4K8

(514) 876-7455
rr, ss, ll

GENETIC DISEASES

National Foundation for Jewish
Genetic Diseases
250 Park Avenue
Suite 1000
New York, NY 10177

(212) 682-5550
rr, bb, pp

GUILLAIN-BARRE SYNDROME

Guillain-Barré Syndrome Support
Group
P.O. Box 262
Wynnewood, PA 19096

(215) 649-7837
(215) 896-6372
rr, ss, ll, bb, pp

HEAD INJURY

The National Head Injury
Foundation
18A Vernon Street
Framingham, MA 01701

(617) 879-7473
rr, ss, ll, bb

HEADACHE

National Migraine Foundation
5252 N. Western Avenue
Chicago, IL 60625

(312) 878-7715
rr, bb, pp

HUNTINGTON'S DISEASE

Also known as Huntington's Chorea

Huntington's Disease Foundation
of America
250 West 57th Street
Suite 2016
New York, NY 10107

(212) 757-0443
rr, ll, bb, pp

Huntington's Society of Canada
Box 333
Cambridge, Ontario
CANADA N1R 5T8

(519) 622-1002
ss, ll, bb, pp

JOSEPH DISEASE

International Joseph Diseases
Foundation, Inc.
1832 Holmes Street
Building E
Post Office Box 2550
Livermore, CA 94550

(415) 455-0706
rr, bb, pp, cc

MENTAL RETARDATION

Association for Retarded Citizens
2709 Avenue E East
P.O. Box 6109
Arlington, TX 76011

(817) 640-0204
ll

Association for Children and Adults
with
Learning Disabilities
4156 Library Road
Pittsburgh, PA 15234

(412) 341-1515
rr, ll, bb

MIGRAINE

National Migraine Foundation
5252 N. Western Avenue
Chicago, IL 60625

(312) 878-7715
rr, bb, pp

MULTIPLE SCLEROSIS

National Multiple Sclerosis Society
205 East 42nd Street
New York, NY 10017

(212) 986-3240
rr, ss, ll, bb, pp

MUSCULAR DYSTROPHY

Muscular Dystrophy Association
810 Seventh Avenue
New York, NY 10019

(212) 586-0808
rr, ll, bb, pp, cc
NOTE: The MDA provides services not
only for muscular dystrophy, but for most
forms of myopathies, spinal muscular
atrophies, some diseases of peripheral
nerves and diseases of the
neuromuscular junction. These
conditions include: Aran-Duchenne
Disease (Adult Progressive Spinal
Muscular Atrophy)
Charcot-Marie Tooth Disease (Peroneal
Muscular Atrophy)
Congenital Hypotonia
Duchenne Muscular Dystrophy
Friedreich's Ataxia
Kugelberg-Welander Disease (Juvenile
Progressive Spinal Muscular Atrophy)

Malignant Hyperthermia
Werdnig-Hoffman Disease (Infantile
Spinal Muscular Atrophy)

MYASTHENIA GRAVIS

Myasthenia Gravis Foundation
15 East 26th Street
New York, NY 10010

(212) 889-8157
rr, ss, ll, pp, mm

See also Muscular Dystrophy

MYOTONIC DYSTROPHY

Muscular Dystrophy Association
810 Seventh Avenue
New York, NY 10019

(212) 586-0808
rr, ll, bb, pp, cc

NARCOLEPSY

American Narcolepsy
Association, Inc.
P.O. Box 5846
Stanford, CA 94305

(415) 591-7979
rr, bb, pp

NEUROFIBROMATOSIS

National Neurofibromatosis
Foundation
70 West 40th Street
New York, NY 10018

(212) 869-9034
rr, ll, bb, pp

PAIN

Chronic Pain Outreach
822 Wycliff Court
Manassas, VA 22110

(703) 368-7357
rr, ss, ll, bb, ee, pp, mm

National Committee on the
Treatment
of Intractable Pain
Friendship Station
P.O. Box 9553
Washington, DC 20016

(202) 983-1710
pp

PARKINSON'S DISEASE

American Parkinson's Disease
Association
116 John Street
New York, NY 10038

(212) 732-9550
(800) 223-2732
rr, ss, ll, bb, pp

Parkinson's Educational Program
1800 Park Newport #302
Newport Beach, CA 92660

(714) 640-0218
ss, ll, bb, pp

United Parkinson's Foundation
360 West Superior Street
Chicago, IL 60610

(312) 664-2344
rr, ss, bb, pp, mm

REHABILITATION

American Occupational Therapy
Association
1383 Piccard Drive
Rockville, MD 20850

(301) 948-9626
rr, ll, bb

Sister Kenney Institute
Referral Department
800 East 28th Street
Minneapolis, MN 55407

(612) 874-4400
rr

The Arthritis Foundation
1314 Spring Street NW
Atlanta, GA 30309

(404) 872-7100
rr, ss, ll, bb, ee, pp, mm

REYE'S SYNDROME

National Reye's Syndrome
 Foundation
426 North Lewis Street
Bryan, OH 43506

(419) 636-2679
24-hour Hot Line Numbers:
(800) 233-7393
(from outside Ohio)
(800) 231-7393
(from within Ohio)
rr, ss, ll, bb

American Reye's Syndrome
 Association
701 South Logan
Suite 203
Denver, CO 80209

(303) 777-2592
rr, ll, bb

Reye's Syndrome Society
P.O. Box RS
7045 Travers Avenue
Benzonia, MI 49616

(616) 882-5521
rr, ss, ll, bb, pp

SEXUAL DYSFUNCTION

Program in Human Sexuality
University of Minnesota
School of Medicine
2630 University Avenue SE
Minneapolis, MN 55414

(612) 376-7520
rr, ss

Sandra S. Cole
AASECT, CSE, CSC
Director, Sexuality Training Centers
National Task Force: Sexuality and
 Disability
Department of Physical Medicine
 and Rehabilitation
University of Michigan Medical
 School
Room E3254
Ann Arbor, MI 48109

(313) 764-5335
rr

SPASMODIC TORTICOLLIS

National Spasmodic Torticollis
 Association
27212 Huntington
Warren, MI 48093

(313) 779-8462
ss, ll, bb, pp, cc

SPINA BIFIDA

Spina Bifida Association of America
343 S. Dearborn
Suite 317
Chicago, IL 60604

(312) 663-1562
rr, ll, bb

SPINAL CORD INJURY

American Paralysis Association
One Lincoln Center
Suite 275
5400 LBJ Freeway
Dallas, TX 75240

(214) 934-3237
rr, pp

Paralyzed Veterans of America
801 18th Street NW
Washington, DC 20006

(202) 872-1300
ss, ll, bb, pp
NOTE: The PVA is able to provide additional services to veterans.

National Spinal Cord Injury
    Association
149 California Street
Newton, MA 02158

(617) 964-0521
rr, ll, bb, ee, pp

Spinal Cord Society
2410 Lakeview Drive
Fergus Falls, MN 56537

(218) 739-5252
rr, bb, pp, cc

STROKE

American Heart Association
7320 Greenville Avenue
Dallas, TX 75231

(214) 750-5300
ll, bb

National Stroke Association
1420 Ogden Street
Denver, CO 80218

(303) 839-1992
pp
NOTE: This organization is less than one year old, and new services are being developed and added.

TAY-SACHS

National Tay-Sachs and Allied
    Diseases Association
92 Washington Avenue
Cedarhurst, NY 11516

(516) 569-4300
rr, ss, ll, bb, ee

TINNITUS

American Tinnitus Association
P.O. Box 5
Portland, OR 97207

(503) 248-9985
rr, ss, bb, pp

TOURETTE SYNDROME

Tourette Syndrome Association
4102 Bell Boulevard
Bayside, NY 11361

(718) 224-2999
rr, ss, ll, bb, pp

Tourette Syndrome Foundation
    of Canada
173 Owen Boulevard
Willowdale, Ontario
CANADA M2P 1G8

(416) 449-2417
rr, ll, pp

TUBEROUS SCLEROSIS

National Tuberous Sclerosis
    Association, Inc.
P.O. Box 612
Winfield, IL 60190

(312) 668-0787
ss, bb, pp

TUMORS

Association for Brain Tumor
    Research
6232 N. Pulaski Road
Chicago, IL 60646

(312) 286-5571
rr, bb

American Cancer Society, Inc.
777 Third Avenue
New York, NY 10017

(212) 599-8200
rr, ll, bb, ee

MISCELLANEOUS

American Lung Association
1740 Broadway
New York, NY 10010

(212) 315-8700
ll, bb

American National Red Cross
17th and D Street NW
Washington, DC 20006

(202) 737-8300
NOTE: Check with the Red Cross concerning services.

National Easter Seal Society for
  Crippled Children and Adults
2023 West Ogden Avenue
Chicago, IL 60612

(312) 243-8400
rr, ss, ll, bb, pp

The Foundation for Brain Research
P.O. Box 754
Cooper Station
New York, NY 10276

(212) 533-8647
bb

Association for Persons with Severe
  Handicaps
7010 Roosevelt Way NE
Seattle, WA 98115

(206) 523-8446
ll, bb

NATIONAL HEALTH INFORMATION CLEARING HOUSE

National Health Information
  Clearing House
P.O. Box 1133
Washington, DC 20013-1133

(800) 336-4797
(703) 522-2590
NOTE: This service of the U.S. Department of Health and Human Services can provide additional possible resources for many conditions, both those that are listed here and others.

NATIONAL INSTITUTES OF HEALTH

National Institute of Neurological
  and Communicative Disorders
  and Stroke (NINCDS)
National Institutes of Health (NIH)
Building 31, 5th Floor
A Wing, Room 16
Bethesda, MD 20014

(301) 496-5751
NOTE: The NINCDS is a resource for many conditions, both those that are listed here and others.

TISSUE BANKS

Brain Tissue Resource Center
Mailman Research Center
McLean Hospital
115 Mall Street
Belmont, MA 02178

(617) 855-3426

National Neurological Research Bank
VA Wadsworth Medical Center
Los Angeles, CA 90073

(213) 824-4301
NOTE: Both of these organizations are involved in procuring and providing tissue for research.

UMBRELLA ORGANIZATIONS

American Coalition of Citizens with
  Disabilities
1012 14th Street NW
Suite 901
Washington, DC 20005

(202) 628-3470
rr, ll

National Health Council
70 W. 40th Street
New York, NY 10016

(212) 869-8100
rr
NOTE: The above organizations have
other societies as their members. While
they provide few or no patient services
directly, they frequently will be able to
refer to an appropriate member
organization.

Index